A History of Organ Transplantation

A History of
Organ

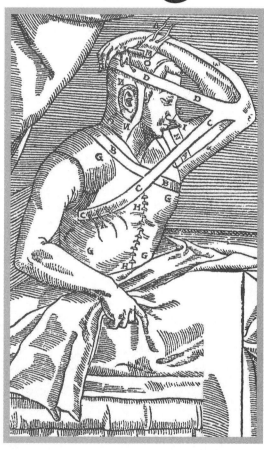

Transplantation

Ancient Legends to Modern Practice

David Hamilton

With a Foreword by
Clyde F. Barker and Thomas E. Starzl

University of Pittsburgh Press

Published by the University of Pittsburgh Press, Pittsburgh,
Pa., 15260
Copyright © 2012, University of Pittsburgh Press
All rights reserved
Manufactured in the United States of America
Printed on acid-free paper
Designed and typeset by Kachergis Book Design
10 9 8 7 6 5 4 3 2 1

Library of Congress Cataloging-in-Publication Data
Hamilton, David, 1939–
A history of organ transplantation / David Hamilton ;
with a foreword by Clyde Barker and Thomas E. Starzl.
  p. cm.
Includes bibliographical references and index.
ISBN 978-0-8229-4413-3 (hardcover : acid-free paper)
1. Transplantation of organs, tissues, etc.—History.
2. Organ transplantation—History.   I. Title.
RD120.6.H36 2012
362.1979´5—dc23   2012008954

Contents

Foreword

DAVID HAMILTON HAS BEEN a senior transplant surgeon at the Western Infirmary, Glasgow, Scotland, and also the first director of the Wellcome Unit for the History of Medicine at Glasgow University. In addition, he is steeped in the lore and the basic science of the field because of his early training under the great transplantation biologist Peter Medawar. Thus, it is no surprise that he has written a history of transplantation that is unmatched in its scope, perceptiveness, and readability.

The masterly account he has crafted comes at an appropriate time, since organ transplantation has now become widely accepted as the best therapy for many otherwise fatal diseases. The surgeon-author of this book has watched and participated in many of the events as the field evolved over the last half century. Having looked back as an informed insider, he has added his historian's detachment and insight to the narrative.

Within living memory, organ transplantation existed only in science fiction. As a handful of surgeons and other dreamers set off in the 1960s "toward the impossible," they met huge challenges. The attitudes of that early time are vividly re-created in this book and will remind future readers that major innovation, clinical or scientific, is never easy and indeed can be a lonely business. Surgical replacement of a diseased organ constituted a paradigm shift. Its success altered forever the practice of several medical specialties while enriching multiple areas of basic and clinical science. Arguably, transplantation created the field of modern immunology rather than the other way around. And it had ripple effects in law, public policy, ethics, and even religion. Not omitted from Hamilton's account is the now-forgotten attitude of many in the medical profession that this journey was futile and should not be attempted.

The momentous scientific events of the 1950s are often taken as the starting point for organ transplantation, but there is a surprisingly long international prehistory, one that is highlighted in this book for its significance. The book is the first to tell the complete story of these earlier times, and this careful account in the first half of the book at last replaces earlier short, patchy, and often patronizing versions. The reader will be surprised at the vitality of the "lost era," as Hamilton calls it, of transplant studies before World War I. Also sharply delineated, analyzed, and explained are the events in the anarchic 1920s, when good science was at a low ebb and the monkey and goat gland transplanters assumed a license to mislead the public.

In the daunting task of taking on the technical challenge of organ transplantation, surgeons formed a fruitful partnership with some of the world's greatest scientists to probe the biology of graft rejection. The author examines this partnership closely and offers the shrewd conclusion that the surgeons were by no means the junior partner in the relationship. The reductionist approach of immunologists and their in vitro models were often misleading, resulting in faulty paradigms. Time and again, surgical empiricism led to unpredicted outcomes and advances that sent the immunologists back to the lab to think again.

Here also is an account, in this niche endeavor, of the so-called scientific method in action. The author is clear that, in surgery at least, there is no single method of discovery but rather a rich variety of methods. In the minor supporting strategies, Hamilton winkles out fascinating examples of good luck, bad luck, serendipity, personal rivalry, and arguments. Adding to his text are extensive scholarly citations that provide a helpful road map into the vast literature on organ transplantation.

As this book clearly shows, developing transplantation as a clinical service was not simply a surgical matter, limited to the attainment of technical success. Hamilton crucially re-creates the multiple influences, helpful and otherwise, that came into play. Transplantation generated a raft of ethical issues, funding challenges, and continuous contact with lawmakers and governments, all of which had national and international nuances.

Running through this book are interesting asides on the use of transplant themes in the fictional literature of the day, a reminder of the public's interest and involvement. Any undue hubris on the transplanters' part meant that nemesis followed—a drop in public confidence and hence a decrease in the donation of organs essential to the service. Nor were the media always supportive. In the aftermath of the transplants of the 1968 "Year of the Heart," as it is called here, there was an international crisis of confidence in transplant circles, one which should not be forgotten.

Throughout, the patients were the heroes, supporting the transplant surgeons from the first and disarming nay-saying critics simply on the grounds that, as patients, they would rather be alive than dead.

Limitations of space preclude a complete consideration in the book's later chapters of recent advances made possible by tacrolimus, multivisceral grafts, composite tissue transplants (e.g., hand and face), and increasing recognition of the crucial role of cellular chimerism as transplanters approach their ultimate goal—tolerance of organ allografts without need for immunosuppressive drugs.

Hamilton acknowledges that the story of transplantation is still being written. Yet, because some of the key professional figures of the early days of transplantation are still alive, this is an important time to tell the story. As noted in *The Puzzle People* (T. E. Starzl, 1992), the pioneers are "working their way one by one to the side of the stage. Passages into the wings are done by steps, minuet style. One device to get there is with a conference at which past contributions and efforts are celebrated by one's friends and former foes . . . ; they resemble the tours from city to city made by ageing baseball stars, some modest and some not, who are in their final season of play. The meetings are not designed to discover why these men did what they did. The secrets are within them, hidden beneath a pile of emotional stones which only they have a right or the knowledge to probe."

DR. CLYDE F. BARKER
Distinguished Service Professor and Professor of Surgery,
*   Emeritus, University of Pittsburgh*
President of the American Philosophical Society

DR. THOMAS E. STARZL
Director Emeritus, Thomas E. Starzl Transplantation
*   Institute, University of Pittsburgh*

Acknowledgments

IN THE EARLY 1970S, I became involved in clinical transplantation, and from that time forward witnessed the work of the transplant pioneers as they contributed to the evolving field. When I developed an interest in medical history, I had more focused discussions with many of the early workers, notably Sir Peter Medawar and Avrion Mitchison at Mill Hill, Tom Gibson in Glasgow, Sir Michael Woodruff in Edinburgh, Leslie Brent in London, and Sir Roy Calne in Cambridge. During my travels, I talked with many notable figures in the United States, including Joseph Murray in Boston, Blair Rogers in New York, and Willem "Pim" Kolff at Salt Lake City. In Europe, there were visits to Jean Hamburger, Marcel Legrain, and Gabriel Richet in Paris. More recently, I asked questions of others, notably Stuart Cameron and Richard Batchelor in London and, in the United States, Norman Shumway and E. Donnall Thomas passed on many helpful insights. Paul Shiels in Glasgow assisted with news from the new world of cellular engineering, and Richard Rettig contributed his unique knowledge of how U.S. political culture influenced the treatment of end stage renal failure.

Assisting with text, Jack MacQueen, Winifred MacQueen, and Harry Hine translated the early Latin extracts, and Sandy Reid in Edinburgh made the first full translation of Yuri Voronoy's pioneering papers on kidney transplantation from the 1930s. Henning Köhne and Anni Schneider made valuable translations of the forgotten German papers of the early twentieth century, and Henri Jacubowicz and Hala Girgis checked and translated the French-language citations.

My wife, Jean, encouraged this endeavor from the start, as did Sir Peter Morris, J. Douglas Briggs, and others in the British Transplantation Society. J. Andrew Bradley at Cambridge read the text at an early stage, and John MacConachie of Lossiemouth was my faithful reader and text editor over many years. Charles Webster and the Wellcome Unit for the History of Medicine at Oxford University gave me space for study during a sabbatical stay there. For written sources, there was great assistance from

London's Royal Society of Medicine Library and its incomparable collection of early journals, particularly of German and French origins, and Jonathan Erlen made the historical collection of the Falk Library in Pittsburgh available to me.

I am especially grateful to Thomas E. Starzl, who supported me as a visiting lecturer at the University of Pittsburgh Medical School. To his unique position in the history of transplantation he adds keen historical insight, and I am in his debt for detailed comments on the text. He also liaised with the University of Pittsburgh Press in publishing this book, and there I was encouraged and supported by the talented staff of the Press, in particular by my editors, Beth Davis and Alex Wolfe, who saw the project through with skill and care.

Introduction
Toward the Impossible

IT IS USUALLY THOUGHT that within the general advance of medicine, tissue and organ transplantation has a short history. Certainly the modern successful era started only in the 1950s, but there was earlier, much earlier, interest. Even the surgical records from 600 BCE contain accounts of plastic surgery, and the question of the use of tissue from donors appears in surgical works of medieval times. And many outside of surgery were interested from the first in the replacement of lost tissue. In medieval times, numerous shrines to the saints Cosmas and Damian and images of those twin physicians showed them transplanting a human leg. In Bologna, word of Gaspare Tagliacozzi's plastic surgery spread, and people widely (and wrongly) believed that he had obtained grafts from living donors and that when the donor died, the donated graft also died. Philosophers pondered deeply on the matter, and this urban myth, too good to be false, spread rapidly throughout Europe and was sustained by the satirists and coffeehouse gossips of London in the early 1700s.

In the 1800s, the public noticed the activities of tooth transplanters, and antivivisectionists protested experimental transplant work in France. In the 1920s, skin and "monkey gland" transplantation gained a new and dubious public fame. By the 1960s, surgeons rode high in public esteem, not least for the new success with organ grafting. The public were amused rather than shocked by the prospect of humanized pig organs in the 1900s, then intrigued by intricate arm, leg, and face transplants, and entranced by the hopes for organs grown from stem cells. The default view of the public, disturbed briefly from time to time, seems to be that transplantation attempts are admirable. Public opinion has a unique day-to-day input in clinical transplantation since transplantation requires organ donors and, hence, the support of the public. When public opinion is alienated, all donations decrease.

Among the interested public observers of transplant history were writers, fascinated by the possibilities and keen on exploiting each new effort.

London satirists in the 1700s found a convenient literary motif in John Hunter's transfer of teeth from the poor to the rich. The London revival of plastic surgery in the early 1800s provided inspiration for the monster in the novel *Frankenstein,* and by the end of the century, the grafting of skin and glands provided a mother lode of opportunities for what was soon to be called science fiction. An early practitioner, H. G. Wells, introduced fanciful transplantation possibilities into his work and thence into popular culture. This genre blossomed as a result of the anarchy in the transplant world of the 1920s. Adding to the gland-graft rejuvenation possibilities, there were tales of head, brain, face, and limb transplants. The inventive authors had license to transfer much else with the tissue—hands donated from dead murderers could prove murderous, brain grafts might be malevolent, and simian characteristics could appear after monkey testis transplants. With good science restored in mid-twentieth century, transplant themes were temporarily absent from the fiction of the day, but the controversies of the heart transplants and brain death in the 1970s encouraged publishers and writers to return to these genres. These novels fed on the new fears of the times, featuring sleazy doctors and organ-snatching gangs, but in the more settled periods that followed, popular nonfiction accounts found success, and positive personal stories of successful organ grafts sold well.

But it was not until the early 1950s that surgeons embarked with growing success on what was widely considered to be an unreachable mission, namely to successfully graft an organ from one person to another. Such grafting was considered to be impossible because the human body almost invariably rejected grafts from either humans or animals, other than in a few special situations. This reaction against foreign tissue, found at all levels of the animal kingdom, seemed so fundamental that no strategy, surgical or pharmacological, could hope to triumph over the problem. Moreover, many members of the medical community respected this relentless, ubiquitous power of the body to reject what was foreign to it, and many medical professionals, even surgeons, believed that to try to stave off rejection was not only futile but also "against nature." The pioneers in organ transplantation thus faced not only a huge biological challenge but also peer opposition and even hostility at times. Although the early transplants of the 1950s and 1960s are now seen as praiseworthy "firsts," that admiration did not characterize opinions at the time. Recognition of the early achievements took time, and that pioneering work finally won acclaim as one of surgery's greatest contributions. Those surgeons who paved the way steadily gained international honors. By the end of the twentieth century, clinical success with organ transplantation between humans was almost complete, having reached the status of a routine, noncontroversial service. Transplantation science efforts did not cease; further ambitions appeared, namely to develop ways to create new human organs.

In writing this account of how organ transplantation evolved, I had two tasks. The first was to provide an in-depth account suited for readers having some familiarity with the practice of medicine. Previous histories of transplantation have suggested that transplant-related activity before the 1940s was "prescientific," or quaint. I believe it is important to recognize important early work, and those who did that work, and to give them their proper place in a more complete historical record. My second task was to be attentive to medical historians' questions and their attitudes. I hope to have placed the history of transplantation in a broader context, avoiding the "upward and onward" idea of continuous progress in medical history so easily created with the benefit of hindsight. In particular, the many unprofitable matters that exercised the minds of those involved in transplantation from time to time are not ignored, nor should the times of hesitation and diversion be forgotten.

Surgical attempts to replace defective human tissue have a long history. As mentioned, manuscripts from the Indian subcontinent in the sixth century BCE describe carefully conducted plastic surgery. The grafting of skin flaps was the most ancient and established procedure for replacing tissue, and from early times, this practice included the possibility that another person could supply the skin graft for the patient in need. Donor-to-patient skin grafting was a goal surgeons began seriously pursuing in the 1600s. When the advance of medicine revealed that disease might result from problems with a specific organ rather than from a diffuse imbalance in body humors, physicians began to harbor wider ambitions for grafting damaged organs. The availability of anesthesia and measures to combat infection in the mid-1800s made such surgery even more promising.

But the simplicity of the ancient challenge contrasted with the complexity of the response and the diversity of the attempted solutions. When surgeons realized in the mid-1900s that the body's rejection of grafted tissue was a form of immunity, they turned to biomedical scientists for help in understanding and dealing with this obstacle to transplantation. The surgeons, normally self-sufficient in their endeavors and usually meeting the largely technical challenges of their work with their own novel solutions, needed assistance. Distinguished biologists willingly offered support, not only to further the surgeons' quest but also to advance their own efforts in attempting to understand the body's most complex and mysterious mechanism, one able to detect the tiniest deviation from its own structure. The "exquisite specificity" of this cell-mediated mechanism was clearly not designed to defeat the surgeon's efforts and explains the biologists' not-so-hidden interest in this combined venture. The joint effort yielded the rewards of not only clinical success for the surgeons but also broad fundamental insights that changed the course of biological science. The enigma of cell-mediated immunity was better understood, and the behavior of the body's defense cell—the lymphocyte—was so closely studied that this bland white cell became the model for investigating many cellular functions. The efforts to make human organ transplantation a reality also brought in hematologists familiar with blood typing, and they successfully unraveled the complexity of tissue types, allowing organs and tissue grafts to be matched to recipients. When tissue types proved to be related to the development of certain human diseases, scientists entered a new era of research on genetic susceptibility.

In joining this common cause of understanding the body's immune response, surgeons brought the scientists' hopes for inducing tolerance in human grafting. Researchers developed an array of immunological lab tests and measurements that could be put to clinical use, but surgeons were not simply the recipients of a one-way flow of information, and they were cautious in accepting all the results from basic science studies since humans might not function like the mouse. Sometimes discovery and enlightenment traveled in the opposite direction—from a clinical setting to the research lab. Surgeons made many unexpected observations of how the body functioned when it needed and received a transplant, and this real-world information sometimes contradicted received wisdom and made immunologists rethink some of their theories. One such surprise was when, after human organ recipients had transplant rejection "crises," viable grafts could be rescued, something never achieved in studies with small animals. Another unexpected discovery was that long-term human graft recipients showed evidence of the grafted tissue adapting to its new environment, which meant that immunosuppression therapy could cease without prompting rejection. Similarly unexpected was the discovery of microchimerism in long-standing human grafts, when some migrant donor cells still mingle with the host cells. The periodic discovery of such clinical novelties was important to the common effort but was especially significant for surgeons. At times of sluggish progress or public concern, transplant surgeons were often urged to "go back to the lab," but surgeons could weather such periods with confidence, knowing that test-tube reductionism and small animal studies were not the only route to success.

The understanding and treatment of other conditions also benefited from the developments in organ transplantation. Immune suppression to prevent organ rejection led to a range of uncommon and unpleasant infections, and, as a result, the many consequences of the low immune responses seen in AIDS patients were not unexpected, and therapies were thus already available. Even the earliest transplants, well before the 1950s, revised basic understandings of human disease mechanisms. In the eighteenth century, when John Hunter's living donor tooth transplants transmitted syphilis even though the tooth and its donor looked healthy, it was realized that serious disease could lie latent in tissues. A century later, the same lesson was taught when the enthusiasm for skin grafting resulted in the transmission of smallpox from donor to recipient. The situation arose again in the 1960s, when human kidneys from donors with previous cancer were transplanted and the kidney promptly began showing latent metastatic cancer deposits.

Even the understanding of human anatomy advanced as the result of surgical work. One might think that the human kidney had been well described for centuries, but when transplant surgeons had to take a closer look, they discovered the descriptions in even the best texts were deficient, particularly with regard to the main blood vessels and the supply to the ureter. Rather than one large artery, often there were two or more small ones—a situation that was of vital interest to the transplanters. Even more striking was the anatomy of the liver. The left and right lobes were an obvious subdivision used in traditional anatomical teaching, but surgical observation revealed that these lobes were not functionally separate. Bold attempts at excising liver tumors or dealing with liver trauma met uncontrolled bleeding or fatal bile leakage. The surgeons had to analyze liver anatomy with fresh eyes in the hope of finding safe surgical paths through the apparently homogeneous organ. Their efforts revealed true planes of cleavage and lobes with their own vessels and ducts. With this knowledge, the surgeons could split a liver and replace the diseased livers of two persons instead of one, or they could remove one lobe from a living donor. Thus, instead of guiding the surgeon's hands, the anatomy books were being rewritten by the surgeon's hands.

No medical endeavor has as many multiple interfaces with other disciplines as transplantation. Legal considerations played a role from the start, especially with regard to the concept of who owned the body of a deceased person. In the 1950s, the law, such as it was, dated back to the grave-robbing scandals of the early 1800s. When corneal grafting became more widespread in the 1950s, however, lawmakers implemented changes to allow quicker acquisition of donated tissues. By the 1960s, when kidney organ donation became possible, further legal changes were needed, and soon further changes had to follow, not without controversy, after brain-death criteria became used in intensive care units, with organ donation following. With rapid medical advances, the law often lagged behind.

Transplantation issues were among the first group of ethical concerns that gained prominence in medicine. Religious beliefs and the broader prohibitions in the ancient Hippocratic Oath had always had some influence on clinical practice, but in the early 1960s fresh ethical issues steadily arose. One of the first issues to attract attention was how to determine who should receive dialysis treatment for chronic renal failure. A new cadre of bioethicists emerged, and, increasingly, the public became involved in medical decision making. With new issues such as kidney donation to relatives and the intense controversies over brain death and heart transplants, bioethics became firmly established as an influence in the clinic. Bioethicists soon began to debate such topics as "equity" and "utility" in the distribution of scarce donor organs, xenografts (from animals to humans), and stem cell use.

By the 1960s, governments and insurance providers had to acknowledge the reality of organ transplantation. Research funding in the United States and local health care budgets in Europe had financed early attempts at organ transplantation. However, when organ grafting became accepted and the number of transplants increased, overall costs rose, particularly when liver transplantation emerged as the highest-cost single procedure in medical care. Each developed nation fashioned its own method of funding transplantation work, and support was often obtained only after tough negotiations and debate.

The practice of organ transplantation has spread across the globe at an uneven pace. Other types of new surgical procedures usually take hold steadily in less developed nations, emerging when finances permit, public awareness increases, and demand grows. In those circumstances, a surgical procedure usually retains its original clinical characteristics. In the case of organ transplantation, however, there is often resistance in less developed nations. In such places, the demand for expensive procedures like transplants may be outweighed by the urgent need to address common infectious diseases. Cultural attitudes and religious teachings on death and donation may mean that decreased-donor organ transplantation is unacceptable.

Wars, hot and cold, have also had their impact on transplantation research and practice. World War I spelled the end of earlier studies in transplantation immunology on what seemed the eve of the birth of human organ grafting. In the 1920s, many physicians seemed to abandon such progressive notions, reverting to an older, holistic style of medicine with Hippocratic attitudes and simple therapy using lifestyle adjustments. Science-based clinical aspirations faded away, particularly in Europe, and experimental organ transplant surgery stagnated. This mood ceased abruptly in the early months of World War II, when pressing clinical issues, notably aviators' severe burns, meant new government attention to the need for progress in this normally mundane matter. Scientists and plastic surgeons undertook new skin grafting studies and attempted to graft tissue from one individual to another. During the Korean War, the artificial kidney machine, controversial to that point, proved its worth and spread from military hospital settings into routine civilian use, as did improved vascular surgical methods.

The cold war led to massive spending on nuclear weaponry and the search for an effective means of protecting humans from radiation. A solution to the latter challenge remained elusive, but the research led to radiation therapies that could be used in transplanting bone marrow cells. This procedure resulted in the first workable methods for successful human organ grafting. Another result of these military studies was the preparation and production of a range of radioactive isotopes, which promptly proved to be powerful therapeutic and investigative tools. For example, isotope labeling solved some immunological mysteries, notably the lifespan and travels of the lymphocyte.

In the Soviet Union, ideology directed scientists' biological research, which meant a thoroughgoing rejection of "Western" genetic research. This faulty, politicized science meant that the Soviets' creditable contributions to immunology, including the first well-conducted human kidney graft, came to an end for decades.

Technological advances, too, played a role in the advance of organ transplantation, but it was an unsung role. From earliest times, apart from slow, long-standing, steady improvements in surgical instruments, perhaps the first major development to affect transplant work was the improved microscope produced in the mid-1800s; Claude Bernard used the new instrument in his important skin graft studies. In the early twentieth century, new techniques for measuring such things as hormones in the blood made endocrinology respectable. That particular advance defeated the promoters of animal sex gland transplants: the grafted glands produced no hormones. Developed in the 1940s, the flame photometer could measure electrolytes, extending the work of clinical biochemistry labs, and the revolutionary AutoAnalyzer of the late 1950s could rapidly yield the numerous lab test results needed for dialysis efforts. By the 1960s, blood gas analysis devices provided the frequent assessment of respiratory function needed for successful long-term respiratory support in intensive care units. X-ray methods largely dating from the 1920s could assess some aspects of kidney function, but, by the 1980s, ultrasound examination revolutionized the management of organ grafts. Added to the impact of this expensive, sophisticated technology was the availability of plastics. Introduced in 1960, the plastic arteriovenous shunt made regular dialysis possible. Cheap, sterile, disposable tubes and containers revolutionized daily life in the lab, and with helpful micro-dispensers, they notably sped up serological testing and the study of isolated cells—which could also now be cryopreserved. New surgical instruments useful in transplant research and surgery included slim, eyeless needles bearing a single fine synthetic suture and the fiber-optic instruments that revolutionized minimally invasive techniques, including laparoscopic kidney surgery.

It may come as a surprise to some that, until the 1980s, the pharmaceutical industry did little to support transplant surgeons' work. In the 1960s, the industry did not involve itself in organ transplantation matters because there seemed to be no promise of a sizable market. Instead, surgeons devised their own immunosuppressive methods using established drugs or variants, even adding their own homemade agents, such as an antilymphocyte serum. When powerful pharmaceuticals such as cyclosporine were developed and marketed, the industry entered permanently and controversially into the life and activities of transplant units, and the earlier surgical innocence was lost. Each new drug that entered the market was expensive, reflecting the huge costs of development and the required clinical trials. Transplant units increasingly accepted the financial and corporate presence of pharmaceutical companies, which could set the conditions and endpoints of any drug trial. These trials began to dominate clinical management in each unit, and the marketing of the new drugs could also be intense.

I became personally involved in clinical transplantation in the early 1970s, and in this account I offer my sense of how organ transplantation developed in the years that followed. It is an account that I hope will offer insights that a historian might miss when trying to reconstruct events only from scattered primary sources.

I Early Transplantation

To EARLY HUMANS, as to all their descendants, the possibility of restoration of lost or mutilated parts of the body was a lively issue. To make good such losses incurred by war, disease or punishment, ancient humans had recourse to local help and healers. But they also looked for supernatural help, because legends told them that such powers could be used to make the injured part whole again. And there may have been an additional imperative to ancient humans to be restored to normal. If after death the body went in a mutilated, deficient state to the afterworld, subsequent resurrection was deemed to be impossible.[1] This belief persists in some cultures to this day.[2]

Ancient Legends of Replacement

Stories of successful magical replacement of lost tissues are found in the themes of folklore from all parts of the ancient world. The tales of restoration of lost limbs or eyes, and even replacement of decapitated heads, are hardly less popular in ancient lore than the raising of the dead or magical cures for paralysis or blindness. These transplant claims are found in the legends of all nations, from Iceland to Africa.[3]

The tales fall into a number of patterns. An arm, hand or leg, or eyes have been lost. The sufferer is in some way worthy of cure, and a priest or shaman successfully restores the necessary part, but, in other stories, less noble forces are at work. In one variant, villagers capture malevolent marauders and cut off their heads, but new heads grow again immediately, and the raiders continue to attack. In other accounts, an attacker's freshly removed head is replaced immediately, but at an angle, resulting in a permanently twisted neck. In other versions, the head is replaced back-to-front, adding to the terror of the appearance of the restored bandits.

Irish and North American Indian transplant stories tell of a juggler given the power to remove his own eyes a specified number of times, and, having exceeded his quota and thus lost his own, he uses animal eyes to replace the lost globes. In a splendid Irish legend about Nuada, an important ruler who loses a hand in battle, there are many familiar themes:

1

According to Celtic custom, no maimed person could rule, and Nuada was removed from power. But who should turn up on his doorstep but Miach, a celebrated physician. After impressing the half-blind doorkeeper by replacing his bad eye with a good one from a cat, they easily gained access to Nuada himself. . . .

Miach had Nuada's own long-since buried hand dug up and placed on the stump. Over it, Miach chanted one of the best known of old Gaelic charms, enjoining each sinew, each nerve, each vein, and each bone to unite, and in three days the hand and arm were as if they had never been parted. . . .

Ever afterwards the poor doorkeeper's cat's eye stayed awake all night looking for mice.[4]

Traditional tales from China even relate to heart transplantation. In one, Judge Lu assists an illiterate man by giving him a new heart "picked in the nether world from among thousands of human hearts." In another, the Chinese doctor Pien Ch'iao exchanges the hearts of two men to "match their energies better" and uses "potent herbs" to ensure success after the operations.[5] Less dramatically, Hua T'o, the talented "surgeon of the Three Kingdoms," is able to remove, wash, and replace defective intestines.[6] Greek legends recount that the Graiai were sea goddesses who lacked teeth and eyes but successfully passed one of each between them for use. On the utopian island described by Iambulus around 100 BCE were tortoises whose blood had a glue powerful enough to reattach severed body parts. In Apuleius's circa AD 160 Latin retelling of the Greek tale *The Golden Ass,* the hero's nose and ears are removed by witches and then replaced with wax.

These early stories feature the first ethical dilemmas of transplantation. In one, a goddess switches the heads of a married man and his brother. Which part, the tale asked, was now the real husband—the body or the head? Less ethically complex was Zeus's action in stitching the doomed, premature baby Dionysus onto his thigh until the child grew bigger and was ready to be born. A later tale, surviving to medieval times and collected by the brothers Grimm, told of a transplant that transferred the donor's personality: a hand transplant from a thief makes the recipient turn to stealing.

Chimeric Monsters

Another class of legend testified to the possibility of fusing tissues from different species to produce hybrid beings.[7] Ancient humans harbored a lively belief in the centaur (half man, half horse) and in other fusions that resulted in dragons, griffins, mermaids, Pegasus the winged horse, the Minotaur, and the Sphinx.[8] Hittite temple carvings depict some fierce composites with the head of a man, body of a lion, and wings of an eagle. The young Hindu god Ganesha, son of Shiva and Parvati, gained a new

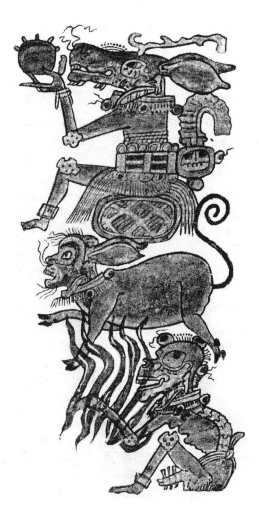

The hybrid "mantichora" shown in Edward Topsell's *Historie of Fourefooted Beastes* (London, 1607), 344. Image courtesy of Glasgow University Libraries Special Collections.

animal head after decapitation by his angry father. Repenting of his act, the father told his servants to obtain the head of the first living being they could find, which was an elephant.[9] In ancient Greece, the fire-breathing Chimera (part lion, part goat, and part serpent) was the alarming creature of *The Iliad* that terrorized ancient Lycia in Turkey before the heroic Bellerophon destroyed it. The unpleasant lamia was a female who was part snake, and the harpies were ugly, winged birdwomen who stole food and abducted humans, while the manticore had a man's head, the body of a lion, and a scorpion's tail. The myths about these creatures suggest that most were aggressive and unpleasant, but others were more kindly, notably Chiron, the wisest of the centaurs, who was teacher and mentor to the young Aesculapius, Greco-Roman god of medicine.

These tales merged slowly into the earliest science-fiction writings, and, in the fourteenth century, Sir John Mandeville's *Travels* (which leaned heavily on the works of Pliny the Elder) told his credulous readers about men with the heads of dogs, men with horse hooves, and lions with eagle heads.

The Power of the Saints

Although such fantastical tales were common across many different lands and cultures, the Christian involvement in tissue replacement in the Western world is perhaps best known.[10] The New Testament is replete with healing incidents because Christ had exhorted his disciples to go forth "two by two, preach, cast out devils and heal the sick." Christ himself, as an act of forgiveness, miraculously replaced the high priest's servant's ear, cut off by Peter during Christ's arrest.[11] Tradition holds that Saint Peter, who witnessed this reattachment, later accomplished a similar restoration of the breasts torn from Saint Agatha during her torture. Thereafter, a number of miracles of hand replacement were taken as credible then, but subject now to skeptical analysis. For example, Saint Mark, late in the first century, was said to have replaced a severed, mutilated hand. A legend from the fifth century holds that Pope Leo punished himself by cutting off his own hand and that Mary, Mother of Christ, appeared to him in a dream and reattached it. When Leo, emperor of Constantinople, falsely accused Saint John of Damascus (AD 645–750) of treason, he then ordered John's right hand to be amputated. This was reported as done, and John carried his severed hand to his oratory and slept, but after sleeping awoke to find the hand replaced and healed. Some cynics immediately accused him of fraud and claimed that the hand had never been lost and that by bribery he had averted the mutilation. John was ordered to show his right hand for assessment at the court, and the surface of the hand showed a convincing scar.[12]

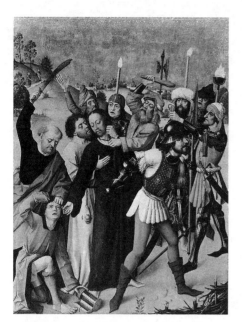

Christ replacing the lost ear of the servant of the high priest, cut off by Simon Peter. From *The Arrest of Christ*, by the school of Dirc Bouts. Image courtesy of Rheininsche Bild-Archiv.

Later Saints' Miracles

Although the cult of cures surrounding Christian saints was to continue, in the next few centuries the pattern of such miraculous intervention changed. Instead of obtaining healing through personal encounters with itinerant holy men, believers began to seek "posthumous" healing from long-dead saints. Religious authorities encouraged the public to visit saints' places of birth or burial to seek a cure. The Church began to invest in shrines to the saints in many churches and cathedrals throughout Europe. If a reputation was gained for healing, it brought pilgrims, penitents, and income to the institution.[13]

Individual saints even became credited with very specific healing powers long after their own deaths. According to the belief, around the year 1150 the spiritual intervention of the twin saints Cosmas and Damian resulted in a successful leg transplant.[14] Little is actually known of the lives of Cosmas and Damian except that they were martyred in Syria during the Diocletian persecution in the second half of the third century. The shrine where the miracle took place was in Rome, far from their homeland (which may have been Arabia), many centuries after their deaths. A written account of the miracle appeared about one hundred years after its supposed occurrence, and thereafter the event gained fame and evoked many paintings and other representations of the event: few other single miracles have such a rich iconography.[15]

The cult of Cosmas and Damian increased from the sixth century onward, and they were elevated as particular patrons of medical practice. Numerous shrines to them were built, and artists generally depict them as physician and surgeon. In Rome alone, three churches were dedicated to them, in that part of the Forum traditionally associated with medicine, and the miraculous leg transplant probably occurred at a church erected by Saint Felix, pope from AD 526 to 530, one filled with brilliant mosaics of the two saints. According to the legend, the worthy sacristan of that church had a cancerous growth of the leg. As it was customary for those seeking healing during pilgrimage to use votive "incubation," that is, to sleep in the sanctuary, the sacristan did so. During the night, the saints appeared to the sacristan in a dream and replaced the diseased limb, using the leg of a recently buried black Ethiopian gladiator who had died the preceding day and been buried two miles away. The cancerous leg was thoughtfully retained by the saints to bury

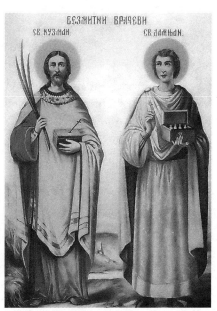

Cosmas and Damian, the twin Christian saints with a reputation for healing, died as martyrs about AD 303, and people visited shrines to these saints hoping to be cured. As in this wood engraving, Cosmas and Damian are often shown as physicians or apothecaries. Some artists depicted them as surgeons. Image courtesy of Wikimedia Commons.

with the donor's remains, thus allowing for the resurrection of a body that was whole.[16]

The story is given with fanciful detail in *The Golden Legend,* Caxton's English translation of an earlier compilation of such miracles. The two saints conferred, and

thenne the other sayd to him, "There is an ethyopyen that this day is buryed in the chirchyerd of saynt peter ad vincula whiche is yet fresshe, late vs bere this thyder and take we out of that moryans flesshe and fyll this place with all." And soo they fette the thye of this dede man, and cutte of the thye of the seke man and soo chaunged that one for the other. And when the seke man awoke and felt no payne, he put forthe his honde and felte his legge withoute hurte, and thenne tooke a candel and sawe wel that it was not his thye, but that hit was another. And when he was well come to hym self, he sprange oute of his bedde for ioye and recounted to al the people how hit was happed to hym, and that whiche he had sene in his slepe, and hou he was heled. And they sente hastely vnto the tombe of the deede man, and fonde the thye of hym cutte of and that other thye in the tombe in stede of his.[17]

Other Christian saints performed similar but less celebrated miracles. In the thirteenth century, Saint Anthony of Padua (1195–1231) was credited with reattaching a severed leg. In Irish hagiography there are also a number of examples of lost tissue replaced after the intervention of the saints. In one well-known account, Saint Ciaran restored the decapitated head of an Irish chief, but with less than perfect alignment, since the head remained twisted thereafter.[18] English pilgrimage sites also reported miraculous tissue restoration. At Worcester in 1200, Saint Wulfstan was said to have cured a man whose eyes and testicles had been removed as punishment. At Canterbury, site of Thomas Becket's martyrdom, a sleeping penitent's liver was taken out, cleansed, and replaced. Becket is also credited with restoring the losses of a cleric castrated by a jealous husband. This event gave the wits of the day their chance for satire:

> Sublustri rutilans allusit abyssus abysso,
> Cura, teste nova, testiculisque novis.[19]

The thrust of the text is that the chaste cleric, though restored, should have no use for new testicles.

In general, these reported miracles and the earlier legends had moral content and served to instruct: the lessons were that divine healing in general, and organ replacement in particular, was possible, but only under some conditions. It was helpful that the penitent's illness or injury was unsought and unfair, but above all, the sufferer had to be worthy and deserving of such intervention.[20] These arguments about who was worthy of such miraculous healing were to reappear when organ transplantation began to be an accepted medical procedure.

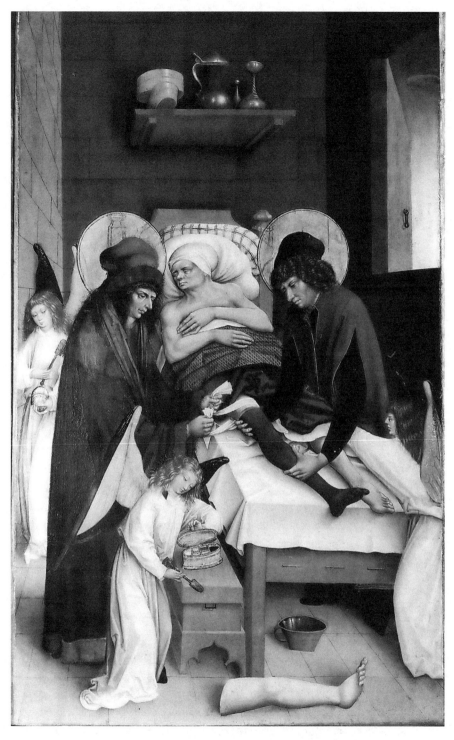

Leonberg's depiction (circa 1500) of the miraculous replacement of a diseased leg by the posthumous intervention of the saints Cosmas and Damian at a shrine to their honor in Rome. Image courtesy of Württembergisches Landesmuseum, Stuttgart.

Decline of Magic

By medieval times, belief in magical cures was in decline, affected by the secular learning and rise of humanism; after all, the texts from ancient Greece carried no accounts of miraculous healing. Fewer individual priests claimed personal powers of healing, and routine visits to shrines began to decline. Stories of the replacement of body parts diminished in frequency, and only modest claims for magical regeneration, rather than transplantation, remained.[21] Supernatural grafting could now be ridiculed, and François Rabelais (1483?–1553), the Renaissance polymath and priest-turned-doctor, could now invoke only secular surgical methods in his satirical description of the successful replacement of a severed head in *Pantagruel* (1534):

Having gone out to search the field for Episthemon, they found him stark dead with his head between his arms all bloody. But Panurge said, "my dear Bullies all, weep not one drop more, for he being yet all hot, I will make him as sound as ever he was." In saying this, he took the detached head, and held it warm fore-against his cod-piece that the air might not enter into it, and the other two carried the body. "Leave off crying," quoth Panurge, "and help me." Then he cleansed the neck very thoroughly with white wine, afterwards he anointed it with I know not what ointment, and set it on very just, vein against vein, sinew against sinew, and spondyle against spondyle, that he might not be wry necked: this done, he gave it round about some fifteen or sixteen stitches with the needle: suddenly Episthemon began to breathe, then opened his eyes, yawned, sneezed, and afterwards let out a great fart.[22]

His use of the antiseptic white wine is laudable, as is his support for speed. Two aspects of Rabelais's surgical mindset are interesting. First, he assumes that reunion of bulky tissues, when placed together, will occur by end-to-end union, notably of the divided blood vessels. Second, he believes that such detached grafts should be kept warm before attachment. These assumptions were durable and were widely affirmed later. The first lasted until the mid-1800s, and the second, namely, the view that for organ grafting "warm is good," lasted until the mid-1900s.

Despite the decline of belief in magical cures, credence in transcendental healing had not entirely disappeared. In late medieval times, a lively belief in the devil intensified, and it was understood that the evil powers of black magic could be called up by some for the infliction, or cure, of disease.[23] Humble citizens thought to be using such aid could attract accusations of witchcraft, and the activities of learned men were also watched. Transplantation of tissues had until then been associated with *acceptable* supernatural powers, but now those medieval surgeons who cautiously attempted even skin grafting had to watch out for their reputations. Gaspare Tagliacozzi, the first known Western surgeon to use con-

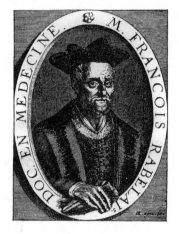

François Rabelais, doctor, scholar, and author, used the myths of head replacement in his epic tale *Pantagruel* (1534). Image courtesy of Glasgow University Library, Special Collections.

ventional methods of plastic surgery, suffered posthumously as a result of gossip from his rivals, who claimed that he had used evil influences.

The Remaining Legacy

One aspect of the age of miracles and magic cast a long shadow over tissue transplantation that extended almost to the twentieth century. The tales of successful human grafting and the belief in hybrid animals meant that the public remained deeply conditioned to believe that transplantation of tissue from animals to humans or from one person to another could succeed. Even though the notion of miraculous grafting was increasingly discredited, the possibility of successful grafting using ordinary surgical methods remained. It was not until the twentieth century that the ancient "default" belief that humans could readily accept foreign grafts was reversed, and then only with difficulty. A paradigm shift to the notion that rejection was the rule following all living grafts—both homografts (from other people) and xenografts (from animals)—was remarkably slow to emerge and difficult to establish.

However, there had also been some early, secular, nonmagical surgical tissue replacements, using skin flaps moved from one part of the body to another (autografts). Skilled operators did these procedures far from Europe, and their methods did not reach Europe until the Renaissance.

Early Plastic Surgery in India

One of the world's oldest medical texts describes plastic surgery. The Hindu Sanskrit text *Suśruta Samhita,* of about the sixth century BCE, describes restoration of damaged ears or noses by methods similar to modern reconstructive surgery.

The tradition is that Suśruta was a surgeon, teaching at Benares in India.[24] His approach to tissue replacement in the face was to create a local skin flap, rotate it to cover the defect, and fix it in place. The operation may have been of some antiquity, and when it was discovered still in use in India in the nineteenth century, it initiated the rapid emergence of plastic surgery in Europe.[25]

The ancient Indian operations were used for those disfigured not only by disease but also by violence or warfare, notably when sword wounds damaged or excised soft tissue from the head and face. In addition, some sufferers had received mutilation in civil feuds or as revenge, or as judicial punishments for serious crimes. Ruthless rulers would deal with threats to their power by mutilating the faces of their opponents, notably by removal of the nose.[26] Such injuries humiliated the victim, equating them with criminals, and would also leave them defective and handicapped in the afterlife.[27] The practice may have been widespread; facial mutilation was common in Chile up to the time of the Spanish colonial period and has persisted to this day in Afghanistan.[28] In Peru, pre-Inca Chimú pottery images placed in the graves of distinguished persons showed evidence of such facial injuries.[29] A Roman fort in Scotland was found to have a collection of human hand and foot bones, doubtless removed from local insurgents to discourage their fellows.

In Asian cultures, a less dramatic deformity of the ear was not caused by punishment but by the use of beautifying heavy earrings or fenestrating ornaments, which intentionally stretched the lobe but could split the thin ring of skin. *Suśruta* gives an elaborate typology of such defects.[30] If local repair of the ear deformity was not possible, the surgeon attempted complete replacement of the ear lobe. The operative detail in *Suśruta* is scanty, but the approach was clear: "A surgeon well-versed in the knowledge of surgery should slice off a patch of living flesh [skin] from the

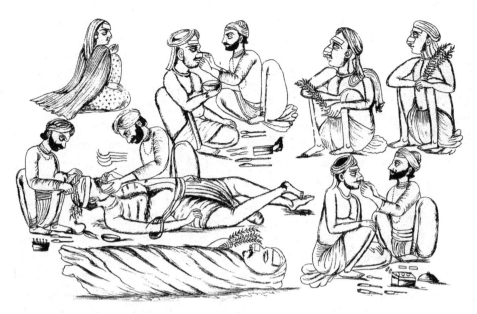

The ancient Indian plastic surgical procedures were illustrated in use late in the nineteenth century in B. H. Baden-Powell's *Handbook of the Manufactures and Arts of the Punjab* (Lahore, 1872).

cheek of a person devoid of ear-lobes in a manner so as to have one of the ends attached to its former seat. The part, where the artificial ear-lobe is to be made, should be slightly scarified and the living flesh, full of blood and sliced off as previously directed, should be adhesioned to it."[31]

The principle involved in the surgery is clear, and the operative detail is convincing. A "rotation" flap was used, namely, one with its base remaining attached in its original position and, hence, still supplied by the original blood vessels. After moving the free end and fixing it, sometime later the base and the original blood supply could be safely severed.

The *Suśruta* is best known for its description of the method of restoring damaged noses. The following passage describes the operation, which was again a rotation flap from the cheek:

Now I shall deal with the process of affixing an artificial nose. First the leaf of a creeper, long and broad enough to fully cover the whole of the severed or clipped off part, should be gathered; and a patch of living flesh, equal in dimension to the preceding leaf, should be sliced off (from down upward) from the region of the cheek and, after scarifying it with a knife, swiftly adhered to the severed nose. Then the cool-headed physician should steadily tie it up with a bandage decent to look at and perfectly suited to the end for which it has been employed.

The physician should make sure that the adhesion of the severed parts has been fully effected and then insert two small pipes into the nostrils to facilitate respiration, and to prevent the adhesioned flesh from hanging down. After that, the adhesioned part should be dusted with powders of Pattanga, Yashitmadhukam, and Rasanjana pulverised together, and the nose should be enveloped in cotton and several times sprinkled over with the refined oil of pure sesamum. Clarified butter should be given to the patient for drink, and he should be anointed with oil and treated with purgatives after the complete digestion of the meals he has taken, as advised in the books of medicine.[32]

The method emphasizes that the flap should be cut accurately and that special bandaging was important. As in other ancient surgical procedures, exotic ointments were used for local application, and postoperative medication and diet were important.

Indian surgical technique was advanced at the time. Those learning the technique practiced suturing on fruit or leather, and models stood in for humans for bandaging practice. The *Suśruta* text shows that student surgeons learned anatomy by dissecting cadavers. It seems that surgery had a high status at the time, and since it was taught together with internal medicine, it is likely that a distinguished and literate man like Suśruta might perform the surgery he describes. In the centuries that followed, however, manual work of any kind became offensive to the higher castes in India, and with their cultural distaste for touching the human body in life or death, the study of anatomy declined, as did the practice of surgery among the learned.[33] Later, when Western colonizers discovered that the ancient Hindu plastic surgery techniques were still in use, the operations were being performed by artisan surgeons associated with the lowly trades of potter and brick maker.

Early Indian surgeons may also have succeeded in transplanting skin without use of flaps. They could use detached skin, that is, "free" grafts, since some Indian texts mention the use of skin taken from the buttock to replace defects elsewhere. This skin is too thick to use unchanged elsewhere on the body, so donor skin was prepared in a special way. A suitable area of the buttock was flayed by a whip, causing swelling and bruising, and the skin was then removed and used. Since skin prepared in this way was fissured and split by the trauma, this perhaps created, in later terminology, a partial-thickness skin graft. This thin layer might heal in and survive, unlike the thick, normal buttock skin.

Later Accounts of Plastic Surgery

These ancient methods used by indigenous healers probably continued unchanged in India for centuries and certainly persisted there until the end of the nineteenth century. It would be surprising if the methods were not in use widely in the Middle East in ancient times, but the many Arabic medical texts are silent on this topic up to medieval times. The techniques are hardly mentioned in the surgical texts of the great Greek medical writers, beginning with the contributors to the Hippocratic collection, written about the fifth century BCE. There is no evidence that such surgery was carried out in ancient Egypt, but later, Alexandrian writers did briefly describe plastic surgical methods.[34] This knowledge must have passed to the Romans, since the surgical techniques appear in the works of the medical authorities Celsus (25 BCE–AD 50) and Galen (AD 129–216).[35] Both writers describe briefly, but vaguely, methods for replacement of lost tissue, and it may be that these methods were merely copied from text to text. Learned medical writers often included operations that were thought to be possible or were in use by the humbler "artisan" surgeons, rather than in use by the learned author.[36] The Byzantine encyclopedists, notably Oribasius, used the same material that had appeared in Galen's work, and it also appears in the works of Paulus Aegineta of Rome, written prior to the Muslim invasion of AD 640. Later Arab surgical works, notably that of Rhazes (circa AD 924), continued to give short references to techniques for addressing deformities. By the tenth century, the caliphate of Córdoba was the most culturally advanced area in Europe, and, under the rule of Al-Hakam II, Muslim scholarship, manuscript collection, and translation flourished. It is significant that plastic surgery is absent from the influential *Chirurgia* section of the thirty-volume medical treatise by Al-Hakam II's court surgeon and physician, Abulcasis (Abū 'l-Qāsim Khalaf ibn 'Abbās al-Zahrāwī, AD 936–1013). It seems that the techniques had not reemerged in the western Mediterranean at that time nor were they featured in the older Muslim texts held in Córdoba.[37] Possible explanations for this absence are that the need for plastic surgery was small or that, in the Western world, attempts at plastic surgical repair were now deplored as vanity and thus cosmesis was left to beauticians.[38] Abulcasis had another constraint on his practice. Distinguished surgeons at the time avoided "capital" operations, which included procedures like cutting to remove bladder stones or for relief of strangulated hernias, because they could have a fatal outcome. There were others in the "medical marketplace" who might offer such surgery—notably the humble local artisan or itinerant surgeons, who, being illiterate, left no writings.[39] They had empirical skills guarded by semisecret trade practices.[40]

The Revival of Plastic Surgery

The Renaissance, starting in Europe in the fourteenth century, led to a hunt for the ancient texts containing the knowledge and wisdom of Greece and Rome. The visual arts were also liberated and reborn. In medicine, the classical manuscript texts were sought and studied anew, and, in Italy, migrant Greek scholars assisted with translation of the works of Galen and Hippocrates. With the introduction of movable type printing in Germany in 1438, wider dissemination of knowledge occurred by books rather than via copied manuscripts. In Italy, soon to be a major printing and publishing center, the new humanism first assimilated and built on the classical medical knowledge and finally began to challenge the revived Galenic wisdom. The surgeon-anatomists were particularly innovative, and, in the north of Italy, the universities at Bologna and Padua both taught surgery; the medical teachers had salaries exceeded only by those of the professors of law. The celebrated Italian surgeons with this new elevated status moved their craft forward and, in doing so, accepted a scholarly obligation to share their knowledge through publication of elegantly illustrated texts.

However, the ancient Indian use of methods of skin grafting by flaps reemerged first in southern Italian practice, not in northern academic circles.[41] The ancient Eastern learning entered Italy via Mediterranean trade routes, and the passage of the Crusaders and streams of pilgrims visiting the Holy Land further disseminated knowledge. Sicily was a central point in these movements of people and information, and it grew to be the major power in the Mediterranean under the rule of Roger II (1096–1154). Economic confidence and a cosmopolitan attitude also aided scholarship, and Roger added distinguished scholars to his court. The need for medical men in the armies of the Crusades grew and encouraged medical teaching in Sicily, which notably flourished under the patronage of Frederick II (1215–1250). The medical school at Salerno—the Schola Medica Salernitana—had a laudable emphasis on empirical clinical study by apprenticeship, rather than a traditional focus on theory and disputation. It may have been medical practitioners or travelers returning from the East or perhaps Sicilian naval campaigns that brought news of old, forgotten surgical skills, including the Indian methods of facial plastic surgery, back to the island. Whatever their route, these techniques probably first appeared in Europe in Sicily in the fourteenth century, and it was the local, craft-trained practitioners who used them.

The Sicilian Surgeons

The first Sicilian surgeons known to offer nose reconstruction (rhinoplasty) were the Brancas, a father and son in Catánia on the east coast of Sicily, opposite Reggio de Calabria in mainland southern Italy. While Branca the elder used the original Indian method of rhinoplasty—using an adjacent flap of skin swung over from the cheek or forehead—the son significantly improved on the older Indian strategy, starting to use more distant flaps of skin, notably from the arm.

The methods were a trade secret, but news spread and interest in the Sicilian activities grew among the elite northern Italian surgeons.[42] A contemporary account by one such surgeon describes his visit with the Brancas and erroneously credits them with developing the rhinoplasty technique that they had actually inherited from abroad. The northerner's account gives a version of the operation, though a flawed one; perhaps the Brancas did not let him see too much:

Branca, the elder, was the inventor of an admirable and almost incredible thing. He conceived how he might repair and replace noses that had been mutilated and cut off, and developed his ideas into a marvelous art. And the son Antonius added not a little to his father's wonderful discovery. For he conceived how mutilated lips and ears might be restored, as well as noses. Moreover, whereas his father had taken the flesh for the repair from the mutilated man's face, Antonius took it from the muscles of his arm, so that no distortion of the face should be caused. On that arm, cut open, and into the wound itself, he bound the stump of the nose so tightly that the patient might not move his head at all, and after fifteen days, or sometimes twenty, little by little with a sharp knife he cut away the flap, which had become attached to the nose; finally he severed it entirely from the arm, and shaped it into a nose with so much ingenuity that it was scarcely possible with the eye to detect the flap that had been added.[43]

This otherwise clear account had a major error in describing the use of the muscle of the upper arm, rather than skin flaps. This important and improbable misunderstanding was to be a persisting source of confusion for two centuries thereafter.

These face or forearm flap operations, performed by humble Sicilian surgeons, were known in Italy for some decades before some of the distinguished university-based surgeons of the northern Italian towns ever mentioned them. The professor of surgery at Padua, Alessandro Benedetti (c. 1445–1525), knew of the work of the Brancas and gave a brief account of it in his text *Anatomice, sive historia corporis humani* (1514). In that book he included some advice regarding care of the new nose after its creation, notably that it should not be roughly handled.[44] This practical detail suggests that he was studying patients who had returned from Sicily after surgery and reported to him. Benedetti was, however, cautious about carrying out novel or heroic operations, sharing the attitude among the elite surgeons at the time that one should seek to avoid professional disaster.[45] It was only Gaspare Tagliacozzi who was prepared to try.

Tagliacozzi's *De curtorum chirurgia*

Tagliacozzi (1545–1599) had studied under eminent teachers in Bologna, notably Girolamo Cardano and Ulisse Aldrovandi. He then set up in that town as a surgeon and teacher of anatomy, soon achieving a reputation for wound management, and he succeeded Giulo Aranzio in the university's chair of anatomy. In 1597, at the age of fifty-two, Tagliacozzi published his first and only book. This famous, beautifully illustrated text, *De curtorum chirurgia per insitionem* (On the surgery of mutilation by grafting), contained a detailed description, based on Tagliacozzi's years of treating many patients, of the theory and practice of plastic surgery.[46] Tagliacozzi graciously made it clear in his text that his inspiration came from southern town surgeons in Calabria who followed in the Branca tradition.[47] But as one of the new academic surgeons, he had to distance himself from the artisan surgeons' approach and claim that his own methods were superior, since they were based on a university training that gave him a sophisticated understanding of the physiology of healing. He gives verbose descriptions of the erroneous biological science of the day and how it applied to surgery, but his faulty theory did not hinder him in copying the Brancas' empirically successful surgery. In some matters, Tagliacozzi may have improved upon the operative technique, notably in measuring and marking the bed and graft, and his text shows minute attention to the details of pre- and postoperative management, together with some timeless, wry asides. When operating, for instance, "the attendants must observe diligently every nod of the surgeon, for many things happen during an operation which need to be indicated by a nod, and not by speech. One must be sparing of words." The best operative environment for carrying out surgery, he wrote, was "two nimble assistants, good light, and all others to leave the room."[48]

Tagliacozzi's patients, as revealed by his text, were wealthy. They came to him due to their loss of a nose, ear, or lip, usually from warfare, violence, or dueling. Increasingly, however, a new reason for patients to seek his help was syphilis, which had spread rapidly from Naples through Europe in 1495. In its tertiary stage, syphilis could erode the inner nose. Tagliacozzi did treat such patients but only after attempts to control the disease with mercury.

Tagliacozzi followed the younger Branca's technique by raising a flap of skin from the upper arm and applying it to the freshened bed of the deficient nose. The numerous illustrations in his book show his attention to detail and that Tagliacozzi had brought to perfection the design of bandaging necessary to hold the donor arm and skin flap firmly in position against the face for

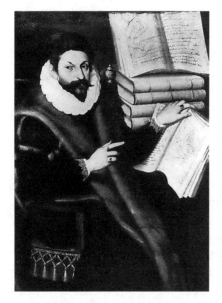

Gaspare Tagliacozzi, surgeon of Bologna, gained a lasting reputation because of his celebrated text on plastic surgery and his manuscript text, shown in the background. He was appointed professor of anatomy in the University (Studium) of Bologna in 1570. Image courtesy of Wikimedia Commons.

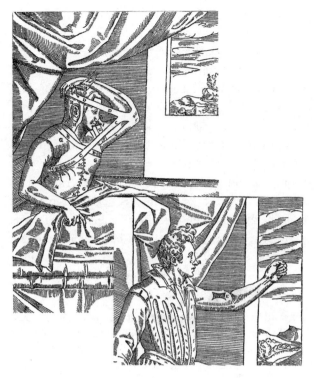

A wood engraving from Tagliacozzi's *De curtorum chirurgia per insitionem* showing the use of a flap of upper arm skin to replace tissue lost from the nose. The important system of support for the arm is shown. This illustration has been used in the seal of the American Association of Plastic Surgeons. Image courtesy of Wikimedia Commons.

some time. He also provided elegant shields to protect the new nose after the surgery.

In his analysis of the mechanism of attaching the skin flap to the nose bed, Tagliacozzi's mindset was markedly conditioned by horticultural practice. The urban Italian savants often owned country villas and had estates to supervise, and there they might use the services of tree grafters.[49] Tagliacozzi freely used their word *scion* to describe his grafts, and the term *insitionem,* used in the title of his book and throughout its text, was a word then used for grafting in agriculture. Tagliacozzi at one point uses the phrase "as in human surgery, as in the orchard," and he transferred two specific technical insights directly from the orchard to his surgical technique. The first was that the grafting of the upper part (scion) of one type of tree or shrub into the root system of another (one more vigorous or disease resistant) required prolonged close contact and fixation. A second strategy from horticulture was the grafting variant of "layering," which meant lowering and burying living limbs of trees or plants into adjacent soil, waiting until a new root system penetrated the soil, and then dividing the original connection to leave a new, freestanding tree.

Although Tagliacozzi's greatest contribution was in autografting (i.e., transferring tissue from one part of the body to another), his name was drawn into a heated debate in the next century on homografting, that is, grafting from one human to another (known as allografting in the later nomenclature). He was incorrectly thought to support the use of human donors to supply a new nose.

Tagliacozzi's text contains nothing to suggest use of another person as a donor, though it is less clear whether or not he was hostile to this idea. In chapter 12 of his book, he dismisses the idea of using another person as a donor, though it seems that some fearful patients had requested doing so, hoping to avoid some of the pain of the procedure. He refused, mainly because of the difficulty of binding the donor and recipient together during the many days required for the graft to heal in. His view was that

no one in his right mind would argue that for some slight gain of beauty and saving of effort we should call the entire fate of the work into danger . . . which certainly happens if we try to perform this operation with the aid of another person. . . . And so no one can fail to see from the difficulty of tying together and from the necessity of inconvenience which two persons tied together encounter, how doubtful, if not entirely vain, will be the outcome of the art. . . . Hence it appears superfluous for us to reply to those who, either in the interests of the appearance of the arm or pandering to their own sensibilities, refuse this operation on their own persons.[50]

These technical objections to using a donor for the operation seemed uppermost in his mind. However, in the final part of the chapter where he makes these objections, there is a remarkable statement that might hint that he dismissed the idea of grafting between humans for biological reasons:

Now let it suffice that judgment in regard to the flap [from another person] is extremely difficult and almost impossible, and that the singular character of the individual entirely dissuades us from attempting this work on another person. For such is the force and the power of individuality, that if anyone should believe that he could accelerate and increase the beauty of union, nay more, achieve even the least part of the operation, we consider him plainly superstitious and badly grounded in physical sciences.[51]

In this passage, Tagliacozzi seems to dismiss the idea of grafting between individuals because of an incompatibility—a "singularem illum individui characterem." This concept of the "force and power" of individuality, elegantly expressed on his part, may be a philosophical stance rather than biological assertion of human individual uniqueness. But it is tantalizingly close to the understanding of the transplantation immunology that emerged much later, and very slowly. One additional scrap of evidence supports this conclusion. The Venetian adventurer Nicolò Manuzzi (1639–1717) settled in India and left a travelogue manuscript, published much later, in which he records that he had seen many natives with restored noses. Manuzzi had acquired some surgical skills and was asked to repair a nose but to use a slave donor for the skin. Manuzzi replied that "it would be of no avail, for being another's flesh it would not unite."[52]

Tagliacozzi died in 1599. There were immediate tributes to his skill, and requiem masses were said in his honor. But shortly after, the old allegations of links between successful transplantation and magical assistance were invoked by his gossipy detractors, who put it about that his surgical skills involved recourse to unacceptable supernatural powers.[53] Helpful "white" magic was acceptable at the time, but the "black" magic of the witches and others was condemned. Tagliacozzi's reputation was restored after an investigation, and a few surgeons, notably his pupil Giovanni Cortesi, felt it was safe to follow his master's lead cautiously, but only for a while. There was sufficient interest in the long and detailed *De curtorum chirurgia per insitionem* for a pirated edition to appear quickly in Venice and then in Frankfurt. Nevertheless, Tagliacozzi's innovative surgery was mysteriously put aside. Remarkably, it was not revived until about 1800.

Tagliacozzi's surgery failed to be incorporated into the routine text-based surgery of the day, and aiding this neglect were some added basic misunderstandings, even about the technical surgical detail. It may be that gossip and academic myths still had greater force and authority in the medical discourse in the early days of printing than did the printed word.

The first continuing misunderstanding of the Tagliacozzi technique was that the nose was to be buried into the arm, rather than a flap raised, and that muscle was used to form the new nose, despite Tagliacozzi's clear engravings showing use of the skin. But the second and more serious misunderstanding of Tagliacozzi's method was that the donor skin for the new nose could be taken from another person. Commentators wrote that Tagliacozzi used slaves or servants as donors of skin to restore their masters' mutilated faces, whereas his text shows not only the opposite but also his hostility to such grafting. This error, with its assumption that such homografts could succeed, was to intrude into the writings on plastic surgery and transplantation for centuries.

Another dampening effect on the use of Tagliacozzi's innovative rhinoplasties was that there was a safe alternative: a false nose could be fitted. Such replacements were known to be in use from earliest times and have

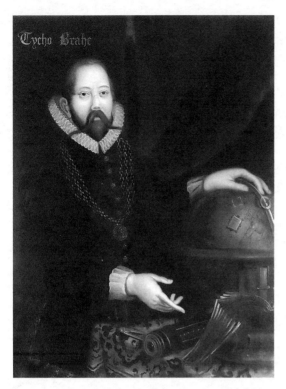

Tycho Brahe, the Danish astronomer, had a nasal deformity as the result of a duel, and he favored a prosthesis, which is detectable in some portraits. Portrait by M. J. Mierevelt, image courtesy of the Royal Society, London.

been found, still in place, on Egyptian mummies.[54] The surgeon Ambroise Paré described a wide range of such prosthetic devices for lost or absent human tissue, and these gold or silver devices were skillfully enameled to give a fleshlike appearance when used to replace eyes, noses, and ears. There were a number of distinguished users of such prostheses. The duke of Urbino (1422–1482) had one, and when Tycho Brahe (1546–1601), the great Danish astronomer, lost the bridge of his nose in a duel in 1566, he opted for a skin-colored metal prosthesis. This device, stolen from his coffin after death, can be seen in some portraits of him. However, having opted for the safety of a prosthesis, it gave him little comfort, and he was never reconciled to his deformity. Brahe became "unapproachable, uninhibited, unsparing and ever vengeful."[55]

The neglect that overtook plastic surgery in general, and Tagliacozzi's work in particular, in the 1600s is perhaps surprising. War was endemic in Europe, war wounds were common, and legal mutilation still existed. In 1637, the Puritan activist William Prynne was branded and had his ears "clipped" off as punishment for antiroyalist pamphleteering, and there were similar mutilations during the unrest in Scotland, mostly removal of hands and ears. But perhaps the switch from swords to firearms as the main weapon in warfare made damage to the nose or ear less common. Also, the virulence of syphilis may have decreased after its rampage around Europe from 1495 onward, and so there were fewer severe nasal deformities. The status of surgery relative to medicine declined, and all forms of cosmetic work may still have been shunned by established practitioners.

The New Biology

Other medical inquiry flourished during the 1600s, however. This period witnessed the rise of investigation by experiment, and no longer was study of the ancient texts seen as the primary means toward progress. From Francis Bacon's teachings in his influential book *Novum organum* came a new method of advancing knowledge to replace the scholasticism of the humanists and their dependence on ancient authority. Instead, data were to be sought and gathered, then observations made and conclusions inductively drawn. But there was a snag in this admirable new emphasis on personal contemporary experience: at first, every experience was given equal weight in the new mood of the times. In the little world of tissue transplantation, every new, flawed tale, from whatever source, was looked at eagerly and believed.

As direct knowledge of Tagliacozzi's original textbook waned (despite the three editions available in print), descriptions of his method were still distorted, and new stories supported the myths about his work. The most damaging claim was that human donors could be used for his nose replacement. One widely believed report claimed that Tagliacozzi had grafted the nose of a slave servant to a nobleman and, after a successful outcome, the grateful recipient granted the slave his freedom. The slave later died, and, it was said, the transplanted nose then also died and fell from the nobleman's face. This tale of the "sympathetic" loss of the grafted nose—an urban myth too good to be false—caught the imagination of writers and philosophers keen to gather all information that might help them understand the natural world. Scholars were steadily dropping belief in miraculous intervention in disease, but now there were other novel influences they could study, forces that could also act unseen. The power of magnets and gravity and the forces influencing the compass were of interest. It was not unreasonable to explain the slave nose donor story as tissue loss at a distance via an invisible force.[56]

The influential philosopher Tommaso Campanella (1568–1639) accepted the slave donor story and then, reasoning metaphysically, concluded that since the human soul was indivisible, the death of the donor inevitably meant death of the graft, no matter how distant from the deceased.[57] This unity of the soul, he went on argue, also meant that grafts could be used to send signals and thus could enable communication between donor and recipient. But the Jesuit polymath Athanasius Kircher (1602–1680), writing in 1643, sternly denounced Campanella's claim for this imaginative use of reciprocal skin grafts: "By pricks inflicted upon themselves according to numbers which had been agreed upon for the various letters of the alphabet, and reciprocally felt, they could speak to each other about anything whatsoever at any distance whatsoever." He then rebuked Campanella: "But away with such foolish absurdities and stupid imaginings of crazy men, whose part it is, lacking true science, to seek glory, which they could not otherwise attain, from dubious and false arts with the aid of the devil."[58]

The old allegation of satanic assistance being needed to achieve graft success is overt in Kircher's denunciation of Campanella. But the tale of the paid slave donor would not go away, and there were hopes that it involved a hitherto unknown force-at-a-distance. Jean Baptiste van Helmont (1577–1644), one of the controversial new Paracelsian physicians who rejected the ancient teachings of Galen and sought to introduce chemical therapy, robustly retold and supported the sympathetic graft loss story, using it as crucial evidence in a new, evidence-based medical world. He also tried to dismiss supernatural influences:

This one experiment [i.e., the slave donor graft] of all others, cannot but be free from all suspect of imposture, and illusion of the Devil. A certain inhabitant of Bruxels, in a combat had his nose mowed off, addressed himself to Tagliacozzius a famous Chirurgeon, living at Bononia, that he might procure a new one; and when he feared the incision of his own arm, he hired a Porter [servant] to admit it, out of whose arm, having first given the reward agreed upon, at length he dig'd a new nose. About thirteenth months after his return to his own Contrey, on a sudden the ingrafted nose grew cold, putrified, and within a few days, dropt off. To those of his friends, that were curious in the exploration of the cause of this unexpected misfortune, it was discovered, that the Porter expired, neer about the same punctilio of time, wherein the nose grew frigid and cadaverous. There are at Bruxels, yet surviving, some of good repute, that were eyewitnesses of these occurrences. Is not this Magnetism of manifest affinity with mumy, whereby the nose, enjoying, by title and right of inoculation, a community of life, on a sudden mortified on the other side of the Alpes? I pray what is there in this Superstition? What of attent and exalted Imagination?[59]

These hidden mechanisms, thought to perhaps be related to magnetism, found a welcome even in the influential writings of Sir Thomas Browne (1605–1682). His influential *Pseudodoxia epidemica, or, Enquiry into very many received Tenents, and commonly presumed Truths,* sought to banish "vulgar errors" and replace them with sound knowledge based on the data-collecting Baconian strategy. He concluded that the slave skin graft had been linked in some way to its donor at death and that "this Magneticall conceit how strange soever, might have some originall in reason."[60]

These unseen forces that were surmised seemed related to another class of influence, one advocated at the time by Sir Kenelm(e) Digby, namely the power of "sympathy." Digby, a polymath, diplomat, traveler, and early member of London's Royal Society, supported attempts to cure injury by transferring the damage away from the sufferer, back to the weapon that had caused the harm. He attempted this transfer by treating the weapon with a "weapon salve" or "powder of sympathy."[61] Digby's most important work dealing with sympathetic medicine was his *A*

Late Discourse Made in a Solemn Assembly of Nobles and Learned Men at Montpellier in France. In the Frankfurt edition of 1661, the work is prefaced by an engraving with some vignettes showing sympathetic power in action. One of these panels shows the rejection of the slave nose graft after the death of the donor, the first illustration, albeit a fanciful one, of homograft skin loss.[62] Many other scholars added new frills to the "learned myth" slave donor story in the 1600s.[63]

The mood finally changed, and attitudes outside of learned circles became more skeptical. The savants' flirtation with these sympathetic powers attracted the ridicule of writers. When Samuel Butler published his mock-heroic tale *Hudibras* in 1663, a satire on the puritanical revolutionary regime that had recently been overthrown, Butler did not spare the fanciful ideas of sympathetic medicine.[64] He used the slave donor story in a modified way, incorporating the idea that the skin was taken in the ancient Indian way, from the flayed buttocks. Word of this technique must have already reached British popular culture from India by an unknown route.

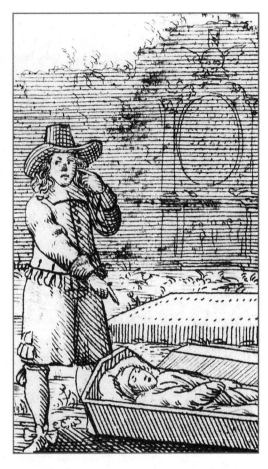

Vignette from the frontispiece to the 1661 Frankfurt edition of Sir Kenelm Digby's *A Late Discourse Made in a Solemn Assembly of Nobles and Learned Men at Montpellier in France* allegedly showing "sympathetic" loss of a living, unrelated donor skin graft to the nose, after the death of the donor. Image courtesy of James Tait Goodrich.

> So learned Taliacotius, from
> The Brawny Part of Porter's Bum,
> Cut supplemental Noses, which
> Wou'd last as long as Parent Breech;
> But when the Date of Nock was out,
> Off dropt the sympathetic Snout.

But the wits missed the point. They assumed that such an operation had occurred, and this assumption helped fix the myth that the innocent Tagliacozzi had indeed used such donors.[65]

Surgical Opinion

Although the European literati of the day can be excused for accepting the claim that Tagliacozzi used human donors, the practical surgeons should have been better informed. One serious student of Tagliacozzi was the Scottish-educated London surgeon Alexander Read, who translated part of Tagliacozzi's *Curtorem* and used it in his own text, *Chirurgorum comes* (1687). Even though he had read the original *Curtorem* text, however, Read thought that Tagliacozzi might have used human donors. Read, also influenced by botanical analogies, reasonably asked "what should hinder a piece of one man's body from being ingrafted into anothers, seeing both are of the same kind, and nothing near as different as one kind of tree is from another . . . ?"[66]

The standard English surgical text of the late 1600s was *Mellificium chirurgiae—The Marrow of Surgery*, by James Cooke (1614–1688) of Warwick. Cooke, after describing the Tagliacozzi operation briefly, repeats all the old misconceptions about it, namely that muscle was used, that the graft could be taken from a donor, and that the graft may be lost when the donor dies:

> The operation being so difficult and painful, besides the necessary preparation for the Work, the Symptoms that fall out, the danger that follows the least neglect, 'tis almost altogether unattempted, yet to satisfy the curious, take somewhat of it here, and then if any have lost a part and like the Operation let them take their Penance. The Nose lost, may be restored both the former ways. To restore it from the Body, it may either be from their own Body, or the Body of others. If the last, let them be sure they can, that such be longer-liv'd than themselves, lest they lose what they have got before they die. To perform this work, remove the Callous Edges of what's remaining of the Nose; after make Incision into the Biceps Muscle of the Arm.[67]

London's Royal Society

The upheaval of the English Revolution and the Civil War of the mid-1600s reinvigorated many of London's ancient institutions, and new radical groupings emerged. One venture was the College for the Promoting of Physico-Mathematical-Experimental Learning, known from 1662 onward as the Royal Society of London, one of the world's first learned academies. The new society was a cooperative venture organized by a group of men interested in advancing natural sciences, and this cooperation was a change from the secrecy exhibited by some savants, notably the still-active alchemists. The society was also largely free of the outside influence of any institution or patron. Some of the European courts had a court "scientist," but his role might be to entertain rather than enlighten; one such appointee, Francesco Redi (1626–1697), the distinguished Tuscan physician, had to put on entertainments for his idle, gossipy Medici courtiers. On one occasion, Redi convinced them that he could replace the head of a praying mantis after its decapitation. His trick was possible because the detached heads adhered strongly to the trunk via the viscous fluid exuded, and privately Redi scorned the court, who "only saw but did not observe."[68]

The members of the new Royal Society acted as peer witnesses of the results of each other's projects, and, in the Baconian spirit of the times, they appointed a "corresponding secretary" to gather reliable, relevant news from abroad. A deliberate attempt was made to banish abstruse discourse and instead substitute functional, plain language. They also resolved not to engage in personal disputes. The Royal Society looked to Bacon's writings not only for his new observational method but also for an appropriate administrative structure for research.[69] The new Baconian research method involved not only observing nature but also testing and taking nature apart, by experiment. "Eyes not ears" were important, and, as the society said, "The want of this exactness has very much diminished the credit of former *naturalists*." Later, the society's motto "*Nullius in verba*"—"nothing upon another's word"—suggested a growing skepticism toward unchecked claims brought to them.

Kenelm Digby's sensible botanical text of 1660 was the Royal Society's first publication, and, shortly afterward, the group turned its novel investigative arrangements toward a study of tissue transplantation. The Royal Society had a remarkable format for its twice weekly meetings. Ideas for investigation were proposed and discussed, with presentations of evidence from all available publications, personal experience, and information from scholars located elsewhere. Having reached a preliminary consensus on the matter at hand, an experimental protocol was then agreed upon, and the project was handed over to a salaried experimenter.

In 1663, the Royal Society turned its attention to skin grafting, one of the procedures they considered would be of likely use. Perhaps one of the members was aware of the dispute surrounding Tagliacozzi's work, and since Butler's poem *Hudibras* had been published earlier that year, this poem may have brought the disputed matter of tissue transplants to their attention. The society organized an experimental attempt at skin grafting (using dogs as subjects) that turned into a muddle and, in the end, a story of high farce. Nevertheless, the independent outlook of the investigators, as well as their attempt to investigate this procedure by experiment, marks a crucial break with the past. It was also noteworthy as the earliest recorded animal experiment in tissue transplantation, and criticism of the society's use of vivisection promptly appeared.

Transplantation was still a sensitive subject for other reasons. Dur-

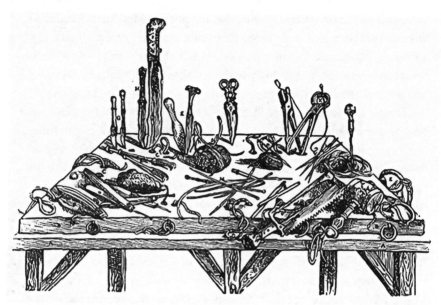

The arrangements for the Royal Society's experimental dog surgery would resemble those in Andreas Vesalius, *De humani corporis fabrica* (1543).

ing this period, a celebrated Amsterdam surgical text by Jobi Janszoon van Meek'ren described the case of a Russian nobleman who had a severe skull injury that was repaired by the use of a rabbit bone graft. The Church threatened to excommunicate the patient because of this implant, so he asked the surgeon to remove the graft.[70] Meek'ren's account came second- or thirdhand from contacts in Russia, so it may have been another unreliable transplant myth.

The impetus for the Royal Society's landmark skin grafting experiment was a proposal by John Wilkins (1614–1672), a founding member and the society's first secretary. According to the society's minutes, on September 16, 1663,

Dr Wilkins proposed the experiment of making a piece of the skin of a dog to grow upon another. Some things were objected against the probability of success thereof, viz., how veins, arteries, and fibres could disseminate themselves and grow into this strange piece of flesh patched on: it being necessary even to the restoring of a separated part to the same animal that there may be left some vessels, and that they join another, and it being hardly conceivable, how the healing can be effected, where the orifices of said vessels do not meet. Others alleged experience and several examples of separated parts healed together again.[71]

This preliminary discussion on the proposed experiment was a familiar clash between theory and empiricism. The theorists could not conceive that new blood vessels could penetrate into the graft, and thus they assumed that successful transfers could succeed only if the arteries and veins of the donor skin made Episthemon-like union directly with the vessels of the recipient. The chances of this happening were slim, as they reasonably pointed out, if only because these vessels were not lined up. The new empirically minded members of the group alleged that grafting had been accomplished in the past, and that was enough for them: experience was as important as theory.

The empiricists carried the day, and all present at the meeting favored a trial, rather than a debate. As a start, they sensibly proposed that instead of grafting from one dog to another (an allograft/homograft), a simpler autograft transplant should be attempted first: "It was ordered hereupon that the experiment should be first with a piece of skin cut from the body of a dog, and sewed again upon the same dog: and Dr Croune and Mr Hooke were appointed curators thereof, and the operator ordered to provide a dog against the next meeting." The members then added some extras to the transplant agenda: "Mr Hooke was also desired to try the growing of hair, and of a cock's-spur upon the head of a cock."[72] Thus, the Royal Society was also preparing to investigate other known types of tissue transplantation, including hair transplants and a spur-to-comb transfer in the chicken, an experiment usually credited to John Hunter's

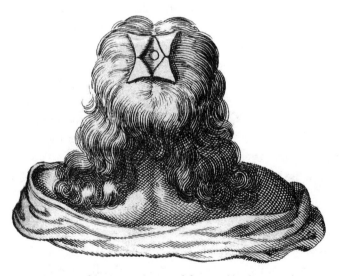

A representation of the Russian bone graft from a rabbit donor to a human patient. From Jobi Janszoon van Meek'ren, *Heel-en Genees-Konstige Aanmerkkingen* (Amsterdam, 1668). Image courtesy of Glasgow University Library, Special Collections.

studies in the next century.[73] On another occasion, human tooth transplantation was discussed briefly at the society, and they carried out some animal blood transfusions.

The dog skin transplant project was handed over to Robert Hooke (1635–1703), the Royal Society's salaried "curator," a talented, disabled man of humble origins who had the responsibility for conducting all of the society's experiments.[74] His talents and patience were regularly stretched by the enthusiasm of the members. Hooke's achievements were considerable, and he can be accorded the honor of being the first experimental tissue transplanter.

A month after Dr. Wilkins proposed the skin grafting experiment on the dog, the society's minutes for October 14 record a delay: "Dr Croune and Mr Hooke having not yet met to cut a piece of dog's skin and sew it on again in order to see whether it will grow; and Dr Charleton, affirming that he had tried this experiment formerly, he was desired to meet on the Friday following with the other two curators at Gresham College, and there to make the experiment together. Dr Hoare promised to bring in an account of a cock's spurs growing on a cock's head."[75]

James Hoare (died 1679) was one of the less active members and missed a place in the history of transplantation by failing to give his promised paper on the transplantation of the cock spur to its comb. Walter Charleton (1619–1707) was an Oxford-educated physician, and, as the translator of van Helmont's text on sympathy and the "magnetick" cure of wounds, he had a direct interest in the matter of the dog experiment. These extracts from the society's minutes show that he claimed previous experience of skin transplantation. However, it is unlikely that a cultured physician of the time would do such manual work, and his role was probably to encourage Hooke to make haste with the experiment.

By October 21, 1663, the experiment had been carried out, but Hooke had encountered a technical problem, one familiar in later attempts. Hooke reported "that as soon as the skin was cut off, it shrunk into half its dimensions, so they could not stretch it out so far as to cover the whole flesh with it, as it had done before. . . . The whole process was ordered to be given, in writing, by Mr Hooke." Hooke was also appointed curator for the ingrafting of feathers upon a cock's comb. There was no update on the dog skin graft project at the society's meeting on November 25, but the members did agree to a further delay until "a warmer season."[76]

Springtime was generally agreed to be a propitious time for surgery. On May 4, 1664, the members gave instructions for a further attempt, and on May 25, Charleton and the dilatory Hooke at last did the surgery. One week later came the sad report that he had met with another problem that became all too familiar to later surgeons: "The dog, a piece of whose skin had been cut off and sewed on again, had got it off: [Hooke] was desired to repeat the experiment at the next meeting, and think upon a way of securing the patch." Even if Hooke had managed to secure the graft, still a further and final misfortune ended the experiment in the next month. The minutes of June 22 explained: "The dog that had a piece of his skin cut off at the former meeting, being inquired after, and the operator [Hooke] answering, that he had run away."[77] There is more than a hint that the put-upon Mr. Hooke, now that the dog was gone, was no longer interested in the project.

A plague epidemic soon afflicted London, and the frightened physicians fled to the safety of the country. In March 1666, it was judged safe to return to the capital, and when the society meetings resumed, they turned instead to another related matter: attempts at blood transfusion. The society may have been energized by the news from Paris in June of that year that the French had carried out a human blood transfusion. Members King and Lower, piqued at the French initiative, and concerned about their priority, then reported a similar human transfusion in November 1667. They ruefully recorded the timeless surgical innovator's lament, claiming that their hesitation and failure to be first was because there were no suitable patients. Also, ethical constraints had arisen: "We have been ready for this experiment this six Months, and wait for nothing but good opportunities, and the removal of some considerations of a moral nature."[78] The blood transfusion they finally performed was into a "feeble-minded cleric" who agreed to be transfused, on two occasions, for twenty shillings. There were no serious reactions.

The Royal Society made no further attempts at skin grafting, studying the cock's comb, or studying tooth transplantation. The distinguished and productive group at the society had failed in their worthy plans for experimental transplantation, defeated in the end by bad luck and technical failures. There may have been sensitivity about further animal experiments, since the society received criticism when Hooke used dogs to demonstrate in public the success of open-chest resuscitation using bellows.[79] Hooke wrote to Robert Boyle, the distinguished Oxford investigator, in 1664 that he had looked for an "anesthetic" to assist the experiment: "I shall hardly be induced to make any further trials of this kind, because of the torture of the creature: but certainly the enquiry would be very noble, if we could find a way so as to stupefy the creature, as that it might not be sensible, which I fear there is hardly any opiate will perform."[80]

Even the plans for further human blood transfusion were put aside. In 1668, a second transfusion experiment in Paris had killed the patient, and the incident produced, in France, the first interdicts on human experimentation. In spite of this precedent, shortly afterward the Royal Society applied to Bedlam, the large mental asylum in London, to use a patient for another transfusion, but the physician in charge declined to cooperate "on a scruple."[81] This, plus the earlier "considerations of a moral nature," were early stirrings of ethical concerns about human experimentation.

Whatever the reason, at the end of the 1600s, the Royal Society turned away from all forms of experimental biology, and, with the medical men among them leaving to form a separate College of Physicians, which did not favor experimental work, the remaining *virtuosi* focused their considerable talents on studies of the physical sciences.

Satire Continues

The matter being undecided, the London satirists were free to continue to ridicule transplantation, and Tagliacozzi was mentioned once again, this time in William Congreve's popular comedy *Love for Love* (1695). In it, the proposal was to transplant new, sturdy legs to a decrepit old man: "Alas, poor Man; his Eyes are sunk and his Hands shrivelled; his legs dwindl'd and his back bow'd. Pray, pray, for a Metamorphosis. Change thy Shape, and shake off Age; get thee Medea's Kettle and be boil'd a-new, come forth with labr'ing Callous Hands, a Chine of Steel, and Atlas Shoulders. Let Taliacotius trim the Calves of twenty Chairmen [sedan chair carriers] and make thee Pedestals to stand upon, and look Matrimony in the face."[82]

Worse still, *The Tatler* of December 7, 1710, at the start of an enlightened century, carried a ponderous essay, "Noses," by Addison in which Butler's lampoon of Tagliacozzi in *Hudibras* was repeated and the Italian surgeon ridiculed. The surgical textbooks of the new century, notably Lorenz Heister's hugely successful *Chirurgie* of 1718, dismissed the Tagliacozzi operation and suggested that an artificial nose would suffice for those disfigured in the way described.

Although the outcome of the transplantation studies in the otherwise progressive 1600s had perhaps been unimpressive, the Royal Society's approach signaled a major shift in attitudes to the study of the natural world. No longer were matters to be decided by study of classical texts or by anecdote. Instead, experimental biology was emerging, and in the following century, two investigators with the new outlook, Abraham Trembley and John Hunter, used their talents to look at tissue transplantation.

2 The Eighteenth Century

THE SUBJECT OF HUMAN TISSUE grafting disappeared from surgical and literary texts in the early 1700s, but some experimentation continued. Two individuals in particular, Abraham Trembley and John Hunter, took an interest in grafting in order to gain insight into the fundamental mechanisms of animal life. Their work focused on tissue vitality, regeneration, and adhesion. Only later did Hunter turn to human studies.

Trembley's Transplants

Of these two noted investigators, the first to achieve fame was the Belgian naturalist Trembley (1710–1784), who in 1736 became tutor to the sons of the Comte de Bentinck in the Netherlands. Trembley added to his duties by carrying out observations on the tiny, lowly forms of life he found in the ponds on the grounds of the nobleman's residence at Sorghvliet, near The Hague.[1] The advances in microscopy at this time, arising from the instruments made and used by Antoni van Leeuwenhoek (1633–1723) in nearby Delft, had immediately revealed that water, particularly stagnant water, might contain "an innumerable company of little Animalcules," as Leeuwenhoek eagerly reported in letters to the corresponding secretary of the Royal Society in London.

With knowledge of this animate pond life, Trembley became particularly interested in one of the bigger varieties, the freshwater coelenterate hydra (polyps), which were just big enough to be seen and manipulated without the use of magnification. In the new spirit of investigation, he went beyond mere observation and, "questioning nature," carried out celebrated experiments. His particular interest was in how each part of a divided polyp could regenerate and how polyp parts could fuse together. When he divided a polyp into two or more parts, the fragments of the original polyp could reunite if he enclosed one part within the other or used bristles to affix the two parts to each other. In other experiments, he found that he could reunite two halves of *different* hydra to make one animal.[2]

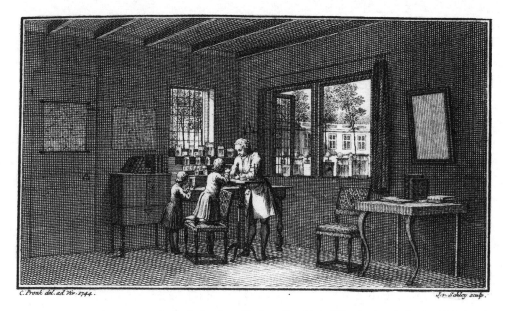

An illustration from Abraham Trembley's *Mémoires* (1744) showing him at work on his famous polyp experiments. Image courtesy of the Wellcome Library, London.

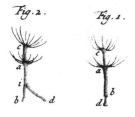

An illustration from Trembley's *Mémoires* (1744) showing his polyp grafts. Image courtesy of the Wellcome Library, London.

Trembley had begun the polyp experiments in 1741, and, when describing them, he encountered reflex disbelief from *"les incrédules,"* as Trembley called them. Accordingly, in 1742, he developed methods to distribute polyps, with instructions for use, so that others could study them; these gifts, plus the "how-to" information, ensured that skeptics would finally believe him. His findings reached the attention of important figures, notably Réaumur, in Paris, and gained Trembley honors in the close-knit European scholarly world of the day. The Royal Society was informed of his results in 1742, and when the polyps arrived in London in 1743, they were distributed to various investigators in England and Scotland. Trembley's technique was demonstrated to an audience of 120 in London, and the Royal Society published his findings in 1743. The society promptly awarded Trembley its Copley Medal in 1743, one year before publication of his famous, elegantly illustrated monograph.[3] At this busy time, there was a priority dispute and an allegation of scientific misconduct when Henry Baker, a London microscopist who had received some polyps via the president of the Royal Society, in 1743 rushed into publication in London a work of his own, prior to the release of Trembley's own account.[4]

The Impact

The primary interest in these experiments at the time was in regeneration rather than grafting. Some individuals, however, did address the wider significance, in a style of inquiry that was characteristic of the philosopher's world, of which the infant subject of biology (as it later came to be called) was still part. The philosophers traditionally assumed that the workings of the animal body were an impenetrable mystery and that the fabric of the body was energized by the soul—a nonphysical life force that resided in central organs such as the brain and heart. But Descartes's controversial materialist and mechanistic view of living matter was gaining support, suggesting instead that the body was simply a series of engines and pumps, also directed from the center.

The behavior of Trembley's polyps did not fit this mechanistic view. If the polyp could be divided repeatedly, and a whole animal could grow from each of the parts, then this was no machine, and critics of Cartesian materialism were thus given hope, and also a problem. Philosophers traditionally associated the life force with the central organs, yet the experiments showed vigorous, surviving peripheral life in the polyp fragments. Thus, the life force of these animals must be diffused throughout its structure and must therefore be divisible. The polyp, "to whom are allotted an infinite number of souls," was embarrassingly more fortunate than humans, "poor star-gazers [who] must sourly drag along with one solitary soul."[5]

Trembley's work also raised hopes that, if bits of polyps could unite, surely detached parts of the human body, God's greatest creation, might be rejoined. There promptly appeared in print stories describing successful reattachment of human body parts, usually ears and noses, and these fanciful anecdotes were taken seriously by some.[6] Popular culture revived the older legends of successful grafting, and traveling quacks made claims for immediately successful skin grafts. Gathering a crowd and apparently cutting off a patch of their own skin, these performance artists, after the initial legerdemain, seemed to replace the skin by applying their infallible (and profitable) healing balsam.[7] Muddled understanding of this matter continued throughout the century, but one influential textbook at last took a stance in 1801 about the grafting of large patches and bits of the body. John Bell in Edinburgh expressed himself with vigor on this matter, saying that "parts which are entirely separated are entirely and irrecoverably dead."[8]

Regeneration Studied

Trembley's work may have encouraged hopes for human transplantation, but it also suggested that regeneration could be a strategy for restoring tissue loss. If the lowly hydra had such powerful regenerative powers, could not similar mechanisms be activated in higher animals and humans? The polyp experiments aroused the interest of the Swiss biologist Charles Bonnet (1720–1793), who showed that the rainwater worm could also regenerate after division into parts.[9] The debate widened when Lazzaro Spallanzani (1729–1799), working in Pavia, found that the snail also had considerable powers of regeneration, as did frog larvae and salamanders.[10]

These experiments indicated that regenerative power was latent throughout the tissues of lower animals. It seemed reasonable that humans should also have this capability. These hopes were repeatedly raised and dashed, and, by the early twentieth century, the scientific community generally accepted the doctrine of August Weismann, which proposed that the greater differentiation and sophistication of higher animals meant a loss of the pluripotent characteristics seen in simpler animals. At the end of the twentieth century, however, this verdict was dramatically overthrown with the discovery and use of stem cells, which had important consequences for clinical transplantation.

John Hunter

The new scientific approach of experiment rather than mere observation made its appearance in the surgical world in the 1700s via the work of John Hunter (1728–1793). After basic education in Scotland, he settled in London, and the fees from his medical practice supported his scholarship and investigative work at his well-organized London dissecting rooms, library, and celebrated museum. He and his brother William and their talented pupils steered surgeons away from their traditional anatomical studies and toward gaining an understanding of pathological mechanisms and the normal workings of the body. The eighteenth century had many distinguished British surgeon-anatomists, notably William Cheselden in London, and Edinburgh had the Monro dynasty and, later, the Bell brothers. But Hunter's anatomy went beyond mere dissection and description and sought clues as to function. His museum was not the usual "cabinet of rarities" but was arranged to show relationships from comparative anatomy. He also conducted his experiments in physiology, as it was called later, notably seeking to understand and identify the factor that, added to anatomical structure, energized the living being and distinguished it from dead or inanimate objects. In doing so, Hunter helped raise the reputation of surgeons from their traditional parity with

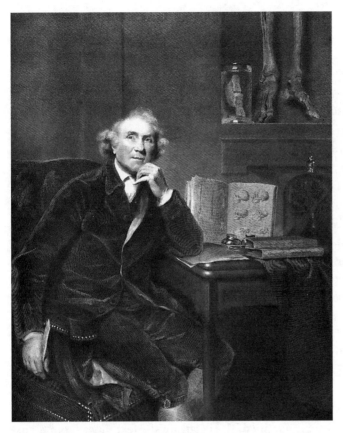

John Hunter, the Scottish-born "father of experimental surgery" in William Sharp's engraving of a portrait by Joshua Reynolds. The image shows a specimen in the top right corner that is suggestive of a successful experimental bone graft; the actual specimen, however, is lost. Image courtesy of the Royal College of Surgeons, London.

artisans working with their hands to a more gentlemanly status, even that of a savant. In particular, this reorientation enabled the London Company of Surgeons to gain status, and, following a change of name to a scholarly "College," they also gained royal patronage. Surgeons had thus finally become prominent in the ranks of medical men. Hunter's famous texts are *The Natural History of the Human Teeth* (1771–1778), *A Treatise on Venereal Disease* (1786), and, published after his death, *A Treatise on the Blood, Inflammation and Gunshot Wounds* (1794).

Hunter's contributions have been closely studied. Regarding his scientific style, one view is that his upbringing during the Scottish Enlightenment nurtured his interest in theory and a liking for hypotheses. Once he began working in England, he added Bacon's data collection methodology to his scientific practice. The English historian Henry Thomas Buckle wrote that "as a Scotchman, [Hunter] preferred reasoning to particular facts; as an inhabitant of England, he became accustomed to the opposite plan of reasoning from particular facts. His natural inclination was to conjecture what the laws of nature were, and then reason from them, instead of reasoning to them. But inasmuch as he was surrounded by the followers of Bacon, this natural bias was warped."[11]

It was hardly warped. Hunter's wide-ranging studies and museum collection gave him material for his speculations, and these two elements together gave Hunter his strong hypothetico-deductive methodology.

Topics of Study

The studies of Hunter that relate to tissue transplantation address three primary issues. One of these was the mystery of tissue vitality, and he conducted a group of experiments with grafts to determine if "life" was present or absent after they were detached. He conducted another series of studies to examine mechanisms of tissue adhesion. Finally, in human clinical work, he made a famous study of tooth transplantation.[12] Perhaps surprisingly, he made no attempt to study skin grafting, in spite of the ancient surgical interest in this topic, nor did he show interest in Tagliacozzi's plastic surgical methods. His brother William, a bibliomaniac and collector, did have Tagliacozzi's book in his great library, but both brothers might have been unaware of the details of the text. It was John's custom—an important one—to ignore previous authorities and their books, particularly those written in Latin.[13]

In two smaller, more arcane matters, not unconnected with later tissue transplantation work, John Hunter's curiosity and insight can also be applauded. He was first to study, by dissection, the puzzle of the freemartin female cattle, an animal well known to country people. The freemartin female born with a male twin is sterile. Later research revealed that in such cases, male hormones pass into the female via fused placentas.[14] Hunter was the first to dissect and show the changes in the internal organs of freemartin cattle. He perceptively concluded that the freemartin was not a hermaphrodite but something else. The study of freemartin cattle almost two centuries later, in the 1950s, helped lead to success in achieving graft "tolerance" and, hence, successful transplantation. Another first for Hunter was when, in a postmortem observation, he reported the absence of one kidney. This solitary left kidney had multiple renal vessels and two ureters, and these kidney anomalies would ultimately be of vital importance in day-to-day surgical transplantation routine and are looked for carefully.[15]

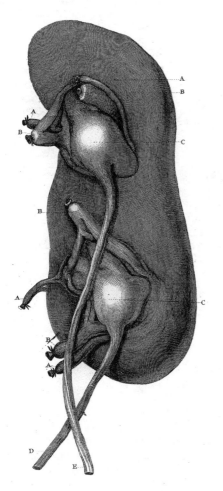

John Hunter was the first to describe congenital absence of one kidney when, in a postmortem examination, he noticed the solitary left kidney, which had duplex collecting systems, double ureters, and extra blood vessels. His observation marked the first awareness of these important variants. From *Medical Transactions* (of the College of Physicians) (1785). Image courtesy of the Royal Society of Medicine Library, London.

Experimental Transplantation

In Hunter's main investigative transplant endeavors, one of his best-known but simple experiments was what he called "the common experiment," namely transplanting the spur of a young chicken from its foot to its comb. This transplanted spur could grow to a length of twelve inches and could have a pseudo-articulation joint with the skull. It was a traditional farmer's trick for producing odd-looking animals, not unlike unicorns, for freak shows or traveling circuses.[16] This diverting and easy experiment had been investigated earlier by the Royal Society. Henri-Louis du Hamel (or Duhamel de Monceau, 1700–1782) in Paris also reported this trick in 1746, adding the first illustration of this successful "free" animal graft and using the word *greffe* for the first time.[17] Hunter was aware of the cock's comb as a

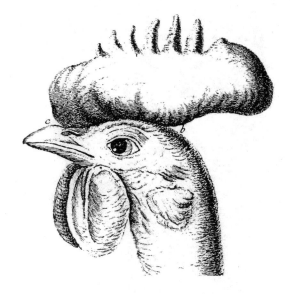

French botanist and polymath Henri-Louis Duhamel (or du Hamel) was one of many who experimentally used the cock's comb as a graft bed, and he prepared the first illustration of chicken spurs growing firmly in the comb. From *Compte rendue de l'Académie Royal de Sciences, Paris,* November 12, 1746. Image courtesy of the Archives of the Institut de France.

recipient site and attempted a related experiment but may not have taken it too seriously. W. Irvine, a doctor from Glasgow who visited Hunter, reported that

he is tomorrow to perform an operation of this kind before several gentlemen. He has procured a couple of Jack Apes. Into the forehead of the one he is to graft the horn of a calf, and into the other the horn of a young deer, and he proposes, as Gavin Pettigrew has long complained of want of money, to send them to him and doubt not that by shewing them up and down the country he will make an immense fortune. The success of these operations depends on there being little time lost betwixt the separation of the part from one animal to the other.[18]

Hunter's emphasis on speedy implantation is admirable, but how serious this proposal was is not clear. If the procedures actually took place, the written record may have been in the many papers lost after his death. These regular demonstrations by Hunter to "several gentlemen" were part of his effort to raise the status of his craft.

Bone Grafts

In other work with bone, Hunter may have been successful in using a bridging bone graft for treating experimental limb fractures. The evidence is from an illustration of a specimen of the bones of a foot, now lost, but shown in the top right corner of the familiar engraving of Hunter by Joshua Reynolds, now held by the Royal College of Surgeons in London.[19] The museum's notes state that "Hunter selected the metacarpal of an ass for many of his experimental investigations into the repair and living reactions of bone. There is a gap in the bone—apparently half an inch or more has been sawn out. At one side of it and crossing the gap, is the 'ossific prop' which I take to be a bone graft."[20]

Gland Grafting

Another Hunter transplantation project was grafting the sex glands between male and female animals. This work arose largely from his interest in adhesion mechanisms, and he showed little interest in the functional outcome of such grafts. In 1771, he wrote, "I have frequently taken out the testes of a cock and replaced it in his belly, where it has adhered, and has been nourished; nay, I have put the testes of a cock into the belly of a hen with the same effect."[21]

Hunter showed that the testes graft "adhered" within the recipient's abdomen, and he prudently looked for clear evidence of a blood supply being established in these gland grafts. To find proof of blood flow, he used either his pioneering method of dye injection of the specimen to show that penetration by blood vessels had occurred, or he ingeniously fed the animals with a dye and showed that the dye was deposited within the graft. Both methods were at the time major innovations in experimental method. His conclusions after grafting cocks' testicles into hens were modest, and he was careful not to claim that sperm production occurred or that the recipients' "femaleness" was altered. He accepted this functional failure, since, in spite of apparent technical success, it had not "altered their natural disposition."[22]

In related experiments using the cock's comb bed for homografts, he had similar failures when grafting spurs of cocks to hens, but he had some success with placing hens' spurs into cocks.[23]

Adhesion and Vitality

To Hunter, adhesion of a graft was not simply the first stage in grafting but the most important element. This was because he assumed that, once a graft had healed in, then it would function thereafter; in other words, he believed the only hurdle to transplantation was attachment. Hunter's general conclusions on the healing-in process of grafted tissue, stated with his usual clarity, were that "the success of the [grafting] operation is founded on a disposition in all living substances to unite when brought into contact with one another, although they are of different structure, and even although the circulation is only carried on in one of them. . . . This disposition is not so considerable in the more perfect animals, such as quadrupeds, as it is in the more simple or imperfect, nor in old animals, as in the young."[24]

Hunter's views are a synthesis of conclusions from his own experiments, his clinical experience, and other available evidence on tissue attachment, notably Trembley's work.[25] In his writings, he attempts an explanation of the "Trembley paradox," namely the ease of adhesion of separated parts seen in lower animals and the difficulty in obtaining the same effect in humans. He simply accepts as others did that the higher animals' sophistication meant a loss of peripheral power which he interestingly noticed was age related.

Plants and Animals

In one thread of thought running throughout his writings, Hunter was mistaken. In his writings on adhesion (and hence on grafting), Hunter's assumptions were the same as those of Tagliacozzi, namely that animal grafting was similar to plant hybridization and, therefore, that grafting between different animals could succeed as well as it did when uniting different species in the plant world. For his grafts, Hunter continued to use the gardener's term *scion*. He remarked in a footnote on this terminology that "since transplanting is very similar to the in-grafting of trees, I thought that term [scion] might be transferred from gardening to surgery, finding no other word so expressive of the thing."[26]

Hunter was not first to use the word *transplant*.[27] *Scion* was a misleading word, and it shackled scientific thinking for a while. Successful grafting in the orchard was known to be the result of direct joining of the nutrient vessels of graft and trunk, thus allowing sap to circulate. Hunter and others were deeply conditioned to expect that any success with animal grafting would involve a similar direct union of blood vessels, after prolonged fixation of the donor tissue to the recipient, thus enabling the blood vessels to unite. However, this assumption that direct vascular union in animals would occur was seriously flawed and served to constrain the theory and practice of transplantation until the mid-1800s.

Vitality and the "Living Principle"

In his transplant work, Hunter addressed a growing interest among naturalists: the nature of animal life and tissue vitality. Philosophers and theologians had no doubts about the explanation; they believed that a "soul" was the key addition to the physical structure of the body; that it maintained life, and that it departed from the body at death. Hunter continued looking for more information, however. He had a number of methods for determining whether a detached tissue was living or dead, and one of these was transplantation back into a host. In his grafting experiments, he examined detached tissues and looked for clues to what he neutrally called the "living principle." A graft that survived had, in his view, retained some "living principle," and if a graft failed, then this principle had departed before it was attached. He concluded that "the living principle in young animals and those of simple construction is not so much confined to, or derived from, one part of the body; so that it continues longer in a part separated from their bodies and even would appear to be generated in it for some time; while parts separated from an older or more perfect animal died sooner and would appear to have its life entirely dependent on the body from which it was taken."[28]

Hunter's empirical findings cannot be faulted. His analysis is that a detached part loses a "living principle" steadily after separation from the donor, but at different rates in different situations. In higher animals, he suggests, there is centralized generation of the "living principle" that is then delivered to the periphery, but in lower animals it is more diffusely stored. The movement of the living principle from the center was, he suggested, via the blood and not the nerves. Once again, he was correct.

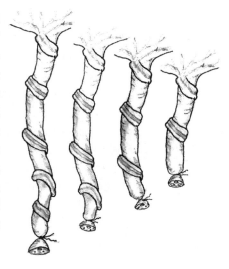

A reconstruction of John Hunter's investigation of the duration of tissue vitality using the contractility of human umbilical cord vessels. The cord was tied at each end and small lengths cut off each day. At first, the distended artery in the released segment contracted after release of the enclosed blood, but after forty-eight hours it failed to contract. This gave Hunter an estimate of the time it took for this tissue to die. Drawing by the author, based on Hunter's text.

With his customary ingenuity, Hunter devised a model to measure loss of the "living principle." He took a length of fresh human umbilical cord and tied it at each end, thus trapping the blood within the distended umbilical vessels. Each day he cut off small segments and retied the remainder, releasing the contained blood in the segment removed and watching to see if the wide but now emptied vessels in this detached segment contracted, which they did promptly on the first day. By the second day, the arteries in the next segment removed failed to contract when emptied, and he concluded that the muscular tissue of the vessels could live for up to forty-eight hours before tissue death. This simple, inventive experiment was the first in vitro study of human tissue vitality.

John Hunter and the Soul

Hunter's works do not address metaphysical issues. For this Enlightenment man, there was no appeal in pondering the role of the soul in his "living principle." He avoided use of the word *soul* and thus steered clear of any theological implications. In using his words carefully, sticking to the facts, and avoiding any transcendental explanation for his "living principle," he attracted neither religious approval nor criticism. Hunter's care was rewarded later when the French post-Revolutionary investigators who followed his teachings and experimental methods declared themselves to be materialists; they were condemned in Britain for this atheism. Hunter, however, was elevated as a respectable British hero, and his findings were sometimes reworked to show that he had identified the God-given soul. The French investigators were also soon condemned for cruelty because of their extensive use of vivisection, while Hunter's own pioneering use of animals was downplayed. Animal experiments in Britain came to a halt and did not reappear until the 1870s, when the continental European dominance in physiology research was so marked that a cautious start had to be made, in spite of intense opposition from British antivivisectionists.

Respiratory Resuscitation

Hunter also took an interest in the process of death in the intact animal or human, being curious to judge when the "living principle" was entirely lost. He taught correctly that in most forms of death, lung function failed first and the heart stopped later. He repeated the earlier experiments of the Royal Society that had shown that doomed animals could be revived if the lungs were artificially inflated with bellows, and, as a result, he was asked to advise the new London Humane Society on methods to revive those "apparently drowned." His advice shows his customary, timeless insight:

I consider that an animal, apparently drowned, not as dead; but that only a suspension of life has taken place. This, probably, is the case in the beginning of all violent deaths, except those caused by lightning or electricity, by which absolute death may be produced instantaneously. . . .

The loss of motion in drowning seems to arise from the loss of respiration. . . . This privation of breathing seems to be the first cause of the heart's motion ceasing; therefore most probably, the restoration of breathing is all that is necessary to restore the heart's action. . . .

Perhaps the dephlogisticated air described by Dr Priestley, may prove more efficacious than common air. It is easily procured, and may be preserved in bottles or bladders. . . . How far electricity may be of service, I know not; but it may, however, be tried, when every other method has failed. I have not mentioned injecting stimulating substances directly into the veins, though it might be supposed a proper expedient.[29]

Astonishingly, Hunter had set out a complete agenda for resuscitation and even sensed that handy containers of "dephlogisticated air"—that is, oxygen—might be of value.

Tooth Transplantation

Hunter's human tooth transplantation studies have a major place in his writings. Hunter was not the first to attempt the procedure, but he was the first to study it and publish on the matter.[30] By the eighteenth century, tooth transplantation was already an ancient skill.[31] A skull in Ecuador dating from the second century shows an example of such tooth implantation, and Albucasis in Spain taught in the eleventh century that lost teeth could be replaced in this way. Later, Paré (1510–1590) recorded a case of human tooth replacement in which he used one from a servant donor, and Henry VIII's regulations for the barber-surgeons of London permitted them to extract and implant teeth. In London in 1663, the Royal Society not only undertook its skin graft project but also resolved to study the matter of tooth transplantation, and it received the description of a lady who had been transplanted with a fresh tooth taken from a "porter" (i.e., servant). The first English-language text to describe such transplants (and to use the word *transplant*) was Charles Allen's *The Operator for the Teeth* (1685). Allen had reservations about using human teeth, and he detailed his methods as follows: "First I would chuse an animal whose teeth should come nearest to those of the Patient; such as a *Dog*, a *Sheep*, a *Goat*, or a *Baboon* . . . and then with the use of suitable Remedies, I do not question in the least but that it would unite to the Gums and Jawbones."[32]

Although Hunter's name is firmly linked with the transplantation aspect of dentistry, Hunter's authority came not from being first to perform the procedure but from his careful study of the matter and his claim that its success was soundly based on known mechanisms. It is likely that he drew heavily on the clinical experience of others in London doing such transplants, notably dentists like his fellow Scot, James Spence.[33] He may also have had access to several late-eighteenth-century textbooks of surgery and dentistry that described methods of tooth transfer in some detail. The need for such published descriptions may have arisen because changes in diet were leading to more tooth decay and thus the need for more tooth transfers, or perhaps concern about the cosmetic defects of missing teeth was growing. The charges for transplantation were about five guineas for inserting a living donor tooth, two for putting in one from a dead donor, and three for inserting a human tooth on a gold bridge.

Donor Teeth

Hunter preferred to use fresh "living" human teeth, since he claimed that these retained vitality when transplanted and thus were whiter and more translucent than teeth used sometime after extraction, which in his opinion remained dull and opaque. The supply of fresh donor teeth came from both willing and unwilling donors. Bourdet in *L'Art du dentiste* (1757) describes the paid donors of Paris as "Savoyard boys, who at the time on account of their poverty, seem to have been used exclusively for transplantations."[34] Hunter was doubtless encouraged by the cock's comb strategy, since he had transplanted a human tooth there with apparent success.[35] However, his human tooth transplants succeeded only as inert implants and served quite well in the medium term if firm fixation was achieved. All the donor cells died or were destroyed early on, as was the case with bone grafts he performed.

Hunter's transplants were attempted only with single-root teeth. The patient's diseased tooth was drawn first and the socket and gums inspected. Hunter advised that the best way of proceeding when planning an extraction-then-transplant was "to have several people [donors] ready whose teeth in appearance are fit."[36] Hunter preferred the donors to be young and female, since the teeth of females are smaller than those of men, and this size difference would help to ensure a snug fit with either the male or female socket. It seems that well-off patients would sometimes bring along their servants as possible donors, a strategy that might avoid the use of teeth from unknown, possibly diseased, donors. A visitor to Belvoir Castle about this time encountered a beautiful peasant woman with a missing front tooth. Asked how this misfortune happened, the woman said that the Duchess Isabella, wife of the fourth duke (of Rutland), had lost the corresponding tooth and "forced me to have mine taken out to replace it."[37] Private soldiers in the armed forces might also be obliged to give teeth to officers. The fee paid for donating a tooth could be generous—up to five guineas. Popular opinion was not always supportive, however, and in England, the artist Thomas Rowlandson (1756–1827) satirized the practice of donating teeth. One of his engravings (circa 1781) shows in detail all stages of the transplant, including the extraction of the diseased tooth from the dentist's wealthy client, the implant, and the use of poor people for the paid donation.[38]

Human teeth taken from cadavers or that had been stored for some time were used if the recipient's socket was unusual in shape or if no human donor was suitable, and Hunter advised that every operator should "have at hand some dead teeth, so that he may have a chance to fit the socket." A reserve store of dead human teeth was easily obtained; teeth could be salvaged from corpses at postmortem examination or offered by grave robbers, who, if a body was found to be unsuitable for dissection, still took the teeth. Scavengers who visited the battlefields of Europe, notably after the Battle of Waterloo, removed teeth from the huge number of

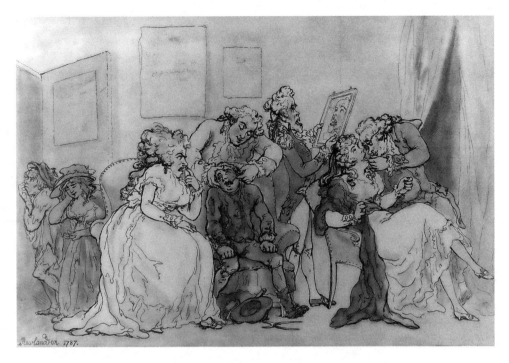

Thomas Rowlandson turned from conventional portraiture to caricature about 1781, and his satirical studies of London caught the mood of the age. This montage shows all aspects of tooth transplantation using paid donors. In the center is the senior dentist, backed by his diplomas and warrants, examining a poor young man as a potential donor for his rich, stressed patient on the right. To the left and rear of the dentist, an elegant recipient is studying his new tooth. Poor young donors are seen exiting left, holding their painful jaws; at least one has been paid. Image courtesy of the Royal College of Surgeons of England.

dead soldiers.[39] These old teeth were sold for about two pounds each to the dentists for making into dentures or for use as transplants.

Tooth Transplants Elsewhere

Because John Hunter dominated British surgery, his authority gave respectability to the procedure of tooth transplantation, and the practice spread. An early advertisement by John Rae, an Edinburgh surgeon-dentist, offered tooth transplantation in that city in 1784.[40] In the previous year, an Edinburgh dentist named Spence had paid two guineas for two donor teeth taken from a young girl, but on hearing shortly after that she needed the money to pay for her parents' funeral expenses, he promptly repaid the fee and re-implanted her teeth. In colonial America, itinerant tooth pullers were prepared to transplant teeth and advertised for donors.[41] The New York *Daily Advertiser* for January 28, 1789, recorded this poignant tale: "In the severe winter of 1783, which was a time of general distress in New York, an aged couple found themselves reduced to their last stick of wood. They were supported by a daughter, who found herself unable to secure wood, fuel or provision. She accidentally heard of a dentist who advertised that he would give 3 guineas for every sound tooth. She decided to do this. On her arrival she made known the circumstances which caused her to make the sacrifice. He, affected by her tears, refused, and presented her with 10 guineas instead."[42]

In America at this time, the peripatetic dentist John Le Mayeur was a tooth transplant enthusiast. Le Mayeur boasted that in the winter of 1785 in Philadelphia he had transplanted 170 teeth, but when a local dentist later claimed he personally had removed 50 of these grafts, using only thumb and finger, the practice began to be ridiculed. Nevertheless, it is recorded that George Washington, who had chronic dental problems, made discreet inquiries regarding Le Mayeur and his claims. Although an enthusiastic report came back, the general himself remained skeptical and decided not to proceed. Instead, the dentist John Greenwood supplied Washington with dentures.

Greenwood is known to have been critical of Hunter, and he wrote this rather sharp marginal comment in his own copy of Hunter's *Natural History of the Human Teeth:* "This [tooth transplantation] is a miserable practice and the recommendation of it shows plainly that the Doctor [Hunter] knew nothing about the nature of Human Teeth. . . . I presume this book was rote in a Great measure to get Money."[43] There is some evidence that this was the case. It was Hunter's first book, and, though the book was strong on theory, he drew heavily on the experience of dentist friends. In addition, Hunter may not have been routinely involved in follow-up on the cases.

Transmission of Disease

Further criticism of tooth grafting arose when there was increasing evidence that disease, notably syphilis, which was widespread at this time, could be transferred with donor teeth from apparently healthy living donors. Hunter noted that local changes resembling syphilis occurred in six patients after tooth transplantation, but the appearances were not typical of syphilis and he considered it was unlikely that venereal disease could lie latent in apparently normal tissues. But he left the matter open and called for further study.

Others in London came to accept that there was indeed a danger from teeth taken from living donors. New care was taken in selecting the donor, and the dentists involved routinely inspected "the tonsils and pudenda" of paid tooth donors. But William Rae, who had lectured on dentistry at Hunter's house in the late 1700s, turned against the operation ten years after Hunter's book was published. Rae gave details of a case of syphilis following tooth transplantation, although not one of Hunter's, noting that

a singular case of this kind happened a few years ago [in 1785] and made a great noise in the world. Mr Hunter says we cannot inoculate the venereal disease by the blood, yet we have many instances of the contrary. A young lady from Southampton came to town to have a tooth transplanted, and being anxious to have a proper one got and perfectly free of any infection, the subject [donor] was examined by some eminent surgeons who pronounced it very safe: the operation was soon performed, and she was soon affected with the venereal disease, which destroyed all that side of her face, and she very shortly died.[44]

It was now concluded that apparently normal tissue could transmit serious, latent disease.[45] In 1786, one year after the case, a presentation at a clinical meeting of the Society of Collegiate Physicians in London affirmed the reality of this complication. A Dr. Lettsom presented two further cases of syphilis occurring after tooth transplantation, and the mode of transmission then seemed certain.[46]

Ethical Concerns

To add to these serious clinical complications, the use of living human donors for tooth transplantation was not without its critics on ethical grounds. Such concerns were first noticed when misgivings were aired at the Royal Society in 1667 about their plans to carry out a human blood transfusion. The phrase "considerations of a moral nature" was used to explain the delay in starting the transfusion. Concerns over the use of living donors for tooth transplantation were more explicit, however. Charles Allen preferred to use animal donor teeth, and he gave his reasons in his 1685 text on dentistry: "I do not like that method of drawing teeth out of some folks heads, to put them into others, both for its being too inhumane, and attended with many difficulties; and then neither could this be called the Restauration of Teeth, since the reparation of one, is the ruine of another: it is only robbing of *Peter* to pay *Paul*."[47]

These early objections to tooth donation for transplantation continued in a small way into the eighteenth century but became prominent after Hunter's advocacy of the operation. William Rae, already skeptical about the clinical results of the treatment, added this view "that it is cruel to take the teeth of a poor creature, whose necessities may induce him to part with it."[48] Joseph Fox, another pupil of Hunter, was appointed to Guy's Hospital as the first hospital dental surgeon, and Fox raised this ethical concern again in his own *The Natural History of the Human Teeth*, published in 1803, when the transplant operation was losing popularity. "I might indeed have observed," he wrote, "that this operation involved in it a defect of the moral principle, as one person is injured and disfigured, in order to contribute to the luxury and convenience of another . . . an injury is done to the moral sense by the operation."[49]

Europe seems to have been less interested in tooth transplantation at the time, and a German dental text took the moral high ground, deploring the "English trafficking in the teeth of living persons."[50] It was almost 150 years before concerns over "injuries to the moral sense" emerged forcefully again in issues surrounding human transplantation, notably at first in the use of living donors.

Later Verdicts

Although Hunter had called tooth transplantation "one of the nicest operations," its popularity waned, discredited by poor results, serious complications, and ethical sensitivities. The verdict by the early 1800s was made clear by James F. Palmer in an aside delivered when he was editor of Hunter's works:

It is unnecessary in the present day to enter into any discussion on the merits of an operation now, I believe, wholly discontinued. . . . The frequent failures which occurred, even in the operation itself, and still more the severe results which very often succeeded its performance at different periods, have very properly induced almost all subsequent practitioners to abandon its employment. Nothing but the sanguine expectations created in an ardent mind, by the interesting results which followed his first experiments, could account for a man of so sound a judgment having followed up a practice so obviously objectionable.[51]

Palmer's analysis is that Hunter's apparent success with his human tooth transplant to the cock's comb, plus his many experiments on adhesion, gave an apparently sound experimental basis to move on to these human transplants. Palmer excuses Hunter's mistakes as the kind of aberration that can afflict an enthusiast with a mission, particularly when backed up by a successful animal model.[52]

Just as tooth transplantation was being abandoned, there was a quite sudden rediscovery not only of Tagliacozzi's plastic surgery text and its technique but also of the similar earlier Indian methods of surgery. Once these methods were reintroduced into European surgery, a host of related surgical operations quickly followed, firmly establishing "plastic surgery" as a new service. These events also had significance for tissue transplantation; consideration of grafting tissue, notably skin, using donors was never far away.

3 The Reawakening

THE ANCIENT CRAFT of plastic surgery was revived in Europe in the early nineteenth century. With the discovery of early Indian surgical methods, which were still in use there, and the realization that Tagliacozzi's works, when read in the original language, had merit, human skin replacement was performed in Europe for the first time in two centuries. The techniques quickly became part of surgical routine.[1]

The awakening began when European colonists in India observed local practitioners performing practical plastic surgery using methods that were long established.[2] The colonists were in India largely because of the East India Company, and through its various commercial agreements with local rulers, large parts of India came under British influence. The soldiers, civil officials, and doctors who came out with the company often had broad scholarly interests, including scientific study and observation of natural history, and they took an interest in indigenous healing methods and those who practiced the healing arts. Europeans thus discovered that local healers still routinely attempted surgical reconstruction of noses damaged by the still-common punishment of facial mutilation. As late as 1769, after the conquest of Naskatspoor, the victorious Gurkha king ordered that the noses of some of the town's inhabitants be cut off. This type of punishment persisted in parts of India until the late 1800s.

The West's "Discovery"

The first Western description of the Indian method of nose reconstruction to appear in print in Europe was published in the *Gentleman's Magazine* issue of October 1794. This particular story had already circulated among Europeans in India the previous year in a printed broadsheet entitled "A Singular Operation." The author of the broadsheet was James Wales, and the operation and the patient were illustrated in an engraving, itself a publishing novelty at that time. The report described the treatment of an Indian bullock driver called Cowasjee who had helped the British Army at Poona; when captured by anti-British insurgents in 1792, his nose

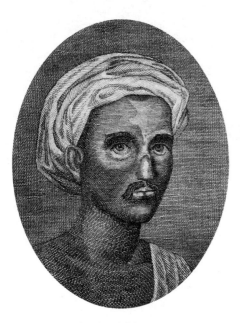

A portrait of Cowasjee from the broadsheet engraved in India describing his nose restoration. This image was used again in the October 1794 issue of *Gentleman's Magazine*.

and one hand were cut off, as an example to other collaborators. After he escaped, the British government's Resident in Poona, Sir Charles Malet, aware that India had skilled surgical empirics, arranged for Cowasjee's treatment by such a practitioner. A new nose was created in the ancient manner by cutting out and rotating a forehead pedicle flap down onto the remaining nose stump. The forehead was, as usual, left to heal by inward growth and contraction of skin from the sides. The operation may have already been copied locally by émigré surgeons; in 1795, an editorial in the *Bombay Courier* praised one expatriate, a Mr. Colly Lyon Lucas, the "ingenious surgeon of Madras," for having taken an interest in local traditional surgery. The editorial writer commented that Lucas had used this "Kooma method" of nose restoration, probably from the 1780s. The mysterious Mr. Lucas can therefore claim to be the first Western surgeon to offer plastic surgery in the modern era.

In Britain, the report in the *Gentleman's Magazine* caught the attention of both lay and medical readers, including the energetic and much-traveled Sir Joseph Banks (1743–1820), president of the Royal Society. Banks had by then revived the Royal Society's earlier interest in natural history, and there was favorable comment in Britain on the skills found in indigenous medicine and on this operation in particular.[3]

At some point unknown, someone noticed that the Indian method was not unlike Tagliacozzi's forgotten technique for nose reconstruction.[4] Credit for the rediscovery might belong to a Dr. Ferriar in England, some Edinburgh clinical lecturers, or an Italian experimentalist. Each may have read Tagliacozzi's original text and then, having seen or heard the story about Cowasjee, realized the surgery's significance. It seems that rhinoplasty was a surgical operation whose time had come.

John Ferriar

In 1798, just as the Indian rhinoplasty method was being recognized and admired, a curious little book by the Manchester physician and scholar John Ferriar (1761–1815) gave the first sign of a reappraisal of the reputation and methods of Tagliacozzi. Ferriar had studied medicine at Edinburgh, and upon moving south, he became prominent in the Manchester Literary and Philosophical Society. Ferriar was also a bibliophile. His book *Illustrations of Sterne* was a commentary on Laurence Sterne's *Tristram Shandy* (1759), a novel that contained a satirical "Treatise on Noses." Ferriar advised:

There is a writer who deserves a higher place in Mr Shandy's library, because his fame has been unjustly and unaccountably eclipsed. I allude to Gaspar Tagliacozzi. . . . He had indeed the misfortune of being too learned for his time. . . . The obscurity under which Taliacotius's brilliant discoveries have remained, is not more remarkable than its cause: it was occasioned by the jest of a Dutchman. The contemptible story which Butler has versified, in his well-known lines [i.e., *Hudibras*] was forged by Van Helmont. . . . It is a disagreeable proof of the neglect of medical literature, that facts, so important to the theory and practice of the art, were so long obscured by silly and unpardonable prejudice.[5]

Ferriar's almost accurate analysis is that, in the 1600s, the story about the demise of the transplanted nose after the death of the distant slave donor, as supported by van Helmont (though not in jest), gave the satirists their opportunity and thus marginalized the more sensible reconstructive surgery. But in Britain, Ferriar seems to have been alone for a while in his support for the Italian pioneer's surgical procedures.

The Edinburgh Influence

When the medical school in Edinburgh was the most prominent in Europe, it was the source of several publications that commended the Tagliacozzi surgical methods. Three Edinburgh academics were behind these publications. The first was the surgeon and anatomist John Bell (1763–1820), who, in his *Principles of Surgery* (1801), gave a balanced account, stating that Tagliacozzi's skin-flap method was workable. The long dormancy in the use of this surgical practice disturbed him, since there was, he said, "nothing unnatural in this [Taliacotian] operation, as this reunion [of skin flaps] . . . is just such as we procure in more difficult circumstances every day. The doctrine, and all the useful conclusions which have flowed from it would not have fallen into such discredit, had it not been for the ignorance of some, who thought to lie the theory into credit, and who undertook to back up this reasonable doctrine of Taliacotius with absurd incredible stories!"[6]

Bell's conversion and conviction could only have come from a study of Tagliacozzi's text, some versions of which were held in Edinburgh at the time.[7] Bell's new enthusiasm for the old skin-flap procedure was combined, as noted earlier, with remarkable scorn for the trickle of claims in the previous decade for re-implantation of separated noses or ears.

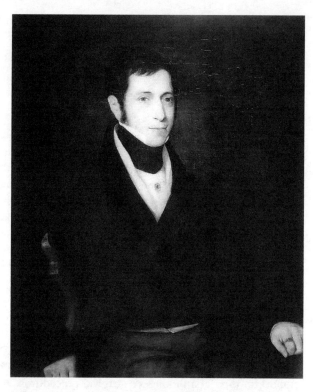

John Bell taught medicine in Edinburgh and, together with Charles Bell, his younger brother, published notable surgical and anatomical works. In his *Principles of Surgery* (1801–1808), John Bell encouraged the revival of Tagliacozzi's skin-flap plastic surgery. Image courtesy of the Wellcome Library, London.

A second teacher in Edinburgh was enthusiastic not about Tagliacozzi but about the Indian operation reported at this time. The distinguished academic James Gregory published and lectured in medicine, and such was his authority that the continental European medical literature mentioned his lectures from time to time. The abstracting periodical *Bibliothèque Britannique,* published in Geneva, offered French translations of the "ouvrages de sçavans de la Grande-Bretagne" and carried an account in 1803, two years after the appearance of Bell's book, of a lecture in which Gregory spoke enthusiastically about the possibility of nose restoration using the Indian method.[8] This article also had an engraving of the operation based on the original in the *Gentleman's Magazine* of nine years earlier, though it differed in some respects. The *Bibliothèque* engraving is cruder, and Cowasjee is shown looking to the right rather than to the left, as in the original, as if copied using a mirror. Although it did not mention Tagliacozzi, the report of Gregory's lecture also helped the revival of interest in Tagliacozzi.

The third Edinburgh savant involved in the revival of rhinoplasty was John Thomson (1756–1846), professor of military surgery. Thomson published his *Lectures on Inflammation,* considered to be an advance on the doctrines of John Hunter, some ten years after James Gregory had voiced his support for the feasibility of nose repair by the Indian method. Thomson's remarkable book has scholarly digressions into the history of surgery, carefully referenced, and a detailed review of the scanty transplantation literature to that date. Thomson boldly joined his colleague John Bell in unqualified support for Tagliacozzi's surgery, which he commended as useful and practical, adding a further apology for the neglect and denigration Tagliacozzi had suffered. When Thomson consulted Tagliacozzi's original text, possibly reading William Hunter's copy when he was in London in 1792, he described with awe his discovery of the "indefatigable and persevering industry by which his [Tagliacozzi's] cures were accomplished . . . never was a surgeon more zealous in his profession . . . the tedious minuteness of no fewer

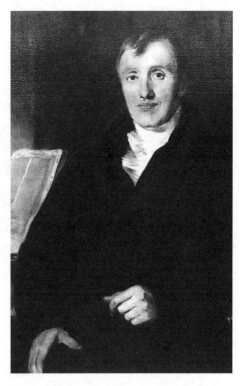

The surgeon John Thomson became professor of military medicine at Edinburgh University in 1806. His textbook, *Lectures on Inflammation* (1813), helped revive the lost teachings of Tagliacozzi. Image courtesy of the Royal College of Surgeons of Edinburgh.

than twenty-five chapters . . . [methods] illustrated and rendered visible to our senses in no fewer than twenty-two plates."[9]

Despite this authoritative pedagogic approval from the Edinburgh scholarly medical community, no surgeon in Britain began to do the surgery Tagliacozzi had described. The antipathy toward the procedure was not easily reversed in Europe, and in Britain, no one wanted to be first: failure could mean professional disaster. Not until 1812 was the first European human nose repair reported, by Joseph Constantine Carpue in London.

In the interim, and appropriately in Italy, there was a revival of interest in experimental skin grafting, stimulated, ironically, by the scholarship coming from Edinburgh.

Giuseppe Baronio's Experiments

The first experimental skin grafts in this new era were carried out in Italy by Giuseppe Baronio (1758–1811).[10] Baronio's experimental work—the

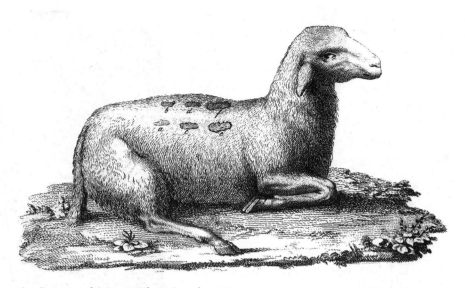

This illustration of skin autografts in sheep from Giuseppe Baronio's monograph *Degli innesti animali* shows a montage of his three successful skin graft experiments using all layers of skin. Image courtesy of the Wellcome Library, London.

first involving skin grafting since the pioneering interest taken by the Royal Society almost a century and a half previously—resembled Hunter's, though Hunter had never carried out skin grafting. As an admirer of Hunter, Baronio claimed that a great growth in natural philosophy was possible by means of the "questa novella arte di osservare, nata per cosi dire a giorni nostril" (this new art of observation, born in our time).[11] The inspiration for Baronio's transplant work came partly from the new awareness of his compatriot Tagliacozzi's original text, but he was also stimulated by the British rediscovery and enthusiasm for the Indian methods.

Baronio qualified in medicine in Pavia in 1780, and although he was a combative, ambitious young man, he failed to obtain a hospital post in Milan.[12] Instead, he obtained some humble employment with the prison medical service, but he soon gained an important patron, Count Anguissola of Milan, who had already supported Alessandro Volta's pioneering research on electricity. Baronio's first interest was in regeneration. He submitted a thesis on the regrowth of limbs in animals, a topic suggested by Lazzaro Spallanzani, Europe's authority on regeneration of tissues and the first investigator to describe the tissue capillaries.[13] Baronio's scientific work then switched from regeneration to transplantation. He repeated the old spur-to-cock's-comb experiments, remarking that such altered animals, including some of his, were still in demand for purchase by traveling circuses. Attitudes toward this old surgical trick could still be hostile, however, since the earlier unease about possible involvement of black magic persisted. Baronio mentions that, though his animals were first exhibited with success in Venice, the subsequent owner of the animals was later forced to leave Corfu because of this "abnormal practice," and he then fled to Russia, where he sold the birds for a good price.[14]

Baronio's introduction to his classic text on skin grafting, *Degli innesti animali* (1804), mentions the publication in London of the Indian methods of nose repair. However, he then credits James Gregory of Edinburgh with making this technique widely known, using Gregory's illustration from the Geneva *Bibliothèque Britannique,* identified by the reversed portrait of Cowasjee. Tagliacozzi's work is mentioned only briefly, with the accolade that his lost methods "would deserve being put into practice again for the good of mankind."[15]

Baronio conducted his experimental skin grafting at his patron Count Anguissola's country estate. Baronio usually worked alone, but he was careful to record the names of those who witnessed his work, hinting at the old suspicions about black magic. In his experiments, Baronio detached large patches of full-thickness skin from one side of the sheep and grafted them to similar-sized defects made in the skin on the other side, holding the grafts in place with bandages and strips of adhesive wax plaster. His fixation technique not only succeeded in maintaining the position of the grafts; as improbable as it seems, five out of six of these thick autografts survived, as shown in his famous composite illustration. His test of successful connection and blood flow in the grafts was to cut into the grafts to look for bleeding; on the eighth day after the grafting procedure, the punctures bled. In other experiments, Baronio attempted grafts between different species of animals, and he reported the failure of large grafts of skin between a cow and a horse and vice versa.

Baronio had been lucky with his thick grafts. He was correct in his overall conclusion that it was possible to transfer free skin grafts from one part of the animal to another part but not between species.

It was an observation in Baronio's nontransplant experimental work that led him close to unraveling the secret of routinely successful free skin grafting, a strategy not understood until sixty-five years later. His mentor Spallanzani had been first to describe normal capillary blood vessels, and Baronio, with this awareness, looked for these vessels as he conducted various studies. He learned that, after a sharp skin wound, the cut blood vessels at the edges of the cleft closed down quickly, never to reopen. During healing, *new* capillary vessels grew across the wound and joined up. In passing, Baronio gave a characteristic rebuke to those who had believed the opposite, "ed in lorvece altri nuovi piu piccoli aperti, che penetrano, ed irrorano la nuova sostanza intermedia formatasi," that is, that "in the immediate union of wounds the blood flow is restored by the joining of one vessel to another."[16]

Baronio did not apparently apply his entirely correct new paradigm to the healing-in of his grafts, namely that the new blood supply to such skin would also be via new ingrowth of capillaries and not direct union— "inosculation"—of graft vessels with the host vessels, as had always been assumed. If he had done so, he would have realized that the thinner the graft, the better the chance of success. This essential step of applying the new theory of capillary ingrowth to the design of grafting procedures was still to be made.[17]

Carpue in London

Joseph Constantine Carpue (1764–1846) made the first new attempt at human nose repair by skin-flap surgery eighteen years after its description in the *Gentleman's Magazine* and more than two centuries after Tagliacozzi's work. Carpue was one of London's surgeon-anatomists and ran the private Dean Street Anatomy School from 1800 to 1830.[18]

Carpue's activities earned him a certain level of notoriety. He was named in the poem *Mary's Ghost*, which satirized grave robbing:

> I can't tell where my head is gone,
> But Dr Carpue can:
> As for my trunk, it's all pack'd up
> To go by Pickford's van.[19]

Carpue gained further notoriety when he joined up with Giovanni Aldini, nephew of the physiologist Luigi Galvani, during Aldini's sensational visit to London in 1803. Aldini and Carpue used an electrical machine to galvanize muscular movement in the corpse of a recently hanged murderer.[20]

Carpue, descended from a wealthy Spanish family, was a Catholic and hence excluded from public office by Britain's Test Act, legislation not repealed until 1828. His only lowly public appointment in London was as surgeon to the Duke of York's Hospital in Chelsea. He was also excluded from fashionable circles in London and marginalized by the College of Surgeons. He perhaps had little to lose in attempting his pioneering, controversial plastic surgery. Joseph Carpue knew Sir Joseph Banks of the Royal Society and heard from him the news about the Indian rhinoplasties. Carpue lectured to his students on the method and demonstrated it on cadavers, delaying attempts on live patients for some time. In his publications, Carpue acknowledges the advice of the Edinburgh surgeon, John Thomson, gained when the Scot worked for a year in London at John Hunter's premises in 1792. Carpue was therefore influenced by two enthusiasts who had knowledge of either the Indian or the Tagliacozzi method, but not both.

In 1812, Carpue finally performed rhinoplasty on his patients using the skin-flap technique. The two procedures he did were carefully recorded and illustrated in his elegant quarto monograph, *An Account of Two Successful Operations for Restoring a Lost Nose* (1816). Carpue's report contains a scholarly review of the subject, and his historical introduction was taken largely from his friend Thomson's *Lectures on Inflammation* (1813).[21]

Carpue's first rhinoplasty case came to his attention when a Captain Williamson, an army officer stationed in Gibraltar, wrote to Carpue in 1814 and asked the surgeon to consider reconstructing his badly deformed nose. The officer's nose had not been injured in war, nor by an accident; the damage was the result of syphilis and the therapy for it some years previously. Williamson had been treated with the routine antisyphilitic drug of the day: calomel, a mercury salt. This drug had some efficacy but was tricky to use, and overdosage could damage the inner nose, leading eventually to loss of nasal skin. This situation was well known to early-nineteenth-century practitioners, and it presented a diagnostic puzzle: was nasal damage the result of continuing, active syphilis or successful but overdone mercury treatment? If syphilis was still active, poor healing resulted, and any surgical procedure would be thwarted and a new skin flap would be similarly destroyed.

In his description of the case, Carpue described the then-current diagnostic test to resolve this dilemma. He made two small cuts into the edge of what remained of the officer's ulcerated, eroded nose and observed the patient for some days. These wounds healed quickly. This favored mercury damage as the problem, rather than active syphilis, and hence the defect was amenable to repair. Carpue explained frankly to the officer that he had never attempted the Indian procedure, but the concerned patient nevertheless agreed to be Carpue's first patient, and the operation proceeded.

As in all operations carried out before the availability of anesthesia, Carpue's surgery was swift and decisive. He followed closely the Indian forehead flap plan, rather than use the Tagliacozzian arm source, and he cut a flap, measured to fit the nose, from the forehead, rotating it down onto the nose bed and attaching it there with a few stitches.[22] Carpue's speedy mobilization of the forehead flap and attachment to the nose bed took a mere fifteen minutes. He divided the flap at its base "some time later," and the residual graft was then judged to be a success. Carpue's powerful patron, Sir Joseph Banks, was still interested in nose and skin repair. Banks wrote to a correspondent, "We talk at present a good deal on both these Subjects. Mr Carpue, a Respectable Surgeon, has actually Re-

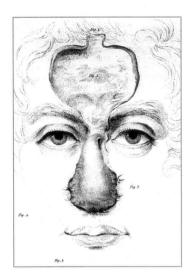

The outcome of Joseph Constantine Carpue's second successful rhinoplasty, taken from his monograph *An Account of Two Successful Operations for Restoring a Lost Nose from the Integuments of the Forehead* (1816). Image courtesy of the Wellcome Library, London.

placed the nose of an officer who Lost his in Spain & promises me to Shew me the Patient within a Fortnight with his new nose."[23]

Carpue's second patient, in 1815, also successfully treated, had loss of the soft tissues and cartilage of the nose as the result of a saber cut.

Lawrence, Mary Shelley, and *Frankenstein*

Carpue's work marked the starting point of modern plastic surgery. It may also have influenced one of the most famous literary works of the day. In London at this time, the surgeon William Lawrence (1783–1867) was part of a loose grouping of some surgeon-anatomist-physiologists who were building on Hunter's views.[24] Lawrence, an outsider like Carpue, is credited with the first use of the term *biologist,* which he included in his lectures in 1819. In an address on the "living principle," he caused a sensation by suggesting that life might not be divinely given and that it was instead a physical mechanism. After accusations of blasphemy, he retracted his statement. One member of Lawrence's loose circle of associates was Mary Shelley, author of the novel *Frankenstein* (1818), the gothic horror story and literary sensation of the day, and Dr. Frankenstein, her creation, was to be the prototype thereafter of the secretive, irresponsible scientist.[25] It is known that Shelley took advice from Lawrence on how Dr. Frankenstein might surgically create a composite monster, and it may be that Lawrence passed on fanciful possibilities from Carpue's London plastic surgery cases, published two years previously. Moreover, when Shelley's group visited Switzerland, where she constructed her story, one of the members present for the interlude was John Polidori, an Edinburgh medical graduate, who might have heard about plastic surgery from his teachers.

Shelley spared the reader the details of the Creature's assembly in her novel, but the surgical hints are there: "I collected bones from charnel houses and disturbed, with profane fingers, the tremendous secrets of the human frame. In a solitary chamber, or rather cell, I kept my workshop of filthy creation. The dissecting room and the slaughter house furnished many of my materials and often did my human nature turn with loathing from my occupation whilst I brought my work near to a conclusion."[26]

The unpleasant hybrid thus patched together was then animated by an electrical machine; as noted previously, Carpue was the London expert in this matter. Polidori published his own book, *The Vampyre,* in 1819, and it was the first in this enduring genre, one not unrelated to tissue transfer, which reached its peak with Bram Stoker's *Dracula* (1897).

Spread of Plastic Surgery

Carpue's surgical-flap method was quickly noticed in Europe, and his monograph on rhinoplasty promptly appeared in a German translation. Plastic surgery then began to develop rapidly. It was an endeavor whose time had come, and the deep-seated resistance and group timidity disappeared with remarkable speed. The German enthusiasm for plastic surgery was a puzzling development because German-speaking thinkers were the origin of *Naturphilosophie* and the Romantic movement, whose antiscience stance rejected the scholarly achievements of Enlightenment thinking and substituted a free-floating theorizing and philosophical stance. Somehow, plastic surgery, a fundamentally mechanistic human endeavor without the slightest hint of the mystical, flourished.

However, the hostilities in Europe and elsewhere also played a part in making plastic surgery more common. Across Europe, those with war wounds or other deformities began benefiting from Carpue's methods. In Berlin, Carl Ferdinand von Graefe (1787–1840) translated Carpue's work for publication in 1817, and he revived Tagliacozzi's technique of using a forearm flap. He described his own increasing surgical experience in his book *Rhinoplastik* (1818), published two years after Carpue's monograph.[27] Von Graefe's text was important, not least because in the title the term *plastic* was used for the first time in surgery. Other German texts soon appeared with reports of new adventures in plastic surgery. Johann Dieffenbach (1792–1847) reported his early surgical experience in *Nonnula de regeneratione et transplantation* (1822).[28] Rivalry between innovative German and French plastic surgeons commenced when the French monograph *Mémoire sur la rhinoplastie* by Jacques Lisfranc appeared in 1832 and marked the first use of the word *rhinoplastie* in a title. In the next several years French texts by Pierre-Auguste Labat (1834) and Philippe-Frédéric Blandin (1836) appeared, the latter reporting eighty-four flap operations.[29] Zeis attacked these two works in his classic *Handbuch der plastischen Chirurgie* as being anti-German and "having all the superficiality of the French character."[30] Italian surgeons had also been quick to follow Carpue, notably Schoenberg in Naples, who published *Sulla restituzione del naso* as early as 1819.

Carpue visited von Graefe in 1834 and recorded his impression of the growing vitality of German surgery, soon to be dominant in Europe, and their innovative specialist clinics. Carpue recalled an incident at von Graefe's clinic:

Another patient was brought in. It was a nose case; an operation for restoring the nose having been already performed on the patient.

Dr Graefe said

"Mr Carpue, I wish to have your opinion on this case, as it is your operation" referring to my being the first to perform the Indian operation, in Europe. . . .

I replied

"Dr Graefe this does you great credit."

He answered

"I did not perform this operation but this young man" pointing to one of his pupils.[31]

Events were following a pattern familiar in surgical innovation then and since. A pioneer reports a surgical novelty carried out with difficulty and only after discussion, hesitation, and conventional advice given not to proceed. Others follow with increasing success, and opposition declines. Other cases suitable for the operation or a variant appear and prove more numerous than was previously thought. With experience, the at-first-heroic operation becomes a routine one, easily learned by trainees unaware of the challenges encountered and surmounted earlier by the pioneers.

Plastic Surgery in America

News of the surgical methods sweeping across Europe reached America via the travels of Jonathan Mason Warren (1811–1867), a young Boston surgeon who was studying in Europe. In 1834, he wrote of his experience to his father, the distinguished surgeon John Collins Warren, who had also visited Europe earlier. Young Warren watched Vienna's Johann Dieffenbach at work "making some beautiful noses at the different hospitals. . . . [He] is still here and I had an opportunity to see him exercise his skill a few days since on two noses both of which he repaired in a very ingenious way. . . . Dieffenbach has operated on about 100 patients for renewing or repairing the nose with obvious success."[32]

On his return home, Warren carried out the first such rhinoplasty in America, in 1837.[33] In 1847, John F. South remarked in his introduction to the American edition of his translation of Joseph von Chelius's surgery textbook that there was general acceptance of the new procedures, stating that "there are few hospital surgeons who have not more or less frequently made new or mended old noses." An international flurry of publications also reported a growing range of techniques for addressing other facial defects and deformities of the body. These methods began to proliferate even at a time when anesthesia was not available, nor antisepsis practiced; the stoicism of the patients, though expected, necessary, and never remarked on, is something to be admired.

But Britain lagged behind in this surgical progress, and rhinoplasty reports in this period were of scattered, single cases—three from Scotland and two from London. Large clinics with concentrations of similar cases were not evolving in Britain. The politics of the time were anti-European, and these Germanic moves toward specialization in surgical matters could be reflexively resisted. "General" surgery—broad mastery of all surgical challenges by all surgeons—was still the British ideal.[34]

Old Misunderstandings

The rediscovery and international spread of plastic surgical methods had two unfortunate effects on attitudes toward transplantation. Success with the flap seemed to encourage the belief that skin was, after all, easily grafted, and more attempts followed with surgeons using large, thick, detached bits of skin. The old tales of re-implantation of entire noses, ears, and skin reappeared, even in scholarly works and respectable journals, and success was once more claimed.[35] Predictably, homografting returned, and the distinguished surgeon-scientist Henri Dutrochet (1776–1847) claimed a successful ear replacement using a paid donor: "The ear of a pariah was therefore bought, cut off and used to replace the ear."[36]

One such case is worth studying, however—that of Christian Heinrich Bünger (1782–1842) of Marburg.[37] He reported in 1822 that his patient was a young girl with extensive destruction of the center part of her face by "lupus"—probably tuberculosis. Although Bünger had experience with the new skin-flap method, he considered the area of the face too extensive to be covered by this method. Bünger stated that "nothing remained open to me now except the Indian method, by which a full separated piece of skin is taken out of the buttocks and transplanted to the nasal stump."[38] Bünger was alluding to the use of flayed skin in the ancient Indian plastic surgery. He placed a free skin graft, perhaps treated to make it thin or fissured, on the raw area, and claimed a good outcome.

Although the skin-flap method was considered a triumph in surgical technique, clinical attempts at routine grafting of large areas of free thick skin or large detached tissues foundered. Slowly, the surgical world reached a consensus that while free grafting of thick skin perhaps ought to work routinely, it did not. Dieffenbach in Berlin authoritatively summarized the view that the temporary connection of a graft by a flap to its base of origin was essential: "The basis of all plastic operations is that separated skin portions grow on fresh wound cicatrixes [scars] at another site, provided they [the grafts] are not deprived of a remaining nerve conduction and blood supply by a narrow nutritive connection."[39]

New Directions

A number of advances in medicine and biological knowledge in the mid-1800s are of relevance to later events, and although they were unrelated to transplantation practice at the time, they can be considered here. The first was the new understanding of the existence and effects of acute and chronic kidney failure, and the second was the demonstration of the phenomenon of dialysis.

A reasonably accurate idea of the functions of the kidney existed from earliest times. Rabelais, himself a trained doctor, summarized medieval thought on the subject via Panurge's thoughts in a rare moment of seriousness in *The Histories of Gargantua and Pantagruel:* "Each member [organ] here bestirs himself afresh to purify and refine this marvelous treasure [the blood]. The kidneys, through the emergent veins, extract from it the bitterness which we call the urine, and by means of the ureters, conduct it down below. There the urine finds a suitable receptacle, the bladder, which at the proper time empties it out."[40]

The early anatomists knew that obstructing the ureters proved quickly fatal. In 1827, Richard Bright (1789–1858) brought a number of his findings together to show that chronic kidney damage was the cause of some fatal clinical conditions, including dropsy. The Edinburgh physician Robert Christison (1797–1882) in 1832 added that in such cases, urea levels rose steadily in the blood. These advances in knowledge were more than just triumphs of clinical pathology. Diseases had been assumed in earlier times to be diffuse disturbances of the body manifesting secondarily in the confusing spectrum of pathological changes seen in the various organs of the body at postmortem. Now the paradigm was changing. Disease was increasingly considered to start in one organ, and from there the effects spread out to produce secondary changes. This new paradigm led to a profound reworking of familiar findings. If disease was localized, treatment might be aimed at the organ, at least at the start. In surgery, this was a highly attractive prospect, since surgery was becoming bolder and would soon, with anesthesia and antiseptics, be able to explore the inner body.

Shortly after Bright's major advance in the understanding of chronic renal failure, acute failure of the kidneys was also being identified, and an effective treatment had its first, tentative, controversial exploration. In December 1831, the first and worst of the British cholera epidemics spread rapidly. In serious cases, profuse diarrhea preceded notable "suppression of urine flow"—acute renal failure. Thomas Latta (died 1833), a surgeon in practice at Leith near Edinburgh, noted that the blood of cholera victims was concentrated and showed little serum above the cells when clotted. The chemists Thomas Thomson (1773–1852), professor of chemistry in Glasgow, and William O'Shaughnessy in London confirmed this dehydration. Latta, learning of the confirmation from the laboratory, reasoned that the sufferers were short of fluid, and he resolved to omit the conventional treatment by bloodletting and enemas and instead "to throw fluid immediately into the circulation." He gave about three to eight pints of saline intravenously using a large syringe, and three out of five patients treated in this way survived, with particularly prompt restoration of urine flow in one case.[41]

There was resistance to such a serious paradigm shift. The distinguished members of the Board of Health in Edinburgh revealed the assumptions of the day by deeming such therapy as "inconsistent with physiological principles." A colleague of Latta recalled that the humble young surgeon met with illiberal opposition in Edinburgh: "Latta is a worthy, but rather obscure man . . . certain worthies attempted to frighten him or bully him that he might not persist in his practice."[42] Latta's treatment by volume infusion replacement was put aside until the rediscovery of its crucial diagnostic and therapeutic value in the early twentieth century.

Totally unconnected with these events was the demonstration, about this time, of the physicochemical mechanism of dialysis, which would be used about one hundred years later in devices to treat acute and chronic renal failure. Thomas Graham (1805–1869), professor of chemistry in Anderson's University in Glasgow, had first described his "Law of Diffusion of Gases" in Glasgow in 1830.[43] Moving to the chair of chemistry at University College London, he turned to look at diffusion within liquids, and, in his classic experiments, in 1861 he showed that a parchment membrane would allow small molecules, including urea, to pass across, while holding back larger molecules,

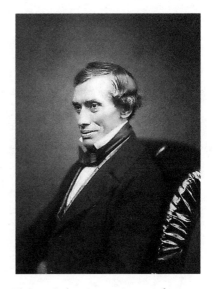

Thomas Graham, at one time a professor of chemistry in Anderson's University in Glasgow, moved to London, and his 1861 paper delivered to the Royal Society described differential diffusion of solutes across a membrane, and for this he used the neologism "dialysis." Image courtesy of Maggs Bros.

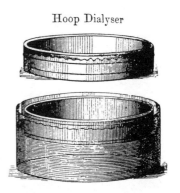

Thomas Graham's first dialysis membrane was made of parchment and stretched across a gutta-percha hoop. Image from *Philosophical Magazine* (1861).

including proteins. This principle, which he named "dialysis," was to be the basis later of the artificial kidney machines of the twentieth century.

It was not until 1869 that routine success with detached skin grafts was obtained. This achievement came from the realization that if the skin used was relatively thin, the grafts would heal in easily. This "split-skin" grafting method had an almost revolutionary effect on the world of surgery, but it was to cause problems when efforts at tissue transplantation by homografting were revived as a result of the new method.

4 Clinical and Academic Transplantation in Paris

G ERMANY WAS THE FIRST nation to nourish and broaden the revival of the old techniques of plastic surgery, but it was mid-nineteenth-century French surgeons who can be credited with finding the simple solution to the problem of grafting detached skin. The solution was for the graft to be very thin, and although this simple discovery may have been an entirely empirical surgical venture, the talented group of biological investigators led by Claude Bernard had some input.[1] As this history has already shown, such surgical advances had important consequences for tissue transplantation from donors.

The Collège de France

Claude Bernard (1813–1878) initially worked under François Magendie (1783–1855) at the Collège de France and then succeeded him. The two men extended the Hunterian experimental methods and proposed that the animal body was understandable in physicochemical terms. This stance was less controversial in the nineteenth century than in the century before, but it was one that still risked censure, and there was now an added objection that the results of reductionist experimentation might say little about integrated animal responses. Bernard's alternative view, and the resistance to it, was outlined with clarity in his classic work *An Introduction to the Study of Experimental Medicine* (1865). He said of the older school that "they assume a vital force . . . making the organism an organized whole which the experimenter may not touch without destroying the quality of life itself."[2]

This stance had elements of the German *Naturphilosophie,* then declining in influence. Its antireductionist view held that the whole was greater than the sum of its parts; it also had hints of the "uncertainty principle"—that observation changed what was being observed. One of Bernard's persistent critics, the distinguished Paris surgeon Gerdy, took another angle in attacking his view; at a scientific meeting, he placed the vitalist's new argument against all biological experiment. They were simply not repeatable and doomed to fail: "You [Bernard] say that the results of experiments in physiology are identical; I deny it. Your conclusion would be true for inert nature, but it cannot be true for living nature. Whenever life enters into a phenomenon, conditions [of an experiment] may be as similar as we please; the result will still be different."[3]

Gerdy's view might excuse some of the earlier thinking and the mindset behind claims for survival of some tissue homografts. If biological responses are not repeatable, then these complex, aleatory responses could mean that at one time grafts might fail and at other times succeed. But Bernard's work firmly established a new way of investigation and soon showed that standardized physiological experiments could indeed give repeatable, quantitative data. The new approach also showed that animal tissue, far from being in a state of flux, had remarkably constant features when chemical or physical properties were measured.

There was yet a further complaint about the physiologist's activities. The Paris experimenters were the first to devote themselves to such work; full-time scientists were taking over from the gentleman amateurs of earlier times. The clinical world reacted by arguing that investigative work should be in the hands of doctors only. This was the view of Oxford's distinguished professor of medicine, Sir Henry Acland, who sought to keep the new physiological studies directed at clinical aims and within the medical profession: "Modern civilisation seems set on acquiring, almost universally, what is called biological knowledge; and one of the consequences is that whereas medical men are constantly engaged in the study of anatomy and physiology for a humane purpose . . . there are a number of persons now engaged in the pursuit of these subjects for the purpose of acquiring abstract knowledge. This is quite a different thing. I am not at all sure that the mere acquisition of knowledge is not a thing having some dangerous or mischievous tendencies in it."[4]

Nevertheless, Claude Bernard's classic studies gained recognition for the new cadre of biomedical scientists, and this success started a lasting turf dispute on where research initiatives should come from and where funding should go. Bernard and the new physiologists faced a further problem in Britain: he was the bête noire of the antivivisectionists, as was Magendie before him, and some lurid and not always incorrect versions of their experiments in Paris appeared in the British antivivisectionist activists' literature. Some of these experiments involved transplantation, and the activist outcry ensured that no similar studies were attempted in Britain.[5] Some time later, in London, there were proposals to establish a research establishment similar to Paris's successful Pasteur Institute. The hope in Britain was to catch up with French and German medical science, but setting up the new institute was blocked by the antivivisection lobby, whose members included aristocrats, clergy, politicians, writers, and even doctors and their wives. Such an institute, claimed the *Star* newspaper, would be "a market garden of disease, an Inferno for innocent creatures, a material danger and a moral horror."[6]

Claude Bernard and Transplantation

For ten or fifteen years, beginning about 1860, Claude Bernard and the world's most innovative biological research laboratory maintained an interest in tissue transplantation, an input that has seldom been acknowledged.[7] Claude Bernard himself had a continuing interest in surgery, and in 1854, at the age of forty-one, he had published a beautifully illustrated surgical text together with Charles Huette, a surgeon from Orléans.[8] This work contained a description of rhinoplasty along with fine, new engravings of the classical nose restoration method. This forgotten involvement of Bernard in clinical surgery explains much and meant that he was part of the Paris surgical community. He was also to assist in a major clinical advance in human skin grafting.

Early Experiments

One member of the research group at the Collège de France was Charles Éduard Brown-Séquard (1817–1894). He and Magendie started tissue transfer experiments when they injected red blood cells into different species to see if they survived. They ingeniously used the characteristically oval red chicken cell corpuscle, which was easily distinguishable from the round mammalian variety, even in mixtures. After these intravenous injections of "discordant," readily identifiable blood cells, the researchers noted that the donated red cells rapidly disappeared from the recipient's blood.[9] They explained the red cell loss on a fundamental incompatibility between the species, a view not yet generally held in biology. In 1875, Leonard Landois (1837–1902), in Greifswald, provided the explanation for the red cell death, showing in simple mixtures in vitro that a serum factor—a natural hemolysin—destroyed the foreign cells immediately.[10]

Brown-Séquard went on to study tissue vitality, seeking the basis of Hunter's "living principle." He studied the contractibility of the human iris in a surgically removed human eye and found responses to light persisting for fourteen days, suggesting that if conditions were right, tissue vitality could be preserved for some time. Using limbs from guillotined criminals, he found that for a period of time he could maintain muscle contractility by perfusion with the blood of the deceased.[11] His limb perfusion studies were continued by Edme F. A. Vulpian (1826–1887) in the Paris group and reported in 1861.[12]

Brown-Séquard's Travels

Brown-Séquard left France when Claude Bernard was instead preferred as successor to Magendie, and he wandered the world, first taking a clinical post in Mauritius, the country of his birth. He then moved to North America, working for a while at the Medical College of Virginia and then at Harvard. He then moved to Britain and eventually returned to the Collège de France in triumph as successor to Claude Bernard. During his time in Mauritius, Brown-Séquard managed some experimental transplant work, as described by his biographer: "Cocks sporting rat's tails on their combs, and other mutilated animals, let loose together in his back yard, began to gain for him the reputation of a sorcerer among the negroes of the community."[13]

This is the last trace of the chicken spur–to-comb experiment. It is also a reminder of humanity's ancient distrust of transplantation; here, persisting in another culture, was the old association of black magic and grafting success.

Bernard's Group

When Bernard was in charge in Paris, he extended his school of experimental physiology at the Collège de France. Importantly, Bernard welcomed clinical hospital staff and clinical ideas to his laboratory. In Bernard's circle were men who seemed to move easily between the clinical world, including surgery, and the laboratory, and who were well known later on through their achievements in clinical areas. These individuals and their area of later specialization included Paul Broca (neurology), Vulpian (cardiology), Georges Martin and Henry Armaignac (ophthalmology), and Paul Bert (respiratory physiology). Louis Ollier was a young chief surgeon at the Hôtel-Dieu hospital, and, in his work on bone growth and grafting, he acknowledged Bernard's influence. Moreover, in his experiments in the mid-1860s, Ollier successfully used small grafts of the naturally thin periosteum, which covers bone, rather than thick bone grafts, to show the fundamental process of bone formation. This simple "thin-is-good" conclusion may have meshed with the important thinking of others in Bernard's lab. Bernard's group may also be seen as the first biological research team sharing a general program of work. Not surprisingly, it was from Bernard's group that the first-ever collaborative biomedical publications appeared; they were the first to contribute papers with joint rather than individual authorship.

Bernard's famous demonstration was of the need for constancy of the chemical composition, temperature, and osmotic forces of the internal environment—the *milieu intérieur*. Less well known is his group's interest in the derangement of this *milieu* when tissue was detached from the body and vitality was ebbing.

Tissue Vitality

Only two approaches to testing the viability of detached tissue had been attempted until this point. The first was the study of contractility of isolated muscle, as in John Hunter's umbilical cord experiment and in the Paris iris and limb perfusion studies. The second approach, also cumbersome, was to transplant detached tissue to another animal and then study the graft's success or failure, as Hunter had done when he investigated the "living principle." To these tests, the Paris group added another—the first microscopy of grafted tissue. Perhaps surprisingly, they took no interest in whether or not grafts survived on recipients for any length of time. Their interest was restricted to the life or death of grafts shortly after removal from the donor.

Paul Bert

Of Bernard's extended group, Paul Bert (1833–1886) had the greatest involvement in the transplant work, and, in the 1860s, he looked anew at the physicochemical events involved in death or in the survival of tissue removed from the body.[14] For the first time in transplantation studies, he used the newly available improved microscopes of the day, and he made a crucial contribution to the understanding of the initial events in "adhesion," as Hunter called it. Bert concluded that in a small graft, the first event was that new blood vessels grew in; the vessels of the graft and host did not rejoin. Bert showed that host capillary vessels appeared and entered into the graft and that these vessels then enlarged and matured. This observation vindicated Baronio's general stance from decades earlier, and Bert had finally buried the long-held assumption that "inosculation" was the first event in free grafting—that the recipient and graft vessels had to join directly, end to end, to rescue and nourish the graft. Bert had thus made a major conceptual advance. It explained, at last, why large, thick skin grafts with attached fat and fibrous tissue and containing small, apparently useful blood vessels did not succeed but that thin ones lacking these vessels did survive.

Bert also used for the first time a new terminology, namely of "homografting" for grafts within a species, and "heterografting" for transplantation across a species gap. It was a sensible and clear terminology used by

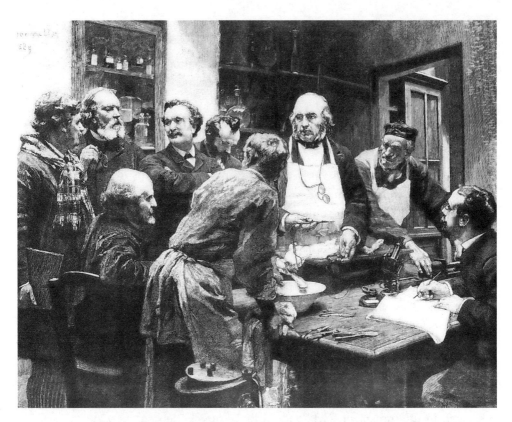

Paul Bert, depicted here (arms folded) in Claude Bernard's Paris laboratory, studied the vitality of tissues separated from the body and published on animal transplantation in the 1860s. Image courtesy of l'Assistance Publique, Hôpitaux de Paris.

careful writers thereafter but ignored by others, causing considerable confusion in the literature of the late 1800s and early twentieth century. The terms *homografting* and *heterografting,* as well as other terms introduced, were replaced in the 1960s by *allografting* and *xenografting.*

Graft Vitality

In other experiments, Bert studied how long a graft could retain its vitality when separated from the body. He took rat tails, exposed them to different temperatures and ranges of oxygenation and humidity, and then transplanted the tails subcutaneously into the same or different rats to study microscopically the survival in the short term of the treated tail tissues. During this work, he made an observation of crucial importance to transplantation and one taken up much later: several days of cold storage of the graft permitted a successful outcome. His intriguing but brief report of a successful fusion of adult rats—a process known as parabiosis—may have been an attempt to prolong graft life.

Bert's work was highly regarded at the time in Paris, and, in 1865, he was awarded one of the prizes of the prestigious Académie des Sciences. Although Bert's publications are difficult to analyze and, judged by later standards, are short on adequate experimental details and data on outcome, his work ushered in a new approach in transplantation studies.

Related Research

Bert's work was later continued in Paris by Georges Martin and Henri Armaignac.[15] In the introduction to his thesis, Martin thanks the local surgeon Leon Gosselin for his support, which confirms that the Paris physiologists had regular contact with the surgeons. Martin established that human skin could be successfully stored for up to five days if cooled and that grafts heated to above body temperature were dead. Martin was the first to discuss these methods of tissue preservation in detail and quotes remarkable unpublished work by Caliste and Pélikan showing that a weak solution of potassium would sustain vitality for lengthy periods.[16]

Another now-forgotten thesis produced during this period in Paris was Paul Broca's *Recherches sur l'hybriditie en general* (1860), which considered the broader question of biological individuality.[17] Like the others, Broca's career followed a surgical-scientist route, in and out of the lab, and he had published a book on surgery for aneurysms four years earlier.[18] Included in this substantial work is an elegant engraving of an arteriovenous fistula at the elbow, caused by damage during attempts at bloodletting, a therapy still in favor at the time. Fistulas of exactly this kind were deliberately created in large numbers a century later to prepare patients for regular hemodialysis treatment.

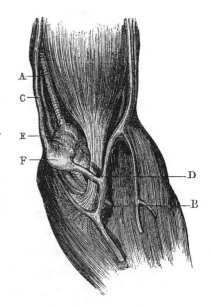

Grafts from Animals

Broca and Bert, influenced perhaps by the midcentury writings of Charles Darwin, advanced a new and important doctrine. They taught that not only were the animal and plant worlds different but that the various species of the animal world were also distinct biologically. There were thus biological barriers to transplantation between species. Bert wrote that

In 1856, Paul Broca described an arteriovenous fistula of the elbow, caused by bloodletting, similar to the fistulas deliberately created in the 1960s for hemodialysis patients. From Broca, *Des anévrysmes et de leur traitement* (Paris, 1856).

animal and vegetable species are separated by peculiar conditions which prevent them from mingling, so that fecundation, grafting and transfusion cannot be performed between beings of different species. These problems are of great interest, which I believe may be attacked and reduced to differences in the physico-chemical properties of the environment.

I have not been able to obtain a graft between animals of different species. . . . I have most often seen more or less rapid elimination. Only a large number of experiments will permit some intrepid surgeon to attempt a graft from a mammal to a human.

Bert also believed that the human races were different species, notably white and nonwhite. His advocacy that intermarriage meant sterility, and should be prevented, did not lead to another prediction, namely, that grafting between humans of different "species" (races) would fail. The cultural baggage of racism did not assist scientific inquiry into the fate of grafts between humans. Much enthusiastic homografting was to follow.

Thin Human Skin Grafts

At the end of the 1860s, a crucial advance in clinical tissue grafting was made at a Paris hospital not far from the laboratory of the Collège de France. Jacques-Louis Reverdin (1842–1929) was a young Swiss doctor newly promoted to the staff from his post as a lowly house-surgeon to Leon Gosselin, a professor at the Hôpital de la Charité.[19] The reasons why Reverdin turned to grafting small bits of human skin, rather than, as of old, using thick, large areas are not clear. It may have been an entirely empirical venture, one in which he was trying to imitate the regeneration of skin sometimes seen from surviving skin pegs or skin appendages, notably after a burn. But there is a possibility that the young man, or Gosselin, was aware of the newer knowledge of biological mechanisms uncovered three years earlier by Bernard's group at the nearby Collège de France, notably that the first event in graft survival is penetration by new blood vessels. Paul Bert's work had by 1866 indicated that skin grafts should be thin, and the word of this approach may have spread. Professor Gosselin might have heard about it, since Martin had thanked Gosselin for encouraging his transplant work with Bernard.

The clinical observation that ensured success in skin grafting, perhaps a simple and obvious one in retrospect, was made by Reverdin in 1869. In treating human unhealed ulcers, he chose to use skin grafts that were small and thin. This new approach was an immediate success and was so reliably successful in other hands that news of it spread quickly. The simple method was copied internationally, and some observers, aware of the historical significance of the new technique, even wrote down their version of the events as they unfolded.

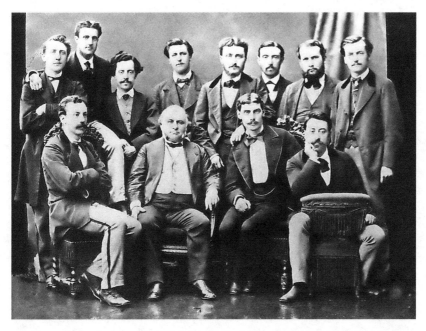

Jacques-Louis Reverdin (*seated, far left*) with Leon Gosselin (*seated, second from left*) and other assistants at the Hôpital de la Charité, Paris, shortly after Reverdin performed his pioneering 1869 skin grafts at the Hôpital Necker. Image courtesy of Sauerländer Verlag.

Reverdin's Work

Paris had an active network of professional and scientific societies noted for the vigor of their discussion and debate. Many groups met weekly and arranged for rapid publication of these presentations in the local medical broadsheets. Reverdin first reported his findings on thin grafts to the Société Impériale de Chirurgie in December 1869, and Bernard assisted him in this effort. Bernard was a member of the society, thus showing his continued interest in surgery, and in elite, limited-membership organizations like this one, members could introduce the work of nonmembers. Bernard did so in Reverdin's case, making it likely that Bernard had encouraged the new human grafting "thin-is-good" method from the start, as a natural consequence of Bert's capillary ingrowth graft insight at the Collège de France or even of Ollier's success with thin periosteum grafts.

Reverdin's patient had a "common" ulcer of the leg ("*pathologie bien vulgaire*"), normally treated by bed rest and dressings. On it he placed thin "pinch" grafts ("*greffe épidermique*" or "*lambeaux cutané*," as he called them)—small, wedges of skin taken from another part of the patient's own body. These narrow little grafts (not the "split-skin" slices used later) were obtained by thrusting the familiar double-edged "bleeding lancet" vertically through the skin below the knee into the tissue beneath. The lancet was turned through 180 degrees and pushed back out of the skin as a second puncture close by, and as the broadening lancet blade emerged, the instrument sliced out a little wedge of skin, usually three to five millimeters wide, full thickness in the middle but thinning out at each edge.

Reverdin recorded that when these little grafts were scattered on the ulcer, they generally healed in. But more importantly, this new skin then spread out. It was "une qualité particulière des ilots développés autour des greffes." The new skin from each *ilot* speedily joined up with its neighbor, eventually giving a full covering, albeit a thin one. Moreover, the new graft skin was pleasingly resistant to superficial infection, and as the *ilots* grew out and coalesced, on their way they cleansed the raw area.

Reverdin's paper was published in brief in two local journals shortly after his presentation. One of these journals also printed the typically robust discussion the young man had to face at the meeting. Senior surgeons identified as Trelat, Guyon, Tillaux, Despres, Le Fort, and Blot spoke in turn, some declaring reflex opposition to such novelty and suggesting that Reverdin should show more "critical sense and humility."[20] Their view was that the skin cover must have come instead from surviving deep host skin appendages, such as hair roots.

Reverdin did not publish his full method and results until 1872, three years later, the delay being due to the Franco-Prussian War, which put Paris under siege until 1871. His final report lists twenty-nine further cases treated by his *méthode*.

Few clinical innovations have been recognized and accepted as fast as the thin-skin graft. Spread by word of mouth and demonstrations at clinical meetings, the grafting treatment was even reported in the popular press. One unusual route was that the news traveled to the German military surgeons involved in the siege of Paris. These surgeons included Karl Thiersch, soon to be an important skin graft proponent, and word soon reached Russia via the surgeon Alexander Yatsenko, seconded at the time to the German army. His home base was the surgical department at the University of St. Petersburg, headed by Nikolay Pirogov, the local rhinoplasty expert. After returning to Russia from the front in 1871, Yatsenko not only made haste to publish a monograph on the technique, *K voprosu o perenesenii ili privivkie otdielennich kusochkov,* but also rapidly produced two papers on skin grafting for the Berlin and Vienna medical journals, thus establishing himself in print one year prior to the publication of Reverdin's full paper.[21] But 1870 certainly was "Reverdin's Year." Many surgeons made modifications to Reverdin's technique, useful or otherwise, and as is usual in such innovation, priority disputes emerged, particularly as the publication of young Reverdin's paper had been delayed.

Of those who took up and supported the new method of human skin grafting, George Pollock (born 1817), an English surgeon, was one of the earliest enthusiasts. Pollock was a well-known medical man in London, being past president of a number of clinical societies, as well as surgeon to the Prince of Wales.[22] Pollock heard about the new French method of skin grafting from a medical student named Wallace Bowles, who had returned to England in late 1869 after having witnessed the first of the Paris skin grafts.[23] The student was present in May 1870 when Pollock, at St. George's Hospital in London, presented an eight-year-old patient with a huge, unhealed ulcer of the right thigh, resulting from a burn. Bowles told Pollock of Reverdin's new method of using a number of small, slim grafts rather than waiting for ingrowth of skin from the side, and Pollock tried the new grafts on the child, with success.

Pollock went on to incorporate an ingenious variant to investigate the possibilities for the new little "pinch" grafts. After applying the first set of grafts from this patient's own body to the leg burn, Pollock also transferred two small grafts from the shoulder of a "black man"—a servant in the employ of a local family. The black skin grafts appeared to grow for a while, and then Pollock reported that they "disappeared." Pollock, on two other occasions, also used small skin grafts taken from his own body; these, he reported, also failed to take. Pollock's success can be admired for his objectivity in acknowledging the loss of these homografts taken from unrelated donors. Many other surgeons and scientists in the next decades were less critical.

Pollock reported sixteen cases using Reverdin's method to the Clinical Society in London in 1871, one year before the delayed publication of Reverdin's full paper.[24] Pollock's status ensured that his cases were widely and fairly discussed in London, and he was pleased at the success of his advocacy. This was aided by the first tissue transplantation story in a newspaper, since "a national daily paper," attracted by the intriguing use of black donor skin, had in May 1870 already carried the story of Pollock's hospital presentation on skin grafting.[25] Many British surgeons were enthusiastic about the new technique, supportive case reports from Bristol and Exeter appeared quickly in the journals, and the topic was a favorite one at medical society meetings that year.

A Growing Need for Skin Grafting

The need for skin grafting was probably greater at this time than earlier or later. One of the most frequently encountered cases in the surgical wards of the time was that of the "common ulcer" of the leg, as in Reverdin's first case. These ulcers could result from the widespread nutritional deficiencies of the times, and there were cases of skin loss from syphilis or tuberculosis or even from varicose veins. The Industrial Revolution had also produced an epidemic of industrial accidents and burns that left a legacy of unhealed skin defects. Warfare in general, and the Franco-Prussian War of 1870–1871 in particular, also resulted in unhealed skin wounds in veterans, notably in the many unhealed amputation stumps. All of these ulcers were potentially treatable by the new method. Moreover, grafting was an economical, speedy alternative to the tedious conventional approach of waiting for the slow, uncertain ingrowth of new skin from the distant edges of the defect.

In Britain, Charles Steele (1838–1914), surgeon to the Bristol Royal Infirmary, commented on his pleasure at having a new solution to the dreary, ever-present challenge of these skin ulcers: "Ulcers thrust themselves upon the care of all surgeons, the private practitioner, the parish and the club-doctor; while the most aggravated and chronic cases continually come under our notice as hospital surgeons. To all, a means of decided and rapid cure, such as transplantation of skin promises, is a matter of congratulation."[26]

Dr. John Woodman, surgeon to the eighty-bed infirmary for the indigent at the Exeter City Workhouse, also realized that his chronic ulcer cases might benefit: "I was much struck with the importance of the subject [skin grafting]; for if this was capable of extension to all, or nearly all, cases of obstinate ulcers, a new era in surgery would commence, in which bad legs, instead of being the bête noir of hospital and workhouse surgeons, would be an object of interest and credit to the surgeon."[27] Those who funded the workhouses were also glad to hear the good news about this quick, economical treatment for a common problem.[28]

The new method had received powerful support from the great surgical events of the previous decade, which included antiseptic measures and anesthesia. In skin grafting, the raw bed for receiving the graft could be prepared and made free from infection, increasing the chances of a "take." The donor area on the patient could be cleansed prior to surgery, thus reducing the omnipresent threat of erysipelas or "hospital gangrene" at the removal site. Furthermore, the excision of skin was painful, and the increasing use of general anesthetics made it less traumatic for both patient and surgeon.

America and Elsewhere

The earliest enthusiast for free skin grafting in America was Frank Hamilton (1813–1886), an important figure in the New York and Buffalo surgical communities. Hamilton had toured and visited all the British and European continental surgical centers in 1843, and, in 1854, he had tried an ambitious pedicle skin flap graft (rather than a free graft) from one leg to another to treat chronic ulcers.[29] He realized the importance of Reverdin's discovery and published quickly on the method at the end of 1870. Others followed Hamilton, and J. J. Chisholm of Baltimore described it further in a North American publication. Luis Muñoz in Mexico, a distinguished surgeon and historian, was also quick to publish, with his case report appearing on December 12, 1870.[30] In the following year, W. H. Hingston of Montreal reported the Canadian experience with the method.[31] Stanislav Zebrowski, at Constantinople's Hôpital Anglais, claimed the first cases treated in Turkey with the new method.[32] In Ireland, the operation was performed regularly in Dublin.

Only occasional resistance to the novelty was encountered. In Edinburgh, traditionally accustomed to innovation but perhaps piqued by the rising reputation of the new European centers, there was criticism. The president of the Royal Medical Society tried Reverdin's method immediately but concluded that the graft merely stimulated ingrowth of host skin from the ulcer edges. He patronizingly opined, "This method of skin grafting is of limited application; and as its result leads to no regeneration of true skin . . . it is an operation which cannot rank with plastic operations proper, and which is not likely to occupy a permanent place in minor surgery."[33]

Reverdin published nothing further on his method after 1872. He later achieved fame in another field, when he may have been the first to describe and explain a major complication after the new operation of total removal of the thyroid gland. As discussed later, this led to attempts at thyroid gland homografting.

The Method Evolves

The international flurry of publications continued, testifying to the routine, self-evident success of the new "pinch" skin grafts.[34] A semenological typology was used, comparing the size of the graft with the seeds from the pea, bean, millet, flax, or barley. Special grafting scissors appeared, designed both to pinch and hold up the skin and to cut a small horizontal graft, rather than a vertical slice.[35] Broader sheets of thin skin soon came into use, and these gave better coverage and a more pleasing cosmetic effect, a strategy that can be attributed to Karl Thiersch (1822–1895); this type of graft still bears his name.[36] However, after World War I, patriotic British surgeons tried unsuccessfully to drop the German "Thiersch" label in favor of "Steele grafts," to honor the Bristol graft enthusiast Charles

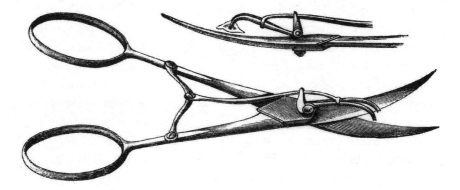

The increasing use of skin grafts led to the appearance of the first instruments designed to remove large, thin slices of skin using a horizontal cut. From H. Beigel, "Über die gynäkologische Verwendung der Transplantation kleiner Hautstückchen," *Wiener Medizinische Wochenschrift* 22 (1872): 573–77.

Steele.[37] The last ironic twist in this evolution of routine free-skin grafting was the realization that, after all, some full-thickness grafts from certain parts of the human body were suitable as free grafts. John M. Wolfe (1824–1904), the Glasgow ophthalmologist, showed that naturally thin body skin, from which all the attached subcutaneous tissue and fat was scrupulously removed, would regularly succeed as grafts. These grafts gave better cosmetic results than split skin and are often used in facial plastic surgery; for such procedures, thin skin is taken from the inner forearm or from behind the ear.[38] Wolfe's name is often eponymously linked to this new method.[39]

The Homograft Era

The new success for split-skin autografting immediately produced one undesirable effect. Its widespread use raised the old question of using skin from other human donors. The "default" view taken by most surgeons and the new scientists was that all humans were biologically alike. Bernard's group had taught that species were distinct, and heterografts (xenografts) failed, but they were silent on the status of grafts between individuals within a species. Indeed, Bert had assumed that in his grafting work all his outbred rats were identical. In clinical skin grafting, if the area to be grafted on a particular patient was large or the patient too young, or too nervous, or too distinguished, the mindset of the day considered it acceptable to use skin from other human donors. Such use of donor skin proved irresistible, since it was widely available, notably from newly amputated limbs, and could be painlessly applied. All over the world, enthusiastic and uncritical homografters began to carpet wounds with such tissue and, in spite of Bert's warning, use of animal skin also had support.

Problems with Homografting Emerge

Perhaps surprisingly, Reverdin's later reports claimed equal success with homograft and autograft skin, and he also tried animal skin. As the enthusiasm for skin homografting and heterografting grew, the *Glasgow Medical Journal* of May 1873, in reviewing the remarkable rise in skin grafting in the previous two years, supported homograft use. The anonymous scholarly reviewer (possibly Sir William Macewen) concluded, based on the many publications on the subject, that all sources of skin grafts gave equally good results:

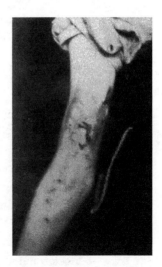

The earliest photograph of tissue transplantation shows a skin graft performed in 1894 by Sir William Macewen. From a casebook held in the Royal College of Physicians and Surgeons of Glasgow.

M. Ollier of Lyon takes his [skin] from limbs amputated for accidents. . . . This proceeding is practised also by Dr Wilson of Greenock. . . . Jacenko (de Kiew) states that he has transplanted tissue from man to man, from man to dog, from dog to dog, but that he failed to transplant from dog to man. . . . Mr Bryant transplanted the skin of a negro on to a white man. . . . M. Philippe transplanted a portion of the skin of a rabbit on to a man with success. Reverdin used a graft from a rabbit and another from a sheep and succeeded in both instances.[40]

The grafting of skin from black donors to white recipients was a niche endeavor reported a number of times, and the success claimed seemed to add some scientific objectivity to the concept of homografting. In fact, the semblance of successful homografting was misleading; the grafts had quickly failed, but the pigment from the dead skin cells remained, thus leading the surgeons to believe the graft had succeeded.[41] Also around this time there appeared the perennial and irresistible idea, one too good to be false, that grafts of fetal or very young tissue had special powers of survival. For the first, and not the last time, some surgeons began to advocate the use, as grafts, of foreskin removed during childhood circumcision.[42]

The practice of homografting had one notable supporter—Joseph, later Lord, Lister, an icon of scientific objectivity. One of his patients in Edinburgh's Royal Infirmary kept a diary and recorded Lister's day-to-day practice about the time of Reverdin's major advances in 1870. One entry in the diary reads,

There was a patient in No. 3 who had a very sore leg from varicose veins. After trying several sorts of treatment Professor Lister said, "There seems to be only one experiment more I would try with this patient and that is if I could get a bit of live skin off a living person (which I suppose I will not get) I would graft it onto the sore on the patient's leg and I believe it would then heal." One of the students, a

Mr Peddie, spoke and said, "Please sir, here's my leg to take it from" (All in astonishment). "Thank you kindly, Mr Peddie. Well then you must go through your operation. Then we will go to the Theatre, gentlemen." Then all went out and soon returned, and Mr Peddie was sent home in a cab. Prof. then grafted it onto Miss Reid's leg and it got on very well every day and did heal, and she was dismissed.[43]

Mr. Peddie was clearly anxious to assist the professor, but some donors elsewhere were less willing. Donors in Germany's hospitals came forward to provide skin grafts only when paid with "a groschen [ten-penny coin] or a bottle of beer."[44]

Obtaining skin from hospitalized donors or from staff may have been quite common, and one such donation in Glasgow led to legal proceedings. In 1878, the *Glasgow Herald* reported a "case of a somewhat extraordinary character" involving a charge brought at the Small Debt Court against a doctor and a nurse involved in skin grafting at the Glasgow Royal Infirmary.

The complainant was the father of a boy treated in the Royal Infirmary for a broken leg. One of the nurses, without the knowledge of the boy's parents, had, it was alleged, taken "a piece of flesh from his right arm in order to graft it onto the arm of another with an unhealed wound." The boy, alleged the father, had suffered pain and disfigurement from this removal of tissue, and damages of twelve pounds were claimed. At the trial, the nurse admitted that she had done this operation and had taken the skin with "a pair of pincers." This, she said, was done at the request of Johnston Herbert. "Dr." Herbert, who proved to be a medical student, when examined, ungallantly denied all knowledge of the events. In his judgment, Sheriff Birnie considered the charge against Herbert "not proven," but he criticized the nurse for proceeding without the family's permission, and she was found liable for five pounds in damages. The sheriff added that he had no criticism of the operation itself.[45]

Lastly, in a famous diary from the late nineteenth century, there is another testimony to the widespread acceptance of skin grafting between persons. The young Winston Churchill, while serving as a newspaper correspondent in the Boer War in 1898, was asked to donate skin to an officer with an unhealed wound:

Molyneux had been rescued from certain slaughter by the heroism of one of his troopers. He was now proceeding to England in charge of a hospital nurse. I decided to keep him company, and while we were talking, the doctor came in to dress his wound. It was a horrible gash, and the doctor was anxious that it be skinned over as soon as possible. . . . He [the doctor] was a great raw-boned Irishman. "Oi'll have to take it off you," he said. There was no escape, and as I rolled up my sleeve he added genially, "Ye've heard of a man being flayed aloive? Well this is what it feels loike." He then proceeded to cut a piece of skin and some flesh about the size of a shilling from the inside of my forearm. My sensations as he sawed the razor slowly to and fro fully justified his description of the ordeal. . . . This precious fragment was then grafted on to my friend's wound. It remains there to this day and did him lasting good in many ways. I for my part keep the scar as a souvenir.[46]

This graft could not have survived.

Grafts from Animals

In addition to these faulty claims for grafts between humans, there was widespread use of animal skin grafts for human patients, and respectable surgeons claimed success with the procedure. Even dog skin was used,[47] and one inventive notion in that regard was the use of hairless Mexican dogs as skin donors. In 1877, the first reported use of pig skin for human grafting came from London. Since the pig was to rise to importance in transplant matters later, this report might be called a dubious "first."[48] Frog skin was in vogue from 1887 to 1893, and its use was popularized by the distinguished surgeon Watson Cheyne, who introduced grafting of the chest wall after extensive removal of large tumors of the breast.[49]

To add to the confusion, there was now no agreement on terminology for the types of graft, and many neologisms appeared. Paul Bert's sensible typology of the 1860s (auto-, homo-, and heterografting) was disturbed when, in 1871, Antonin Poncet (1849–1913) and other surgeons in Lyon, a medical center beginning to rival Paris in grafting and other matters, introduced the terms *hetero-epidermic* and *zoo-epidermic*, while others were already using the more attractive *xenograft*.[50] Further confusion came when others introduced the term *isografting* for homografts, claiming validation from the classical languages. When the word *homogeneous* was used for autografts, the confusion in the literature was complete.

Assessing Graft Survival

An exasperated commentator on this era of transplantation, particularly the use of animal donation, stated in a later review that "it is difficult to draw conclusions about the application of frog skin grafts. . . . It seems unlikely that they [the surgeons] purposely lied. Probably the optimistic view about frog skin was based on misguided observation."[51]

The reasons for this "misguided observation" or frequent self-deception, even among celebrated surgeons, are not difficult to find, and they explain the inexplicable claims of the individuals involved. Judging the success of a skin graft is surprisingly difficult. Both then and today, the process requires an awareness of the pitfalls, plus a detached attitude on the part of the observer, and a refusal to accept any preconceptions about success.[52] Skin grafts generally heal in at first and survive, and homograft skin survives for about seven to fourteen days, or even longer in ill or malnourished patients. This early "take" and survival was often judged to mean a successful graft, and if the patient was gone from the hospital, follow-up of surgical cases not being routine at the time, the matter seemed decided. The early workers expected either immediate failure or continued success, and they apparently found other alternatives difficult to contemplate. After all, had not John Hunter proposed that the initial adhesion of a transplant was crucial?

When surgeons did notice loss of a homograft some time after successful healing in (a process now known as rejection, caused by the immune system's reaction), they reported this as a puzzling "erosion," "ulceration," or "disintegration." This loss did not fit any known mechanism at the time. The delayed loss might be attributed to infection, or a proud surgeon could blame clumsy dressing changes during his absence. Moreover, if grafts fail slowly enough, the patient's own skin has time to grow in from the edge of the wound, spreading under a dead or dying graft.[53] These ever-open traps for those judging skin grafts were to mislead some inexperienced or uncritical observers for a century, certainly until the 1950s.

Special Cases—Bone, Cornea, and Blood

Some tissue grafts did survive because of special dispensations, and these successes buttressed the faulty claims for skin survival. Surgeons had already begun bone grafting, with undoubted clinical success.[54] Louis Ollier, who had moved from Paris to Lyon and further strengthened the vitality of surgery there, pioneered the procedure in Lyon, and Macewen later followed suit in Glasgow.[55] The success of bone grafts was due not to the survival of transferred cells but to the inert bony implant that provided a site for the ingrowth of host cells.[56] Corneal grafting was another procedure that had success at this time, but only because no blood vessels nourish the cornea and host cells cannot reach corneal grafts and cause rejection.[57] Blood transfusion was another special case, since random successes at transfusion had been achieved because, as it was later discovered, the number of blood types was low and the majority of people fall into two type categories.[58]

Adding to the uncertain verdict on skin homografting, these special types of grafts, not affected by the "rules of immunology" to be uncovered later, also encouraged the use of yet more fragments and slices of tissue homografts to replace human deficiencies, real or alleged.[59] The many types of homografts used—retina and choroid from the eye, spleen, fallopian tube, fat, and uvula—seem ridiculous now. But of lasting significance, and worth examining as a special case, was the similarly mistaken enthusiasm for grafting slices or lumps from the testes or ovaries or from the pancreas, adrenal, and other glands.

Gland Grafting

The uncovering of the role of the glands and their hormones proceeded rapidly in the late nineteenth century, and recognition of problems resulting from underactivity of these glands was a major advance at the time. Addressing these gland deficiencies was an obvious goal. The idea that gland grafting might succeed in this was an important change in surgical ambition, a shift from simple plastic surgery and restoration of physical defects. To alter the body's general constitution, and even the patient's personality, was a heady goal for surgeons to add to their more mundane life of "cutting and stitching."[60] However elegant the grand plan, the activities of most of the gland grafters were to result in an embarrassing period of bad science and flawed surgery, one that persisted to the 1930s.

The gland homografts were placed below the skin or at even deeper levels in the body. There was scholarly debate on the best site for implantation, and the consensus was that "deep was good"; surgeons often placed them in the abdomen, almost as a tribute to John Hunter. The gland-graft surgeons conspicuously failed to heed the earlier finding that thin grafts were desirable, and they reverted to the older bad habit of implanting large bits of tissue, such as whole lobes of thyroid, large parts of pancreas, entire testes, or whole ovaries. Judging survival of visible skin grafts was difficult enough, and beset with problems, but the grafting of bits of organs deep within the body where, unlike skin grafts, they could not be observed, gave even less chance of critical analysis of outcome. If the disease ran a variable course, as did many glandular deficiencies, spontaneous improvement could be credited post hoc to a benefit from the graft. When hopeful patients encounter a charismatic surgical enthusiast with a new treatment, a balanced verdict is possible only if objective criteria of success are available. Objective criteria of success were distinctly lacking in gland grafting.[61]

One encouraging development in the study of tissue grafts was not as helpful as it might seem. Use of microscopy in biology and medicine was increasing, and Paul Bert had been first to study grafts in this way. When samples of the allegedly surviving gland grafts, human or experimental, were examined under the microscope, a complex mass of cells was found. The microscopists of the day, charitably inclined when venturing into this unknown area, often reported to the optimistic surgeons that much of this living tissue was not unlike the tissue of the original graft. Thus, gland homograft survival claims were often said to be supported by microscopy. In fact, however, most of the cells observed in the graft were the host's own scavenger cells and white blood cells attacking the foreign tissue.

One of these gland homograft attempts at the end of the nineteenth century is of particular interest. Thyroid deficiency was recognized in the late 1800s as the cause of not only childhood cretinism but also adult myx-edema (with symptoms of hypothyroidism such as fatigue and mental impairment) and the syndrome resulting when too much of an enlarged thyroid gland was surgically removed, known as cachexia strumipriva. This detective work earned Theodor Kocher (1841–1917), a Swiss surgeon, his 1909 Nobel Prize, which was somewhat controversial since Reverdin, of skin-grafting fame, also claimed priority in these findings.[62]

The matter would be neatly rounded off if thyroid replacement could cure these three types of deficiency.[63] Since skin homograft success was hardly in doubt at the time, considerable efforts were made in thyroid transplantation, aided by the ready supply of fresh thyroid tissue removed from other surgical patients. But thyroid deficiency of all kinds can run a variable course, characterized by times of spontaneous improvements. Proper assessment of these thyroid grafts' function was difficult.

Success was first reported in 1884 by Moritz Schiff (1823–1894), then Heinrich Bircher in Aarau in 1889, and then Theodor Kocher.[64] The pioneer in Britain was Victor Horsley (1857–1916), the distinguished London surgeon. Better known later for his innovative surgery of the brain and spinal cord, he was virtually the only person in Britain who did some animal experimentation and was leniently dealt with by the antivivisectionists. Horsley preferred to use sheep thyroid glands to transplant into his patients.[65] Horsley's and others' flirtation with heterografting has been decently minimized by their biographers.[66] The vogue for thyroid grafting in the decade 1880–1890 was only partly put aside when, in 1891, George Murray isolated the hormone produced by the thyroid gland. Chemical replacement of this hormone was to be the first consistent success in endocrinology, not only revolutionizing the treatment of thyroid deficiency but also giving promise for treatment of other endocrine deficiency diseases. And the success of the hormone therapy occurred regardless of which species the substance was extracted from, since most species made the same hormone. This discovery had an unfortunate effect, however, since it reasonably suggested that the glandular cells of all animals were also similar, and this legitimized the continuing use of animal gland grafts.

Sex Gland Grafting

Efforts at sex gland transplantation already had a long history. John Hunter had attempted transplantation of the testes but did not claim any functional success. Encouraged by the apparent success of skin and thyroid ho-mografting in the confident late 1880s, surgeons could not resist the lure of sex gland transplantation.[67] Human ovarian grafting seemed suitable for many ills—notably infertility and a mass of ill-defined sexual and gy-necological problems with notoriously variable courses and susceptibility to cure by suggestion. In surgical work, there was a steady supply of hu-man ovaries available for grafting since the increasing surgical confidence of the time had led to routine and increasingly radical abdominal surgery, notably the removal of the uterus and undiseased ovaries.

One pioneer in this murky area of human ovary transplantation was New York surgeon Robert T. Morris (1857–1945).[68] His publications and memoirs give enthusiastic accounts of his ovarian transplant work, for which he, ahead of his time, required "a written expression of willingness to take risk."[69] In particular he claimed to restore fertility and that preg-nancies followed the grafting procedure. Feeling he had a place in his-tory, he entered on a vigorous dispute with other ovary grafters, notably B. F. Church in California, who also claimed to be first to attempt human ovarian transplantation.[70]

Legal and Ethical Issues

Had these ovarian grafts survived and pregnancy resulted, the implica-tions would have been considerable, not only for treatment but also be-cause the ovum had come from the donor, not the mother. International interest in Morris's work followed, and this interest initiated a spurious ethical debate, briefly anticipating later concerns in the field of assisted human conception.[71] Professor John Halliday Croom of the University of Edinburgh noticed Morris's claim for pregnancy following human ovar-ian grafting, and when Croom discussed the situation at an Edinburgh medical society, he raised broader questions. Who, he asked, was the real mother of the child—the recipient, or the donor of the graft? Was the child even illegitimate? There was also the matter of consent to do-nate. He took a stern view and opined that the donor's ovaries properly be-longed to the donor's husband and that consent thus lay with him.[72] This premature ethical debate on ovarian transplantation brought in, for the first time, nonclinical commentators, and the first outsider to publish on these issues was Rabbi Yaakov Gordon of London, in 1907. He can thus be called the world's first medical ethicist.[73] He was not in a position to challenge the clinical claims for success made by the transplanters, how-ever. He accepted the claims and went on to explore the consequences that naturally followed.

Ovarian grafting seemed to fade away in the early twentieth century without any obvious criticism or moment of confident dismissal. But testis transplantation, which came later, was to have a high profile in the 1920s.

Disease Transmission

In spite of the clear warning from the eighteenth-century experience that syphilis could be transmitted via grafted teeth from apparently healthy donors, this ancient lesson had been forgotten. With the increasing use of human skin homografts, this unpleasant and eventually fatal venereal infection was again found to be transmitted. Skin grafts were also found to transmit tuberculosis. Even smallpox could be transferred from a donor who was apparently well but actually incubating the disease. H. D. Schaper bravely reported a disaster in 1872, when donor skin was taken from a limb amputated from a patient who was incubating smallpox and the skin then used for grafting four patients. It caused death from smallpox in one of the recipients and serious illness in two, with one recipient unaffected.[74] The danger of disease transmission by a graft, thus relearned in the late 1800s, was destined to be forgotten again until new incidents appeared during the rise of kidney grafting in the 1960s.

More Literary Attention

In the late 1800s, literary attention to transplantation themes, largely unexploited since the *Tatler* took an amused interest in 1710, reappeared, and satire again seemed appropriate. Edmond About's 1862 Paris novel *Le Nez d'un notaire* described the solicitor's loss of his nose in a duel. A new nose is offered by a poor but handsome man, and the donor and recipient were bound together for a flap transplant, and high drama follows.[75] The folk fairy tales collected by the brothers Grimm, still selling well at this time, told of successful grafting of cat and pig organs. But in 1896, when H. G. Wells made transplantation a central theme in his novel *The Island of Dr. Moreau,* this new genre of disturbing science fiction introduced sinister transplantation possibilities into popular culture and simultaneously attacked animal experimentation. In the novel, the irresponsible biologist Moreau is assisted in a secret island laboratory by a Scottish surgeon, disgraced and exiled for his earlier vivisection experiments. A castaway discovers the pair at work making humanoid animals. Moreau explains to the new arrival that his mission was to go beyond Dr. Frankenstein's patchwork plastic surgery: "You forget all that a skilled vivisector can do with living things. . . . You have heard of a common surgical operation resorted to in cases where the nose has been destroyed. . . . These creatures you have seen here are animals carven and wrought into new shapes. You begin to see that it is possible to transplant tissue from one part of an animal to another, or from one animal to another, to alter its chemical reactions and methods of growth."[76]

An old admirer of Wells, Sir Peter Chalmers Mitchell, the secretary of the Zoological Society of London, reluctantly criticized Wells's book and the science in it, but only in part. The eminent zoologist's critique reflected the biological views of the times. Mitchell believed Wells had erred in describing use of animal tissue for the monsters created, since Mitchell thought that only homografts were successful: "Those of us who have delighted in the singular talent of Mr Wells will read this [book] with dismay. His central idea is a modeling of the human frame and endowment of it with some semblance of humanity, by plastic operations upon living animals. . . . A multitude of experiments on skin and bone grafting and on transfusion of blood shows that animal-hybrids cannot be produced in these fashions. You can transfuse blood or graft skin from one man to another; but attempts to combine living material from different creatures fail."[77] The flawed understanding of the day is clear in this distinguished biologist's book review.

Fortuitously, one advance in the acknowledging of human individuality was the increasing use of fingerprinting in criminal investigations.[78] It was now accepted that each person's print was unique. Support for human diversity may have been emerging in other spheres, political and literary, perhaps resulting from a concern for the loss of personal identity and autonomy in an increasingly industrialized and materialist world. This emphasis on the importance of individuality may have subtly assisted the appearance, shortly afterward, of the same view in transplant matters.

Fin de Siècle

In the early 1900s, one major technical advance was to change the course of surgical history and result in significant developments in transplantation. Until this time, human and experimental grafting involved only detached bits and slices of tissue. But after the turn of the century, workable ways of rejoining blood vessels emerged, thus restoring blood flow, and, as a result, "vascularized" grafting of whole organs became possible. Assessing outcome became easier and more exact. After surgery, an organ graft either had blood successfully flowing through it or it did not, and if flow was restored, an organ like the kidney either functioned or it did not. Observer enthusiasm, which had plagued skin and gland grafting, could play no part. One important finding emerged conclusively: homograft organs failed at about a week after grafting, and xenografts had even shorter lives.

5 The Beginning of Organ Transplantation

A T THE START OF THE TWENTIETH CENTURY, the new methods of blood vessel surgery allowed experimental and human organ transplantation to commence, and some order returned to the understanding of tissue transplantation. Increasingly, the famous European surgical centers took up tissue grafting studies and did so carefully and critically. With increasing confidence, surgeons and scientists concluded that animal-to-human grafts always failed, and there followed a slow acceptance that most homograft transplants, from human-to-human or between experimental animals, did not survive. The haphazard use of homograft slices and fragments of graft tissue was slowly, though reluctantly, abandoned.

The new experimental transplant work was carried out mostly in the academic units and surgical clinics of Germany and France, which led the way during this period of expanding medical knowledge and practice through the innovative structuring of European university medical schools. These developments brought in eager visitors from elsewhere, notably Britain and the United States, who, on their return, tried with varying levels of success to transfer the lessons from the continental European institutional structures. The major clinical surgical advances made at this time were based on bolder exploitation of the opportunities offered by anesthesia and the aseptic approach.

Also at this time, the science of immunology arose, and the concept of the immune system had its origin in the observation of antibody responses, that is, a chemical "humoral" defense against dangerous microorganisms. Researchers soon discovered other cellular defense mechanisms and made important observations that led to what was later called transplantation immunology.

In the late 1800s, the famous clinics in the German-speaking nations, notably Vienna's academic surgical units, which Theodor Billroth and Eduard Albert headed, were the center of the surgical world. Stable politics and economic success underpinned solid organizational support for clinical medicine and research, and the university departments and their salaried appointments were crucial in this era. University departments of physiology and pathology also flourished and had both excellent facilities and a culture of innovation. Clinical care was organized in large, well-staffed, well-funded units, and the posts of professors, eagerly sought, were the most prestigious in the profession. For the chairs of surgery, "the university authorities had sought and found men of whom the promotion of science may be expected . . . not only famous in the field of practical surgery, but also in areas of physiological and pathological research."[1]

Learned German societies flourished, and their journals were read throughout the world. By 1874, Germany had two specialist surgical journals well before any similar specialized publications appeared elsewhere. In the Western world, it was increasingly accepted that some understanding of the German language and time spent in Germany would be helpful, even essential, for a successful medical career. In some places, however, particularly in England, medicine could remain an individualistic calling with success measured in worldly, not scholarly terms, based on the vagaries of private practice carried out largely outside the medical schools.

In this period of expansion, these European surgical units carefully considered the question of tissue transplantation. This cautious approach involved taking a skeptical look at the earlier skin homograft survival claims, and when methods of blood vessel surgery appeared, some of the pioneers attempted experimental, and even human, kidney and gland transplants.

Vascular Surgery

Until this time, in dealing with the damage to large vessels and blood loss, the choice was limited to tight compression, heat-sealing by cautery, or ligature.[2] The new clinical challenge was to repair cuts in vessels or join the severed ends to allow blood flow to continue. There had been sporadic early attempts at direct stitching of a leaking vessel. In 1759, a Yorkshire surgeon named Hallowell tried to deal with the common problem of damage to the main artery at the elbow as a result of bloodletting. In such cases, the vein had been the target but had been missed. Knowing the risks of simply tying off this important artery, Hallowell instead explored the area. Controlling the recent, clean-cut laceration in the artery, he placed a pin transversely through the two lips of the wound and, in the manner of the times, tied a figure-of-eight thread around the pin—

the tailor's or farrier's stitch—neatly closing the rent. This suture and pin worked free safely some days later. William Hunter took an interest in Hallowell's procedure and communicated it to a London medical society.

The New Methods

New methods of repairing blood vessels were first reported and improved on by Nikolai Eck, who in 1877 used over-and-over silk stitches to join two large abdominal vessels, the portal vein and vena cava, in a procedure that still bears his name.[3] The year 1882 has been identified as the year when modern vascular surgery began because it was at the Eleventh German Congress of Surgery that year when attendees heard a number of important papers on the subject.[4] However, it was still thought that, although joining human blood vessels might succeed in the short term, the repair was doomed to fail because of vessel wall weakness causing a bulging aneurysm that would later rupture. The first successful human end-to-end arterial suture was accomplished in Chicago in 1897 by John Benjamin Murphy (1857–1916), who made a strong overlapping repair of a femoral artery badly damaged by a gunshot wound in the groin.[5]

Vascular Studies in Europe

There were many European centers involved in devising new vascular surgery methods, notably in Vienna, Bucharest, and especially at Lyon in France.[6] The technical challenge was an obvious one, namely, to join blood vessels without leakage, infection, aneurysm, narrowing, or clot formation. No anticoagulants were available to prevent clotting, and the challenge in that area was correspondingly greater. Despite the use of finer silk and finer needles, a needle of any size still had an eye, and a bulky, damaging double loop of suture material passed through the walls of the vessel. The merits of stitching fully through the wall or only partially through were debated, as was the choice between inverting or everting the two edges, and whether to use multiple single stitches or one continuous over-and-over stitch. For a while there was no consensus on the best method. But when this tight end-to-end union was achieved, with difficulty, and flow restored, the feared weakness, bulging aneurysm formation, and delayed rupture problems proved less troublesome than predicted.

Regular success with smaller vessels was not achieved, and for these a radically different expedient was followed for a while. The new approach involved using hollow stents or similar inner tubes to link the vessels, with the two cut vessels pulled over and secured, as pioneered by Robert Abbe (1851–1928) in New York in 1894 using glass, by Max Nitze (1848–

1906) in 1897 using ivory tubes, and by Erwin
Payr (1871–1946) in Graz.[7] In 1901, Payr opted
for absorbable magnesium stents.[8] From time to
time, this stent strategy was revived in various
forms.

The stents were a temporary diversion. With
experience, surgeons began returning to direct
suturing of smaller vessels when better materials were found. In France, Briau and Villard,
surgeons in Lyon, had worked on vascular suturing, and, in 1896, the head of the surgery department, Mathieu Jaboulay (1860–1913), with
Briau, had been first to publish good results
from small blood vessel suturing. They used
single "interrupted" sutures penetrating all layers of the vessels, and everting the edges if possible.[9]

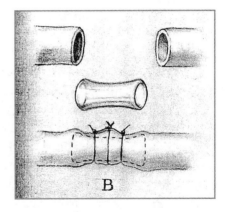

The various early approaches to vascular suturing included Erwin Payr's method (circa 1900)
of joining blood vessels with tubes of absorbable magnesium metal. This cumbersome but
workable technique was the first to be used with
routine success for smaller blood vessels, and
it was used in Emerich Ullmann's dog kidney
transplants of 1902. Illustration from the *Western
Journal of Surgery, Obstetrics and Gynecology* (1957).

Alexis Carrel

The credit for a lasting success in surgically joining blood vessels usually goes to Alexis Carrel (1873–1944), who issued the report of his studies
from the innovative milieu of Lyon.[10] It is Carrel's method, as described in
his paper in the journal *Lyon Médicale* of 1902, that is often taken both as
the origin of modern blood vessel surgery and as the start for organ transplantation.

Carrel had graduated from Lyon in 1893 and then had begun four
years of training toward a career in surgery, also becoming about this time
a "prosector," that is, an anatomy teacher. He did his blood vessel studies
in the anatomy department and not in the surgery department headed by
Professor Mathieu Jaboulay. Carrel was doubtless aware of Jaboulay and
Briau's interest in the topic and their publication on newer methods of
blood vessel stitching.

Carrel did not use Jaboulay's method, however.[11] He instead began
using over-and-over continuous stitching, also putting the stitches only
partially through the vessel wall, rather than through all layers. This approach was later abandoned, even by Carrel, in favor of Jaboulay's original
through-and-through stitching. However, Carrel had found better needles, considerably thinner and finer, and used finer suturing material—
"coton d'Alsace, No 500." A technique he devised was to "triangulate" the
vessel, thus holding the vessel open and keeping the back wall clear of
the stitching in front—a still-useful standard strategy in coping with a

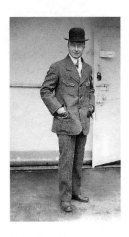

Alexis Carrel trained in surgery in Lyon and, while there, studied the techniques of vascular surgery. In the United States, he eventually settled at the Rockefeller Institute in New York and won a Nobel Prize in 1912 for his experimental transplantation studies. Later, he moved into tissue culture, while still encouraging other transplantation work at the institute. Image from the George Grantham Bain Collection, Library of Congress.

difficult end-to-end anastomosis. The "Carrel patch" was useful in similar situations but came later. Carrel had exceptional surgical skill and persistence and had increasing success with vascular surgery on small vessels.

Carrel's famous 1902 report was restricted to a description of his not entirely new blood vessel surgery technique, but the text shows that he was planning to move on to organ transplantation. Of his stitching method, he said it was merely today's prelude to tomorrow's routine gland transplantation: "Simple curiosité operatoire aujourd'hui, la transplantation d'une glande pourra peut-être un jour avoir un certain intérêt pratique." Apparently, it was still a priority in the surgical world to graft endocrine glands, reflecting the persisting clinical interest at the time in dealing with glandular deficiencies. Seven years later, Carrel retained this hope. Speaking at a Pittsburgh symposium on thyroid disease, he opined that "the ideal treatment of hypothyroidism and athyroidism would be transplantation of thyroid substance. On the success of this therapeutic [sic], vascular surgery may have a considerable influence."

After publishing the 1902 paper on his vascular repair technique, Carrel remained in Lyon for two years more and published little else on this subject. In 1904, at age thirty-one, he was unsuccessful in a competitive examination for a career surgical post in Lyon. Perhaps his publication of his variant on vascular stitching offended those with a long-standing interest. To add to this career turmoil, Carrel entered into a public controversy over faith healing and a miraculous cure he claimed to have witnessed at Lourdes. Lyon's professional class had anticlerical views at the time, and his public statements about miracles were hardly prudent for a young man seeking promotion and may have counted against him.[12]

Marginalized in Lyon, he left for North America in 1904 and after a while embarked on a vigorous program of experimental transplantation, building successfully on the European experience. He remained a lifelong critic of French surgeons, French surgery, and French attitudes, and he was not made welcome on any return trips to his homeland.

Experimental Organ Transplants

During this period of trial and error in the suturing of blood vessels, attempts at experimental organ transplantation were also made. In 1902, using the Payr stenting method, Emerich Ullmann (1861–1937) reported the first technically successful experimental organ transplant.[13] Ullmann, then age forty, had studied in Vienna and obtained a post at the famous Second Department of Surgery of the Vienna Medical School. Ullmann's paper showed that he managed to remove a dog's own kidney and join renal vessels to the blood vessels of the dog's neck. Some urine flow resulted, but few details of this operation are given. The animal with its graft was demonstrated to one of the regular weekly meetings of the celebrated Vienna Medical Society on March 1, 1902, and the technical achievement generated favorable comment at the time.

It was a busy year for organ transplantation. Also in 1902, another Vienna doctor, Alfred von Decastello (1872–1960) of the Second Medical Clinic, carried out dog-to-dog kidney transplants using stents at the Institute of Experimental Pathology.[14] Later in the same year, Ullmann carried out a dog-to-goat kidney transplant, and, to his surprise, the kidney passed a little urine for a while.

Neither Ullmann nor Decastello continued their transplantation research, instead moving on to other topics, as the research style of the times was to take a wide interest in all matters on the fast-growing edge of surgery. However, Ullmann did return to the subject of transplantation when he gave an address to the International Society of Surgery in 1914. In his address, he, like others at the meeting, dismissed hopes for success with homografting. Decastello also had moved out of kidney transplantation research and instead joined the expanding Vienna work under Karl Landsteiner (1868–1943) on the newly discovered human blood types. Decastello was one of the doctors whose blood was "grouped" or "typed," and his name appears in the famous table of cross-agglutination in the 1901 paper. He is also remembered for later discovering the AB blood type. The role of blood types in the outcome of transplantation was soon to be an important theme.

Technical Advances

After Ullmann's pathbreaking work, kidney transplantation techniques matured in the first decade of the century. In his 1905 experimental kidney transplants, Floresco in Bucharest reported important modifications, such as inserting the ureter into the bladder after placing the kidney in its usual high position. He had two other "firsts." He was first to use anticoagulation in transplantation, testing leech heads (hirudin), peptone, or helicorubin to prevent clotting.[15] Secondly, he used saline (Locke's solution) to flush blood from donor kidneys and then showed that the procedure did not alter subsequent kidney function. In 1907, Rudolf Stich

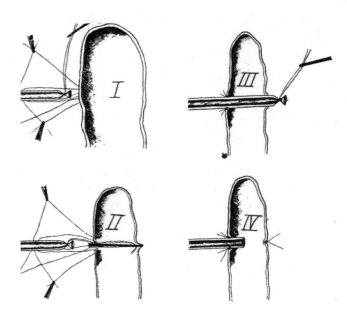

Johannes Henricus Zaaijer, who in 1907 used the pelvic position for experimental kidney transplantation, devised a method of bladder insertion. From J. H. Zaaijer, "Dauerresultat einer autoplastischen Nierentransplantation bei einem Hunde," *Beiträge zur Klinischen Chirurgie* 93 (1914): 223–27.

at Breslau was the first to position a kidney graft deep in the pelvis, an approach later familiar to those performing transplant, both human and experimental.[16] Johannes Henricus Zaaijer used the same method the following year. Meanwhile, Carrel was in Chicago and then New York regularly, grafting animal organs.

The Lyon Human Kidney Xenografts

Beyond Vienna, others also took up studies in organ grafting, and Théodore Tuffier, the Paris surgeon, remarked in 1907 on the dominance of the subject in the literature and on the widespread interest in transplantation: "la transplantation des organes sont à l'ordre du jour."[17] Transplantation was still the "order of the day" in the Lyon department, and Jaboulay, after a flirtation with thyroid gland slice grafting, continued with a major interest in vascular surgery.[18] He was now confident enough to use his vascular surgery expertise in a human kidney transplant.

Jaboulay, in 1906, at the age of forty-six, carried out this first attempt at human kidney transplantation.[19] Jaboulay's operations involved two patients, both dying from chronic renal failure. He used a pig's and a goat's kidney, respectively, transplanted to the patient's arm or thigh; this choice of animal donors was still acceptable according to the attitudes of the

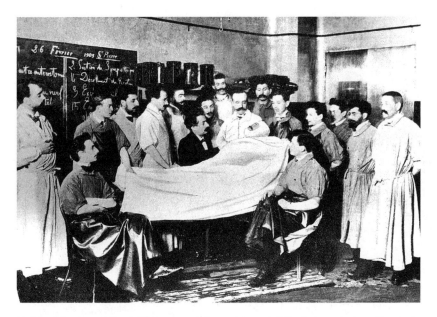

Mathieu Jaboulay and his staff at Lyon, ready for work in 1903. This photograph shows the surgical dress of the era and the operation list for the day.

day.[20] In the first case the pig kidney was joined end-to-end to the divided brachial artery at the elbow over a "ferrule," that is, a variant on Payr's tubes. The kidney worked immediately, passing 1.5 liters of urine with good urea content before the artery clotted on the third day. The second kidney also functioned for three days. Jaboulay had success in this matter: none of the human kidney transplants in the next few decades ever produced urine.

Ernst Unger's Cases

More is known of the third and fourth attempts at human kidney transplantation, both carried out in 1909 by Ernst Unger.[21] Unger (1875–1938) set up his own clinic in Berlin in 1905, and, in the years that followed, he and his group carried out more than one hundred experimental kidney transplants, studies supported by the Countess Bose Foundation, which was the first known grant-supported transplantation research. Unger's work was reported in a series of long, detailed publications, and he used Paul Bert's useful terminology, namely auto-, homo-, and heterograft. An early publication contains the first illustration of experimental kidney transplantation.[22]

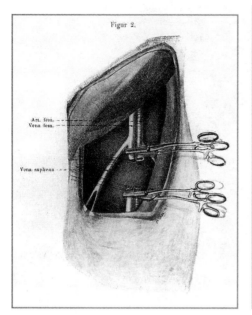
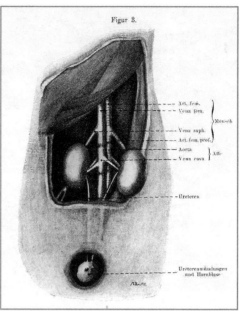

Ernst Unger's pioneering monkey-to-human transplant in 1910 used *en bloc* pig-tailed macaque monkey kidneys with the aorta and cava joined to a gap in the femoral vessels in the upper thigh. This anatomical position was used in some of the sporadic attempts at human homografting until the 1950s. This is the first illustration of a human kidney transplant operation. From E. Unger, "Nierentransplantationen," *Verhandlungen Berliner Medizinsche Gesellschaft* 41 (1910): 72–86.

Unger's Human Xenograft

The illustration came from a report describing surgery involving a young female patient terminally ill with renal failure. Both kidneys from a *Macacus nemestrinus,* pig-tailed macaque, were grafted en masse, that is, using the donor aorta and vena cava, to the girl's thigh vessels. Unger's published paper contained drawings of the operation, marking another first—the first illustration of a human organ transplant.[23] The operation was well planned and carried out with confidence. There was simultaneous surgery on donor and recipient and minimal delay in inserting the kidneys— a "warm time" of about fifty minutes. It seems that on this occasion Unger was unlucky. In spite of a fresh kidney graft, no urine was produced and the patient died thirty-two hours later. Perhaps the patient's terminal condition and multiple metabolic and cardiovascular derangements meant poor flow in the transplant. Professor C. Benda, a Berlin pathologist, reported on the transplant and was able to claim another first for this operation: the first microscopic study of a human organ transplant. He described a lymphocyte infiltrate and mitotic figures in the kidney tubules, and although there was some necrosis and *"abgestossen,"* meaning "repulsion" or "rejection," he considered the damage *"reparabel."*[24]

Unger soon moved on to other interests. Thereafter, although his main contributions to surgery were in the area of esophageal resection, he returned to the subject of grafting in 1930, contributing a long review on organ transplantation methods to a multiauthored book devoted to research methods.[25]

These human xenograft failures were consistent with growing experimental evidence that there was after all a barrier of some sort to the use of animal organs, contradicting the early enthusiastic reports from the skin and gland slice grafters. A necessary step backward was then taken. This time, single animal kidneys were taken out and retransplanted as autografts, with long-term success, notably by Zaaijer.[26] This achievement negated concerns that a functioning transplanted kidney shifted to a new position in the pelvis and deprived of its nerves and lymphatics would steadily deteriorate. Others in Jaboulay's Lyon department continued transplant research. Two members of his team, Villard and Perrin, published a paper in 1913 that marked two "firsts"—a photograph of a long-standing successful experimental autograft kidney, and a photomicrograph of its well-preserved histological appearance, showing *"substance rénale bien conservée."*[27]

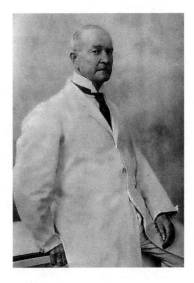

Eugen Enderlen was trained in pathology in Munich and later was a surgeon in Würzburg. He was first to carry out a vascularized human organ homotransplant, performing technically successful thyroid lobe homografts in three patients. Enderlen was the German surgeon-general during World War I and headed the surgical clinic in Heidelberg thereafter. Image from *Langenbeck's Archives of Surgery* (1933).

Human Homografting Commences

The use of animal organ grafts to human patients had failed. For a while there remained hope for grafting from human donors, and the first human vascularized homografts were attempted. Perhaps unexpectedly, these were not kidney gland grafts but thyroid and testis grafts. Endocrine transplants had not yet lost prominence on the surgical agenda.

The first homograft attempt was reported in 1909 in Würzburg as part of a large joint study by the surgeon Eugen Enderlen (1869–1940) and his colleague, the pathologist Max Borst (1869–1946).[28] They had extensive experience in experimental transplantation and now moved on to carry out human-to-human thyroid grafts. The three patients were thyroid-deficient cretins aged eight, eighteen, and twenty-five, and Enderlen used

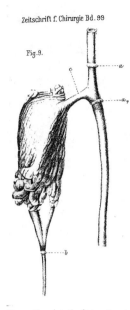

Zeitschrift f. Chirurgie Bd. 99

Fig.9.

Operative detail of Max Borst and Eugen Enderlen's successful experimental transplantation of dog thyroid lobes using vascular connection of the donor thyroid vessels to the recipient neck vessels. They used a similar approach in their pioneering human thyroid transplants, the first vascularized human homografts. From M. von Borst and E. Enderlen, "Über Transplantation von Gefässen," *Deutsche Zeitschrift für Chirurgie* 99 (1909): 54–163.

thyroid lobes with tiny attached vessels removed from other cases at surgery. He attached them to the patient's arm vessels. It was a considerable technical feat, assisted in the first case by using donor "Carrel patches"—as they were called later—from the donor carotid artery and facial vein. The authors reported that all the grafts had obtained a good blood supply, but they were in little doubt about the final outcome: "With neither of the children were we able to detect changes in their growth or increase in their intelligence. . . . We can assume that homoio-transplantation is at best very uncertain, if not impossible."[29] They added to their report a remarkable engraving of the thyroid lobe and its vascular connections in their dog grafts.

Hammond and Sutton

Two years later, another gland graft was reported, and though rather mysterious, it has to be considered the second human vascularized homograft. It was a bold attempt at a human testis graft carried out by Levi J. Hammond and H. A. Sutton in 1911 at the Methodist-Episcopal Hospital, Philadelphia.[30] The patient had presented with a tumor in one testis, necessitating removal of the gland. The other testis was still present, but the surgeons believed replacement of the lost gland should be attempted. The donor of the gland graft had died from a ruptured liver, and "shortly after" death, the testis and cord with vessels were removed and put in warm storage at forty degrees Fahrenheit for nineteen hours, a temperature that, if accurate, would have promptly killed the graft. It was then inserted as an organ graft, with its tiny vessels joined to the spermatic artery and vein of the donor at the groin. Fine needles and linen thread were used, and the testis was reported to flush with blood before placement in the normal position. The testis was deliberately left partly visible in the scrotal wound, and after twenty-three days the graft was alleged to be perfusing normally with blood. But by one month after the operation, the doctors reported that it had atrophied. The authors make no mention of how they acquired the remarkable technical skill required for the operation, and there is no evidence that they ever used it again.

By about 1910, investigators were in agreement that human organ grafts carried out by joining the blood vessels of donor to recipient failed, and experimental kidney grafts worked for a while but did not survive more than eighteen days. It also seemed to most investigators that previous claims for the success of slices of homograft tissue transplants into humans were likely to be wrong.

As European scientists reached these conclusions in the first decade or so of the twentieth century, the United States was able to claim its first transplant investigator, William S. Halsted (1852–1922). Halsted was an admirer of the work of the great German surgical centers,[31] and he traveled in Europe and initiated an exchange of junior surgeons. His careful studies concluded, as had those of his German heroes, that gland homografts did not succeed. Halsted's gland grafting model at Johns Hopkins School of Medicine in 1909 was to graft slices of dog parathyroid gland to the dog spleen. Halsted found that autografts of the dog parathyroid gland survived but that homograft slices did not.[32]

Halsted's Law

Halsted qualified his findings by stating that the autograft gland slices survived only if the recipient's own parathyroid glands had previously been removed. Although this assertion was never confirmed, it was elevated to a general principle, such was Halsted's status in the world of surgery at the time.[33] "Halsted's Law" suggested that gland grafts would succeed only if the recipient's body needed the output of the gland, that is, if the patient's own glands were no longer functioning or present. Unfortunately, this "law" was soon applied beyond autografts to gland homografts, and the myth persisted until the 1950s that homograft gland survival could result if there was a deficiency of the relevant hormone. Halsted never made this claim for homografts; his correct view was that such grafts were uniformly rejected.

Alexis Carrel in America

After Alexis Carrel's career ended in controversy in France around 1904, he had gone first to Montreal to give a paper at a French-language medical conference. Carl Beck then recruited him to join the Beck Surgical Clinic in Chicago as a surgeon. Beck had trained in surgery in Vienna, and, being fluent in five European languages, he was familiar with the French medical literature in general and papers on blood vessel surgery in particular. Beck had pioneered the use of diagnostic x-rays in surgical practice in America and had also attempted experimental kidney transplantation in Chicago.

But Carrel's clinical work did not go well. With Beck's help, he was able to take up a salaried post in Chicago in the well-known physiology department under George M. Stewart, who had trained in Edinburgh.[34]

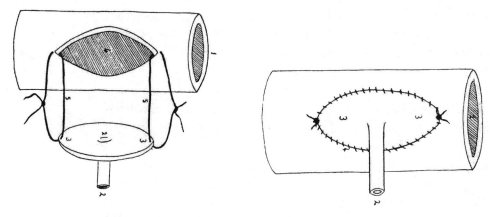

This illustration of the famous "Carrel patch," an ever-useful device in vascular surgery, appeared in a joint paper by Alexis Carrel and Charles C. Guthrie, "Anastomosis of Blood Vessels by the Patching Method and Transplantation of the Kidney," *Journal of the American Medical Association* 47, no. 20 (1906): 1649.

There, Carrel was put under the supervision of a young graduate, Charles C. Guthrie (1880–1963), since Carrel's earlier interest in vascular surgery seemed to match Guthrie's interest in using similar methods to join divided ends of bowel.[35] The two young men (Carrel was thirty-two, Guthrie, twenty-five) discussed vascular surgery techniques, and Guthrie suggested that it would be better to revert to Jaboulay's method, in particular that the stitches should, after all, fully penetrate the walls of the blood vessels. The two cooperated closely and productively from 1905 to 1906.

The two men showed energy, persistence, and attention to detail in all aspects of their evolving vascular surgery technique and its application to organ grafting. The vessels to be joined were now held and controlled with new clamps more suitable for small vessels. Exceptionally fine, straight needles with silk were used, although these still had the awkward double loop through the eye. The operative area and vessels were flushed regularly with saline, asepsis was strict, and the thread, surgical gloves, and vessels were lubricated with petroleum jelly. About this time, they added another regular technical improvement for dealing with small vessels— the "Carrel patch." When this patch was used, the donor artery was not stitched directly but was used still attached to a sizable cuff cut from its larger vessel of origin.

The men's scientific output during this short period of collaboration was remarkable. The unworldly but productive Guthrie needed Carrel's ambition and drive, while Carrel needed not only Guthrie's energy but also his help with the preparation of their scientific papers in English. Between them, in just over one year, they published twenty-one papers on experimental transplantation, and Carrel wrote five other papers on his own. In this yearlong effort, the two were breaking with the European tradition of maintaining broad surgical research interests and instead had settled into a pattern of in-depth, longer-term work on a single subject.

Carrel was careful to bring their successes to the attention of the leaders of American surgery. When the American Surgical Association met in Chicago, a number of surgeons were invited to Stewart's laboratory, and Carrel gave them a demonstration of their organ transplantation methods. At the time of the surgeons' laboratory tour, Carrel gave the local newspapers a vivid account of his achievements and the possibilities for organ transplantation.

Carrel's research prominence was rewarded in 1906 with two invitations to head other departments: the first was from Western Reserve, and the next from Cleveland. He was also considered for chief of surgery at Harvard but did not get the appointment, since the Boston insider's dismissive but also complimentary verdict was that Carrel was "nothing but an expert Sew-er."[36] The Harvard job went instead to Cushing. Carrel shortly afterward was appointed, perhaps more appropriately, as head of experimental surgery at the new Rockefeller Institute. He was not alone in this interest. In the South, Rudolf Matas (1860–1957) was pioneering surgery to repair aneurysms of large vessels, a significant problem among the local black population.[37]

After Carrel's move to New York in 1906, he and Guthrie worked separately but continued to correspond.[38] Together and apart, they not only gained experience with blood vessel and kidney transplantation but also had short-term success with vascularized grafts of the spleen, small intestine, and thyroid. They even achieved a degree of short-term success with dog hearts transplanted to the blood vessels of the neck. It was abundantly clear that homograft organs did not survive for long, and it was not long before Carrel started to look for ways to prolong graft survival.

Charles Guthrie's Studies

Guthrie's own contributions from this period are less well known but important nonetheless. One important finding was that cooling the grafts prior to transplantation protected them. He also extended his joint work with Carrel to include experimental transplants using the heart, lung, and limbs, and he even carried out a "two-headed dog" experiment. Another significant finding was that, while most tissues died steadily in storage, even in the cold, blood vessels were different and could be used successfully quite a bit after harvesting. Although the cells of such vessels had died, the more robust noncellular tissue survived and allowed the graft to function as a simple inert conduit. This finding led to a highly successful strategy, one used when human arterial surgery started in the 1950s.

In 1912, to the delight of Americans, Carrel was awarded a Nobel Prize for his work on organ transplantation. It was the first Nobel for an American and emphasized the emergence of American scientists on the world stage.[39] The Nobel Prizes had been instituted in 1901, and Carrel was favored over the other distinguished nominees at the time, namely J. N. Langley, Charles S. Sherrington, Otto Loewi, and John B. Murphy, America's other pioneer of vascular surgical methods.

The American and French newspapers gave ecstatic accounts of Carrel's research, including claims that he could graft organs from one animal to another. Added to this fanfare was the startling claim that Carrel's colleague Jacques Loeb had "created life in the laboratory" and thus the idea that Carrel was growing organs in tissue culture to meet the needs for surgical replacement. These claims also appeared in the speeches at the Nobel awards ceremony in Stockholm, and much of the content of the confused orator's remarks clearly derived from media sources rather than the scientific literature.[40] These fantasies were not unwelcome. The Rockefeller Institute, as a medical charity, necessarily had a keen sense of public relations and the need for good news, and Carrel continued to assist the management in this matter by making himself available to the press. Rapid publication by the staff was encouraged. The usual route was via short papers, published most notably in the *Journal of Experimental Medicine,* a Rockefeller journal, and advance copies were given to the press.

Charles Guthrie's Complaint

By 1909, Guthrie had been increasingly concerned that Carrel was publicly taking the credit for their joint organ transplantation success. The placid Guthrie, now a senior figure at the University of Pittsburgh, was angry enough to write a letter complaining about Carrel's actions to the journal *Science,* which had accepted their earlier papers.[41] Such a public complaint about a scientist is unusual, and Guthrie repeated these complaints in the introduction to his remarkable book on vascular surgery published in 1912.[42] Guthrie continued to have reservations about Carrel and to dispute Carrel's Nobel Prize, and he even challenged Carrel's data. His efforts were to no avail: the unworldly Guthrie was soon forgotten.

Alexis Carrel Diversifies

Carrel had added to his organ transplant studies in 1910, when he entered vigorously into tissue culture work. Once again he courted controversy,

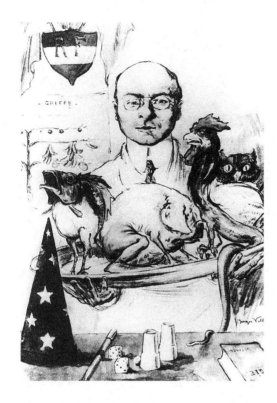

About the time Alexis Carrel won his Nobel Prize in 1912, the French magazine *Chanticlair* depicted him as a magician, capable of hybrid creation by cross-species transplantation.

and there were complaints from scientists already in the field on matters of Carrel's priority and courtesy to others. His fame then and since in this new endeavor of tissue culture conceals a continuing interest in transplantation at the time, and he gave visiting researchers some important joint transplant projects. When Ragnvald Ingebrigtsen (1882–1975) visited in 1912 from Norway, the two men coauthored an apparently visionary paper, claiming identification of antigraft antibodies.[43] On his own, Carrel explored two opposite methods of prolonging the survival of tissues. He was the high-profile authority on tissue culture and increasingly could keep cells alive for long periods in what he called "actual life" by culturing cells at normal body temperatures. The alternative was what he called "latent life," that is, cold storage, and Carrel borrowed data and insights from Guthrie's continuing Pittsburgh work in this area. In a visionary lecture at the American Medical Association meeting in June 1912, Carrel pointed out for the first time that, after death, the different body organs died at different rates. He then turned to compare two possible methods for organ preservation for later use: "While the preservation of a tissue in active life is better in latent life, it is also very much less safe. The technic [tissue culture] is more complicated and the danger of infection very much greater. The more active the metabolism of a tissue, the more sensitive are the cells to external influences. Therefore, for the preservation of tissues used at present in human surgery, the cold-storage method is simpler and more practical and must be used."[44]

Carrel set up a little-known and little-used prototype tissue bank containing, among other things, chilled noncellular tissue like periosteum, bone, cartilage, and tendons and urged their use on the reluctant surgeons. They showed no interest.[45]

Carrel was also exploring the idea that there might be ways of matching tissues. He had given another project to Ingebrigtsen, his Norwegian visiting fellow, that involved observing the relationship of blood types, which had recently been discovered, to homograft blood vessel survival in cats. Accordingly he "blood grouped" the cats and then transplanted their carotid arteries, but with inconclusive results from this creditable project.[46]

The Way Ahead

Carrel was also watching the work, in an adjacent laboratory, of his Rockefeller colleague James Bumgardner Murphy (1884–1950), who was reporting some very important findings regarding graft loss and also seeking methods to prolong graft life. These studies by Carrel, Murphy, and others elsewhere have been largely forgotten but were so numerous and perceptive that this period in the early twentieth century might be called the "lost era" of transplantation immunology. These many insights were confirmed much later, and this forgotten body of work can now be looked at closely.

6 The "Lost Era" of Transplantation Immunology

AWARENESS OF the phenomenon later called "immunity" existed in ancient times.[1] After epidemics, those who recovered from the disaster seemed naturally protected from future outbreaks of the illness. Possibly in India or China, early peoples learned to induce a state of immunity to smallpox by inoculation—placing a small amount of material from mildly affected patients onto scratches in the skin of others at risk, who later usually did not experience the full effects of the disease. The strategy was observed in use in Turkey in the early 1700s and was brought back to Europe and used with success. To add to this method, Edward Jenner later became aware of the protective effect of cowpox against smallpox.

In the effort to explain immunity, the first contributions from the laboratories were unhelpful. Louis Pasteur believed that the difficulty in growing microorganisms outside the body for any length of time meant that these bacteria required "growth factors," which, when exhausted, meant that the organisms failed to thrive. This theory he applied to the intact mammalian body, arguing that organisms invading the body ran out of an essential nutrient and died, rather than succumbing due to a defensive response of the body.

The Humoral School

This "exhaustion" or "athrepsia" theory of immunity was put aside after Emil von Behring and Shibasaburo Kitasato's crucial demonstration in 1890 of the appearance of protective circulating antitoxins in cases of diphtheria and tetanus. It was accordingly proposed that, in general, microorganisms assaulted the body via a toxin (antigen), and the body defended itself by an antitoxin (antibody), that is, a chemical, "humoral" mechanism. On a second exposure to the toxin, production of the antibody was found to be faster and greater. This "secondary response" and the "memory" involved were taken as the hallmarks of an immunological reaction.[2] Paul Ehrlich (1854–1915) usefully broadened the role of the antibody, suggesting that it could appear as a response to many invaders, indeed any protein, not just the familiar pathogenic microorganisms that dominated clinical work at the time.[3]

Cellular Immunology

This "humoral" school was not unopposed. An alternative view emerged to suggest that cellular mechanisms—phagocytes and other scavenging cells of the newly identified reticuloendothelial system—were involved in the defense of the host, and Elie Metchnikoff (1845–1916) and his followers vigorously advocated this proposal. The debate over the roles played by these defense mechanisms proceeded in Europe in a partisan and chauvinistic way, lining up French scientists (cellular supporters) against Germans (humoral mechanism advocates). The view that Metchnikoff's cellular system was the primary and only defense mechanism lost ground steadily, and, as a compromise, Metchnikoff's phagocytic system was later accommodated into a dual partnership, one part (humoral) with specificity and memory and the other (cellular) without those attributes. This harmony was blessed with the joint award of the Nobel Prize in 1910 to Ehrlich and Metchnikoff.

Immunology and Transplantation

We can admire these contributions of Ehrlich to basic immunology, but when he changed direction to study reactions to tissue transplantation, his contribution was initially less than helpful. In 1903, Ehrlich plunged into a study of the behavior of tissue transplants, using the newly described transplantable mouse tumors. This leap overlooked a crucial first step, one that later became obvious: thoroughly studying the immunology of *normal* mouse tissue acceptance or loss.

The existence of these animal tumors had been known for some time, but their study was to cause decades of difficulty in understanding immunological responses to normal tissue grafts. In 1806, the Medical Committee of the Society for Investigating the Nature and Cure of Cancer, based in London, defined the aims of its proposed research.[4] The committee reported that "it is not at present known whether brute creatures are subject to cancer, though some of their distresses have a very suspicious appearance. When this question is decided, we may inquire what class of animals is chiefly subject to cancer. . . . As establishments are now formed for the reception of several kinds of animals, and as the treatment of their diseases has at length fallen under the care of scientific men, it is hoped that the information here required may be readily obtained."[5]

The first comprehensive study of animal tumors was by Edwards Crisp (1806–1882), a London physician, and, in 1854, he provided the first description of a mouse tumor.[6] The first report that some of these animal tumors could be transplanted and grown in another animal of the same species came twenty-five years later, when Mstislav Alexandrovich Novinsky, working in the veterinary department at the University of St. Petersburg, reported the transfer of a dog tumor. However, credit for the first such effort usually goes to Arthur N. Hanau (1858–1900), the Swiss lecturer in pathology, and his 1888 description of a transplantable squamous carcinoma from a mouse.[7] Three years later, Henri Moreau in France published the first illustration of a similar tumor.[8]

The finding that some tumors could be transplantable within a species seemed of relevance to cancer in general, and the experimental use of the mouse for studies of tumor growth was a particularly attractive one, as A. Borrel astutely forecast in 1909:

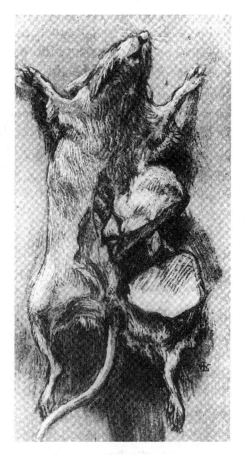

An illustration of Henri Moreau's transplantable mouse tumor appeared in his paper of 1894, "Recherches expérimentales sur la transmissibilité de certains néoplasmes," *Archives de Médecine Expérimentale* 16 (1894): 677.

In the mouse the evolution of tumors is rapid, and because of its diminutive size every inch of this little animal, including all the organs subject to metastases, can be minutely explored, tumors recognized in their very earliest stages, and prepared in their entirety for microscopic study. As the mouse lives but three years at the most, and produces many generations of descendants, the question of heredity can be submitted to experimental investigation under definite and fixed conditions. One year of observation in the mouse is as good as a hundred years in man. Cheap to buy and easy to maintain, mice can be housed by the thousands in a small space, and hamlets, villages, and cities of them subjected to conditions the most diverse, so that investigation into the cause of cancer has at last become a reality.[9]

These intriguing tumor grafting models had apparent relevance to human cancer. When tumors persisted, they could be maintained for study by transfer from animal to animal, even in the not yet fully inbred strains that existed. This persistence mimicked the behavior of human cancer. On the other hand, there were situations in which the tumors failed to thrive and even regressed, and it seemed to give hopes for a "cure of cancer." A huge literature on tumor transplantation was to emerge, and for decades it greatly exceeded the modest number of studies on normal tissue transplantation. "Any old mice and any old tumor" could quickly produce apparently exciting results. Much later, Peter Medawar looked back and summarized the problem, acknowledging that

prodigies of labor were performed. . . . But these early investigations suffered from three grievous conceptual handicaps which continued to haunt research on transplantation long after they had been given what we can now see to have been an entirely adequate burial. . . . These were that out-bred animals were being used, secondly that tumor loss was not considered to be due to the reaction to normal, i.e. non-tumor, antigens on the graft, and thirdly that natural immunity was not considered to be a quickly acquired primary response. . . . Nearly everyone who supposed that he was using transplantation to study tumors was in fact using tumors to study transplantation—not always to very good effect.[10]

Some of the early tumor experiments, though voluminous and flawed, were important in increasing understanding of the normal homograft response. Soon it was agreed that second grafts of the same tumor were lost more quickly than the first, clearly pointing to an immunological mechanism being at work.

Jensen's Sarcoma

At the turn of the century, the Danish biologist Carl O. Jensen (1864–1934) found a mouse sarcoma that could be transplanted from mouse to mouse if the transfers were made quickly enough. He reported that mice of different "races" (that is, the early, partly inbred strains of that time) differed in susceptibility to the transplanted tumor, and his model gave reasonably reproducible results. By measuring the dimensions of the tumor lumps beneath the skin, Jensen could quantify the vitality of the transplanted tumor tissue. Even with this crude system, he suggested that an immunological response was involved in tumor loss.[11]

When Ehrlich began doing cancer research, he also used the Jensen mouse sarcoma, and one of his first findings was to confirm an observation of Jensen's that "second set" grafts of the same tumor to the same animals were usually lost more rapidly. But in explaining these findings, Ehrlich surprisingly revived an "athrepsia" nutritional theory of graft loss: "It would be possible to imagine that the resorption of the tumor might be the result of an active immunization. . . . I do not, however, consider it permissible to accept these immunological explanations . . . [as] a produc-

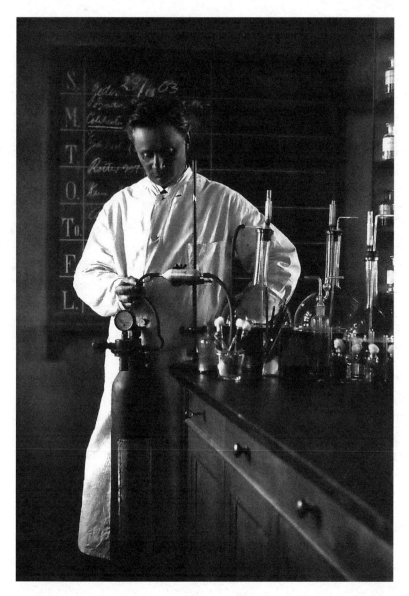

Carl O. Jensen at the Royal Veterinary College in Copenhagen first reported regular transplantation and transmission of a mouse breast tumor, leading many to begin experimental transplantation of cancer. Image courtesy of the Royal Veterinary and Agricultural College, Copenhagen.

tion of antibodies has not been proved. A far simpler and more natural explanation of all these phenomena is afforded by my concept of athrepsia."[12]

So Ehrlich laid aside the immunity theory of graft loss. The "no antibody, therefore no immunity" mantra was a plausible but blinkered standpoint and was to hinder transplantation immunity studies later. Ehrlich stuck to his unhelpful view and advocated it until the time of his shared Nobel Prize in 1910. But others had already supported an immunological view of tumor graft rejection.

Schöne's Contribution

It is in the work of Georg Schöne (died 1960), one of the new young German "scientific surgeons," that the origins of modern transplantation immunology can be seen. Schöne had spent time in Ehrlich's laboratory. For unknown reasons, he stayed out of the intriguing cancer studies there and instead did the dull experiment of transplanting skin, rather than cancer fragments, between the mice. He was doubtless aware that many practicing surgeons claimed that such homografts could survive, but he found instead that these normal tissue grafts between the mice always failed. Convinced that this consistent failure signified a basic principle, he moved on to look at why these homografts failed. Schöne continued pursuing this question after his time with Ehrlich, and, working in Marburg in 1912 and later in Greifswald, he added a crucial finding: he confirmed that a second graft of homograft normal tissue failed even faster than the first, as Ehrlich had found with tumors.[13] But Schöne was bold enough to dispute the analysis of his distinguished mentor, proposing that the faster tempo of tissue loss meant that there was an immunological explanation, instead of the nonimmunological athrepsia. In his writings, Schöne even used the phrase *"transplantations immunitat"* for the first time, and he can now be given the title of the first "surgical transplantation immunologist."

Another surgeon, Erich Lexer (1867–1937) of Vienna, supported Schöne's findings and explanation of the graft failures, dealing a further blow to any lingering hopes that unaltered human homografts might succeed.[14] Lexer's blunt verdict was that the earlier claims for homograft survival were "the result of erroneous observation" and that grafts were uniformly "expelled by a violent reaction." An active response to the graft was what Lexer had in mind. Lexer's use of the word *reaction* marked a crucial change in mindset, since the terms used until then for any graft loss were rather passive—for example, "melting away" or "resorption." *Reaction,* a word Schöne also used, had the same active dimension that the word *rejection* was to have when introduced in the mid-twentieth century. Lexer concluded that graft loss followed a host reaction to "irritation of a foreign proteid" and that loss was proportionate to genetic difference, being greatest with race differences but lower with grafts between distant relatives and lowest of all with grafts between individuals within a family.[15] Georg Perthes had found the same in 1917, and thus both men recognized a genetic factor controlling transplantation mechanisms.

Further support for this view came when American surgeon H. L. Underwood recounted that, in treating a patient with extensive burns by performing multiple homografts over three weeks, the last set had "melted off." He suggested that graft loss was similar to the "active immunity acquired in the course of an infectious disease." Underwood's patient had been treated four years earlier, in 1910, and he may have written his paper after hearing of the "immunity" theory of graft loss.[16]

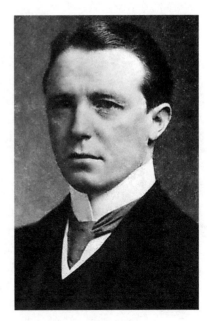

Ernest Bashford's annual reports to the Imperial Cancer Research Fund recorded his group's important findings on lymphocyte function. Image courtesy of the Royal Society of Medicine Library, London.

Agreement in Britain

In London in the early decades of the twentieth century, tumor transplantation work at the Cancer Research Fund laboratories started, and at first the researchers' analysis followed the Ehrlichian athrepsia line. But the group, led by Ernest F. Bashford, soon shifted to support an alternative, immunological cause of tumor loss.[17] Bashford's group confirmed the more rapid loss of second grafts of the same tumor in mice. His group also reported that, if the recipient animal had a prior graft of normal tissue from the tumor donor, the tumor would fail to grow, just as in the secondary graft response, thus showing that tumors shared antigens with normal tissue.[18] They then made the first careful microscopy studies on the cellular changes in the grafts and were impressed by the invasion by lymphocyte and plasma cells.[19] Since they found no antibody to their tumor grafts, Bashford's group, notably C. Da Fano, was the first to favor a primarily cellular mechanism of tissue graft destruction. Thus, by about 1913, the various research institutions (if not in some less critical clinical surgical settings) had reached a consensus that homografts in general did not survive and that loss was the result of some form of transplantation immunity.[20]

Rockefeller Institute Work

As the research community reached this important agreement on what caused homograft and transplantable tumor loss, Peyton Rous joined the Rockefeller Institute in New York in 1909. He and his pupils were to establish a solid foundation for transplantation immunology, including the role of the lymphocyte. Rous made the remarkable discovery that a virus caused a particular type of tumor in chickens, and this work received rather delayed recognition with a Nobel Prize in 1966, when Rous was eighty-seven. A bonus for researchers was that the Rous sarcoma could be transplanted.

James Bumgardner Murphy (1884–1950), one of Rous's group, took up this research and succeeded in unraveling much of the response of the body to tumor and normal homograft tissue; his work anticipated many of the key findings in transplantation immunology later in the century.[21] Murphy joined Rous in 1911, and, casting around for a way of keeping their important sarcoma virus alive after extraction from the tumor, they found they could propagate the virus in chicken's eggs—that is, in the most convenient embryo available, which, like all embryos, lacked immune responses. This strategy was thereafter to be a standard method in virological studies. Murphy then showed that the Rous sarcoma tumor itself would also grow easily when implanted into the yolk sac of these chicken embryos, and the graft could be viewed by placing a transparent window on the egg. This useful bit of lab methodology had turned into a powerful biological and immunological test bed. Murphy exploited it to the full and neatly showed that the chicken embryos could be given power to "resist" the tumor implants if adult chicken spleen cells (mostly lymphocytes) were also added to the embryos. This elegant experiment clearly showed a role for the lymphoid system in graft "resistance," as he called it. This theory was strengthened by findings at another anatomical site, this time the adult rat brain; Murphy confirmed Japanese work that sarcoma tumor grafts would grow within the adult rat brain, identifying it as a "privileged site" protected from immunological attack. If he added host lymphocytes to the tumor implant in the brain, the tumor graft was destroyed.[22]

Spleen Enlargement

Murphy also noted an odd finding in his chick embryo model, one of immense historical importance. His was the first observation of the graft-versus-host (GvH) reaction, as it was to be called much later. Whenever adult lymphocytes were added to the embryo, the embryo spleen would greatly enlarge; nonlymphoid cells did not cause this enlargement. Mur-

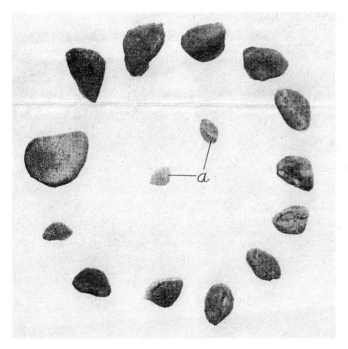

James Bumgardner Murphy clearly described the marked splenic enlargement in the chick embryo (normal spleens shown in the center) after grafting of adult homograft tissue. This effect was later rediscovered and recognized as the graft-versus-host response. From J. B. Murphy, *Monographs of the Rockefeller Institute for Medical Research* 21 (1926): 1–168.

phy described the impressive effect carefully, but he could not explain it, handicapped as he was by the teaching of the time that the lymphocyte was a nonmotile cell and thus could not have traveled freely within the embryo.[23] Had he broken out of the then-current paradigm of belief in the static lymphocyte, he might have realized that the grafted adult lymphocytic cells were attacking the defenseless embryo.

Over the next few decades, others assiduously studied this splenic enlargement in the chicken embryo. Unable to contemplate that the added lymphoid cells could migrate and cause the effect, researchers instead erected a safe and acceptable explanation based on humoral mechanisms, namely, that the adult lymphoid cell graft released vague "organ specific growth factors" that stimulated the embryo spleen.[24] Awkward findings were uneasily accommodated until the paradigm collapsed: the bland lymphocyte's well-concealed ability to travel at speed within the body was finally detected in the 1950s. At that point, the graft-versus-host attack was swiftly recognized.

As a side issue, Murphy had also shown that the host embryo cells were attackable, that is, they had the antigenic features of an adult graft. In spite of this, the prominent idée fixe in the transplant world then and thereafter was that embryonic and fetal cells were immature, and some faulty claims for prolonged fetal graft survival had resulted. Murphy's chick embryos were clearly already endowed with a full array of transplantation antigens.

Murphy's Analysis

Murphy eventually gathered together all of his findings about the lymphocyte. His review of his experimental work in rats showed that resistance to malignant tumors, transplanted or spontaneous, is closely associated with the lymphoid tissue.[25] He thought that the lymphocytes gathering in the rejected graft were part of a systemic response, and he noted cell divisions of lymphocytes in the local draining lymph nodes. Murphy had mostly worked with the lymphocyte response to tumor grafts, but from other work he discovered that the lymphocyte was responsible for immunity to tuberculosis, thus prophetically putting the host response to tuberculosis into what was later called the cellular immunity class.[26] In Norway, Ragnavald Ingebrigsten, just back from working with Carrel at the Rockefeller Institute and doubtless aware of Murphy's work, broadened this view and showed that tissue lymphocytes were also prominent in experimental kidney transplant loss.

More Immunological Studies

Murphy's contributions were substantial and perceptive, but many other investigators were also exploring aspects of the immune response and cellular immunity, reporting many of the core findings that were then forgotten until transplantation immunology gained renewed attention in the 1950s. This body of knowledge did not go unrecognized when it first appeared. The investigators were established scientists working in major institutions, their reports appeared in the important journals of the day, and they were aware of and quoted each other's work. The studies in what we can call the "lost era" were broad and included investigation of the thymus and its function, lymphocyte behavior, manipulation of the immune response, autoimmunity, and serological studies.

Bursa and Thymus Examined

The "lost era" had a good, even spectacular, start.[27] In 1900, at Edinburgh University, the embryologist John Beard (1857–1924) correctly described the thymus gland as the origin of the body's lymphoid cells.[28] Beard's paper is extraordinarily prescient: it explained not only the function of the thymus but also why simply removing the adult gland would not have any deleterious effects. Beard stated clearly that the thymus, which has a bulky presence in the young animal's chest, in early life had quickly finished populating the peripheral lymphoid tissues, and thus thymectomy after this point would show no ill effects. He employed a powerful colonial metaphor in characterizing his view of thymus function:

The thymus is the parent source of all the lymphoid structures of the body. . . . The thymus is an example of an organ which after assuming function in early life atrophies at a later period. . . . It no more ceases to exist in later life no more [sic] than would the Anglo-Saxon race disappear were the British Isles to sink beneath the waves. The simile is a real one, for just as the Anglo-Saxon stock has made its way from its original home into all parts of the world, and has set up colonies for itself and for its increase, so the original leucocytes, starting from their birth place and home in the thymus, have penetrated into almost every part of the body, and have there created new centres for growth, for increase, and for useful work for themselves and for the body.[29]

Beard was nominated for the Nobel Prize in medicine in 1906. Others considered that year were Camillo Golgi and Santiago Ramón y Cajal (the winners), Joseph Lister, as well as Paul Ehrlich and Elie Metchnikoff, the eventual 1910 winners. Beard's nomination listed his embryological "apoptosis" (programmed cell death) work and his proposal for the role of the thymus gland. Beard's work was soon forgotten; awareness of it would have prevented sixty years of late, fruitless adult thymectomies and the resulting dreary view that the thymus had either no function or "something to do with growth," as the textbooks taught until 1960. It was only then that Jacques Miller showed the profound deficit caused by very early removal of the gland in mice, namely depletion of the T lymphocytes.

Beard's work was matched in France by Jolly, who, with neat historical symmetry, proposed in a series of publications up until 1914 that the bursa of Fabricius, the large lymphoid gland found in the pelvis of birds, also had a role in the origin of some of the white blood cells, later known as the B lymphocyte when the bursa's function was revealed in 1956.[30]

Lymphocyte mobility was suggested in 1885 by the German anatomist Walther Flemming, who opined correctly that the cell might reenter the bloodstream via the lymph nodes and lymphatics; he had noted that the lymph emerging from nodes was much richer in cells than the lymph entering it.[31] Arthur Biedl and Alfred von Decastello in 1901 performed an experiment that made this lymphocyte migration route seem likely: after tying off the thoracic duct in a dog, they found that circulating blood lymphocyte levels fell to a quarter of normal. In 1909, Benjamin Davis and A. J. Carlson in Chicago managed to insert a tube into the dog thoracic duct, and the fluid draining from it contained a high level of lymphocytes.

To explain this puzzle they raised the possibility of lymphocyte recirculation.[32] These studies were not revived until the 1950s, when these striking earlier empirical observations were made anew and the reality of lymphocyte recirculation was reestablished.

Cellular Roles

In 1891, the St. Petersburg scientist Trapeznikov, temporarily working in Metchnikoff's laboratory at the Pasteur Institute, reported a pioneer "cell-excluding chamber." This was in effect a "millipore" device, which provided a helpful means of untangling the elements of the immune response because it allowed antibodies and fluids, but not cells, to pass. He showed that anthrax spores were protected from normal destruction for up to forty-five days if the organisms were placed within his fine *"sac de parchemin,"* a parchment container, and the organisms retained their virulence on removal from this protection.[33] No fewer than five German papers before 1914 had demonstrated cellular transfer of tuberculin sensitivity.[34] A German respiratory physician even managed to transfer human tuberculin sensitivity temporarily to the skin of those who had previously tested negative using material extracted from the positive test sites in other patients.[35] In Britain, a Manchester doctor accurately described and explained the "delayed sensitivity" to the industrial chemical dinitrochlorobenzene; he correctly blamed "a form of immunity": the chemical was later used as a standard test of cell-mediated immunity levels.[36]

Lymphocytes Studied

Studies in New York produced useful antisera directed against lymphocytes.[37] These antilymphocyte antibodies were made and studied most notably by Simon Flexner and his pupil Bunting at the Rockefeller Institute.[38] By 1917, Alwin M. Pappenheimer Jr. at the New York College of Physicians and Surgeons had made an antihuman-lymphocyte serum and had assayed it in vitro using trypan blue exclusion, just as was done during the important 1960s revival of interest in such serum production.[39] His serum was active on whole-body responses, and a similar serum was prepared and imaginatively used against myeloid leukemia by Gustaf Lindström in Stockholm.[40]

Murphy used Carrel's tissue culture system to demonstrate that spleen cells in vitro would inhibit tumor cell proliferation.[41] In 1922, Carrel, together with Albert Ebeling, suggested that cultured white blood cells produced immunological stimulants, a discovery that later gained Carrel the additional title of "patron saint of cytokines."[42] These techniques also re-emerged in the 1960s.

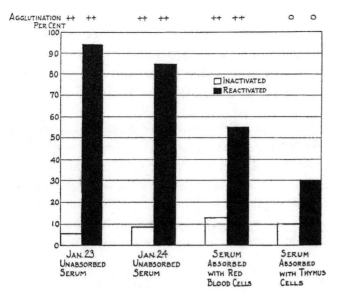

In 1917, Alwin M. Pappenheimer prepared impressive antilymphocytic sera active against human and rat lymphoid cells. From Pappenheimer, "Experimental Studies on Lymphocytes: II. The Action of Immune Sera upon Lymphocytes and Small Thymus Cells," *Journal of Experimental Medicine* 26, no. 2 (Aug. 1917): 163–79.

Immunotherapy Starts

The finding that immune responses were involved in tumor graft destruction led logically to attempts to boost general immune reactivity, with hopes for the success of "immunotherapy" for cancer, to use the later term. It was the ever-seductive idea that there were ways to control or eliminate cancer by specific or nonspecific stimulation of host responses.[43] This belief built on reports from William B. Coley, who in the late 1890s made persistent claims that the "toxin" he obtained from the bacteria causing the erysipelas infection would cause regression of human sarcomas.[44] Coley was an experienced surgeon with an interest in sarcomas, and his claims were taken seriously then and since.

From 1910 to 1920, other researchers made similar worthy attempts using extracts of patient's tumors to stimulate a host immune response. A crude serum used by J. W. Vaughan in Detroit in 1910—his "Vaughan residue"—was claimed to be effective against human cancer. At Cornell in 1912, Arthur Coca (1875–1959) tried a similar approach—his "Coca-Gilman emulsion"—and he can be admired for his careful studies and for admitting the lack of success of his vaccine against human tumors.[45]

Murphy, at the Rockefeller Institute, and others noticed a late effect of irradiation in animals—a rebound in the white cell count, above normal—and it was suggested that radiotherapy did not act directly on the tumor but by stimulating the lymphocyte response. Murphy found the same effect in human patients, and he embarked on a trial of this method in breast cancer patients, but no results were published.

One cautionary and mysterious behavior of experimental tumors was noted at the Rockefeller Institute. Simon Flexner, while immunizing against rat sarcomas and looking for rapid rejection, could often demonstrate instead a paradoxical "promoting influence," obtaining not accelerated loss of grafts but rapid growth, the phenomenon later called tumor "enhancement."[46] When this phenomenon was redescribed in the 1960s, the goal of this beneficial "enhancement" was eagerly sought for organ grafts, but without success.

Autoimmunity

This "lost era" also saw the first recognition of what was later to be called autoimmune disease. Researchers identified a self-directed antibody in the rare disease paroxysmal hemoglobinuria, in which the patient's own red cells are attacked. These studies were made independently by John Eason in Edinburgh and by J. Donath and Karl Landsteiner in 1903.[47] Even the important Coombs antihuman globulin test, announced in 1945, was effectively described during this "lost era," in 1908, by the eminent Italian serologist Carlo Moreschi (died 1921). Landsteiner noted and praised the importance of Moreschi's test at the time. Although Robin Coombs's name has been safely attached to this important test, he belatedly discovered Moreschi's earlier paper and then graciously acknowledged the Italian scientist's priority.[48]

The First Immunosuppression Work

The most remarkable feature of this remarkable time was the emergence of a clear understanding of workable methods of suppressing the immune response as a practical strategy for allowing grafts to survive. One of the earliest efforts (ultimately unsuccessful) was the work of Ferdinand Sauerbruch and M. Heyde, who, followed by Georg Schöne and B. Morpurgo in Turin, attempted parabiosis, that is, surgically joining two animals together, hoping to modify them to accept reciprocal grafts after separation, as already reported by Paul Bert.[49] Although these efforts failed, marked spleen enlargement was observed in one partner, another early demonstration of the graft-versus-host response.

The most important lead came again from James Bumgardner Murphy. With his clear understanding that "resistance" to tumor grafting re-sided in the lymphoid system, he sought methods to prolong the life of tu-mors in adult animals by removing lymphocytes. The modalities he used were irradiation, removal of the spleen, or both; he then tried a second ap-proach, one chemical in nature, which was to treat the host with the toxic substance benzol. His successful results make him another unsung pio-neer of immunosuppression.

Murphy's interest doubtless came from contact with and encourage-ment from his Rockefeller Institute colleague Carrel. Carrel's laboratory was close by, and Carrel and others had made it clear that since homograft kidneys did not survive, some intervention was needed to sustain graft function. Carrel was watching Murphy's experiments closely.

Use of Radiation

Wilhelm Röntgen's finding of the penetrative properties of x-irradiation in 1895 led to immediate and widespread use of x-rays as a diagnostic tool. But tissue damage caused by irradiation became apparent from 1905, most notably in the skin, but also in the lymphoid system and the bone marrow.[50] This led to experimental studies on irradiation's effect on im-munity, and, in 1908, Erich Benjamin and Erich Sluka noted that total body irradiation would reduce the antibody responses.[51] Ludvig Hektoen (1863–1951), at the John McCormick Institute for Infectious Diseases in Chicago, from 1916 onward showed depression of antibody formation af-ter external radiation or internal use of radium.[52] At the Rockefeller Insti-tute, Murphy took up the study of this effect, and from 1915 to 1922, he published steadily on radiation effects on lymphoid tissue and grafting, and, along with surgeon J. J. Morton, of Rochester, New York, he showed that irradiation prolonged the life of rat tumor grafts.[53] Two other of his observations were not rediscovered until the 1960s. Morton showed that irradiation would allow growth of tubercle bacilli in naturally immune animals.[54] Not long after, shielding of limb bone marrow was shown by Morton to protect against lethal radiation.[55]

The director of the Rockefeller Institute, Simon Flexner, was aware of the significance of Murphy's irradiation work, and in one of his annual re-ports for the institute he stated that Carrel, in doing his organ transplan-tation studies, had taken up Murphy's ideas. Flexner went on to state that in unpublished work, Carrel "found that in animals damaged [by irradia-tion or benzol] transplantations could be accomplished which in healthy animals were absolutely unsuccessful." It is needless to say that these re-sults have a fundamental bearing on the problem of transplantation.[56]

Use of Chemical Immunosuppression

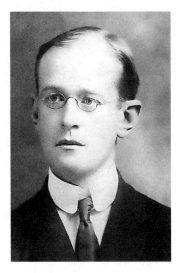

Glanville Yeisley Rusk, the unwitting "father of chemical immunosuppression," trained at Johns Hopkins and settled in California, eventually heading the University of California Department of Pathology at San Francisco. Image courtesy of UCLA Archives.

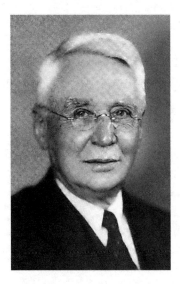

Ludvig Hektoen of the John McCormick Institute for Infectious Diseases, Chicago, showed the suppressive effect of benzene and toluene on bone marrow function and found that these chemicals would reduce antibody formation. Image courtesy of Rush Medical College Archives.

Irradiation was not the only agent found at this time to affect lymphoid tissue and thus cause immunosuppression. Benzol (i.e., benzene) was synthesized in the late nineteenth century for use as an industrial solvent and soon found to be dangerous. Investigation of illness and deaths in those exposed to the chemical showed low blood counts and damaged bone marrow.[57] Laurence Selling, the first to investigate these hazards, worked in Germany and then at Johns Hopkins.[58] In 1910, he and others showed experimentally that benzol had a useful differential action, affecting the white cell series rather than red cells.[59] Benzol was soon found to make animals susceptible to a variety of pathogens, including tuberculosis.[60]

Soon after, Glanville Yeisley Rusk (1875–1943), working in the University of California Medical School, showed in 1914 that benzol would suppress antibody formation.[61] This finding was confirmed by Ludvig Hektoen at the McCormick Institute and by several others.[62] The chemical toluene also suppressed antibody formation.[63] The inventive Murphy at the Rockefeller Institute was also involved and showed that the life of his experimental cancer grafts was also prolonged by benzol and toluene use. Benzol's capacity to damage lymphoid tissue was used intelligently for a while after its use in 1912 as the first, but forgotten, attempt at chemotherapy for lymphoid cancer.[64] A substantial literature, mostly German, emerged on this use of benzol, administered to recipients in olive oil. Frank Billings, a Chicago physician, in 1913 was the first in America to use the chemical to treat leukemia.[65] This promising treatment, incorporating a new idea, came to an end in the 1930s because it was discovered that benzol itself caused leukemia; it was quickly put aside.[66]

Murphy had shown two separate means of experimental immune suppression—radiation and chemical—and microscopy revealed that both methods reduced lymphocyte infiltration of grafts. This finding further convinced him that the presence of the lymphocytes in the graft was not a secondary event. To him,

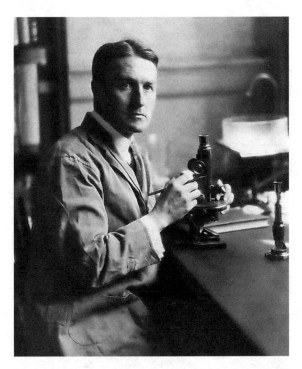

In 1919, Edward Bell Krumbhaar was first to report the toxic effect of nitrogen mustard on the blood and bone marrow. Image courtesy of the University of Pennsylvania Archives.

the lymphocyte was the key player responsible for tumor or homograft destruction.

Nitrogen Mustard

Yet another immunosuppressive agent appeared at this time: nitrogen mustard, used as a poison in World War I. The biological effects of this poisonous chemical came to light when the German army made the first combat use of mustard gas, at Ypres in 1915.[67] E. B. Krumbhaar (1882–1966) and Helen Krumbhaar, two American military doctors sent to the front, did a thorough study of the acute effects of this poison, and they noted that surviving soldiers had significant bone marrow changes and lower white cell counts. Those patients affected had difficulty resisting infection.[68] With this information, Ludvig Hektoen in Chicago, already aware of the suppressive effects of benzol, extended his interest in the immunological aspects of the chemical, showing that administration of a watery solution of mustard gas also depressed antibody formation in experimental animals.[69]

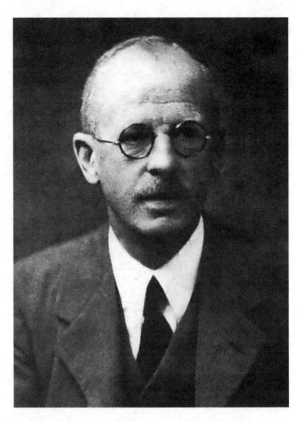

Using blood from cattle that had been transfused with cells from other cattle, British veterinarian Charles Todd produced a serum that reacted only with the red cells of the original donor. Image courtesy of the Royal Society, London.

Another inventive approach involved attempts at blocking the reticulo-endothelial system, namely the fixed scavenging phagocytes of the body, to suppress transplantation immunity. In 1913, J. Golanitzky found a modest suppressive effect with trypan blue, a dye taken up in macrophages. Low-key interest in the idea continued through the 1920s, and later.[70]

Tissue Matching

Far away, in Cairo, a British veterinarian named Charles Todd (1869–1957) even explored the possibility of "matching" individuals. Todd took blood from cattle injected with blood cells from other cattle, and, by mixing the resulting sera with cells taken from still other cattle to absorb some antibodies, eventually produced a serum reacting only with the red cells of the original donor. Landsteiner praised Todd's attempt at "matching" during his Nobel Prize lecture in 1930; the work earned Todd a fellowship in

London's Royal Society. He carried on the work, unnoticed and unquoted, at Mill Hill in London, though in 1957 his obituary memorialized him as the "pioneer of the study of individuality." In revealing the complex antigens found on cattle red cells, his methodology and analysis had uncanny anticipation of the later tissue-typing methods used to match donor and recipient for organ transplantation.[71]

The New York Meeting

A remarkable stock of useful knowledge on many aspects of surgical transplantation and transplantation immunology was available in the literature of the early 1900s, and much of it was presented at a major surgical conference in 1914. In that year, the prestigious International Society of Surgery opened its fourth triennial meeting in New York in style. The president of the United States was expected to speak, but dealing with the threat of war in Europe kept him away. The delegates were welcomed instead by Mayo Clinic cofounder William J. Mayo, and he outlined the three core topics for this gathering: gastroduodenal ulceration, methods of amputation, and tissue transplantation. Transplantation was still clearly "*l'ordre du jour.*"

The invited speakers in the transplantation section were Emerich Ullmann of Vienna, M. Hippolyte Morestin from Paris, Erich Lexer of Jena, M. E. Villard from Lyon, and they were joined by the local Nobel Prize hero, Alexis Carrel.[72] The proceedings were published, summaries of these speakers' papers given out ahead to the press, and the information was widely reported in international medical journals and mainstream publications. Ullmann, the pioneer of experimental kidney transplantation, said that "the hopes raised 15 years ago on the future of transplantation of tissues had only partly been realized. Heteroplastic [xenograft] transplantation seemed to meet with anaphylaxis while homoplasty [homografting] encountered the biochemical properties of the individual."[73]

Lexer also spoke, and he did not have to repeat, in this company, his well-known view that human homografts regularly failed: "In all my experiments I have found that, although autoplastic transplantations were always successful, homoplastic transplantations invariably proved unsuccessful. It is probable that by using animals closely related, such as mother and son, for instance, better results could be obtained."[74]

The *New York Times* carried a long interview in which Carrel gave important additional data. The article reported that

the investigator [Carrel] also described several experiments in grafting or transplantation carried on by Dr. James B. Murphy of the Rockefeller Institute. Here is one of them: Dr. Murphy attempted to discover how a homoplastic [graft] or heteroplastic grafts could be made to develop indefinitely on its host. In these new experiments he grafted on to rats a mouse tumor which had never taken on rats previously (having extirpated the spleen from the rats). Next he studied the effect of benzol, which has the power of diminishing the activity of leukocytes (white blood corpuscles).

In rats injected with benzol he found that the duration of the life of the mouse tumor was longer and that resorption did not occur before fifteen days: but although the results were positive the action was too small to be of any use.

He next attempted to use Röntgen rays, and the action of this treatment was very pronounced. The mouse tumor developed very rapidly and extensively on rats exposed to the Röntgen rays, and after thirty-five days this tumor is still growing. It is too soon to draw any definite conclusions from these experiments. Nevertheless it is certain that a very important point has been acquired with Dr. Murphy's discovery that the power of the organism to eliminate foreign tissue was due to organs such as the spleen or bone marrow, and that when the action of these organs is less active a foreign tissue can develop rapidly after it has been grafted. . . .

We are now able to perform transplantations of organs with perfect ease and with excellent results from an anatomical standpoint. But as yet these methods cannot be applied to human surgery, for the reason that homoplastic transplantations are almost always unsuccessful from the standpoint of the functioning of the organs. All our efforts must now be directed toward the biological methods which will prevent the reaction of the organism against foreign tissue and allow of the adapting of homoplastic grafts to their hosts. . . .

The outlook is by no means hopeless. . . . The principles of immunity, which yield such brilliant results in other fields, would seem worthy of being tested in this case.[75]

Carrel's Road Map

Carrel's intuition and genius are evident in the article that resulted from this interview, and he outlined an entirely reasonable agenda. Carrel knew that the surgery of organ transplantation was soundly established. Carrel also realized that the mechanism of "reaction" against organ transplants was via the lymphoid system and white blood cells and that this reaction could be manipulated. He also hinted at a phase of "adaptation" of a graft after the initial acceptance. Carrel had it in mind to use the "principles of immunity" to thwart rejection, and he knew from his colleague Murphy's work that use of irradiation or benzol treatment was a useful start. But this "road map" was not taken up until almost forty years later.

The New York meeting at which Carrel spoke was followed by the outbreak of war. Bravely, the organizers urged the members to plan ahead for assembling again in 1917, but the International Society of Surgery was never to reconvene, and surgical science, particularly in Europe, entered a period of decline. The next invited lecture on organ transplantation given to a large general surgical meeting was not until 1948.

Transplantation Immunology Dies

In summary, both in Europe and in America, there had been excellent "lost era" studies on the lymphocyte, lymphocyte movement, fetal unresponsiveness, privileged sites, immunopotentiation, antilymphocyte sera, lymphocyte culture, cellular transfer, serological individuality, autoimmunity, and immunosuppression by radiotherapy and chemical treatment. Surgical skills gained in experimental organ grafting meant that a solid platform of reliable knowledge had been erected to allow progress in extending the survival of organ transplants. These contributions came from established investigators in famous institutions and were published in the leading journals.

A grand denouement looked likely, but this failed to emerge. The promising transplantation studies and Carrel's "road map" simply and mysteriously disappeared from the surgical agenda after World War I, and Carrel and Murphy moved on to study other matters.[76] The many gains were abandoned, and the insights of "lost era" were forgotten. Much later, when studies resumed, most of the lost and forgotten information was innocently rediscovered.

With good transplant science sidelined in the 1920s, "bad science" returned, and the work of uncritical enthusiasts flourished unchecked. For a decade, the lack of rigor seen in the nineteenth century reappeared, and there was a deplorable return of the age-old belief in the success of homograft tissue grafts, notably gland grafts. At times, these claims were to verge on quackery.

7 Anarchy in the 1920s

T HE IMPRESSIVE GAINS in transplantation immunology research and the technical expertise developed in experimental and human transplantation were largely forgotten in the wake of World War I. War, which often gives birth to medical advances, was in this instance the assassin. Although academic studies in mainstream humoral immunology, particularly in antibody structure, continued to progress, these were increasingly unrelated to clinical needs, especially with regard to tissue transplantation. This research trajectory veered sharply away from the "lost era's" immunological developments with transplant applications, and this gap has broad importance in medical history.[1]

The war in Europe certainly played a role in this premature death of transplantation immunology by curtailing research and development in once powerful but now defeated Germany.[2] The postwar financial reparations demanded by France and Britain hit hard at all levels of German society. Germans were excluded from medical congresses for some years after 1918, and, in any case, the great German and Austrian surgical societies no longer met and their famous journals ceased publication or shrank in size. In demoralized Vienna, once the center of European medical research, the old vitality had gone, and fraudulent research claims, some involving transplantation, appeared. In 1923, Theodore Koppányi (1901–1967) claimed to have successfully transplanted whole rat eyes.[3] His Vienna department became notorious the following year for his friend Paul Kammerer's claims for the acquired characteristics of midwife toads, shown to be fraudulent in 1926, when it was revealed that the animals had been tampered with to suggest Lamarkian inheritance. Shortly thereafter, Koppányi settled in the United States with the assistance of surgeon R. T. Morris, who claimed to have successfully grafted human ovaries. In the early 1920s, Koppányi continued to claim restoration of sight in rats after eye transplantation, but then he became a respected academic pharmacologist and teacher at Georgetown University.

The great innovative German and Austrian surgical centers were no more. Around 1920, Erwin Payr, the proud but humbled German pioneer of vascular surgery, wrote to William Halsted, saying that

the war has destroyed a nation which was capable to excel [sic] intellectually in any area for 50 years or more. . . . Our science is heavily threatened by poverty. Perhaps people will start writing poetry and philosophize again, at least they don't cost anything. Undoubtedly technology, the natural sciences and medicine are finished if we don't get help. . . . Things are bad for us. We don't have the necessary financial resources to obtain priceless foreign literature. We have trouble feeding and keeping the experimental animals. Because of the retributions demanded by our opponents we are being threatened by total poverty.[4]

Britain and impoverished France also had difficulty supporting medical research in the postwar period. There was little money for travel, hence poor dissemination and sharing of knowledge, and internationalism in science came to an abrupt end. Although the prewar American medical scientists had been confident in their command of European languages, many being, in any case, multilingual emigrants from Europe, the postwar home-born generation of American clinicians contained few accomplished linguists. In the United States and elsewhere, with Germany and the German scientists out of favor, this lack of language skills seemed to justify the marginalization of older German medical literature.

In addition to these changes in financial and cultural circumstances, policy at the highest levels in biomedical science shifted. Professional scientists were encouraged to concentrate on basic biological research rather than applied studies. It was a reductionist philosophy that favored new biochemical methods over studies on the integrated response of the whole animal. Understanding subcellular biochemistry was thought to be the way forward, and the rhetoric was that, although this policy would not be particularly fruitful in the short term, it would pay off later with benefits in understanding, curing, and preventing human disease. This exciting but distant vista of a total understanding of intracellular mechanisms made tissue and organ transplantation attempts seem unsophisticated and elicited patronizing attitudes that dismissed such research as empirical, that is, not soundly based on an understanding of basic biology. The blunt weapon of radiation and the crudity of benzol use for obtaining graft survival now seemed unattractive. Attempts at organ transplantation should have to wait patiently for yet-to-be-uncovered basic science.

Research Philosophy at the Rockefeller Institute

This shift in research philosophy was vividly apparent at the Rockefeller Institute. The institute's new research star was the biochemist Jacques Loeb (1859–1924), who firmly advocated this reductionist view of medical research.[5] Loeb's philosophy is featured in his own writings and appears in the novel *Martin Arrowsmith* (1925), which author Sinclair Lewis based on the Rockefeller scientists and their work. Paul de Kruif, a research worker at the institute and later an author of best-selling books on medical research, had briefed Lewis about attitudes at the Rockefeller Institute. Loeb, contemptuous of previous policy, rejected applied research with dogmatic fervor. He declared that "medical science is a contradiction in terms. There is no such thing. You should begin with chemistry of proteins."[6] The Loeb view was that even immunology had to be reduced to the laws of mass action and that the future of immunology would lie not in the complex, unpredictable, and difficult-to-standardize experimental model—that is, the living organism and animal experimentation—but in the study of chemical reactions in test tubes.[7] Loeb urged clinicians to drop any pretensions of being scientists and to concentrate instead on healing the sick. Relevant to this proclamation was the popularity of William Osler's teachings and example. The view of this physician was that research was only a "leaven" added to the mix of clinical practice. As in making bread, this leaven from science was an important but only a small component of the healing arts.[8]

At the Rockefeller Institute, no longer was clinical relevance or patient need a factor in the choice of projects, as had been the worthy original remit of the institute. Immunology was not neglected, but it now involved study of the chemistry of antigens and antibodies. The 1920s and 1930s were a time of other successes, notably Oswald Avery's fundamental work on the pneumococcal capsule and its transformation. But much had been lost. The stars of the "lost era"—Alexis Carrel and James Bumgardner Murphy—were little heard from, but were still there, and their new colleague Karl Landsteiner showed no interest in studying tissue groups, which would have been an obvious next step had there been any momentum in the organ transplant effort. Carrel's new "holistic" projects on cancer languished, and Murphy's nonimmunological studies went nowhere.[9] Carrel's fame as a Nobel Prize winner meant that he received many pleading letters offering or seeking organ grafts. His secretary sent back a form letter indicating that he declined to be involved. In the United States, the only biologist interested in tissue transplantation in the 1920s was Leo Loeb in St. Louis, brother of Jacques Loeb.

Changes in Britain

In Britain, a very similar postwar shift in policy also occurred at the state-funded Medical Research Council (MRC), set up in 1901 to promote research into common medical conditions, notably tuberculosis. After the war, the MRC took the new view that useful knowledge would come mainly from biochemists and physiologists. The new policy, described using botanical metaphors, was that the seeds planted by basic scientists would grow into great fruit trees, from which others less gifted could pluck the fruit. Moreover, there should be no "attempted purchase of practical fruitfulness before its time."[10] This statement was a warning to impatient, empirically minded surgeons that they must wait for good news to be handed down from academia—research was "too difficult for doctors." There did follow a successful age of British basic biomedical science, rewarded by Nobel Prizes, but the promising prewar work on the role of the lymphocyte from Ernest Bashford's group did not continue. In London, what passed for immunological research were Almroth Wright's nonspecific cellular phagocytic mechanisms and his famously quirky "opsonic index."[11]

There was also an antiscience mood in Europe. Some considered that the German defeat was a judgment on that country's emphasis on value-free science, on their neglect of liberal humanism, and on their extensive use of experimental animal research, a verdict heartily supported by the influential British antivivisection movement. Elite London physicians took an ultra-Oslerian stance, lauding a holistic approach to medical care and claiming it to be a mystical personal art carried out with minimal aid from the laboratory and with considerable assistance from the *vis naturae medicatrix*—the healing powers of nature.[12]

In Britain, it was not a time to attempt, or even consider, kidney transplantation in dogs.

Surgeons' Hubris

Hastening the demise of transplantation studies in the 1920s was an element of complacency in the surgical world. The impressive growth of clinical surgery thanks to anesthesia and asepsis had now leveled off, and the lull may have prompted surgeons to take stock of their craft. At Johns Hopkins, William Halsted expressed sorrow for the young surgeons who now, he said, had no challenges to tackle. Lord Moynihan, the dominant British surgeon of the time, was even clearer in his assessment, saying in 1930 that "we can surely never hope to see the craft of surgery made much more perfect than it is today. We are at the end of a chapter."[13]

It is tempting to conclude, as did S. P. Harbison, the Pittsburgh surgeon and historian, that this curtailment of research in transplantation and vascular surgery was because "the great surgeons dropped the ball," since they had no ambition to catch it.[14] But on each side of the Atlantic, both scientists and doctors seemed to have agreed that the clinicians should confine themselves to their central role—treating patients. In the world of surgery, only at the Mayo Clinic was there any interest in organ transplantation and, influenced by the dogma that innovation should come from laboratory science, this interest was tentative and limited.

Homografting Returns

Some old ideas, long buried but not fully dead, crept into the neglected area of tissue transplantation in the 1920s. Notable was the revived view that homografting might, after all, succeed. In addition, conservative physicians espousing a holistic view of health and disease had also revived the concept of "diathesis"—the idea that there was a unique, individual host response in disease. These physicians taught that human reactions to illness varied from time to time and person to person and were so different that there could be no rigid classification or description of diseases and no standard therapies. It required no great extension of this view to accept the possibility that skin homografts might be accepted at some times and rejected at others.

Whatever the reason, human skin homografting was back in favor, and no one was prepared to contradict new claims for success. In spite of the emphatic verdict to the contrary by Georg Schöne, Erich Lexer, Alexis Carrel, and many others in the prewar years, there lived again the old doctrine that, with a bit of luck, and surgical skill in particular, grafts of skin or glands from one human to another could succeed.

Colebrook's Skin Grafts

One apparently thorough study of skin grafting, reported after World War I by a talented British military surgical group, aided this revival of claims for the possibility of skin homografts. In an article in the *Lancet* in 1919, Captain Leonard Colebrook (later a mentor of Peter Medawar) and Alexander Fleming, a distinguished military surgeon, called for the wider use of skin grafts in coping with the legacy of open, unhealed war wounds.[15] Surprisingly, this included advocacy of the use of homograft skin, obtained from donor limbs amputated for other reasons. They claimed regular success with these homografts and accordingly supported their more general use, but they had fallen into the old observational traps.

Postwar American Work

In the United States, there was a new uncertainty about homograft outcome, even in Baltimore, where Halsted, now fairly senior, was perhaps less influential. There, John Staige Davis abandoned his Johns Hopkins mentor Halsted's prewar verdict that homografts universally failed. Davis was aware that this was the settled European view, but he was now prepared to contradict it. He recalled that Lexer, "at the 1911 meeting of the

German Surgical Congress, made the statement that iso-skin-grafts [homografts] were never successful, and that none of them ever lasted longer than three weeks. I cannot agree with him, as I have seen a number of permanently successful iso-skin-grafting."[16]

Others in the United States had plenty of opportunity to revisit this use of homografts. Following the war, there was a legacy of unhealed wounds, malunited fractures, and other chronic medical problems among the many American veterans who returned from the European conflict. One thousand American doctors had been drafted in 1917 to serve with the forces in Europe, and after the armistice in 1918, the military retained some surgeons to deal with the aftermath. One of these was Fred Albee (1876–1945), a surgeon at a veterans hospital in Colonia, New Jersey, one of a network of American "Reconstruction Hospitals" established in the early 1920s to address the needs of patients maimed in industrial accidents and wartime service. In the two-thousand-bed facility in New Jersey, the volume of cases available encouraged study and innovation, and Albee developed an expertise, in his case in the use of bone grafting, as described in his standard text on the subject.[17]

Many attempts at skin grafting took place in these hospitals filled with wounded veterans, and Captain Harold Shawan, of the U.S. Army General Hospital at Detroit, shared in the revival of homograft use. From the European conflict he brought back not only experience with skin grafting but also a familiarity with the new methods of blood transfusion. He meshed these two topics for a study of the effect of blood typing on success and failure in skin graft work. But his interpretation of the results was wrong.

Blood Types and Outcome

For Shawan's skin grafting and blood type studies at Detroit, the patients and skin donors were grouped using the new typing sera or matched by a simple direct test between donor and possible recipients. Shawan believed that his homografts survived for variable times, and from his results he concluded that success and failure in skin grafting simply followed the rules of transfusion. In particular, those with blood type O were considered to be "universal skin donors"—those whose grafted skin would survive indefinitely on the recipient. Shawan's paper, however flawed, may be admired for introducing the term "biological compatibility" to the transplantation discourse, where it remains to this day.[18]

In Baltimore, Davis held the view that blood grouping aided transplantation outcomes, but in 1927 he decided he had erred in that view. He then explained that he had not personally studied the 550 grafts he reported but had instead relied on a risky review of others' cases, using the patients' notes. But at the Mayo Clinic, there was similar enthusiasm for skin transplant "matching."[19]

This belief had faded by the 1930s, with the appearance of more careful observation and better science. However, this denial of the influence of blood groups on skin grafting had a curious effect in later years. The pioneer human kidney transplanters of the 1960s ignored blood groups and were not prepared for the crucial importance of such typing in human organ graft work; it came as a surprise.

With these optimistic reports from reputable sources and awareness of successful blood transfusion, skin grafting became a favorite operation in the United States, notably with small-town surgeons, and their local medical journals and newspapers shared this enthusiasm. Surgeons were then at the peak of their public esteem, and they and their work were always newsworthy. The new vogue for skin grafting between humans was second only in popularity to reports on removal of the appendix from important persons, and the new skin grafting operations were regarded with awe, particularly when noble and notable donations were made by relatives and friends. This use of multiple donors made some sort of sense. Tiny grafts could be taken under local anesthetic from the many donors, and this removed the concerns, clinical and ethical, of giving a general anesthetic to a single person simply for the purposes of donation of larger areas of skin. Multiple grafts might also increase the chances of random matches, but they also increased the risks of transmitting disease. In the absence of offers from such donors, surgeons could always use some spare skin taken from the edge of their operative incisions, and they also had access to skin from amputated limbs.[20]

In one notable case, the plight of a badly burned young girl was mentioned in the local newspaper in Gary, Indiana, and, as a result, a number of local citizens volunteered to donate skin to cover her burns. Among the volunteers were a local newsboy named Willie Rugh and a local Gary physician. But there was one unusual feature. Willie Rugh's offer was to donate the skin from his crippled, polio-damaged leg, and, to get the skin, the surgeon proposed to amputate the leg, and he performed the surgery on September 30, 1912. This altruistic sacrifice of skin caught the imagination of the American public, and the *New York Times* was quick to applaud Rugh's selfless action. There was no word about the transplanted skin, but Rugh, the donor, reportedly suffered a "relapse," and his death from "surgical complications" was soon announced. Contributions toward a memorial came in from all over America, and the gravestone is found in the Gary Cemetery to this day. Amid the media interest in the donor, there was no report about the fate of the skin grafts.

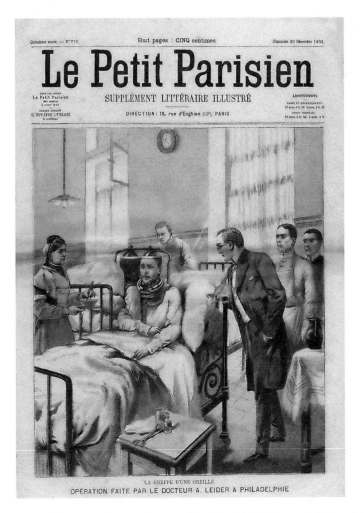

Quinzième année. — N° 776.

Huit pages : CINQ centimes

Dimanche 20 Décembre 1903.

Le Petit Parisien

SUPPLÉMENT LITTÉRAIRE ILLUSTRÉ

DIRECTION : 18, rue d'Enghien (10e), PARIS

ABONNEMENTS

PARIS ET DÉPARTEMENTS
12 mois, 4 fr. 50. 6 mois, 2 fr. 25
UNION POSTALE
12 mois, 5 fr. 50. 6 mois, 3 fr

LA GREFFE D'UNE OREILLE
OPÉRATION FAITE PAR LE DOCTEUR A. LEIDER A PHILADELPHIE

In 1903, the return to the use of homografting included a "Tagliacozzian" attempt at ear grafting in Philadelphia in which a donor and recipient were bound together until the graft was united. Image courtesy of the National Library of Medicine.

In this early twentieth-century revival of the use of homograft skin, the other ancient, attractive, too-good-to-be-false notion reappeared that *young* tissue was accepted more readily than tissue from mature donors. There was now a revival and vogue for the use of young, thin skin, and the most widely available source was the human foreskins removed in large numbers from young boys. The surgeon Frank Ashley of Brooklyn "kept a bank of such foreskins, storing them in a refrigerator or even embedding them in ice cubes for use later."[21] Others considered that warm storage was best. In New York, surgeon Hugh Baldwin's method of short-term

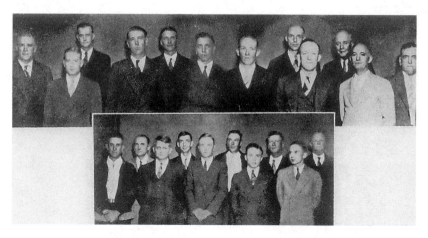

Multiple grafts for a single patient using skin from donors had support in the 1920s. Image from the *Annals of Surgery* (1942).

storage of skin had something of Carrel's tissue culture methods: "The removed redundant skin was put in salt solution and then placed on an ordinary radiator, while the operator went to the opening baseball game of the season. Returning at six o'clock, Reverdin grafts were placed on a large ulcer involving a child's abdomen." Every small graft took, he said.[22]

So complete was the reversal of history at this time that some surgeons attempted Tagliacozzian "slave-donor" transplants. In Chicago in 1903, an ear donor was paid five thousand dollars and bound with an earless recipient for many days. After the ear graft to the recipient was sufficiently healed, the two were then separated. The final outcome was not announced.[23]

Only an occasional public commentator was critical of such grafting in the 1920s, but the authoritative *American Mercury*, the current affairs journal edited by iconoclast H. L. Mencken, commented on the mood of the times in 1925 and took the view that a scientific mistake was being made. He lamented that this was a period of poor clinical science: "Often, when the newspapers report a child badly burned by accident, with a great loss of skin, they add a tale of heroism about the victim's family and friends, with the names of playmates who have offered to sacrifice skin for the sufferer, estimates of the number of square inches needed, and other harrowing details. On recovery, the whole thing ceases to be news, and we hear no more of it. Unfortunately, such thrilling tales of self-sacrifice are almost invariably untrue."[24]

One perceptive American surgeon, Emile Holman, who had trained with Halsted at Johns Hopkins, also broke ranks to deplore the wave of uncritical homografting. He remarked dryly in 1924 that "iso- or homo-skin grafting is frequently employed by the profession to the wondering delight of the credulous laity, who enjoy contributing small squares of skin as sacrificial offerings on the altar of self-inflicted martyrdom. It is a procedure which has captured the imagination of the public. . . . That such grafting is most often a failure seems little known."[25]

In contrast to this very public altruism, there was still evidence of a market, however ill defined, for the purchase of donor skin and other tissues. The Illinois General Assembly proposed legislation to outlaw such sales after reports that testis grafts might be sold. Gland grafting was indeed back.

Gland Grafts in the 1920s

The return to skin grafting apparently legitimized the revival, in this "daft decade," of the closely related earlier belief, decently forgotten since the early 1900s, that the grafting of slices and bits of endocrine glands could also be successful. But while the errors and excesses of the skin homografters of the 1920s were eventually forgiven (and omitted from their obituaries), a more serious fate awaited some of the gland grafters of the 1920s. Public and professional ridicule was to result, and the label of quackery was to stick, sometimes appropriately.

The Testis Transplanters

The testis gland had always been suspected of being responsible for the masculine features of the adult male. Proof of the existence of hormone secretion from the testis had been announced, wrongly and prematurely, in 1889, after Charles Éduard Brown-Séquard, one of the innovative "transplant group" at the Collège de France, studied an extract from the testis that he claimed had stimulating effects on muscle power and general vitality, notably in himself.[26] Shortly thereafter, others used the same approach, but with other glands, and obtained two undoubtedly potent extracts: the hormone of the thyroid, prepared in 1891 by George Redmayne Murray, and adrenaline, obtained from the adrenal gland in 1895 by Sir Edward Albert Sharpey-Schafer.

By the start of the twentieth century, more gland extracts were available. Some of these, like the adrenal and thyroid preparations, had powerful and undoubted actions and gained a legitimate and permanent place in the pharmacopoeia.[27] Others, like the still-marketed Brown-Séquard testis extract, were more controversial and less respectable. This muddle regarding glandular therapy led to Herbert Evans's famous remark that endocrinology had experienced "obstetric deformity" at birth.

Accordingly, with the testis extract increasingly discredited, transplantation of this gland was still viewed as a possible alternative therapy for alleged testicular deficiencies.[28] In the anarchic 1920s, as in the case of the skin grafters, it seemed that the gland transplanters had a new freedom and renewed license for their activities, unchecked and free of scientific censure.

The best-known gland grafter of the 1920s was Serge Samuel Voronoff (1866–1951), a Paris surgeon who was to become famous and rich through his advocacy of testicle grafting. He was not, however, the pioneer of such testis transplants. Levi Hammond and Howard Sutton had reported the first testis homograft in 1912, and, in 1913, Victor Lespinasse, a Chicago surgeon, claimed successful use of slices of human testis in a patient who had suffered the loss of both testicles. In 1914, a number of similar transplants for testis loss were reported by G. F. Lydston (1858–1923) from Chicago, author of a standard work on urological surgery. Using the testes taken from human cadaver donors, including executed criminals, up to seventeen hours after death, he claimed good results.[29]

Both Lespinasse and Lydston continued testicle slice homografting into the 1920s and also began claiming success in treating the effects of aging and a broad range of male ills. Lespinasse extended his indications later to include attempts to reverse homosexuality and "sexual perversions." These American publications on testis transplants had little scientific or public prominence—at first.

In Britain in 1923, the testis transplant revival was respectable enough for a London surgeon, Kenneth M. Walker, to use as his subject for the prestigious invited Hunterian Lecture to the Royal College of Surgeons of England.[30] After organizing the army's blood transfusion work during the war, he turned his civilian career toward testis transplants to treat senility. He could neatly and appropriately link his topic to John Hunter's own famous gland experiments. Walker used grafts taken from human testes removed because of their ectopic position—that is, the glands had failed to descend properly into the scrotum.

Other surgeons in Britain also participated in this gland-grafting enthusiasm, including Hamilton Bailey, then a young man and later author of best-selling surgical texts. While holding the prestigious post of Gillson Scholar of London's Society of Apothecaries, he published his improved technique for testis implantation.[31]

Serge Voronoff

It was the work of Serge Voronoff that was to make testis transplantation at first well known, then notorious, and finally comic.[32] Voronoff was educated in Paris, and in the 1914–1918 war he had won praise for his work in the French military hospitals, which included some conventional bone grafting. By 1917, he had completed some animal experiments, including some apparently successful testis gland grafts from young sheep to old rams.

Voronoff then started testicular transplants in human patients but failed to obtain human donor testes regularly. He turned instead to the anthropoid apes, rationalizing this choice of donor on evolutionary closeness. He quoted the new findings on the closeness of the blood types between humans and apes and added that "recent work" showed that blood grouping influenced transplant outcome. He also claimed success in grafting valuable stud racehorses if they showed a declining urge to mate, and he neatly used this claim to counter criticism that human suggestibility was involved in the success of his clinical work.[33]

Between 1920 and 1924, Voronoff grafted human patients with monkey testis tissue for the defects of age or virility, grafting large gland slices and adding them to the usual scrotal contents. His early work was written up and published as orthodox medical papers and was put together in conventional monographs. Skilled in public relations, he became a familiar celebrity, and, always quotable, his activities were followed closely by the *New York Times*. At this time he remained within the realms of orthodox medicine as a well-known, though controversial, surgeon. In France he taught others his technique, and his faithful collaborator Louis Dartigues, later president of the Société des Chirurgiens de Paris, also wrote up their methods in long, illustrated monographs.[34]

While Voronoff's star rose, he was much traveled, and on his triumphal, well-publicized American tour, there was a brisk priority dispute over who had "discovered" testis transplantation. Voronoff vied with Lydston for the title, and the latter, who was indeed the pioneer, and said so, had a tantrum on the occasion of a lecture by Voronoff in Chicago.

Others in the United States, often holding conventional posts, began gland-grafting work as well, using human donor tissue, and Voronoff was banned from using animal donors in Britain. By 1924, Max Thorek, the respected American urological surgeon, could report a series of ninety-seven testicular slice transplants, and he admitted few failures.[35] Others sought to outdo him, notably H. L. Hunt in New York, who eventually reported his experience with a few hundred cases listed in papers published initially in respectable journals, notably *Endocrinology*.[36] But even Hunt was outdone by Leo Stanley (1928–1965), a surgeon at the San Quentin State Prison in California; he claimed "thousands" of grafts on the inmates, work also published in outline in *Endocrinology*. His project did have the merit of a constant environment and excellent follow-up.[37] On the

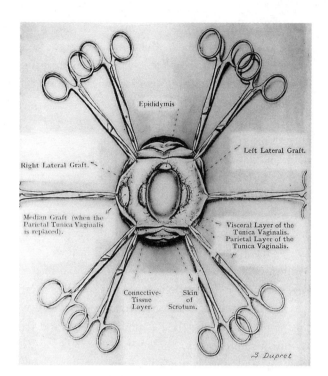

Serge Voronoff's conventional monographs show the surgical detail of the monkey testis slice implants and their position on the recipient testis. From Louis Dartigues's *Technique chirurgicale des greffes testiculaires . . . méthode de Voronoff.*

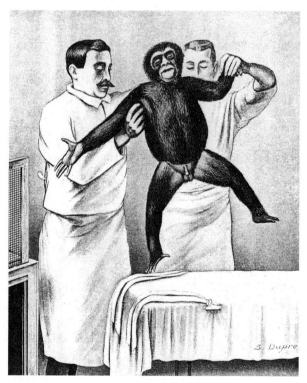

Voronoff's gland-grafting surgery was illustrated and published in conventional texts and also in his colleague Louis Dartigues's book, *Technique chirurgicale des greffes testiculaires . . . méthode de Voronoff* (1923). The text includes this dubious first—an illustration of the details of xenograft donation.

academic side, testis transplantation had some support based on the personal experiments of R.G. Hoskins, editor of *Endocrinology*, performed at the Laboratory of Physiology, Ohio State University.[38]

Other Gland Grafts

Less high-profile claims for other gland grafting also appeared. Ovarian grafting continued to be in favor in the United States, and the gland grafters, dismally ignoring the basic tenet of free grafting (i.e., that the graft had to be thin) often used an entire gland. The distinguished Athens surgeon Skevos Zervos proudly announced his "orchometer," which weighed and measured the entire testis before implantation. In France, the author of the monograph *Les Greffes chirurgicales,* commenting in 1922 on the local surgical enthusiasm for ovary grafts, noted that they were done with "une ténacité extraordinaire de la part des physiologistes et de quelques chirurgiens."[39]

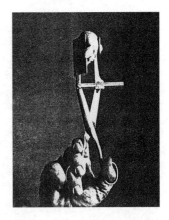

An Athens testis transplanter, Skevos Zervos (1875–1966), took pride in assessing the dimensions of his experimental whole testes grafts in an "orchometer" device prior to implantation of the gland. From his text *La Transplantation des organes* (1936).

Also irresistible for a while was the attempt to treat the adrenal deficiency in Addison's disease with human adrenal gland grafts. The distinguished British surgeon F.C. Pybus reported success in 1922, and in one case he neatly used blood type O fresh donor adrenal in the hope of having "universal donor" tissue.[40] The British surgeon Frank d'Abreu reviewed this growing niche literature on transplantation to treat Addison's disease and can at least be admired for stating that it was pointless to graft fragments thicker than two millimeters.[41] The alleged blandness of fetal tissue, the old idea, had also returned to favor, and fetal pancreas grafts were irresistible in a quick, cheap, and easy strategy for treating diabetes.[42] In the murky world of private rejuvenation clinics, the use of fetal cells was touted as a modern and scientific strategy, and, for the first but not the last time, sheep embryo thymus cells were transplanted at Paul Niehan's high-profile Swiss clinic.

Brinkley's Goat Glands

The gland-grafting surgeons' weakness was enthusiastic self-deception, but there were also genuine transplant quacks about, and one had a very profitable business in rural Kansas. "Dr." John Brinkley (1885–1942) briefly attended but did not graduate from an accredited medical school, and he skillfully promoted his clinic and goat testis transplants as a cure for many male ills and deficiencies.[43] Marketing his product by mail and radio messages, he became rich from the volume of work at his single-

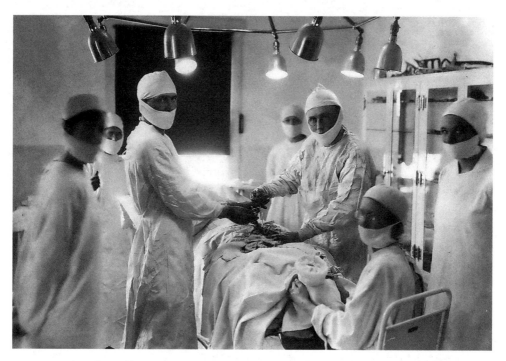

John Brinkley at work in his well-equipped surgical hospital. Image courtesy of the Kansas State Historical Society, Topeka.

operation clinic. He also boosted his income by franchising his snake-oil remedies. In the immunologically disordered medical culture of the 1920s he was unassailable, and supportive patients and politicians protected him, but he met his nemesis in the 1930s, as described later.

Transplantation in Fiction

In this anarchic decade, a frivolous element was seldom absent, perhaps matching the *mentalité* of society in the directionless 1920s. One feature of the times was that popular culture fed strongly on transplant matters, and publishers wished to join the action. Editors of the periodical literature, responsible and otherwise, also hastened to join in. Some of the fiction of the times also featured transplant matters, poignantly assuming that the surgeon's claims were correct and that homografts and grafts from animals could succeed.

In general, surgeons were depicted as miracle workers and only occasionally as Frankensteins. Laboratory immunology, notably Almroth Wright's "stimulation of the phagocytes," was given respect by George Bernard Shaw's play *The Doctor's Dilemma,* and as noted, Sinclair Lewis praised the Rockefeller Institute scientists in *Martin Arrowsmith*. Gland grafters were occasionally satirized, as in Bertram Gayton's ribald novel *The Gland Stealers* (1923) and in Thomas Le Breton's *Mr. Teedles, the Gland Old Man* (1927).

The 1920s saw a flurry of science fiction writing with improbable transplant themes, thriving on the questionable surgery of the day. Monkey gland injections that simianized the recipient are the theme in Conan Doyle's *The Case of the Creeping Man* (1927), and surgical creation of ape-men appeared in the silent horror film *A Blind Bargain* (1922), based on Barry Pain's Wellsian science fiction novel *The Octave of Claudius* (1897). Edgar Rice Burroughs's readable story of a brain transplant surgeon on Mars appears in *The Master Mind of Mars* (1928), and the idea of brain transplants was milked for fanciful stories elsewhere, notably Anthony Cox's *The Professor on Paws* (1927) and Noëlle Roger's *Le Nouvel Adam* (1924), which featured a transplanter at the Collège de France improving the race with intracranial gland transplants. Gaston Leroux (famous for his *The Phantom of the Opera* of 1911) published *Le Machine à assassiner* (1924), featuring a brilliant surgeon switching human brains. The Russian novelist Aleksandr Beliaev's *Golova professora Doula* (1925) was a head-preservation-by-perfusion-plus-transplant novel, eventually published in the West as *Professor Dowell's Head* (1980). The plot of the 1925 film *The Monster* involved surgical plans for soul transplants.

Other popular themes were the yet-to-come hand transplants, which, like brains, would carry on the life and work of their previous owner, as in Arthur Train's earlier *Mortmain* (1907), and, when taken from a murderer, the new hands predictably auto-strangle the recipient.[44] Single hands grafted from black donors might fight with the white recipient's good one. Carrel's work may be the subject of George H. Doran's *The Talkers* (1923), and uncontrolled eugenic transplantation is featured in Victor R. Emanuel's *The Messiah of the Cylinder* (1917). Periodical literature and pulp fiction magazines such as *Weird Tales* carried many short stories exploring the science fiction consequences of transplants.[45] No one mined the literary possibilities of face transplants, however.

More serious was the literary and political use of gland grafting by the Soviet novelist Mikhail Bulgakov, who, having been a medical student under the talented Ukrainian surgeon Vladimir Shamov, produced his political satire *Heart of a Dog* in 1925.[46] In this novel, the attempted humanizing of a dog by human pituitary and testis grafts clearly ridiculed the nation's revolution and socialist attempts to hurry human evolution. Judged to be subversive, the authorities banned the novel, and it emerged sixty years later, in more relaxed Soviet times.[47]

In Britain, popular interest in transplantation was muted. Instead, the more febrile periodicals latched onto the fictional possibilities arising from tissue culture, notably dramatizing the worthy press releases from the Strangeways Laboratory in Cambridge. Journalists for the mass-circulation sensationalist magazine *Tit-Bits* portrayed the work of the lab in a sinister light, alleging that monsters were being made and babies grown in test tubes.[48] In this disorderly time in the transplant world, bad science had let popular culture run riot.

Serious Studies of the 1920s

Well-conducted transplant studies were carried out only in two centers. The first was the immunological work of Leo Loeb at the Washington University School of Medicine in St. Louis. The other was the Mayo Clinic, which carried out some cautious experimental kidney transplants.

In the 1920s and into the 1930s, Leo Loeb (1865–1959) kept up a solitary, sustained interest in transplantation immunity and built on the earlier view of homograft rejection mechanisms.[49] He was the "missing link" between the studies of Schöne and Lexer on skin homograft loss and the Bashford/Murphy stance on the primacy of the lymphocyte, and the later revival of these views in the 1950s. But events have conspired to deny Loeb this credit.

Born in Germany, he was the younger brother of Jacques Loeb, the distinguished Rockefeller Institute scientist. Before emigrating, Leo did transplant studies that included important work on skin and tumor grafting.[50] He had early input on the new tissue culture methods, and he gained fame in linking spontaneous mouse cancer with ovarian control.[51] Loeb also encouraged experimental science in pathology departments across the United States.[52] Locally, he influenced the innovative surgical school at Washington University, particularly the work of the plastic surgeons James Barrett Brown and Earl Padgett, who were to be important in the early modern period of clinical transplantation.

In spite of his experience with tumor transplant work and against the mood of the day, in about 1917, Loeb, like Schöne, turned instead to a study of the transplantation of normal tissues in outbred rats. In this pursuit he had an additional agenda, beyond the study of grafts, rather like John Hunter. Hunter had used transplantation to probe the mystery of tissue life, while Loeb used transplantation to demonstrate tissue recognition mechanisms. He emphasized that the homograft reaction was not primarily to thwart surgical ambitions for transplantation but was instead a fundamental, highly sensitive recognition mechanism of some sort.[53] Even in later years, other investigators often missed this grander view.

Loeb's extensive studies involved placing small, thin tissue slice homografts snugly beneath the kidney capsule of recipient rats. This site allows immediate location of the graft for later examination. His judgments on graft survival were based on microscopic findings, not appearance, thus avoiding the notorious pitfalls of looking at skin grafts. He quantified the homograft response not by measuring survival time but by grading the host cellular response, judged microscopically, to the various donor tissue slices. The cellular invasion of the grafts came from the kidney, not from the connective tissue outside the impervious capsule. Loeb's experimental model of tissue transplantation had strengths and weaknesses. In his hands it proved quite sensitive, and he drew up a numerical scale for the intensity of local cellular ingrowth.

In this long-term project, he raised, addressed, and partly answered many of the fundamental questions regarding tissue transplantation, publishing his findings in 1930 in a long, important article in *Physiological Reviews* when he was sixty-five. The most obvious histological lesson was an old one, pathetically ignored by the surgical human gland grafters at this time in the 1920s, namely, that only the outer few millimeters of any nonvascular graft implant survive, hence the pointlessness of grafting tissue any thicker.[54] Importantly, he agreed with Murphy, Bashford, and the earlier "lymphocyte school" on the importance of that cell in graft loss. His conclusion was that "as to the action of the lymphocytes, there is no doubt that they actually help destroy the transplant. It is largely by these means of the cellular reaction on the part of the host tissues which set in motion the destruction of the homoiotransplant."[55]

Intrafamilial Grafting

Although Loeb was well aware that a growing number of inbred laboratory animals were available (he had a noteworthy role in their development), at this stage in his studies he continued to use ordinary outbred laboratory rats and studied the pattern of graft survival within outbred families. In brother-to-brother or sister-to-sister grafts, the usual vigorous outbred homograft response was seen in one-quarter of the animals, with a moderate response in one half, and a much lower cellular reaction in the remaining quarter, with their transplants surviving very well without much cell ingrowth, even up to forty days. This pattern indicated that there was genetic control of graft loss and pointed to a single chromosomal region being mainly responsible. Loeb assumed that this was the case and, "in the case of transplantation from child to mother . . . the graft would lack one half of the chromosomes and therefore the corresponding chemical groups present in the cells of the graft."[56] Loeb did not take this remarkable insight further, since he was not a geneticist, nor closely associated with the early geneticists, for good reasons, as explained below.

These same 25:50:25 percentage strengths of intrafamilial graft responses were uncovered again when human living-related donor kidney transplantation started in the 1960s and the genetic basis was quickly shown by tissue typing. This ratio can be called "Loeb's Law" and was initially crucial in picking a living-related kidney donor within a family. Other Loeb proposals anticipated later findings. He showed that xenografts were lost via an antibody response, that there are organ-specific antigens, and that each organ had its own speed of rejection, notably, that a kidney was more antigenic than a liver. There might also be a weak response when using male grafts for female recipients. He also suggested that the fetus was a form of homograft but that it was protected in some way. Loeb further showed that, when grafted, dead donor tissue not only failed to survive but also gave a poor lymphocyte response. The protein of the dead cells alone seemed insufficient to stimulate a reaction, a puzzling finding that long remained ignored and unexplained. Since the graft had to be alive, Loeb emphasized that the cellular metabolism of the *graft* had an active role in the response. Loeb correctly highlighted a crucial feature of tissue incompatibility, and his explanation still reads well.[57]

The Search for an Immune Mechanism

While Loeb was in no doubt that lymphocytes were involved in homograft loss, he noted that others had reported accelerated rejection of "second-set" skin grafts and had reported this himself in 1918.[58] But Loeb showed no interest in using his own model to do this experiment, since he did not measure survival times, and indeed a *lesser* degree of ingrowth of sensitized lymphocytes occurs in second-set homografts. It is likely that to Loeb, clear proof of an immunological response was not important, though his later critics thought otherwise. To him, the powerful discrimination of the graft reaction was a constant surveillance system in which primary and secondary responses were perhaps only peripheral phenomena. In any case, others had reported positively on the matter.

Loeb had used inbred animals in some of his other work, but not in his rat transplant studies; he may have been trying to mimic the human outbred situation. But, perhaps after being urged to switch to the precision of inbred animal use, he began doing so, starting slice graft work anew in inbred rats. The origins and growing importance of these animals in the biological sciences are significant elements of the transplant story from the 1920s.

Inbred Animals in Laboratory Use

The emergence of inbred animals was a crucial development in the history of not only experimental transplantation but also genetics and biology in general. From 1910 onward, Loeb and others had begun to seek supplies of closely related mice or rats in order to maintain their important tumor lines.[59] He and others obtained their laboratory animals from mouse fanciers, and Loeb went to the dealer and breeder Abbie E. C. Lathrop (1868–1920), of Granby, Massachusetts, a small town ten miles north of Springfield.

Mouse fancying was an ancient pastime. Albino and other tame mice emerged as pets in eighteenth-century Japan, and the important Japanese "waltzing" mouse arrived in the West in 1890.[60] They had to be closely inbred to maintain their curious neurological defect. Beginning about 1900, Lathrop bred small animals, notably mice, for sale to collectors and other breeders. From time to time she noticed tumors in her animals, and in 1908 sought the advice of the pathologists known to her through their animal purchases. The most enthusiastic response came from Loeb in St. Louis, and he encouraged her to report and study any tumors she found and, later, to carry out her own experimental studies. Thereafter, she published scientific papers with him on these experiments and observations; she was often first author, with the work

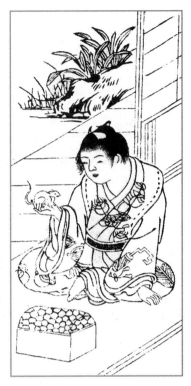

Mice were first tamed in Japan in the eighteenth century, and these partly inbred "fancy mice" found favor as pets elsewhere. From Chôbei Zeniya, *Chingan-Sodategusa* (Japan, 1787).

done largely at Granby.[61] In this series of experiments, they made the crucial observation that in mice susceptible to breast cancer, pregnancy accelerated the tumor onset and ovarian removal delayed it.[62] Prior to her early death from pernicious anemia, Loeb graciously wrote in 1918 that "she for a period of more than ten years collaborated with us in our work on heredity of cancer. . . . Adverse conditions having made it impossible for her to acquire that scientific knowledge which she had always desired, she aided us most conscientiously."[63]

Far from being merely a "talented pet-shop owner," as one customer, the geneticist C. C. Little, patronizingly called her, she is a neglected pioneer among women in science.

Starting with these commercially supplied animals, biologists sought to develop their own strains by inbreeding. They were faced with considerable difficulties and discouragement, especially the sentiment that

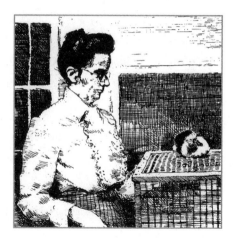

Fig. 7.8. Abbie Lathrop, a Massachusetts animal breeder and supplier, was an early pioneer in the methods of inbreeding and husbandry of laboratory mice. She worked with Leo Loeb on studies of mouse tumors. From Herbert C. Morse, *Origins of Inbred Mice* (1978), courtesy of Academic Press.

these efforts would be futile.[64] Biologists believed, with some justification, that as the number of generations of brother-sister inbreeding increased, it was inevitable that undesirable but inconspicuous recessive characteristics would be matched, revealed, and amplified, with harmful effect. The animals produced, it was confidently predicted by the naysayers, would eventually be too defective to survive, or be too infertile to breed, or even that unknown mechanisms for preserving diversity would thwart these attempts. This was nature's response to incest, it was plausibly argued. A more telling point was that, once developed, the inbred animal's reactions might not be a faithful witness to the biology of the outbred animal.

Many attempts by these early pioneers at creating such mice failed just in the ways anticipated. After some generations, the mice did indeed often show serious abnormalities and sterility, and entire frail colonies could be lost to infectious disease caused by mild pathogens. The first few successful strains developed in this period were the chance survivors of many attempts. It was C. C. Little (1888–1956), the geneticist and pupil of W. E. Castle at Harvard, who by 1911 had developed at Boston and Washington the "DBA"—the first reasonably robust and convincingly inbred mouse. Little had probably started with partly inbred "silver fawn" mice supplied, as usual, by Abbie Lathrop.[65] Lionel C. Strong also claimed to be the first to develop such mice, his being the widely used A strain mouse.[66]

C. C. Little and Transplantation Genetics

Loeb's successes might have been remembered, and his occasional misdirected analysis accepted with the usual historical charity, had he not been one of the many targets of the combative C. C. Little. In a classic genetics experiment with Ernest Tyzzer at Harvard in 1916, Little had contributed to the excitement of that new science. They had cross-mated two types of inbred animals, one of which was susceptible to a transplantable tumor. They showed that all the offspring (called F1 hybrids) were found to be susceptible to this same transplanted tumor.[67] The sentiment of the day led to the view that the hybrid shared the "genetic susceptibility to cancer" of the parent.[68] In fact, the F1 hybrids made from two inbred strains merely lack immunological reaction against *any* tissue from either of the two inbred parents.

In the already confused world of cancer studies, the thesis that susceptibility to cancer is inherited seemed to be sustained. After Little's findings were published, he obtained a research position at the Station for Experimental Evolution in the Carnegie Institution for Science in Washington, DC. The Washington institution also ran the Eugenic Records Office, an organization in Cold Spring Harbor, New York, that has not attracted the admiration of historians.[69] In the anarchic 1920s, the debate on genetics was broadening, and scientists were proposing a genetic basis for a wide range of human defects, notably insanity, epilepsy, alcoholism, criminality, feeble-mindedness, and other afflictions. The conclusion proposed by some was that such defects could and should be removed from the human race by the general application of eugenic measures, including controlled breeding and even surgical sterilization of the afflicted.

Little, with the results of his mouse studies, easily and confidently added cancer to this list with the bold suggestion that a simple hereditary mechanism could promote tumor growth in humans. Little and the Eugenic Records Office began to employ field-workers to seek out and make family studies of human cancer—all kinds of cancer. The field staff eagerly sought evidence—largely anecdotal—of a cancer trait, and, not surprisingly, many alleged "cancer pedigrees" were found. The field-workers reported the good news back to Little's department in Washington.[70] Little then announced that, in mice and humans, "it may be concluded that a tendency to the formation of tumors is clearly inherited. The fact of inheritance is clear."[71] Charles Davenport, the director at the Washington institute, and Little, his colleague, together proposed that human cancer could also be eliminated from the population by controlled selective breeding, compulsory sterilization, and immigration controls.[72]

When Davenport was later removed from his position, Little turned against the work of the Eugenic Records Office and blamed the erroneous notion of "cancer families" on "over-ardent eugenic field workers." Little left research and moved to senior academic appointments, but, never free from controversy, he was twice forced out from senior posts. He eventually returned to mouse breeding, setting up the famous Jackson Laboratory in Bar Harbor, Maine, a private institute for the study of genetics named after its patron, Roscoe B. Jackson, who took holidays locally.[73] It produced and sold inbred mice for scientists all over the world and still does so.[74]

Little and Loeb

In the 1920s, Little had been prepared to lecture others on the way ahead in biology. He made rambling attacks on a number of American scientists, and in this campaign he used the declamatory style more suitable for the unpleasant discourse in the world of eugenics. In 1924, it was Leo Loeb's turn to endure Little's wrath, and in a strange paper in the short-lived, poorly regarded *Journal of Cancer Research,* Little devoted himself entirely to a polemical appraisal of Loeb's entirely sound kidney-slice transplant work.[75] Little's review is superficial and shows no clear understanding of Loeb's work. He scorned the idea that the pattern of graft survival times within families (and particularly the 25:50:25 ratio) reflected genetic relationships, and he rejected all non-inbred experimental animal work as useless. He also dismissed Loeb's interest in the puzzle of the fetus as a homograft by saying that the fetus survived because it had no antigens to react against. He warned medical professionals not to take Loeb's data seriously.

Loeb and some of the others who had received the same treatment from Little did not reply to these attacks, and Loeb had especially good reasons not to respond. The excitable Little remained involved in the still-powerful eugenics lobby, and Loeb was an immigrant German Jew, a mild-mannered man who had already experienced European political intolerance. Loeb's talented biologist brother Jacques had encountered blatant anti-Semitism in New York in his professional life and Leo may not have cared to brush with Little. But others who attracted Little's displeasure, notably Maud Slye, did so and kept up a vigorous debate with him.[76]

In the period after Little's broadside, which did both short- and long-term damage to Loeb's reputation, he felt it necessary to switch to the use of inbred rats, which Little had insisted was the way forward. Loeb moved from his outbred rat kidney transplant slice studies and in 1926 started to use inbred Wistar rats, the famous albino variant of the otherwise unpleasant *Rattus norvegicus,* inbred to forty generations and supplied by the Wistar Institute in Philadelphia.[77] Mathematically-minded geneticists had used their "formulae for inbreeding" to come up with forty as the number of generations required to produce a thoroughly inbred animal.[78] Loeb trusted the geneticists and their confident calculations, and this confidence led to a substantial error, which, though later recognized and corrected by Loeb himself, was remembered and held against him for decades.

Nonidentical Identical Rats

Loeb was puzzled to find that when slice-grafting in his usual way between rats at the fortieth generation in the inbred line, he often found a modest lymphocyte reaction and loss of grafts. Assured by others that the animals at this stage were identical, Loeb now felt compelled to propose that, since these "identical" animals rejected grafts from each other, this suggested that another, finer mechanism of discrimination existed that could separate out even individuals within a mature inbred line. Loeb proposed a superindividuality beyond and above the usual genetic mechanisms; this would mean that there was a difference even between identical twins. He took this position in his otherwise prescient review in *Physiological Reviews* in 1930; it was the only substantial work to that date in the literature on transplantation. His text was difficult to follow, burdened with his own arcane typology (including "homoiotransplant" and "syngenesiotransplant"), which, although a brave attempt to bring order to the chaotic terminology of the day, merely clouded it further. He also omitted his careful and convincing experimental data on the grounds that it was already published elsewhere. When dwelling at length on the baffling challenge of the mysterious, nongenetic superindividuality, he lapsed into the almost forgotten German *Naturphilosophie* mode.

In the late 1920s, Loeb had done relatively little transplant work, perhaps discouraged by its reception, and contented himself with publishing his reflective overview in 1930. In the interim, he instead published on tissue culture and worked on his important ovarian physiology studies. But he returned to transplant projects in the 1930s possessed of a new insight, and he then continued to contribute significantly in calmer scientific circumstances as described later. However, in spite of his perceptiveness and his honored status in other disciplines, Loeb's place in the history of transplantation immunology has been uncertain, even denied.

Mayo Clinic Experimental Transplants

There was a steady intermittent interest in experimental kidney transplantation at the Mayo Clinic in the 1920s, but these studies are not prominent in the written histories of the clinic.[79] Frank C. Mann (1887–1962) was the clinic's director of experimental medicine from 1918 through to the 1930s. Mann encouraged young research fellows to do experimental transplantation work, and these studies were mixed in with other projects.[80] His transplant interest may have been prompted by the earlier work of local surgeon J. C. Masson, who had an interest in skin grafting and blood grouping but had moved on to other projects at the clinic.

The decline in interest in human kidney transplantation at this time did not mean that serious kidney disease was uncommon. Instead, deaths from chronic kidney failure were more common at this time than later, and in America, deaths from "chronic nephritis" rose to a peak in the 1920s, before declining quite markedly. When the first successful treatments by regular dialysis and kidney transplantation became available in the 1960s, deaths from renal failure had fallen to one-fifth of the peak level in the earlier twentieth century.[81] Dealing with renal failure was therefore an all-too-common aspect of routine clinical work in the 1920s.

The first serious attempts to address renal failure were not in transplantation but in the effort to make and use artificial kidney machines. John Abel, who joined the Johns Hopkins pharmacology faculty in 1892, made a dialysis device in 1912 using Thomas Graham's chemical principle of dialysis. Abel's "vividiffusion" apparatus was constructed using collodion tubing as the membrane, and to prevent clotting of the blood inside, he used hirudin, an anticoagulant chemical extracted from leeches.[82] Although Abel's priority was to use the apparatus for physiological studies, he did consider later that it might be of value in treating cases of poisoning, particularly after Heinrich Necheles and Georg Haas tried this approach for the first time in a patient.[83] Abel presented his apparatus at an international conference in London in 1913, and in its coverage of the event, the *Times* gave the device the name that stuck: "An Artificial Kidney."[84]

Renal Function Tests

In Baltimore, one of Abel's collaborators on the vividiffusion work was Leonard Rowntree (1883–1962). Rowntree can be credited with the first renal function test, which came from an earlier serendipitous observation in 1911 that the purgative phenolsulfthalein (PSP) was excreted by the kidney, and he showed that urine output levels related to the severity of kidney failure.[85] After Rowntree moved to the Mayo Clinic in 1920, he introduced another useful test. That test, performed in 1923, showed, again by chance, x-ray visualization of the kidney, pelvis, and ureter after therapeutic injection of sodium iodide.[86] At the Mayo Clinic, Rowntree's PSP test, plus increasing use of blood urea nitrogen estimations, permitted easy assessment of renal function.

This chemical, quantitative approach to disease was itself a novelty.

Although unchallenged later, in the early twentieth century it offered a new, controversial paradigm, one resisted by those who espoused the holistic approach and claimed that bedside judgment, not a laboratory measurement, was the arbiter of disease severity and prognosis. In 1928, Lord Horder, the powerful English physician and medical politician, could say of the emerging clinical laboratories that "materials are dumped in these places much as coals are dumped at our houses. I suppose such places are necessary; anyway they seem to have come to stay. I do not patronize them myself."[87]

In the management of kidney disease, a standard text of the 1930s did note the paradigm shift and commented on the controversial transfer of authority from the doctor to the clinical laboratory: "In the chronic types of nephritis . . . a prognosis may indeed be attempted on purely clinical grounds—albuminuric retinitis usually suggests a termination within two years, and the patient rarely survives the onset of uremic vomiting by more than a few months—but a blood urea gives added certainty."[88]

In the early 1920s, the Mayo Clinic's "scientific" approach may have been unusual and kidney transplantation seen as slightly distasteful. But by the end of the 1920s, the conservative, more holistically oriented physicians were on the defensive, and their claims that prognosis was an art rather than a science were less confident.

Frank Mann's Group

Mann's clinical team used a diversity of transplant models—kidney, heart, and adrenal grafting. They started their varied transplant studies in 1918, beginning with thyroid grafting and picking up where others had left off, but they did not build on the positions already reached by Carrel and by those working in Europe. The Mayo team's varied efforts ceased in 1933 with Mann's own work on heart transplantation, which he performed using Carrel's earlier model.[89] Mann and his colleagues used dog kidney transplantation studies from time to time, however, perhaps because of the clinic's interest in renal function tests. They did their first such kidney study in 1918, conducted by Carl Deederer, and Carl S. Williamson (born 1896) followed up with another study in 1923.[90] Williamson again showed that homograft kidneys invariably failed and that cross-species grafting failed immediately as a result of intravascular coagulation.[91] He was followed by Kenji Ibuka, who in 1926 also studied the same model of dog homograft kidney loss, as did Patrick P. T. Wu some time later.[92]

Mann's additional position as head of the Pathological Anatomy Department led him to use microscopy to study failed organ grafts. He confirmed Loeb's finding of "an extensive lymphocytic infiltration ultimately destroying the transplant."[93] But he did not emphasize this finding, and at times he seemed to show some support for Ehrlich's earlier athrepsia explanation of graft loss. Although he did not try liver transplantation, Mann was first to describe the coagulation defect following total removal of the liver, a problem that was to plague the pioneer liver transplanters much later.[94] Mann was an expert in the procedures of liver removal and making the Eck fistula, and he studied the metabolic consequences thereof. After this work, he published extensively on the new liver function tests, measurements that were to be standard thereafter and have stood the test of time.

Clinic Attitudes

The Mayo Clinic studies hardly extended the conclusions reached by Carrel and, in spite of many years of effort at the Minnesota facility and routine use of technically successful grafting, the researchers signally failed to explore any of the forms of immunosuppression suggested by Carrel, notably radiation or benzol. These were hardly hidden proposals, since the strategies had been published and Carrel had made them known widely in the scientific and lay press in 1914, and Carrel was still working and available at the Rockefeller Institute. Something held Mann back from making further progress.

The first factor was that Mann himself commented on the necessity of retracing their steps and confirming the many early experimental findings in kidney homograft loss, because the decade of the 1920s was muddled by the unhelpful activities of the skin and gland homografters. He wrote that, "owing to the claims of certain surgeons, with particular references to implantation of sex glands, the procedure [homografting] often is considered successful," and Rowntree also severely criticized the gland-grafting claims then current, calling them "myths."[95] The second major constraint on the Mayo surgeons' ambition was the mindset of the day, namely, the lofty advice given to clinicians to await enlightenment from basic science studies. It seems that the talented Mann poignantly accepted his humble place in the hierarchy of investigators. He wrote that "the successful transplantation of a healthy organ for a diseased one awaits the discovery of those biological factors which prevent the survival of the tissues of one individual when transplanted into the body of another individual, together with the development of methods for holding their action in abeyance."[96]

Mann apparently believed that his role was not to make further empirical surgical attempts at prolonging the survival of organ transplants but to wait until scientists elsewhere had gained a full understanding of graft loss. Carrel's "road map" was not to be used until all junctions were identified and the tank was full. With the mandate to reestablish the old doctrine, go over the old ground, and await advice from the learned, it was not time for Mann to press forward. These considerations may explain the Mayo group's almost inexplicable caution.

Harvey Stone's Claims

Another study proved to be a step backward. Mann took an interest in one researcher's claim to have made a graft nonantigenic and thus nonreject-able. This strategy for avoiding graft loss was reported in 1933 from the Johns Hopkins School of Medicine, where the surgeon Harvey B. Stone, mentor to William Longmire, later chief of surgery at UCLA, announced that human thyroid and parathyroid gland slices kept for a while in tissue culture would survive when transplanted.[97] The human patients treated with Stone's gland implants had thyroid or the more serious parathyroid deficiency after thyroid removal. These claims were widely publicized and seemed at last to be a triumph in a decade of gland-grafting attempts. Mann repeated Harvey Stone's work, this time using adrenal gland grafts in rats. Mann, however, found no positive effect, and his analysis was properly cautious.[98] This was the last involvement of the Mayo Clinic in transplant studies for decades.

As the chaotic 1920s came to an end, better science and common sense was to return to the often disordered world of transplantation. But there was a lasting legacy. Because of the frivolous events, many looking back later thought that there could have been no proper studies of trans-plantation before this "prescientific" time in the 1920s. By the 1950s, when transplantation immunology strongly revived, almost three decades and a second world war had intervened since the vitality of the "lost era" in the early 1900s. This innovative period was historically isolated, far away behind the bad science of the 1920s.

8 Progress in the 1930s

B Y THE EARLY 1930S, after the muddles of the previous decade, the prewar European experimental transplant work was revived in small ways. There was some activity in Lyon.[1] In Germany, there was a modest restoration of studies on immunosuppression. In the Soviet Union, there was impressive innovation in blood transfusion, corneal grafting, and tissue transplantation. In the United States, after the uncritical skin and organ grafting of the 1920s, good surgical science was quietly gaining some ground. In his St. Louis laboratory, Leo Loeb returned unostentatiously to build on his solid earlier immunological achievements by detecting and correcting a flaw in his earlier work, and by the 1930s, Loeb had helped the talented local surgeons to restore sanity in the disordered field of skin grafting. At the Jackson Laboratory in Bar Harbor, George Snell started to unravel the daunting complexity of what was later called "tissue typing," as did Peter Gorer in London.

But the first significant event in the field during this decade was that the fringe transplanters, who had a good run in Europe and America in the anarchic 1920s, were at last marginalized.

Serge Voronoff's Nemesis

Serge Voronoff, the monkey-gland transplanter, met public disapprobation and ultimate disgrace around 1930. His claims for monkey-to-human surgery took time to be discredited, such was the laxness of clinical science in the 1920s. His downfall was thus delayed until after one of his characteristically high-profile ventures, this one in French Algeria, where he started to gland-graft the scraggy indigenous sheep. Voronoff was at the height of his fame when he embarked on this large-scale testis transplantation program with French government support. He claimed that the grafts from young donor sheep had rejuvenated older animals and improved their wool production. But then he went too far, stating that this effect was transmitted to offspring and thus was a permanent genetic change. Such claims were, and are, a serious matter, contradicting Mendelian genetic

154

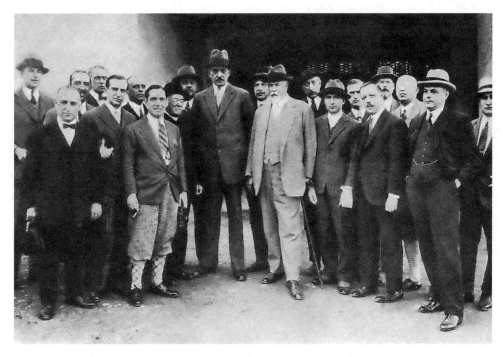

Various nations sent veterinarians to Algeria in 1927 to assess Serge Voronoff's claims to have permanently rejuvenated the poor-quality local sheep using testis grafts. Voronoff is the tall figure in the center. From Serge Voronoff, *Greffes testiculaires* (Paris: Doin, 1923).

orthodoxy, and an international group of veterinarians was asked to visit Algeria; reporting back to their governments, they did so charitably, having been charmed by the ever plausible statements of Voronoff. One of the British investigators pointed out the bad science he practiced, notably the absence of *"témoins"*—control groups of nongrafted sheep—and the convenient exclusion of "failures" in the grafted animals.

Shortly after the delegation's visit, however, came a publication in 1931 by Henri Velu (1887–1973), director of the French Colonial Veterinary Service in Casablanca in neighboring French Morocco, reporting on a similar project with better design and methods. Velu found that the sheep testis grafts were promptly destroyed, ascribing this loss elegantly to a "personal individuality"—a terminology perhaps taken from Leo Loeb, and, interestingly, he attributed the mechanism of graft loss to *"cellules migratices"* in the host, a blood-borne, not a local cellular reaction.[2] At a stormy scientific meeting of veterinarians in Paris in 1931, Velu had to contradict the claims of the distinguished and powerful Parisian establishment, who had supported Voronoff's Algerian project and who were well aware that not only their reputation but also that of the French government was at stake. But Velu courageously held his ground against the gibes that he was an unpatriotic cynic with little experience in such work—unlike the distinguished Voronoff.[3]

The final blow to the supporters of testis transplantation came from biochemical measurements. In Chicago in 1930, Carl Moore developed an assay for the testis hormone. Studying grafted animals, he showed that the gland homografts produced no hormone and were not only dead but had not retained any significant store of hormone.[4] Voronoff's star soon faded, and to add to his scientific reverses, he may have transferred disease to his grafted patients, since monkeys carry some dangerous viruses. But popular belief in the possibility of rejuvenation persisted as ever, and the demand from clients continued. The marginalized, charismatic fringe practitioners in private clinics instead offered revised therapies, notably with fetal animal cell injections, and when these were banned by the regulatory authorities, freeze-dried extracts of secret origin were substituted.

John Brinkley's Decline

Voronoff's weakness was self-deception, but Brinkley's Kansas quackery was cynical and overt. As his claims for goat-gland grafting began to look ridiculous, Brinkley's three fraudulent medical degrees attracted the attention of the newly tough American regulatory authorities, and in 1930 they acted. The memorable court judgment in the trial, which prevented him from practicing and closed his large, profitable transplant clinic, labeled him as "an empiric without moral sense who had perfected and organized charlatanism until it is capable of preying on human weakness to an extent quite beyond the invention of the humble mountebank."[5]

Brinkley's activities were perhaps not entirely irrelevant to the revival of orthodox transplantation immunology in the early 1930s. Brinkley's defense lawyers at his trial in Kansas City enthusiastically quoted the dubious 1920s claims in the conventional medical literature by American testis homograft enthusiasts like Max Thorek, G. F. Lydston, and H. L. Hunt, who claimed success with human skin and gland homografts. With some rhetorical assistance, these allegedly scientific papers gave apparent respectability to Brinkley's testis grafts.

But among the expert witnesses brought in by the prosecution to testify against Brinkley was the respected University of Kansas professor of surgery, Thomas Orr, who dismissed Brinkley's claims. It was in the American Midwest, and particularly in nearby St. Louis and the Mayo Clinic in Rochester, Minnesota, that an increasingly firm stand was emerging against the dreary, revived claims for human homograft skin success. It is possible that Brinkley's excesses and his trial had focused the attention of these midwestern surgeons and scientists on the need to restore order in the matter of tissue grafting.

Loeb's Further Work

Leo Loeb, the St. Louis immunologist, had some discouragements in the muddled 1920s. He did establish most of the key concepts of cellular immunology, notably that a reaction to homografts was the rule, that this was under genetic control, that the lymphocyte was involved, and much else. But after the bizarre attack on his results, conclusions, and even his probity by C. C. Little, he had moved away, with success, onto other, non-transplant work, perhaps also because he was unable to go beyond his major enigmatic finding: that the inbred rats provided for him would reject grafts from each other.

Loeb, soon after publishing his lengthy review on superindividuality, realized he had made a mistake. He had used rats at the fortieth generation of inbreeding, taking others' confident assurance that uniformity had been reached. But as he proceeded to study rats inbred beyond the fortieth generation, Loeb noted that the puzzling homograft responses between the allegedly identical rats were diminishing. When he grafted Wistar rats beyond generation sixty, they failed to show any lymphocyte reaction between siblings.[6] There was no need now to support his proposed extra mechanism: the rats in his early experiments were simply not inbred. Relieved of his problem findings, Loeb dropped his fussy extra level of uniqueness and was content to return to conventional genetics. But his retraction came later and was not as prominent as his *Physiological Reviews* paper, which many continued to quote.

The Wistar Institute and Inbreeding

With Loeb's surprising discovery, Helen King at the Wistar Institute agreed with Loeb that stringent new requirements had to be met when inbreeding for transplantation work or for any demanding genetics studies. Many more generations were required, and this had not been noticed in simpler genetics experiments.[7] She and Loeb were now naturally curious about the quality of the inbred laboratory animals then available commercially, notably those supplied by C. C. Little's Jackson Laboratory in Bar Harbor, including the popular and hardy CBA mice. By 1943, using his graft test for inbreeding, Loeb and King had reported on the quality of many of the famous commercial lines then available. Among Little's Jackson Laboratory mice, some strains were inbred and some were not. The most homogeneous was the pioneer A strain mouse line, whose members generally accepted grafts from each other, and the worst was the AKA line, which generally showed a brisk graft response to intrastrain grafting. This unacceptable situation had not been noticed in less demanding, nontransplant genetics work, nor was there any checking of inbreeding, other than looking at the mice and trusting the breeding records. King and Loeb called for increased vigilance. Mistakes in the breeding rooms seemed to have been common, and any such mistake could cause a disaster in the supply that would mislead users and annul years of work.[8]

Loeb's Test

It was obvious that there needed to be some means of testing lab animals to guarantee an adequate degree of inbreeding, and graft acceptance ultimately became the only guarantee. "Loeb's Test," as it might be called, became indispensable in detecting and guarding against any catastrophic flaws in the supply of inbred animals. The kidney capsule model was cumbersome, and simple ear skin grafting took its place.

There was a fine irony in the fact that Loeb's graft test system now had a central role in the new mammalian genetics. A "whole animal" response was now acknowledged to be superior to any sophisticated test-tube or chemical assessment. This concession of the mouse breeders and geneticists to Loeb, the homografter, doubtless happened slowly, and is nowhere recorded, perhaps through embarrassment at the situation revealed. If Loeb felt a certain schadenfreude at this turn of events, to which he was entitled, he did not mention it. Much later, DNA testing supplanted Loeb's Test for routine quality control in commercial inbreeding, but his older graft test still gives the ultimate discrimination, and skin grafting is still required to check the difference between very closely related strains.[9]

Loeb probably had a direct and beneficial effect on surgical mindsets in the 1930s. In St. Louis, colleagues, medical students, and local surgeons took note of Loeb's efforts to show the ubiquity and regularity of the homograft response, and his consistent principle enabled the surgeons in turn to be confident enough to contradict the claims made by uncritical human skin and gland grafters.

Evarts Graham was the distinguished chief of surgery at Washington University in St. Louis, and his interest in research led to the gibe that he was a "mouse surgeon."[10] As chief of pathology, Loeb, the local rat surgeon, and C. C. Guthrie, now in the Physiology Department, could also influence the two generations of local plastic and head and neck surgeons trained by Graham. In the first-generation group was Vilray P. Blair (1871–1955), whose authority in head and neck and plastic surgery derived from his experience treating the wounded in World War I.[11] Blair's pupil in St. Louis, James Barrett Brown (1899–1971), joined Blair as a close collaborator, and the two did extensive human skin grafting.[12] Also trained by Blair was Earl Padgett (1893–1946), who devised the first successful dermatomes, which still bear his name, for cutting large sheets of partial-thickness human skin for grafting.[13] Padgett's coauthored textbook on skin grafting shows Loeb's important influence on the local surgeons, and Padgett's memoirs pay tribute to Loeb, referring to Loeb's monograph on transplantation as "my Bible."[14]

The interest of the St. Louis surgeons in skin grafting led them to criticize the widespread, uncritical use of human homograft skin then in vogue, and their criticism reflected Loeb's stance. By 1932, Padgett had reported that all his attempts at human skin homografting had failed and that claims to the contrary could be "relegated to the realms of mythology."[15] This publication by Padgett was based on one of his lectures to small midwestern medical societies, visits known to eminent city practitioners as "beating the bushes."[16] At one level, this lecture circuit had the declared objective of informing country practitioners on recent advances, but the meetings had the added agenda of seeking surgical referrals. On his travels, Padgett may well have had regular updates from small-town surgeons on Brinkley's rural Kansas transplant quackery, thus reinforcing the need for better science.

George Snell and Leo Loeb

George Snell (1903–1996) can perhaps be added to the list of innovators in the St. Louis "homograft network" influenced by Loeb. Snell spent a year in St. Louis when he was between his well-described posts with Hermann Muller at the University of Texas and his final, famous position at the Jackson Laboratory in Bar Harbor. According to his book *Search for a Rational Ethic,* in 1933–1934 Snell was an assistant professor in the Zoology Department at Washington University, where he instructed others on research methods and taught courses such as "Evolution, Heredity, Eugenics, and Genetics." It was at this time that Snell switched from fruit fly work to the more difficult genetics of mice and rats, likely having been influenced by Loeb, who worked at the nearby medical campus. After he moved to Bar Harbor, Snell began to transplant skin in mice and used Loeb's characteristic, arcane, but precise transplantation terminology, such as "homoiotransplant."[17]

Loeb's Lost Legacy

Loeb's influence has not received any prominent mention in later histories of transplantation. The likely reasons are the complexity of his discourse, the temporary diversion caused by his inadvertent use of poor-quality inbred rats, and C. C. Little's gibes. All of these factors have discouraged study of his perceptive, original, and detailed findings, which built on the Schöne-Lexer-Carrel-Murphy lymphocyte-based understanding of homograft loss.

The marginalization of Loeb may have started in the late 1930s, when Howard Florey, at Oxford, preparing unsuccessfully for a major assault on the mystery of the lymphocyte, looked, perhaps only briefly, at Loeb's long, flawed article in *Physiological Reviews*. Dismayed and repelled by the complexity, Florey became further irritated when he read that inbred animals rejected each other's grafts; he passed his concern on to his student Peter Medawar, and Medawar and his group shared this disdain thereafter. In the small world of those interested in transplantation, opinion soon began to lean, wrongly, toward antibodies as the mechanism of graft loss. There was no longer any need to master lymphocyte-leaning Loeb's difficult but prescient writings.

Human Kidney Transplants

Between the European attempts at human organ grafting by Ernst Unger and Mathieu Jaboulay in the first decade of the century and the revival in the 1950s, only one surgeon attempted human kidney transplantation. On April 3, 1933, a Soviet surgeon performed the first human-to-human kidney transplant. This attempt may have been related to other developments in Soviet surgery, notably their pioneering corneal grafting and blood transfusions. The Soviet Union was less affected by World War I than the nations of western Europe, and Soviet surgical science showed considerable vitality until the 1930s.

Voronoy worked in Kharkov, Ukraine, in the surgical department headed by the talented Professor Vladimir (Vasili) N. Shamov (1882–1962), who achieved major innovations in blood transfusion methods and who had been first in the Soviet Union to store blood, using citrate as an anticoagulant.[18] Shamov also encouraged tissue transplantation studies in his department; he had attended the International Society of Surgery's 1914 congress in New York, at which transplantation featured prominently. He visited many American and European surgical centers thereafter. At Kharkov, he noted in 1928 (as had John Hunter) that the blood of the animals dying suddenly did not clot, and this effect was confirmed in Moscow by the talented and energetic surgeon Sergei Yudin (1891–1954), then in charge of the huge Sklifosovskiy Institute, which was responsible for all the emergency surgery in the city.[19] He had considerable need for urgent blood transfusion, so he exploited the resource readily available in his hospital institute's emergency room: recently deceased patients. "Many [accident victims] arrived late at night, and it was difficult at times to find suitable [blood] donors at once. At the same time the ambulances bring to the Institute cases with trauma and heart failure so severe that they die in the receiving room or even on the way. Under these circumstances it would be possible almost any day to procure fresh cadaver blood of a suitable group."[20]

Yudin then set up an organization in Moscow to obtain cadaveric blood in this way, and this source was to be important in the Soviet Union thereafter. It was the world's first civilian blood bank. Use of the blood was sensibly delayed until the presence of any transmissible disease was ruled out by postmortem examination and other tests. The deceased donors also provided corneas for Vladimir Filatov's pioneering corneal grafts in the Soviet Union in the 1930s.

It is highly likely that there was a similar donor organization at the hospital in Kharkov, Ukraine, and its presence may have made it possible to obtain the donor kidney for the historic transplant operation. The ease of obtaining tissues after death in the Soviet Union at this time contrasted with the resistance to such donation elsewhere, since only after World War II was donation seen as noble and altruistic in the West. It is possible that the earlier Soviet collectivism either encouraged voluntary donation or allowed routine removal of tissue after death without legal formality.

Transplant Pioneer Yu. Yu. Voronoy

Yu. Yu. Voronoy (1895–1961) received his medical education in Kiev, and his formative years seem to have been from 1926 to 1931, when he was a young member of the surgery department in Kiev under Shamov.[21] In 1923, from Shamov's department, Elanskii published on the relationship between blood types and human skin grafting and, like others in the West at the time, reported a benefit.[22] This interest in blood typing methods also led to an interest in the laboratory techniques of agglutination and other antigen-antibody reactions. Another interest of the department at that time was human testicular transplantation, the procedure still taken seriously in orthodox circles elsewhere in the mid-1920s, and Shamov performed seven such transplants.

Voronoy was therefore working in a department interested in blood transfusion, immunological methods, and tissue transplantation.[23] In 1932, Voronoy published an article in German, translated as "On the Problems of the Role and Significance of Specific Complement-fixing Antibodies in Free Transplantation of the Testis."[24] The title and the text show that Voronoy had detected complement-fixing antibodies following transplantation of testis slices from dog to dog, and this obscure report is the first claim for the existence of such antibodies following tissue transplantation. This paper shows that he had the insight and laboratory skills to explore further the proposal that homograft loss was occurring via an immunological mechanism.

Voronoy then turned to studies of kidney transplantation in dogs, and again an antibody was detected, though some of the data are puzzling. However, Voronoy's thorough approach to the immunology of transplantation can be admired.

In 1931, Voronoy moved to Kherson, in southern Ukraine; the move involved a promotion that gave him new responsibilities for emergency surgery and acute medicine. In his new post, he encountered patients with acute renal failure as a result of taking corrosive sublimate (mercuric chloride), a common form of self-poisoning. He decided for a number of reasons that such a patient might be treated with a kidney transplant. If successful, the kidney would, in the short term, produce urine flow, which would not only relieve the acute kidney failure but might also eliminate the mercury. At postmortem examination of these suicide cases, Voronoy had noted splenic and lymph node shrinkage. He reasoned that, in patients with this type of poisoning, a transplant might last for a longer period of time than usual because of this "reticulo-endothelial atrophy," and he thus considered that he had found a method of such suppression, of sorts. He was doubtless aware of the German work, mentioned above, on the immunological effectiveness of reticulo-endothelial blockage.

It was Voronoy who performed the first human-to-human homograft kidney transplant, in April 1933. Details of Voronoy's operation were published in the Soviet Union and Germany, and, in 1936, the Spanish journal *El Siglo Médico* reprinted the report on the surgery in its section of international reviews.[25] This important Soviet contribution to transplantation, although published in Russia, Germany, and Spain, was not noticed elsewhere until the early 1950s. Even the left-leaning cadre among the pioneer European kidney transplanters missed the original notice of Voronoy's historic transplant. Voronoy's work did not come to the attention of most in the Western scientific and surgical community until the thorough literature search made for David Hume's classic 1955 paper on human kidney transplantation.

In his introduction to the full article published in Russian, Voronoy ridiculed the earlier attempts at human kidney transplant operations using animal donors. His operative findings, postoperative course, and pathological studies, given in unusual detail for his day, are worthy of extensive quotation in translation:

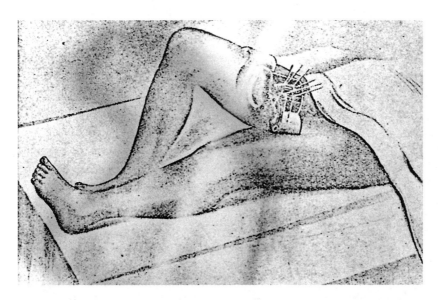

An illustration showing the thigh position Yuri Voronoy used in his pioneering human homograft transplant. From Ü. Woronoy, "Die Immunität bei Organtransplantation: I. Mitteilung: Über spezifische komplementbindende Antikörper bei freier Transplantation der Testes," *Archiv für Klinische Chirurgie* 171 (1932): 361–85.

Female patient B., 26 years, was admitted to hospital on 31st March [1933] suffering from poisoning by corrosive sublimate 24 hours previously: in this suicide attempt, she swallowed 4 grams of undiluted sublimate. On admission, the patient was complaining of spasmodic pain in the abdomen and small of the back. She was in a semi-conscious condition, interrupted by spasms of pain and convulsions. The patient had marked stomatitis, and occasional fibrillary twitching of the muscles was observed. The pulse was tense and slow. Urine was not excreted and on catheterisation, not one drop was obtained. The patient was treated by intravenous transfusion of a 5% glucose solution, enemas and an appropriate diet.

However, on the next day her condition did not improve. In the next 4 days the patient did not excrete any urine.

Dr. Yu. Yu. Voronoy decided to carry out on her the operation of transplantation of a whole cadaveric kidney.

The donor used was a 60-year-old man who was brought into hospital with a fracture of the base of the skull and who died in the receiving room; the kidney was taken out 6 hours after death. In fact the blood groups of the donor and the recipient did not coincide: whereas that of the patient was 1 (O) that of the corpse was 3 (B).[26]

However, Dr. Voronoy decided that, as the blood of the universal donor, the mass of the blood of the recipient flowing in the tissues of the transplanted kidney would not be agglutinated. So it was decided, despite the difference in blood groups, to carry out a kidney transplant. Besides, there were no other opportunities to obtain a donor kidney.

The first clinical transplant in the world of a kidney taken from a corpse was carried out by the Soviet surgeon Yu. Yu. Voronoy on 3 April 1933. At approximately 21.00 hours in the evening, Dr. Voronoy carried out in the patient poisoned by sublimate a transplant of a cadaveric kidney into the right thigh into its middle third on the anteromedial aspect, corresponding to the course of the blood vessels.

Thus took place this really historic operation. Operating under local anesthesia, the surgeon separated out the femoral artery and vein. After this, the right kidney was removed from the corpse after ligation of the pedicle, two ligatures were put on the renal vein and artery and also on the ureter; the blood vessels and ureter were divided between ligatures; the kidney was taken out together with its capsule and transferred to the operation wound of the patient. A bed for the kidney was prepared in the soft tissues with complete covering of the organ by prepared skin flaps. Then at 1.5 cm. above the ligatures, temporary vascular clamps were put on the vessels of the transplant, the parts of the vessels with the ligatures were cut off, and the vessels gaped open in the new site. On the proximal end of the femoral artery and vein in the wound were placed temporary clamps and on the distal ends, tight ligatures. After this, the blood vessels in the wound were cut through and the surgeon proceeded to suture the renal and femoral arteries and veins. For this Yu. Yu. Voronoy utilized, as in previous experiments, the modified vascular suture of Carrel; for example, instead of forceps he employed sterile pieces of cork and also double needles. He led the ureter out through a cleft in the skin of the thigh and gently pierced it by two thin sutures. In the skin were placed knotted sutures and in the corners of the wound two strips of rubber.

In this way the delay before transplantation of the donor kidney to the recipient was over 6 hours.

When the vascular sutures were put in, the blood circulation to the kidney was renewed, and the blood supply good: this was confirmed by the capillary blood ooze from the external surface of the ureter, the capsule of the kidney and several other places injured at the time of extirpation of the kidney from the cadaver.

On the operating table a little peristalsis of the ureter and sudden excretion of a drop of urine was seen but as Dr. Voronoy noted[,] . . . "these occurrences died down towards the end of the operation, despite quite clear pulsation of the renal vessels, but these circumstances did not distress us." It was a fact that he always observed in his experiments on dogs such a "pause in function" after transplantation and this pause lasted from several hours to whole days and then regular secretion of urine began. The pause in function (anuric phase) depended, in the opinion of Yu. Yu. Voronoy on "a reflex to the transplant."

During the operation the patient's condition was unchanged. No anaphylactic phenomena or specific intoxication were observed. On testing, the blood concentration of mercury remained exactly 1.5 mg.%.

The night after the operation, the patient's condition improved somewhat, the vomiting ceased and the cramps stopped. On the morning of the 4th of April she complained of strong thirst. The operation site showed no oedema or infiltration in the region of the wound and the skin flaps were in good condition. An occasional peristalsis of the ureter was noted and excretion of a drop of transparent urine. Towards the end of the first day after the transplant, with the aim of strengthening the reticulo-endothelial "blockade," and diminishing the concentration of mercury in the blood, venesection was done and a massive transfusion of blood of donor Group 1 (O) given.[27] Before this however, analysis of the blood for mercury was carried out and it appeared that during one day after the transplant the concentration of mercury had sharply diminished and was found to be only 0.15 mg.%

After bloodletting (700ml) and transfusion of citrated blood (400 ml) peristalsis of the ureter became more vigorous and some blood-stained urine appeared. But when the patient developed anew her agitated state and the vomiting and cramps returned.

On the second day after the operation, the 5th April, the patient became significantly worse, and sometimes fell into an unconscious state. From the ureter of the transplanted kidney was excreted drops of blood-stained varnish-like urine (as before, the patient's own kidneys were not functioning and were not excreting urine at all).

After a catheter had been placed in the transplanted ureter, 4–5 c.c. of urine was successfully collected after an hour. Investigation of the urine showed a large quantity of albumin, 2–3 leucocytes per field of view, erythrocytes little changed, individual ones leached. Sheets of the epithelium of the kidney showing fatty change were found. The epithelium of the calyces was also separated in layers with epithelial and hyaline casts—3–5 per preparation; here and there were found crystals of neutral phosphoric acid. The concentration of urea in the urine was exactly 1.8 g/l.

On the evening of 5th April at approximately 21.00 hours, the excretion of urine from the transplanted kidney stopped. At 21 hours 40 minutes the patient expired.

In this manner, after the transplant operation with the new transplanted kidney, she survived 2 days, a little over 48 hours.

At autopsy significant degenerative changes were found in the parenchymatous organs, especially in the kidneys, liver and spleen. In the mucous membrane of the stomach and bowel there were inflammatory changes, but without any large necrotic areas. There were some changes in the muscle of the heart and in the cavity of the heart there was liquid blood almost without admixture of clots.

Examination of the site of the transplantation did not show any significant abnormalities. The bed for the kidney in the soft tissues showed a clear outline and the kidney itself showed fibrinous adhesions to the bed, but at its poles were seen traces of hematoma.

The kidney was increased in size and one section was a cherry red in color; the contours of the pyramids were seen; in a calyx was the bloody mass which was being excreted from the ureter. The vessels of the kidney at the site of the sutures were patent.

Microscopic examination of sections of the transplanted kidney and also of the patient's own organs was done in the Kharkov Institute of Pathological Anatomy by Academician N. F. Melinkov-Razvedenkov. There were established significant but irregular degenerative changes. Above all, the patient's own kidneys were injured—here were noted acute changes of the glomeruli, tubules and endothelium of the vessels; but there were also fresh mitoses observed—the occurrence of regeneration in the epithelial cells. There was also noted in the remaining organs, besides degeneration, signs of regenerative process. Especially acutely injured were the cells of the reticulo-endothelial system, where in the spleen for example, on a background of weak lymphoid proliferation, no signs of productive change of the reticular apparatus could be noted.

In the transplanted kidney the pathological changes were reminiscent of the change in the recipient's own kidneys, although they were more acute and more extensive. Significant desquamation of the epithelium and granular disintegration of it stood out separately and also a more acute degeneration and regeneration of the endothelial cells: this led to coagulation of the erythrocytes and in places to formation of delicate mural thrombi. In the extensive loops of vessels of the Malpighian corpuscles were apparent accumulations of hemolyzed erythrocytes and even granular disintegration of them.[28]

In *El Siglo Médico*, an editor's summary of the operation adds important detail, including the fact that Voronoy had checked the donor for tuberculosis and syphilis.

The thoroughness of this account is in contrast to the usual brief reports of earlier human and experimental organ transplants. Voronoy's surgical technique, in particular his confidence with the vascular surgery of organ grafting, was based on his earlier experimental experience. His general management and laboratory backup, particularly the prompt estimates of mercury levels in the blood, are impressive. The description of the transplant operation vividly re-creates the now-familiar events in the operating theater, notably the pleasure of seeing immediate blood flow into the kidney, the painful wait for kidney function, and the false hopes raised by even a few drops of urine. Reassuring blood flow was noticed in the exteriorized end of the ureter the next day, and occasional peristalsis was also encouraging. His technical success with the operation was confirmed at postmortem examination. Voronoy can be admired for attempting a modest exchange transfusion, not only to reduce the mercury content of the blood but also to perhaps diminish the immunologic attack on the grafted kidney.

Analysis of the Transplant

There are three likely reasons for the failure of Voronoy's pioneer human homograft. First, to use later terminology, the donor kidney was damaged by having remained in the body of the deceased for a prolonged period, a "warm time" of six hours and then remaining at presumably ambient temperature for an unknown period before implantation. Like others at the time and even later, Voronoy considered that warmth maintained vitality. He also knew from his dog transplants that the kidney would not work immediately but could regain function eventually. Sadly, events overtook this possibility, and the patient died before any recovery of function could occur.

Second, the kidney and patient were mismatched as to blood type; a blood type B donor organ had been put into a type O recipient, inviting but not ensuring immediate rejection. Rejection did not occur in the operating room, and the normal appearance of the ureter in the next two days, together with the findings at postmortem, suggests that Voronoy was lucky that the kidney had survived major damage in the short term. Voronoy knew of and accepted the blood type mismatch.[29] Voronoy knew that opinion had changed to the view that blood typing was of no benefit in prolonging human skin graft survival and thus could reasonably be ignored in kidney grafting. The pioneer kidney transplanters of the 1950s took a similar attitude and corresponding risk. It was not until the 1960s that the need for blood type compatibility in kidney grafting became apparent.

Reverse Incompatibility

Voronoy did address the blood types of donor and recipient, but he approached the issue in another way. The possibility of "reverse incompatibility" had been an active, but unfulfilled, fear in these early days of blood transfusion; the fear was that not only would donor kidney cells be attacked by the host but also that the residual donor serum in the graft would damage the *recipient's* blood cells. In Voronoy's account of the kidney transplant, he was clearly concerned about such a humoral graft-versus-host reaction, or "reverse mismatch." Since Voronoy's patient was type O and lacked blood type antigens, he knew that he had at least excluded this possible reverse transfusion reaction and any possible secondary kidney damage.[30] Voronoy indicated that he would have preferred to have a complete blood type match between donor and recipient, but his reason for using this kidney was timeless and understandable: he had a doomed patient, and there was only one kidney available for transplant.

The academician/pathologist's carefully described postmortem and histological changes in the transplanted kidney are the first account ever of human kidney homograft rejection. The changes probably represent a mixture of warm damage to the donor kidney before transplantation and some hyperacute rejection from the blood group mismatch. Graft damage from the remaining mercury in the blood stream may have added to the picture. The patient's illness and the short survival of the kidney precluded any cellular infiltrate.

Voronoy has an honorable place in the history of transplantation. It seems that he had prepared well for his bold, well-conducted, and carefully reported human kidney homograft operation. In addition, he realized that graft loss was an immunologic event and that, for graft survival, reduction of the host response was needed. His laboratory training in experimental surgery and his familiarity with serological methods also mark him as a surgical transplantation scientist. It is interesting to speculate on what might have been the outcome if Voronoy had had a fitter patient, a blood-type matched kidney, and a prompt transfer of the organ from donor to recipient: he might have obtained early urine flow. Also, if the recipient had lived longer, even this kidney with its reversible damage might have shown function later.

Transplants Elsewhere

There may have been failed kidney transplant attempts similar to the Soviet case about this time. They may have been controversial, badly planned, and thus unpublished. A paper presented in 1934 at the Charaka Club, an elite group of New York doctors, pronounced a flippant verdict on one similar case, again involving mercury poisoning. The mood at the club was clearly hostile:

This was the period of human woe when bichloride of mercury first became a popular method of suicide, well but falsely advertised as a method of *painless lethalis* by the yellowest of newspapers ever jealous for a beat in their stupid competition for news. One large hospital in New York saw a young lamb put to bed with a would-be suicide to have the lamb's kidney sewn into the circulation of the human sufferer in order that this organ of a healthy animal might substitute its function for that of the damaged kidneys of the poisoned human until the crisis of the toxic dose had passed. The result was prompt and quite in accord with the well-known law of nature that differences of species were exclusive to successful transplantation. The resulting deaths in this case were first, the kidney of the lamb, then, the lamb; and third and last, the would-be suicide, who at no time had any rational treatment whatever.[31]

Carrel Reemerges

Alexis Carrel had moved away from transplant work in the 1920s, when reductionism and the chemistry of antibodies held sway. Carrel was not suited to such an approach. Instead, he was increasingly influenced by interwar concerns on eugenics and Western decline, and he set up a huge animal laboratory to study nature and nurture, aging and nutrition. Uncharacteristically for him, however, these studies had not gone well.[32] In 1935, he published his book *Man the Unknown*, a best seller with a mix of messages on physiology, racial improvement, mysticism, and the need for authoritarian government. He proposed remedies for the alleged deterioration of the peoples and institutions of the West, via race improvement, education, and changed conditions of work, measures to be brought in by unelected savants like himself. The book failed to impress either the scientific world or serious-minded reviewers, but it was a huge international publishing success, assisted by the support of the *Reader's Digest*. Carrel spoke about his social ideas on public occasions, but his conservative stances and eugenic leanings started to irritate the new Rockefeller Institute leadership.[33] But shortly afterward, perhaps having regained confidence or having heeded the criticism, he returned to transplantation studies. A supportive factor was that, by the late 1930s, there were also growing doubts about the reductionist strategy for medical research, which had banished applied surgical studies from agendas of the national research institutes. The new cadre of professional, full-time biomedical scientists had been given their chance to show that innovation was best left in their hands for delivery later to the clinic. But nagging doubts now appeared. Even at the Rockefeller Institute, in spite of much important work, the expected outcome from their impressive fundamental research—curing or preventing common disease—had not materialized.[34] Applied research began creeping back into favor in the 1930s.

Carrel started testing a perfusion machine in an attempt to keep organs alive for extended periods, as an extension of his earlier tissue culture work. Carrel's claims for the new machine attracted immediate publicity, not only because he gained a new colleague who was already world famous but also because the device helped confirm his earlier claim to keep chicken heart cells beating indefinitely in tissue culture. This cellular "immortal life" was later shown to be dubious, but the perfusion project seemed a logical development.[35]

Organ Perfusion

A few organ perfusion methods had already been devised by physiologists.[36] In the early 1880s, Henry Newell Martin (1848–1893) at Johns Hopkins had used a system similar to the earlier organ perfusion apparatus made in Germany by Max von Frey and had managed to obtain short-term function of mammalian hearts isolated from the body. In 1914, Alfred Newton Richards and Cecil Drinker devised a better organ perfusion apparatus at the University of Pennsylvania.[37]

Carrel's new project was a characteristically public one, especially because his collaborator was the famous aviator Charles Lindbergh (1902–1974). Lindbergh, a skilled engineer, was puzzled that no pump was available to use as a heart substitute, and he took the initiative in contacting Carrel. The two became close friends, perhaps because they had many political views in common. Carrel's own attempts to make such a machine had been plagued by infection arising in the perfusion fluid, and Lindbergh devised a closed, sterile pumping system. Lindbergh's role was as the perfusionist, handing over the tissue for study by Carrel, who claimed that thyroid gland lobes survived for many weeks in the machine's small organ chamber. This work is still controversial, and later experts were unimpressed by Carrel's tests for tissue survival, namely, fairly well preserved microscopic appearances. Crucially, he did not claim to have preserved a few tiny kidneys sufficiently for them to produce much urine, and he made only one test on a fetal heart, which was inconclusive.

But in discussing the perfusion machine, Carrel presciently, and timelessly, listed the criteria for successful organ preservation:

The life of the perfused tissue depends on many factors. The fluid must be free from floating particles that may act as emboli. If blood is used there should be no agglutinated corpuscles. The temperature, the osmotic pressure, pH of the fluid, the pulse rate, the maximum pressure and the minimum pressure have to be exactly adjusted. The chemical composition of the nutrient medium and its oxygenation are of capital importance. Moreover, it is imperative that the organ be free from all bacteria. Even if all the conditions save one are satisfactory the result of the experiment is utter failure.[38]

The two perfusionists appeared on the cover of *Time* magazine in 1935, but shortly afterward, Lindbergh left for Britain, and Carrel did not follow through on this organ culture work. Carrel was now increasingly out of favor with the Rockefeller Institute's new director, Herbert Glasser, who was, ironically, a former colleague of C. C. Guthrie, who had quarreled earlier

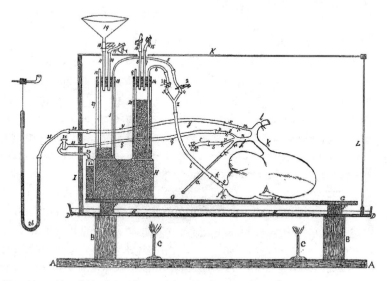

In the 1880s, Henry Newell Martin, working at Johns Hopkins, used a perfusion apparatus to study the mammalian heart outside the body. From *The Physiological Papers of H. Newell Martin* (1895).

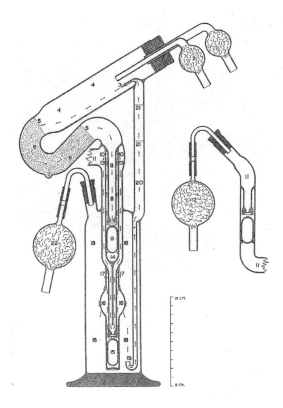

Charles A. Lindbergh, the famous aviator, took up research in the Rockefeller Institute laboratory of Alexis Carrel. He designed a new sterile organ perfusion pump, as shown in this illustration from A. Carrel and C. A. Lindbergh, *The Culture of Organs* (New York: Hoeber, 1938).

with Carrel. Carrel retired in 1939 and moved to occupied France, where he headed a sociology institute in Paris, lavishly funded by the collaborationist Vichy government, with the remit to improve the French nation. Carrel died in 1944 in occupied Paris before much was accomplished, and allegations of his collaboration with the Nazis were not pursued thereafter.

Interest in organ preservation by perfusion did not reappear until the mid-1960s, when the needs of the newly successful human kidney transplantation service meant that organ perfusion and preservation returned to research agendas.

An End to Confusion

By the end of the 1930s, some order began to appear in clinical transplantation circles. There was now a retreat from the renewed idea that unmodified homografts could survive, largely as a result of a stance taken by the St. Louis surgical school under the influence of Leo Loeb. When he had been unknowingly using incompletely inbred rats, Loeb had wavered on whether identical human twins would reject each other's grafts, but Loeb

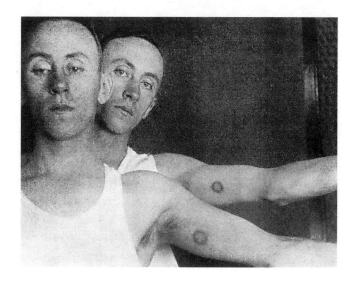

James Barrett Brown successfully grafted skin from one identical twin to the other in 1937. From J. B. Brown, "Homografting of Skin: With Report of Success in Identical Twins," *Surgery* 1 (1937): 558–63.

had found his error and corrected it. After that problem was solved and corrected, Earl Padgett and James Barrett Brown in St. Louis went back to work on the twins issue and reported that skin grafts exchanged between twins were indeed successful. This simple finding, apparently self-evident in retrospect, was essential in signaling the end to a decade of confusion.[39]

However, others outside the perceptive surgical units still had lingering affection for the use of homografts. And one very old idea was to make one final, embarrassing, high-profile appearance. Astonishingly, in 1940, a Washington surgeon, R. E. Moran, attempted the "slave-donor" procedure, attributed to Tagliacozzi in the 1600s. Moran joined a young boy to his badly burned but blood-type compatible cousin using a pedicle skin flap. The graft failed, and serious complications and litigation followed. The case became celebrated in the medico-legal worlds, but not because of the deplorable surgery. The legal action, reported as *Bonner v. Moran,* was on the grounds that proper permission from the young donor's family had not been sought. This famous case established the necessity for informed consent for surgery, particularly in children.[40]

With World War II imminent, a further rapid readjustment of research attitudes and high policy was about to occur. The practical needs of war were once again to influence the debate on the best way of procuring innovation in medical science, and practical surgical projects would return to favor. While Britain fought the war, a short-term surgical research study on a common injury, carried out in a busy hospital burns unit, was to be important in the development of transplantation immunology.

9 Understanding the Mechanism

THE EMERGENCE of a new and lasting interest in tissue transplantation is usually dated to 1943, the year of publication of a reinvestigation by the surgeon Tom Gibson and biologist Peter Medawar. Entitled "The Fate of Skin Homografts in Man," this *Journal of Anatomy* paper emerged from studies at the Royal Infirmary in Glasgow.[1] The conclusion from this careful work reaffirmed that homografts in general did not survive and that the mechanism of graft loss was an immunological one, a view now regarded as self-evident but one that was not yet widely accepted then. Their central finding was that after loss of a first set of skin grafts, the survival time of a second set of grafts taken from the same donor was shorter than on the first attempt. This change in tempo showed that an immunological mechanism was at work. The study was so carefully described, and with such convincing detail, that, together with Medawar's later extensive studies in experimental animals, the wider surgical and biological worlds were prepared to accept the paradigm.

This study of skin grafts had been stimulated by the pattern of combat injuries among members of the British Royal Air Force in World War II. Some American plastic surgeons were posted to Britain in the early phase of the war, and, as a result, they also took up an interest in skin homografting and transplantation in general, studies that were to continue long after the war was over. These plastic surgeons were to influence and sustain the revival of tissue grafting studies in the United States.

Wartime Burns

World War II brought a new degree of central direction to Britain's affairs and new priorities in medical research. In this collectivist atmosphere, the national research interests were diverted toward matters of immediate clinical use. And it was from a government-directed study of a mundane type of injury, one of little intellectual interest in peacetime, that insights of considerable consequence into tissue transplantation arose. The problem of burns was of interest to the wartime government because of the number and severity of such injuries suffered by the armed forces in this war. Increased mechanization of warfare, including aerial combat, meant that fighter pilots often suffered burns from fires in the aircraft's single engine, often situated in front of the cockpit. The Battle of Britain and aerial battles over France resulted in about four thousand burn cases, of which six hundred were severe. Earlier naval accidents also had serious fires, notably in the HMS *Furious* disaster, and in a fire involving a North Sea convoy in 1941. When the *Lancastria* was sunk during the Saint-Nazaire evacuation of British troops from France in 1940, large numbers of service men were also badly burned.

After the Battle of Britain, involving a defensive aerial conflict fought on the south coast of England in August and September 1940, British pilots who suffered burns required not only emergency treatment but also plastic surgery, and various military and civilian hospitals in southern England provided such treatment.

The British Medical Research Council (MRC) organized a new War Wounds Subcommittee, which prioritized the study of burns, and the council also launched a journal called the *Bulletin of War Medicine*. For the war effort, the MRC's "basic science only" policy was forgotten; trauma surgery, a lowly Cinderella among the glamorous specialties, quickly rose to prominence.

For assistance, a Burns Subcommittee turned to Oxford University in June 1941. J.M.Barnes, at Oxford's Radcliffe Infirmary, was appointed to be a research "burns officer," and it was agreed locally that he have charge of all burns cases admitted to that hospital. Barnes and Peter Medawar, as well as Jean Taylor (later to be Jean Medawar), had earlier been brought in by Howard Florey, the talented Australian head of the university's Department of Pathology, in his plan to make a concerted investigation of the mysterious lymphocyte.[2] Barnes was to study the enigmatic thoracic duct outflow, and Medawar and Taylor were to study lymphocytes in isolation. An additional experiment was to study the effect of total surgical removal of the lymphoid tissue in the rat. After inconclusive results from the lymphocyte studies and concerns about both the completeness and unpleasantness of the rat surgery, this grand project on the lymphocyte came to nothing. Only decades later did Florey and James Gowans successfully revive this interest.

Florey instead moved on to his celebrated work on inflammatory responses, and when war started, he assisted in the triumphant Oxford penicillin research.[3] Medawar had also moved away from the lymphocyte work, looking at growth-promoting substances, notably in attempting to increase the regeneration speed of peripheral nerves.[4]

Via his link with Barnes, Medawar was interested in the treatment of burns after an incident in Oxford in 1940 during the Battle of Britain, which he later described:

Early in the war, an R.A.F. Whitley bomber crashed into a house in North Oxford with much serious injury and loss of life. Among the injured was a young man with a third degree burn extending over about 60% of his body. People burned as severely as this had never raised a medical problem before—they always died: but the blood transfusion services and the control of infection made possible by the topical use of sulfonamide drugs now made it possible for them to stay alive. Dr John F. Barnes, a colleague of mine in Professor H. W. Florey's School of Pathology, asked me to see this patient in the hope that being an experimental biologist I might have some ideas for treatment. With more than half his body surface quite raw, this poor young man was a deeply shocking sight; I thought of and tried out a number of ingenious methods, none of which worked, for eking out his own skin for grafting, trying to make one piece of skin do the work of ten or more. . . . I believe I saw it as my metier to find out why it was not possible to graft skin from one human being to another, and what could be done about it.[5]

Barnes gave Medawar a little task. Medawar was to write a report to the new Burns Subcommittee of the MRC on the controversy surrounding one form of burn management, namely, the use of tannic acid as an immediate form of treatment. This unpleasant substance, used to harden leather, was applied to the burns, and the area was then dried with a hair dryer.[6] This "tanning" procedure was an attempt to create an impenetrable layer on the surface of the burn, hoping to exclude infection and limit fluid loss. It was also believed to fix the illusive "wound toxins" alleged to be responsible for the sometimes serious systemic consequences of burns.

This dubious method was widely used to treat burns among civilians, but when "tanning" was in regular use during the war, increasing criticism of the method emerged. The new pattern of burns among the Battle of Britain pilots affected primarily the face and hands, and experience with the use of tannic acid on eyelids and fingers showed that it led to troublesome skin contractures later. Eyelids were deformed, spillage onto the eyes damaged the cornea, and tight bands of scar tissue could form around finger bases. Moreover, it was now realized that absorption of tannic acid could damage the liver.

At the MRC War Wounds Subcommittee, Medawar's report on tannic acid was considered. It was the first time that the group had had direct contact with him, and they were impressed.[7] Shortly afterward, the mood turned against the use of tannic acid, and official government advice to military surgeons then recommended the use of simpler dressings.

After the Battle of Britain and its flood of casualties, the German plan for invasion of Britain was postponed, and Hitler turned his attention to the east instead. The major air battles over Britain ceased, though bombing continued. New military burns were now encountered much less often, and, late in 1941, the MRC received a cautious report on the burn studies at Oxford. In the first year of the MRC study at Oxford, only twenty-five cases of burns of more than 10 percent of body surface had been admitted. The only success to report from Oxford was the first exciting use of its laboratory's new penicillin, applied topically to these cases, with success.

During this difficult time, Medawar soon had an opportunity to study burns at the military hospital at Basingstoke, forty miles due south of Oxford. There, the MRC's man was one of the council's favorite scientists, Leonard Colebrook (1883–1967), the distinguished bacteriologist, who had studied under Almroth Wright. Having published on skin homografting of unhealed wounds from World War I injuries, Wright was an expert in the study of hospital infection in general, and of antibacterial therapy in particular. He had also written the classic early studies on the use of sulfonamide drugs, notably prontosil.[8]

In the early part of World War II, Colebrook was in France, but after evacuation from Dunkirk, he was posted to Basingstoke to study the treatment of burns in the wards of the Plastic Surgery Centre at Rooksdown House, Park Prewett Hospital. There, the senior London surgeon Harold Gillies (1882–1960) headed one of three British units set up in 1939 to deal with civilian cases from air raids on London and casualties from the army and navy.[9] Gillies's reputation came from his experience in World War I when, together with T. P. Kilner, he had dealt with the severe facial wounds resulting from trench warfare. His 1920 text, *Plastic Surgery of the Face,* based on his World War I experiences, was a classic. By 1923, Gillies and Kilner had completed the treatment of all the World War I veterans. For plastic surgery they managed to obtain an occasional hospital bed, and they made a start on private cosmetic surgery. In the 1930s, they were joined by two younger men, Archibald McIndoe (1900–1960) and Rainsford Mowlem, bringing Britain's total number of plastic surgeons to four.[10] In World War II, McIndoe was in charge of one of the other wartime hospital units, at East Grinstead, where the Royal Air Force injured were treated.[11]

At Gillies's unit at Basingstoke, Colebrook pursued his favorite research on infection of burns and the use of antibacterial agents. He also began to seek help with his earlier interest in the use of human homograft skin, for which he had lingering affection. In August 1940, during the Battle of Britain, he had again written to the MRC about his old favorite treatment and that he considered it important once again "to get all knowledge we can about skin grafting, which I used a good deal and wrote about in the last war." Colebrook seemed unaware that the surgical world had accepted the stance taken by Loeb and the St. Louis plastic surgeons that homografting was useless. However, there had been no comparable studies in Europe.

Colebrook looked for help and contacted Medawar at Oxford.[12] Visiting Basingstoke, Medawar obtained leftover human skin from Gillies, and his work with it resulted in a paper describing a method of splitting the two layers of skin, thus providing areas of epidermis alone.[13] He tried to make extra skin by subdividing and culturing fragments or scraping cells off to make an epidermal "soup." Gillies commented that the methods produced no visible tissue on a burn, at least "not to the eyes of a senior surgeon."

Also working with Gillies at Basingstoke was John Marquis Converse (1909–1981), an American plastic surgeon who had been educated in Paris and was working with the Red Cross there before escaping France when the war began. He then joined the Volunteer Surgical Unit of the American Hospital based at Basingstoke, headed by a New Yorker, Philip Wilson Sr. James Barrett Brown (1899–1971), of the distinguished St. Louis surgical group, became chief of plastic surgery for the U.S. Army, arriving first in Scotland by a hazardous Atlantic convoy sea journey in May 1942, before traveling to England, after a few weeks' stay.[14]

This British wartime work later influenced both of these American surgeons. When Barrett Brown returned from Europe after the war, he set up nine units to do plastic surgery, plus head and neck work, notably at Valley Forge General Hospital. Converse continued with his interest in transplantation of tissues as a result of his time in Britain, and for almost two decades after his return, he had a major influence on American transplantation research, a period in which it was closely associated with plastic surgery.[15]

At Basingstoke, Colebrook was primarily interested in infection and skin grafts to treat burns. But Colebrook and the MRC were frustrated in moving ahead with these plans since they no longer had new combat burn cases to treat and the numbers of civilian cases at Oxford were still low. With this dearth, they took advice on where a large number of such patients might be observed. The answer came back that their base should be in Scotland, in Glasgow's largest hospital.

Glasgow Burns Unit

Specialist surgical units in Britain were few, but the Burns Unit in Glasgow Royal Infirmary had evolved in the 1930s as a result of local need. By the 1940s, it treated one thousand burn cases per year, of which two hundred were severe.[16] On the research side, the hospital bacteriologist Robert Cruikshank had made important observations in 1936 on the role of streptococcal cross-infection in burns.[17] Local biochemist David Cuthbertson had made crucial observations on the metabolic response to injury. The MRC sounded out its contacts in Glasgow, notably Cuthbertson, but found that the surgical side of the Royal Infirmary "lacked a scientific outlook." The "visiting surgeon" to this nonacademic unit in the early 1940s was a Mr. Alfred Clark, who seldom attended, as was the style in pre–National Health Service times.[18]

The MRC finally determined that a young surgeon named Thomas "Tom" Gibson (1915–1993), who had "sound judgment and [was] able to assess results critically," was working in a unit headed by Charles Illingworth on the other side of the city. The MRC signed him on as a fellow, and he started work in March 1942.[19] Gibson later recalled some of the attitudes about homografting in those days. Some months before moving to his new post, he had witnessed the use of human foreskin grafting, persisting from the 1920s, and used in patients with chronic leg ulcers:

At this time there was an astonishingly widespread belief that they [homografts] were as good or almost as good as autografts. When I had been Resident with the Professor of Medicine [Sir John McNee] a year or so previously, he had in his ward a lady with a large gravitational ulcer. To graft this, I was sent to the Out Patient Clinic of the Sick Children's Hospital on their "circumcision day" to collect the snipped off foreskins in a "Thermos" flask. After a dash back to the ward the foreskins were opened out and applied to the ulcer. Without exception they all came away with the first dressing. "Ah! Infection!" the Professor said.[20]

After setting up his MRC unit in Glasgow, Colebrook reported back that, at last, he had plenty of burns to study. The main thrust of the new unit's research was infection and the development of new therapeutic creams, as part of the eternal search for the best means of treating fresh burns.[21] In March 1942, Colebrook managed to get some penicillin, and the first supplies of plasma that arrived were quickly exhausted. Gibson at this time also helped produce an instructional film on the treatment of burns.[22]

Gibson was busy with skin grafting, and although he was personally skeptical about homograft survival, his director was not. This situation gave the surgeon a chance to experiment and observe regular loss of such grafts. Perhaps curious about the mechanism, Gibson carried out a crucial "second set" grafting well before Medawar's arrival, and he published details of the case much later.[23] The unit soon had some visitors, notably Harold Gillies from Basingstoke, who toured Scotland, including the salmon rivers, and reported to the MRC on the Scottish surgical units and the shifting policy on burn treatments:

It is evident that the tan [tannic acid] diehards like Learmonth [professor of surgery in Edinburgh] and Wilson [professor of surgery in Aberdeen] are beginning to slough under the edge of their crusts. It is almost universally felt that the severe treatment meted out to that Aberdeen convoy of severe cases [of burns] was not justifiable. There is grave doubt in most people's mind of the value of plasma treatment. The visit to the Glasgow Royal Infirmary Burn Unit made a deep impression on me. No plasma is ever given, no general anaesthetic ever administered. . . . The absence of shock was a very noticeable feature. They never have any late deaths.[24]

This was a bizarre and misleading report from a senior, conservative London surgeon—commendably antitanning, but also antiplasma and antianesthesia, which were both routinely used in the unit.

Another reported visit to the burn unit is an intriguing one and gave rise to one of the research priority disputes that emerged after the Gibson-Medawar work gained renown.[25] After Brown arrived in May 1942, he spent a professionally profitable three weeks in Glasgow, just after Gibson's "second set" experiment. Much later, when the Gibson-Medawar work gained fame, Brown's supporters suggested, and still do, that Brown had been first to suggest the second set study.

At this time, with Gibson installed and busy with skin grafts, Colebrook kept in touch with Medawar in Oxford. Medawar still had hopes of finding ways to expand the area of donor skin, and it seems he had also resolved to do a careful study of homografting. He then wrote to the MRC asking for support, and the secretary wrote to Colebrook in Glasgow, reporting that "I have been speaking to Medawar about his skin homografts and although he is not very optimistic, he would like to make a more extended trial than is possible at Oxford. . . . It was obvious that he wants to work with you. It would be good to get the question of homografts settled."[26]

In order to accomplish his research goals, Medawar needed access to a busy surgical unit that handled skin grafts and had a staff willing to try homografting in a manner suitable for scientific study of graft loss. The Glasgow Burns Unit suited his purpose well. Gibson was grafting burns regularly, with both autografts and homografts, happy that his director still took the view that these grafts were an ethical therapy. Colebrook himself was still trying to link homograft loss to infection, and he reported "five or six grafting experiments each week." His diary records some setbacks: "Homografts on Cheshire, Jean Murray, and Rourke all appeared to be taking well. . . . But later after about three weeks the new epithelium, which had almost covered Cheshire and Rourke suddenly began to disappear without any change in the bacterial flora and in a few days all was gone."[27] The grafts had in fact been rejected. Colebrook agreed to have Medawar work at the Glasgow Burns Unit for two months.[28]

Medawar's Support

Medawar was prepared to do all the necessary laboratory work himself, as no help was available, and he obtained money to buy extra equipment for tissue fixation, microtomy, and staining. He arrived on July 1, 1942. On July 2 there was a meeting of the group—Medawar, Gibson, Colebrook, and John Blacklock, a pathologist.[29]

Colebrook listed the plan for Medawar's research visit:

1. Do stored or mucinase-treated homografts last longer than untreated ones?
2. Can cell suspensions of donor skin give more extensive skin cover?
3. Are amnion, or blister skin or frozen section grafts useful?
4. A study of regular biopsy of skin homografts at intervals after grafting.[30]

This agenda included ideas relating to autograft skin use from Medawar's unfinished Basingstoke studies, to which he added the study of homograft skin biopsies. No second set grafting was planned at this meeting. It seems that it was Gibson who interested Medawar in that topic when the chance to study another case appeared soon after.

The new case was a badly burned twenty-two-year-old woman who had nearly died after admission and remained unwell for some time.[31] Forty-one days after admission, the large granulated area was judged ready for grafting. More importantly for the study, Gibson found a donor of skin in the patient's family, and this brother was not only willing to give skin on one occasion under general anesthesia but to repeat the donation about two weeks later.

Numerous grafts—autografts as well as homografts—were applied not as sheets but as multiple "pinch" grafts, and these were sampled for Medawar's microscopy study. The overall result was clear, but the detail of their "second set" study is more complex than sometimes described. The first set of grafts was lost between fifteen and twenty-three days. The "second set" of homografts was placed, not after the first set was lost, but instead at two weeks after the first grafting. This second set was also lost at the same time as the longest survivors of the first set. The second set thus survived eight to ten days.

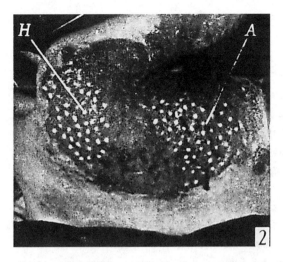

This photograph of Gibson and Medawar's multiple skin grafts shows the first and second set homografts (H) and autografts (A) in place on the large burn and available for regular biopsy. From T. Gibson and P. B. Medawar, "The Fate of Skin Homografts in Man," *Journal of Anatomy* 77 (1943): 299–310.

The histological features Medawar described in detail in "The Fate of Skin Homografts in Man" indicated that, during graft loss, the first set of grafts showed little cellular infiltrate and the second had even fewer cells. The conclusion was that an accelerated pace of second set loss had been demonstrated and that an immunological response was being observed. As a tribute to the Gibson-Medawar analysis, accelerated cell-mediated responses in general are often termed the "second set" reaction.

The Gibson-Medawar Report

Three mysteries still surround the results Gibson and Medawar reported in their historic 1943 paper. The first is that first human skin homografts usually survive for only ten to twelve days, and the much longer time noted in this study suggests that either the patient and her brother had an identical tissue match (Loeb's Law sets those odds at 1 in 4) or that the still-debilitated, burned, untransfused patient at six weeks after admission was a poor immunological reactor as a result of the ordeal.[32] Second, the unimpressive cellular infiltrate reported in the grafts was very unusual and also suggests some recipient immunosuppression or fortuitous matching. Third, the early application of the second set of grafts before the loss of the first set is quite unlike the usual late testing for immunological memory.

In the discussion section of their famous 1943 paper, Gibson and Medawar outlined the two rival theories of transplantation immunity then current. They first cited Loeb's support for a lymphocyte-mediated mechanism of attack. They wrongly assumed the attack on the graft to be a local tissue reaction, not a blood-borne mechanism, the authors being deeply conditioned by the view that lymphocytes did not move about in the body. They contrasted this cellular explanation with the second option—an antibody response. Since they found little cellular infiltrate in the first set of grafts and none in the second set, they concluded, not unreasonably, that "no evidence was found that the breakdown of foreign skin epithelium was brought about by or accompanied by a local reaction on the part of lymphocytes or other mesenchymal cells. The accelerated regression of the second set of homografts suggests that the destruction of the foreign epidermis was brought about by a mechanism of active immunisation. Our results are not inconsistent with the idea that the mechanism responsible for the liquidation of homologous epithelium is humoral rather than cellular."[33]

Gibson took this further and recalled later that he started to look for the antibody: "I injected my buttocks at intervals with finely chopped skin from the same donor and with the help of a grumpy and less than cooperative bacteriologist tried to fix complement with a mixture of skin and my own serum. I was saved from more such foolery by being conscripted into the Royal Army Medical Corps."[34]

Colebrook remained unconvinced about the findings and conclusions of his young colleagues and persisted in his belief that infection rather than rejection was a general cause of skin graft loss. In Colebrook's final detailed report to the MRC two years later, there is no mention of the skin graft work, nor was the now famous *Journal of Anatomy* paper of 1943 listed. In Colebrook's book on the treatment of burns, published much later, in 1950, he was still in denial, repeating his advocacy for homografting.[35]

After his research trip to Glasgow, Medawar returned to Oxford, and he and Gibson wrote up their paper in the *Journal of Anatomy*.[36] The paper makes clear that Gibson had done an earlier "second set" experiment and that Gibson was responsible for the analysis suggesting that active immunity was involved.[37] This was an intriguing, creditable, and productive partnership of the laboratory and the clinic at the dawn of the rapid growth in studies of transplantation immunology, one in which surgeons and scientists were to form a close and long-lasting relationship. The genesis of the project was a clinical problem—the need for successful skin grafts—along with the need for a new look at the old claims for successful homografts. A pragmatic surgeon (Gibson) gained the assistance of the scientist (Medawar), each making contributions from their own skills and disciplines to make important advances via individual agendas. The old-fashioned views of their director were of service on this occasion, rather than a hindrance.

Tom Gibson's Career

The subsequent concerns and careers of Gibson and Medawar differed. To Gibson, the plastic surgeon, their careful work was the final proof that donor-to-patient human skin grafting was, as they both suspected, of no immediate utility. Unlike the visiting American plastic surgeons, Gibson turned his attention and talents to other matters, and in doing so he shared the negative attitude in British plastic surgery circles at that time regarding the future of transplantation—namely that tissue incompatibility and graft rejection were basic biological mechanisms that could not be thwarted. The contrast with the views of American plastic surgeons and their journals at the time is striking.

However, in Glasgow, Ian McGregor (1921–1998), one of Gibson's surgical assistants, did take up this unpopular theme while working with Raymond Scothorne (1920–2007) in the Department of Anatomy at the University of Glasgow.[38] The department had studied cartilage, bone, and corneal grafting, and McGregor made important experimental observations on the reactive changes in local lymph nodes adjacent to rejecting skin grafts, identifying the important cellular proliferation in what was later called the thymus-dependent area.[39]

Medawar's Career

To Medawar, the zoologist, the Glasgow experience was also final and convincing evidence that homograft skin was doomed to be lost through an immune response. But, back in Oxford, he decided that unraveling and understanding the homograft response was a major intellectual challenge, so he abandoned his studies on nerve regeneration.[40] Medawar then submitted to the *Bulletin of War Medicine* in 1943 a short review on the "homograft problem," including an assessment of the literature on the subject. As before, he dismissed Leo Loeb's cellular/lymphocyte theory of graft loss and highlighted the St. Louis scientist's unfortunate terminology.[41] Medawar dismissed, on very flimsy grounds, Loeb's correct insistence on the role of the lymphocyte since lymphocytes were notably absent from the Glasgow patient's skin grafts.

Medawar for many years thereafter attributed graft loss to an antibody. There was some pressure to do so, since, if reemergent transplantation immunological studies were to gain respectability in the immunological big tent, the entry ticket was an identifiable antibody. True, there were other puzzling instances of "missing antibody," conspicuously so in tuberculosis and some skin allergies, but these gaps might be ignored as mysteries awaiting detection of a more subtle antibody. Medawar soon dominated thinking in transplantation immunology, and those now attracted by the subject bowed to his choice of an antibody-mediated mechanism as the basis of the homograft response. But this lasted only for a decade, before the Murphy-Loeb cellular explanation was revived and accepted.

Controversies over the Gibson-Medawar Paper

When the Gibson-Medawar *Journal of Anatomy* paper began to achieve recognition as the starting point of the modern era of tissue transplantation, and particularly when Medawar was awarded a Nobel Prize in 1960, some muted controversies arose over the events plus claims to priority.[42] In Britain, some of Gibson's surgical colleagues believed that he had been written out of the story. In America, others claimed that Converse had been Medawar's mentor in matters immunological. Another view was that James Barrett Brown, the St. Louis surgeon, upon arriving in England from the United States, had suggested the second set experiment to Medawar before Medawar went to Glasgow. A more interesting assertion is that Brown encouraged Gibson to proceed when Brown passed through Glasgow in May 1942 on his way south. Brown and his colleague Frank McDowell had advocated this "second set" test of transplantation immunity in a lecture they gave in the United States about that time. However, the chronology of these contacts, and other evidence, leaves the surgical priority in publication with Gibson. McDowell also informed his associates that Medawar's Nobel Prize had been an error; he had apparently forgotten that the award was instead for Medawar's later demonstration of immunological tolerance.

Medawar in Oxford

In 1943, Medawar applied for a Medical Research Council grant to study "why grafts are lost," and the council decided to support him as a scientist of promise. There was no further opportunity in Oxford to study human burns, and Oxford professor L. J. Witts had pulled out of this link with the MRC since "he found the [burns] work irksome." Medawar's work was thereafter entirely experimental. As a scientist, though, he had been unusually close to the surgical need and the surgical wards, and clinical relevance in his studies remained important to him.

Scientifically, it was solitary work for Medawar. As the only scientist with this interest, he patiently set the agenda and methodology for the growth thereafter of transplantation immunology. Academic immunol-

UNIVERSITY COLLEGE LONDON
DEPARTMENT OF ZOOLOGY

Telephone : EUSton 7050
Professor P. B. Medawar

GOWER STREET WC1

27 Oct

My dear Tom,

Your letter has just arrived, and I'm answering it at once, because none has given me such pleasure. Although under the terms of the Nobel Foundation the award has to be for some one specific thing, in this case tolerance, I know that what lies behind it (in my case) is the work we started together in those old days at the Royal Infirmary — and I do want you to know how clearly I understand my deep obligation to you for giving me my first insight into the _real_ problem we were facing, and my

A letter from Peter Medawar to Thomas Gibson in 1960, after Medawar was awarded a Nobel Prize, recalling their earlier work. Image from the Thomas Gibson Papers, courtesy of the Library of the Royal College of Physicians and Surgeons of Glasgow.

ogy at the time meant study of antibodies, and an exciting immunological milieu was developing in the 1940s, resulting from discoveries revealed by hapten chemistry and the fruitful "lock and key" models of antibody action.[43] Studying skin graft rejection and pointing to its cause as being an immune reaction with no known antibody seemed to be a relic from the prescientific era. From the immunologists came calls to "find the antibody." Medawar was later to say that development and acceptance of transplantation immunity was inhibited by the "tyranny of the antibody," a despotism that he accepted for a decade or more.[44] In continuing with the study of the messy business of skin graft rejection in outbred rabbits, he was also shunning the conventional wisdom offered from the immunology labs, namely, to use inbred animals, or better still, become respectable and adopt reductionist models in simple "test tube" situations.

In his relative isolation, Medawar could proceed with painstaking, unhurried scholarship. As he conducted his experimental work, he wisely showed little interest in the special cases of bone or cartilage grafts, nor was he distracted by the "privileged sites," where grafts could survive in seclusion, topics that would divert the attention of other researchers. Medawar stuck to the use of outbred animals and used the awkward "second set" re-

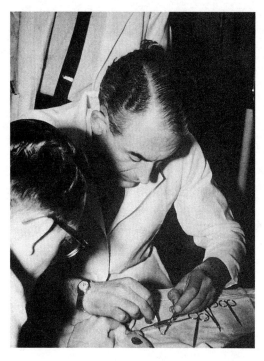

Peter Medawar's experimental skin grafting work, which arose from his earlier interest and experience with practical surgical problems, was unusual for a scientist at that time.

sponse to detect the presence or absence of tissue antigens, concluding that in rabbits at least seven were responsible for rejection.[45] He added the important findings that all tissue could immunize to future skin grafts, and hence that the antigens responsible were found in most cells of the body. His work during this period was described in a number of papers, since there was no obvious journal to take such publications. The *Journal of Anatomy* had taken the Glasgow paper largely because it was the usual publication place for Oxford work, and for a while Medawar submitted his papers to this prestigious journal. As time passed, his papers began appearing in a variety of general biology publications; significantly, they did not appear in any of the serology-leaning immunological journals. Nor did Medawar's early scientific papers cite any work published in prestigious outlets like the *Journal of Immunology*. There was no need to—there were no transplantation papers to quote.

Medawar at Birmingham

Medawar's research continued at Oxford until 1947, when, at the age of thirty-two, he moved to the University of Birmingham as professor of zoology. There, Medawar formed a small research group, and the first colleague to join him was Rupert Billingham. At this time, Medawar's applied transplantation research briefly ceased, perhaps meeting an impasse when he cautiously suggested that "free antibody is not a sufficient explanation of the regression of skin homografts."[46] However, the transplant work continued in Oxford, carried on by his pupil, Avrion Mitchison, who was soon to make fundamental contributions and restore the Murphy-Loeb proposal of the lymphocyte as the main effector in graft rejection.[47] In 1950, the Birmingham group returned, with success, to Medawar's original interest in "actively acquired immunity." About this time he started, perhaps reluctantly, to use inbred mouse strains.[48]

Medawar also added lasting precision to the discourse of transplantation. "Actively acquired immunity" was the helpful term he regularly used to explain tissue loss. The literature of the early 1950s still had numerous terms in use for graft loss, such as "disintegration," "absorption," "necrosis," "destruction," "sloughing," "death," or "dissolution," and Medawar used "breakdown" until 1951. At the first conference on transplantation, held by the New York Academy of Sciences in 1954, the committee proposed standardizing usage in the literature and chose "disintegration" for skin graft loss and favored "arrest" in reference to vascularized organ grafts, but these words did not find favor. Instead the use of "rejection"—with its powerful, helpful metaphor of an active, even sad and regrettable response—crept into regular and permanent use by the transplant community in the early 1950s.[49]

Immunology Expands

A small group interested in transplantation biology began to emerge in the early 1950s, but they had neither lineage nor organizational cohesion. They had no regular meetings, no dedicated scientific society, and no journal in which they could routinely publish their work. Some, like Medawar, had zoology training but were not conventional zoologists; others were pathologists but not active in mainstream pathology. These pioneers were soon joined by still other specialists, including hematologists and surgeons, who turned away from respectable mainstream interests. Members of this scattered group, though pursuing immunological studies, were not regarded as career immunologists, and they therefore had awkward positions in academic departments and a barely respectable niche in the life sciences.

But infectious diseases, the traditional area for immunological research, were declining in the industrialized nations, and the new antibiotics sharply reduced mortality from them. The immunologists had to widen their horizons, and this new area of transplantation began to attract some research workers. But in America, in the interim, it was the plastic surgeons who kept up the interest in tissue grafting.

Involved Surgeons

The American plastic surgeons who had visited Britain during World War II, notably James Barrett Brown and John Marquis Converse, had taken back with them an interest in skin homografting, Converse returned to New York in 1946 and set up a transplantation laboratory at New York University, obtaining the aid of the philanthropist Aida Breckinridge, who was already supporting a drive to encourage eye donation, after death, for corneal grafting. Another influential East Coast plastic surgeon was Herbert

Conway (1905–1970), who had military experience in the Pacific war and, after settling at the New York Hospital, began publishing on skin graft rejection in 1951. Another active institution was the Halloran Hospital at Staten Island, where Blair Rogers and Darrel T. Shaw treated many veterans. While transplantation research in America was closely associated with plastic surgery for some time, ironically, human skin in the end proved to be the least amenable human tissue for transplantation, and it was not used routinely until long after kidney, liver, and heart grafting was routine. Converse made attempts, all unsuccessful, to draw leading American serology-leaning immunologists into this field and was rebuffed even by the Rockefeller Institute, earlier made famous by Carrel and Murphy.

In 1949, Blair Rogers (1923–2006) joined Converse in New York, and they expanded the experimental work on homograft rejection at Columbia University.[50] Converse and Rogers initially opposed the acquired immunity hypothesis, claiming that Medawar's animal model was flawed, and they could not confirm the second set phenomenon in humans. The difficulty was that rejection times were normally fast, quite unlike the slow-paced rejection that aided the Gibson-Medawar study in a badly burned patient. However, Rogers persevered, and, in difficult skin grafting studies with human volunteers at Bellevue Hospital in New York from 1950, he concluded that second grafts from the same human donor were indeed lost more quickly than the first grafts. Rogers worked hard to maintain some professional links with the surgeons of the Soviet Union, notably those active in organ grafting, and, in this unpopular action at this difficult time, Eleanor Roosevelt encouraged and assisted him.

The American journal *Plastic and Reconstructive Surgery* emerged in 1946 and had an interest in transplantation from the first. Converse served on the council of the New York Academy of Sciences, and, through his advocacy, the historic biennial transplantation conferences of this society began in 1954. Rogers and Converse served as coeditors of the proceedings, a role they fulfilled well into the era when transplantation had moved into the sphere of general surgeons.

Thus, the situation in America was the mirror image of Britain. Each nation had strength in either transplantation biology or transplant surgery, but not both. For a while, continental Europe had strength in neither area.

Another link in the American evolution of transplantation studies also came from concerns about noncombat burn injuries. In Boston in 1942, a fire in the crowded and ill-designed Cocoanut Grove nightclub killed 498 people, and a further 114 badly burned survivors were treated at the Massachusetts General Hospital nearby.[51] One of the doctors involved, Francis D. Moore, was later chief of surgery at the nearby Peter Bent Brigham

Hospital, where and he and George Thorn made classic studies on metabolic changes in disease, including acute and chronic renal failure, and obtained an early supply of the new steroid hormones.[52] They supported the early use at Brigham of Willem Kolff's artificial kidney, and Moore encouraged the famous attempts at human kidney transplantation there, which began in the 1950s.

General Surgeons and Transplants

In Britain in the early 1950s, Medawar's first and strongest surgical supporter was Michael F. A. Woodruff (1911–2001), a generalist surgeon then working in Aberdeen and later moving to the chair of surgery in the University of Edinburgh. In the United States, William P. Longmire Jr. (1913–2003) was the first in mainstream general surgery to take up transplantation studies.[53] Longmire had trained at the Johns Hopkins School of Medicine under Harvey Stone, who had attempted parathyroid grafting in the 1930s, and the two had begun publishing on skin grafting in 1947.[54] In 1951, Longmire moved to California and was a founder of the new medical school of the University of California at Los Angeles. He opened a research laboratory in the Beverly Hills area with enthusiastic fundraising assistance from Hollywood celebrities, and one of the first appointments, to a lowly post, was Paul Terasaki, soon to be a distinguished pioneer in tissue typing. Longmire helpfully clarified the language and the muddled thinking of some at this time. He firmly distinguished between what he called "homostatic" grafts—namely, transferred tissue in which the inert matrix usefully survived but the cells were lost (bone, cartilage, and fascia, for example)—and the "homovital" grafts, that is, those in which the cells survived and might be subject to rejection.

The Swiss Twins

The growing acceptance among biologists of the view that there was invariable rejection of homograft skin was now reflected in a legal judgment. In 1947, Sir Archibald McIndoe, a plastic surgeon, was asked to consider the puzzle posed by three six-year-old children in the Swiss town of Fribourg. The parents of a pair of nonidentical twins had noticed that another boy in the town had a striking resemblance to one of their twin boys. It turned out that all three had been born in the same hospital on the same day, and it was possible that the three had been mixed up. McIndoe showed that one of the two nonidentical twins and the third boy would accept skin grafts from each other. The court accepted that this could only mean that they were indeed identical twins.[55] This new view of human individuality also found its way into the literature of the time.

Naomi Mitchison, the novelist and mother of Avrion Mitchison, influenced by the distinguished scientists in her family, used such a situation in a short story published in the *Rationalist Annual* of 1945.[56] But no other writers of fiction were still using transplant themes. Good science had temporarily denied popular culture access to the ever-useful mother lode of literary possibilities arising from surgical claims for successful grafting. This rich seam was to open again later, however.

Myths Decline

Although the new dogma of universal homograft failure was entering into routine discourse, some scientists still had a lingering affection for the old testament, notably, that endocrine glands might be exempt from rejection. Even at the elite CIBA Foundation conference on transplantation in 1954, there were claims that tissue culturing of human parathyroid glands could make them immunologically bland by eliminating surface antigens, and the tolerant audience also had to listen to an embarrassing account of human ovary homografting.[57] But when claims for survival of testis homografts were made, this finally irked some members at the gathering. This gland-grafting paper was given by Ruth Deanesley, a coworker of A. S. Parkes at Mill Hill, both of whom were distinguished endocrinologists, better known later for developing the first methods for storing frozen cells.

Parkes told the assembly that he had found that testis homografts in outbred rats would survive indefinitely if their own testes were removed first—Halsted's mythical law—and this improbable claim annoyed William J. "Jim" Dempster, one of the new young British surgical transplant scientists. The exchange went thus:

> DEMPSTER: I presume these homografts were destroyed at some time.
> DEANESLEY: Why do you presume they were destroyed?
> DEMPSTER: Well, it's generally the case.
> DEANESLEY: But the testis homograft has the benefit of the host's anterior pituitary secretion, and grows so actively that it seems to laugh at immunological reactions.

Medawar privately rebuked Parkes after the meeting for making these improbable claims.[58]

Tedious Rebuttals

Medawar and his colleagues were regularly diverted from their own priorities to take on the tedious task of disproving such dubious claims for methods of prolonged graft survival. As well as dreary gland-grafting claims, other regular reports requiring attention were that fetal tissue, young tissue, or grafts that had been tissue cultured would not be rejected.[59] The journal *Plastic and Reconstructive Surgery* accepted such articles until 1959, as did Boston's respectable *New England Journal of Medicine*.[60] The final, long-awaited end of gland grafting as a special case came with the stern call for better science from a Boston surgeon at the Peter Bent Brigham Hospital in 1962.[61]

Eliminating such claims was important. Plans for progress in the 1950s could finally move from looking for any special dispensations to instead facing up to the difficult task of dealing with homograft rejection. The first hint that the homograft response could be modified came as the result of the availability of the precious first supplies of steroid hormones.

Steroids Emerge

Yet another influence of World War II on the development of successful transplantation was the isolation of hormones from the adrenal cortex. Rumors, never confirmed, circulated during the war that the Germans had successfully extracted these hormones, and a fanciful story came via intelligence sources in Poland's resistance that use of these hormones enabled Luftwaffe pilots to fly at very high altitude without using oxygen.[62] This matter was of wartime concern, and the National Research Council in the United States accepted the effort to isolate such hormones as a top priority. Edward Calvin Kendall's partly purified compound E had been isolated from the adrenal gland before the war. The Merck pharmaceutical company successfully continued the work, and, by 1948, it had obtained nine grams of cortisone, at a reported cost of $14 million.[63]

Two grams of this precious substance were given to R. G. Sprague of the Mayo Clinic, where Kendall worked, to treat cases of adrenal insufficiency. Philip S. Hench and Howard Polley, also doctors at the Mayo Clinic, then persuaded Sprague to give them one hundred milligrams of cortisone for treating a patient with rheumatoid arthritis, and the dramatic, immediate effect on this patient is one of the best-known "breakthrough" stories of modern medicine. It had extensive media attention in September 1948, and Hench's innovation earned him a Nobel Prize in 1950.[64] Broader indications for steroid therapy soon emerged, and wide use commenced when regular supplies became available.[65]

Production delays meant that cortisone was not available outside the United States until 1952. British physicians and scientists regarded the publicity accompanying the appearance of the new preparation with distaste, and they did not welcome a public debate on allocation of expensive, scarce, novel drugs. The medical profession and the British government accordingly approached the cortisone matter with caution. The Merck Company in the United States, aware of Britain's difficulties in making payments in dollars, and perhaps influenced by Hench's anglophile leanings, then gifted one kilogram of the steroid to Britain, agreeing that, "in view of the public clamor, no announcement would be made."[66] A joint Medical Research Council/Nuffield Foundation committee allocated the discreet supply of cortisone to those in Britain with an interest, including a rheumatoid arthritis study. When the results came through, conveniently for the authorities and the conservative physicians, this trial of cortisone in this disease appeared to show that the steroid was no more effective than aspirin. The *British Medical Journal* seemed pleased and declared that "at first high hopes were held that we had in our hands the clue to the mechanism of many obscure diseases and that we could give sufferers from them permanent relief. This prospect is fading rapidly."[67]

Criticism of both the design and analysis of the arthritis trial followed immediately in the correspondence column of the journal. But in the short term, the antisteroid mood served to lower the expectations of patients and assisted the cash-strapped postwar British National Health Service budget.[68]

Steroid Effects

But the British scientists not involved in the controversial arthritis study found that their small allocations of the gifted cortisone had some powerful biological effects. Medawar's group now returned to transplantation studies with new hope, and, joined by P. L. Krohn, an endocrinologist, they found that cortisone could prolong experimental rabbit skin grafts. American users like John Morgan in Longmire's California surgical group found the same. To add to this, unconfirmed claims were made at this time that adrenocorticotrophic hormone (ACTH), the hormone stimulating the output from the adrenal cortex, could prolong human skin graft survival indefinitely.[69] Others found that cortisone reduced antibody formation.[70] It also annulled the tuberculin skin reaction and increased susceptibility to tuberculosis in animals.[71] Other work showed that it accelerated the growth of experimental tumors.[72] Perhaps the most provocative finding was another observation from Longmire's unit in 1952, when he and Jack Cannon (born 1919) added to Morgan's findings and showed that cortisone given to newly hatched chicks would not only prolong the survival of skin grafts but that, even when the cortisone therapy was withdrawn, the grafts would survive in the longer term.[73] This, they commented modestly, was a phenomenon "which up to the present time has not been found in homograft experiments on mammals and humans."[74]

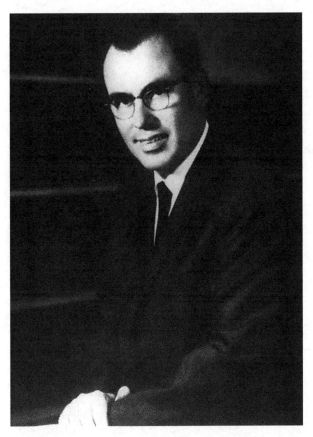

Jack Cannon, one of William Longmire's productive group at UCLA, showed that cortisone use in newly hatched chicks would greatly prolong the survival of skin grafts. Image courtesy of Thomas Starzl.

In clinical work, steroids found an important place in the treatment of a wide range of human diseases, including some serious kidney afflictions. Interestingly, at this time steroids were given in short, sharp courses only. Prolonged, continuous therapy did not fit the mindset of the day. This view derived from the holistic hope that the body needed only temporary assistance to allow its self-righting mechanisms to act and "reset" the body, thus effecting an internal cure. But when this limited-intervention paradigm was seen to fail, prolonged treatment was reluctantly accepted—signifying a major shift in attitude.

From 1951 to 1956, Medawar's group continued to publish careful work on the action of cortisone and related compounds on homograft skin rejection but still found only modest effects.[75] Krohn, working with Medawar, showed that steroids would not prolong skin graft survival in monkeys. At this time, Medawar and Woodruff reluctantly concluded, wrongly, that humans "belong to the class of poor reactors to steroids." By the mid-1950s, they had stopped studying cortisone effects on transplantation, if only because something more exciting had turned up.[76]

The steroid verdict was uncertain. In any case, the modest prolongations of graft survival in experimental animals were not considered of any "clinical relevance." A few days' gain in organ graft survival was not seen as a sign of hope warranting further studies. The assumption was that prolonged survival, obtained by one agent, possibly after a short course, would be of interest only for use in humans. The powerful and crucial effect of steroids in human transplantation, when used empirically in combination with other drugs in 1963, was to be a surprise.[77]

Immunological Tolerance

The other factor behind the waning interest in the use of steroids was an accident of history. In 1953, Medawar's group discovered a quite different, very powerful, and specific mechanism for obtaining lasting success in transplantation, namely immunological "tolerance." It was to revolutionize the approach to experimental transplantation and give hope for human organ transplantation. The apparently trivial, nonspecific effect of steroids, short lived and species variable, was no longer a research priority.

But there had been a revival of experimental organ grafting before and during the enthusiasm for steroid use and well before the discovery of immunological tolerance. Added to this, some surgeons in Boston, Paris, and elsewhere had also gone ahead with a series of attempts at human kidney transplantation in the early 1950s.

10 Experimental Organ Transplantation

A T THIS TIME IN THE LATE 1940s, some surgeons renewed their interest in experimental organ transplantation, attempting to transplant not only kidneys but also the heart. As described earlier, these efforts had started in Europe before World War I and largely ceased when the war began, but the growing interest in transplantation immunology now encouraged another look. Organ and tissue preservation now became important, and in clinical work the artificial kidney found a routine place in treating acute renal failure.

Four groups began experimental kidney transplantation studies, two in Paris, one in Denmark, and one in London. In Paris, the physician Jean Hamburger's unit reconvened after the war and reported on their experience in 1947.[1] The other group in Paris included the surgeons René Küss, J. Oudot, and J. Auvert.[2] By the early 1950s, this laboratory experience had prepared both French groups to attempt human kidney transplantation.[3] But the most detailed experimental studies were done elsewhere—by Morten Simonsen and William "Jim" Dempster.

Morten Simonsen

In Denmark, Morten Simonsen (1921–2002) started kidney grafting in 1948. Newly qualified from medical school in Copenhagen, he was fulfilling a necessary house-surgeon post in Ålborg before looking for a full-time research post. He had developed an interest in organ transplantation after a medical student friend died from chronic renal failure, and Simonsen persuaded a local surgeon to help him with some kidney grafting experiments in dogs. Simonsen then obtained a post in the university department of bacteriology in Copenhagen and continued with this unusual type of work, reporting it from 1949 to 1953. He confirmed the old finding that transplanted kidneys worked well for a while, then failed. He found that a second kidney homograft from the same donor was rejected more promptly than the first and thus supported the "acquired immunity" theory, then regaining favor, and, like others, he hoped to find the missing antibody responsible for graft loss.

Simonsen also had some extra information. He was aware of the pioneering finding by Astrid Fagraeus in Stockholm in 1947 that plasma cells were the likely producers of antibodies, and he found plasma cells (and lymphocytes) not only markedly in the rejecting kidneys but also in the host spleen at the time of graft loss. He noted that "in experiments with successive transplantations from the same donor this proliferation was even more pronounced. Adherents to the plasma cell theory for antibody production will hardly hesitate to interpret this as a sign of antibody production against the homotransplant." Although Simonsen had faith that an antibody might be found, he had some doubts and pointed again to the puzzle that some human diseases also showed clear evidence of an immune response, but without a responsible antibody: "The weakest point in the theory of acquired immunity [in explaining graft rejection] is that it never has been possible to demonstrate the active antibodies by serological means. This is a shortcoming that transplantation biology shares with eczematous allergy."[4]

Simonsen, like others at the time, was unaware that Loeb had solved the problem. Later Simonsen discovered the Murphy-Loeb work and graciously made belated amends. But the sentiment of the day, as taught by physiologists, was that lymphocytes and plasma cells were immobile, confined to the bloodstream or connective tissue. To explain the florid reaction in the graft, Simonsen resorted to a tortuous explanation. He suggested that the lymphocytes in the failing graft came from within, that is, they were *donor* lymphocytes. He proposed that these "passenger" lymphoid cells in the graft were activated and reacted against soluble *host* antigens in the blood reaching the kidney. Simonsen was wrong, and he was absolved from this error later when lymphocyte mobility was at last recognized and the simpler host invasion explanation resulted.

Simonsen's suggestion was not in vain. He went on to show later that this kind of destructive mechanism did exist elsewhere and that this graft-versus-host (GvH) reaction was important. Ironically, this component of the immune response, prominent later in clinical bone marrow transplantation, was not a major clinical feature of human organ transplantation, but had a more subtle role.[5]

William Dempster at Hammersmith

Also involved in experimental organ transplantation in the early 1950s was William J. Dempster, a surgeon in London at the Royal Postgraduate Medical School at Hammersmith Hospital, an institution then at the height of its international reputation for research and postgraduate teaching. "The Hammersmith" was a conspicuous and not uncontroversial institution, and, in the late 1930s, it had been the first place in London to start to produce clinical studies of merit, employing only full-time, research-minded medical staff who did no private practice. The school helped develop liver biopsy, cardiac catheterization, the heart-lung machine, and cardiac surgery, and it had a high media profile when separating conjoined twins. The hospital also had experience with an artificial kidney gifted to it by Willem Kolff in 1946, and the hospital's own medical regimen helped in some cases of acute renal failure.

Hammersmith's kidney transplant research was carried out some distance from London, at the Buckston Browne Research Farm at Down in Kent, an estate that had formerly been Charles Darwin's family home. This surgical facility was built in 1931 as a necessary response to the Medical Research Council's scarcely concealed coolness toward clinical research at that time. The Institution for Surgical Biological Research, as it was known then, had a cautious program of animal experimentation, and it aimed to restart surgical studies after the long European hiatus in such work.[6] In this research effort, the institution benefited from the steady decline in influence of the previously powerful British antivivisection movement, whose activities and membership had almost disappeared by the end of World War II, paradoxically at a time when there was a huge increase in animal use by biomedical research departments, the pharmaceutical and cosmetic industries, and by government entities conducting secret nuclear and biological warfare research. The public accepted at this time that animal experiments aided the rapid advance of medicine.

Transplant Work

Dempster had trained in vascular surgery under René Leriche (1879–1955), the celebrated French surgeon who had moved from Lyon to the Collège de France in Paris and had a clinical unit at the American Hospital at Neuilly. Fluent in French, Dempster could maintain links thereafter with the important developments in transplantation in France. Dempster had an unusual post at Hammersmith, which involved full-time surgical research and no clinical care of patients. In this situation, he was understandably an advocate of the philosophy that clinical challenges were to be solved first in the laboratory and then applied to the patient, a theme running through his 1957 text, *An Introduction to Experimental Surgical Studies*. He based his own transplantation work on this plan and considered that only after experimental laboratory work by scientists, notably himself, had solved the basic problems should attempts at human kidney grafting follow.

His experiments in the period from 1950 to 1955 were similar to Simonsen's, namely kidney grafting in dogs, including the first attempts to prolong survival of organ grafts. Like Simonsen, he confirmed the findings of the early 1900s that dog homograft kidneys reliably showed immediate function and that a "second set" behavior was seen in second kidney grafts. He initially supported the Medawarian explanation of "acquired immunity" then developing in Britain. Dempster also noticed the marked lymphocyte and plasma cell infiltration in the damaged rejected kidneys. Like Simonsen, he shared the assumption of the day that lymphocytes did not move or migrate, and with his thinking thus constrained, he also assumed that the intense cellular reaction in the kidney came from the cells of the graft rather than the host. Dempster wrongly joined in with Medawar in the chorus of disapproval of Loeb, writing that "the [host] lymphocytes, which have so often been ascribed a major role in the death of foreign epithelium or transplanted tumor, cannot have any part in the actual destruction of the graft."[7]

Radiation Studies

With the arrival of cortisone, there were hopes for impeding the homograft response. Dempster made the first attempts at immunosuppression in experimental organ transplantation. Hammersmith Hospital researchers in London were one of the groups to obtain some of the early supply of cortisone from the United States, and together with Bernard Lennox, Dempster studied the hormone's effects on experimental transplantation. In work confirmed by others in the United States, he found that the cortisone had little or no effect in prolonging rabbit skin grafts or dog kidney transplants.[8] He also at last revived the study of radiation in homograft research, forgotten since the Murphy-Carrel road map was drawn up in 1914. But irradiation of the recipient dogs would prolong the kidney graft survival for only a few days, an effect that was again assumed to be of no clinical relevance.[9] He was unfortunate in his choice of model: dogs do not show the human pattern of response to radiation.[10]

Dempster steadily turned against an immunological theory of graft loss, since the graft changes did not seem to fit an immunological event, and he could not find an antibody against the graft. To add to this puzzle, radiation and cortisone seemed to suppress and damage almost all the systems of the body except the reaction against grafts, which added to the special aura of mystery around the "homograft problem" and its apparent invincibility at the time. Dempster distanced himself scientifically and professionally from the growing Medawarian orthodoxy in London, looking instead for nonimmunological mechanisms.[11] Dempster believed there was no immediate way forward and said so frequently during the next decade. In his surgical post in the middle ground between the laboratory and the clinic, his warnings against human organ transplant attempts, based on his considerable experience, seemed authoritative and were listened to, for a while.[12] He noted that others had found a modest effect of cortisone, but he dismissed any prolonged human use because of undesirable secondary effects. But Hammersmith's failure to move forward and take up empirical innovation in human organ transplantation during this otherwise highly successful time for the hospital "has to be accounted as one of its failures by any critical historian."[13]

Early Experimental Heart Transplantation

Unnoticed then and forgotten later, experimental heart transplantation resumed in the early 1950s. But while the experimental kidney transplanters often had continuing contacts with the new immunologists, the American and Soviet heart transplant efforts remained in a world apart.[14] These early experimental efforts are often seen as merely the modest, hesitant preliminaries to the separate, momentous events in 1967. Such an assessment, however, conceals one huge debt owed by the entire transplantation community to the early heart transplanters: the heart surgeons were first to realize the value of cooling the graft prior to transplantation.

Alexis Carrel and Charles Guthrie had been the pioneers of experimental heart transplantation in the early part of the century, and Frank Mann's group at the Mayo Clinic did further work in the 1930s. The challenge was taken up again in the late 1940s by the resourceful and energetic Moscow surgeon Vladimir P. Demikhov (1916–1998) and in the studies of Emanuel Marcus at the University of Chicago Medical School. This work was done before the availability of the heart-lung bypass pump, hence it was simply not possible to operate extensively on the heart, much less remove and replace it; thus, experimental heart transplants, as in the Carrel era, were instead "auxiliary grafts" attached to major vessels elsewhere in the body, with complex rerouting of the blood.

Starting in 1946, Demikhov had attempted numerous such accessory heart and heart-lung procedures on dogs, with technical success from 1949.[15] His tasteless, well-publicized transplantation of a dog's head and neck may have concealed his conventional skills with experimental heart transplantation. Demikhov also used the remarkable new Soviet blood vessel stapling machine for his various thoracic grafts. Designed by the Soviet engineer V. F. Gudov and developed by P. I. Androsov at Moscow's innovative Research Institute for Experimental Surgical Apparatus and Instruments in the mid-1940s, it was the forerunner of the surgical devices that later found widespread international use. Following Demikhov's lead, Emanuel Marcus also tried the many variant heart and lung procedures, and the typology of auxiliary heart positions still bears his name.[16]

The pioneer experimental cardiac transplanters, almost unnoticed by the kidney transplant community, were routinely cooling the detached donor organ. But this strategy, regarded as self-evident later, was reached by a rather tortuous route.

Cooling the Graft

Cardio-thoracic surgeons at the time had started cooling the entire body to allow for more adventurous procedures, including experimental transplantation. The new use of cooling in human surgery was gaining adherents. In 1953, E. J. Beattie's group and Henry Swan (born 1913) in Denver showed that "general refrigeration" would protect the spinal cord of experimental animals from damage during the clamping of the thoracic aorta. Wilfred G. Bigelow (1913–2005) in Toronto suggested total body cooling to allow surgeons more time while doing major vessel and cardiac surgery. In 1950, he explained the general approach and predicted its use in transplantation. In hypothermia, he wrote, "the oxygen requirements of the tissues are reduced to a small fraction of normal. . . . Such a technique might permit surgeons to operate upon the 'bloodless heart' without recourse to extra-corporeal pumps, and perhaps allow transplantation of organs."[17]

Bigelow reported on dog trials but had few survivors, and his "blasphemous" proposals about inducing hypothermia to perform surgery raised "intense interest and strong doubts" at the American Surgical Association meeting in 1950. In January 1953, it was instead John Lewis and Henry Swan in Denver who, after much experimental work, courageously carried out the first direct surgery on the human heart assisted by hypothermia. They had up to fifteen minutes' safe operating time on the open heart, starting what was called the "First Ice Age" in cardiac surgery.[18]

Also in 1953 came a historic report from Wilford Neptune (born 1933), a young surgical resident in the innovative cardiac unit of Charles P. Bailey (1911–1993) in Philadelphia. Bailey had started to use general hypothermia in human operations but stopped after bad results. Neptune continued with the hypothermia experimental studies and received help from a newly arrived British physiologist, Brian Cookson. They used the usual hypothermia procedure in the recipient dogs to give surgeons fifteen minutes' operating time after clamping the major vessels. Then they added two novelties. The first innovation was to preserve the donor organs by cooling the donor dog via total hypothermia. The second was that, after the recipient heart and lungs were removed, donor heart and lungs were transplanted to the normal position, marking the first effort of its kind. They had good short-term functional results.[19]

In cardiac surgery, the practice of general hypothermia did not last for long. By the mid-1950s, the new bypass pump perfusion was available both for experimental and human work. But the cardiac surgeons had learned a lesson in experimental heart transplantation, and though the recipient was no longer cooled, the "cool is good" assumption found favor with respect to the donor heart. Simple surface cooling was judged to be insufficient, and the cardiac surgeons now flushed the graft via its arteries after removal, using a chilled, heparinized perfusion fluid and immersion in ice thereafter. These fluids of high potassium content were already in use for bypass surgery cardioplegia—arrest of the heart during bypass. It was some time before these two strategies—cooling and perfusion—reached clinical organ transplantation.

In a classic 1957 paper on organ cooling experiments in dogs, Watts Webb and Hector Howard at the University of Mississippi School of Medicine reported that they had removed and then replaced the same "refrigerated" heart after eight hours outside the body, thus pointing the way forward for organ transplantation: "[The] demonstration that the heart can be maintained viable and functional for periods of at least eight hours in a nutrient medium has been of great value to us in experimental work in cardiac and cardiopulmonary transplants. When the problems of immunology are solved and transplantation becomes a clinical possibility, it will presumably require several hours for obtaining the heart, preparing the recipient and total implantation. The practices outlined above would seem to make cardiac transplantation completely feasible as far as this time element is concerned."[20]

In the late 1950s, two pioneers, Thomas Starzl and Norman Shumway, also agreed that cooling was useful in their liver and heart transplant experiments. Both had trained in cardiac surgery under John Lewis at Northwestern University in Minneapolis (and later at Chicago), and Lewis was using hypothermia.[21] Those transplanters without cardiac surgery experience hesitated for a while, since flushing and perfusion were thought to be damaging. Simonsen had not cooled his donor kidneys, and Dempster wrote that "on no account should the [donor] kidney be flushed with saline."[22] Hamburger and others, including Francis Moore, taught that cold perfusion of the donor kidney was unnecessary and might even be harmful.[23] As late as the early 1960s, Moore merely surface-cooled his experimental donor livers to fifteen degrees Celsius.

These prohibitions and the alleged danger of perfusion may have dated back to a few experiments with kidney perfusion with simple solutions half a century earlier, notably Guthrie's unpromising experience, and the warnings were handed down almost as a folk memory or learned myth. The unfortunate "warm is good" mantra and the deep-rooted affection for keeping the donor organs warm also had ancient lineage, perhaps relating to Carrel's tissue culture methods. Routine cooling and perfusion did not come into clinical kidney transplantation until the mid-1960s.

Tissue Banks

The value of cold storage of some simpler tissues had been accepted for some time since Carrel advocated it. Blood and corneas were known from the late 1930s to survive surprisingly well for many days at near zero temperatures, and similar preservation of skin in the cold for days for late grafting had also proved possible. Jerome P. Webster, the biographer of Tagliacozzi and mentor to Blair Rogers, is credited with this innovation in 1944, which well served the increased need for skin grafts to treat injuries during World War II.[24]

Cooling began playing another role in tissue replacement at this time. By the 1950s, it had become apparent that many useful tissue grafts, like bone and blood vessels, were successful only as noncellular scaffolds, with the donor cells being lost. Preserving cells within the grafts was thus no longer a concern, and since there was therefore no need to use the grafts quickly, the donated tissues could be kept when frozen. These inert tissue grafts proved to be quite resilient. Fears of infection of any kind—notably contamination at donation or from disease in the donor—could be reduced by testing and use of a strong toxic storage antiseptic like merthiolate, later replaced with sterilization by irradiation or ethylene oxide.[25]

Many "tissue banks" storing human material for later clinical use appeared in the 1950s. The first successes were with stored human arteries, and these misleadingly named "homografts" had a widespread, but forgotten, role in the rise of routine major arterial surgery, notably for aortic aneurysms, until the advent of grafts made of artificial material in the early 1960s. Heart valves, bone, fascia, and particularly the brain's covering (dura mater) also began to be stored. The best-known service was offered by the pioneering U.S. Navy Tissue Bank at Bethesda, set up in 1950 by George W. Hyatt (1920–1993), and during the Korean War it routinely collected tissues during postmortem examinations on service members. In Britain, a similar bank emerged in 1953 at St. Mary's Hospital in London and at Leeds, based on the needs of vascular surgery, and many other tissue banks, some with niche specialties, also appeared.[26]

The relatively simple service provided by these noncommercial tissue banks grew independently of the early events in organ transplantation. But in one important matter, the early banks were the first to deal with a difficult issue, one that awaited organ transplantation later: the legal aspects of tissue donation.

The tissue banks prompted little public debate or controversy. But, in the early days of the banks, some legal commentators noted matters of interest and concern that were later to be prominent in medico-legal and ethical discourse. One perceptive study from the University of Detroit law faculty pointed out the informality of the procedures used in 1955 to obtain donor material:

The full realization of the [surgical] techniques, those known now and those that may be discovered in the area of tissue transplantation, will certainly require greater amounts of donor tissue than have been available in the past. In the nature of things, medical personnel working in this field generally look to those who have recently died as the most frequent source. At the present time there is no routinized, common procedure by which such tissue is obtained, rather various individuals are using diverse methods. Some individuals have obtained the written consent of the nearest of kin as well as routine postmortem authorization before removing tissue for transplantation purposes at the time of necropsy. Others have obtained only the necropsy authorization.[27]

Ominously, the authors quoted cases in which successful claims had been made by relatives when organs had been removed at postmortem and retained beyond the immediate purposes of making a diagnosis.[28] In the earliest such case in the United States, *Palenzke v. Bruning,* the court had ruled that "no-one had the right to remove parts of the body and, without the parent's consent, throw them into a privy vault. Such conduct violates every instinct of propriety, and could not fail to outrage the feelings of the kindred of the deceased."[29]

The Detroit legal commentators went on to note that, although it was common practice to retain specimens that were useful or interesting to the doctors, it was risky, however high-minded the motives. They observed that the surgical community, then considered beyond reproach, might not be aware that a legal swamp was close at hand. Later, there was indeed outrage when some less honorable "privy vaults" were discovered.

To complicate matters further, from ancient times the dead body was not considered a property owned by anyone; seeking permission for deceased donor donation was therefore not a simple matter. It was far from clear who was legally in charge of the body after death.[30] Even the deceased person's wishes during life were not legally binding. While it seemed reasonable for the next of kin to take the ownership role, this procedure was not enshrined in law. As a result of these legal stirrings, the arrangements for gaining permission to use tissue from cadavers tightened up, and various legislatures in the United States soon introduced laws ensuring that permission be obtained from relatives after the donor's death and encouraging those wishing to donate tissue to make a written gift during life.

Artificial Kidneys

As experience with experimental kidney transplantation grew, progress in another form of kidney replacement—the use of the artificial kidney—was a feature of the early 1950s. The increasing need came from rising numbers of cases of acute renal failure. Historically, "suppression of urine" had always been thought to be merely one of many secondary manifestations of serious illness, and many battle casualties in World War II developed renal failure. Following the German air raids on Britain, however, acute renal failure came to prominence as one aspect of the "crush syndrome," which could develop in otherwise well patients whose trapped limbs had just been released from beneath rubble.[31] Other novel causes of well-defined acute kidney failure emerged, notably following use of the newer sulfonamide drugs or after mistakes in blood typing for the expanding transfusion service. The mindset changed to consider that treating acute renal failure might not be futile.

There had already been isolated attempts to use an artificial kidney in human patients.[32] The earliest machines of the modern era were constructed in Europe by Willem Kolff in occupied Holland and by Nils Alwall (1904–1986) in Sweden.[33] After the war, Kolff donated a number of his early machines to various centers in Europe and North America, and, in Boston, the interested surgeons and physicians, encouraged by George Thorn, built one from Kolff's drawings.

The early Kolff machines were awkward to use. Though Hammersmith Hospital had received one of Kolff's prototype machines in 1946, the staff encountered difficulties with it, and they were not convinced of its routine place in the therapy of acute renal failure. Instead, in 1949, Hammersmith's head of medicine, Graham Bull, together with Geerd Borst in Amsterdam, devised a high-calorie, protein-free dietary and fluid regimen for use in renal failure patients. It proved useful and effective in mild, acute failure, notably in sulfonamide toxicity or blood transfusion reactions, prior to the spontaneous revival of kidney function.

At Boston's Peter Bent Brigham Hospital, John Merrill (1917–1984) persevered with experimental work using an improved Kolff-Brigham kidney machine that had plastic instead of rubber tubing, helped by Dr. Carl W. Walter, a staff surgeon with engineering skills. But Merrill was seen as

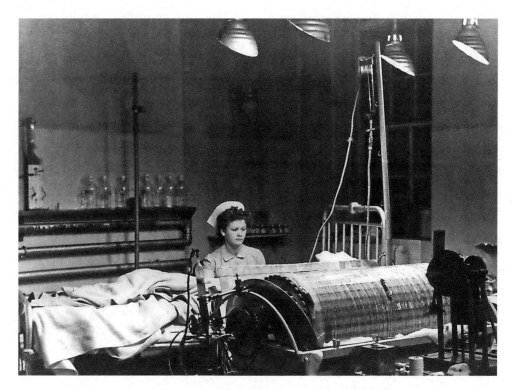

An early Kolff artificial kidney in use at Hammersmith Hospital, London. A sausage-skin dialysis membrane was used, as plastic tubing had yet to be developed. The machine was difficult to use, so the hospital continued to use its "conservative regimen" to treat acute renal failure. Image courtesy of Graham Bull.

maverick, and conservative-minded physicians offered little support for his work.[34] A visitor to Boston at the time recalls that "John was considered an outlaw by the members of the 'salt and water club.' They denied him any of his contributions, even the usefulness of the artificial kidney in acute uremia—particularly in New York."[35]

The authority on kidney function at that time was Homer Smith, the luminary of the "salt and water club"—the group that sought to describe kidney disease through its disordered physiology and to treat kidney failure through a fluid and diet regimen. Smith was dismissive of the artificial kidney, and his influential text *The Kidney* (1951) praised the "Bull regimen," named for Graham Bull.[36]

Merrill in Boston acknowledged the mood of the day in stating that, if nothing else, he could prepare kidney failure patients for any necessary surgery and anesthesia, and his dialysis would allow comatose patients to revive and take their special diet.[37]

Holism in Retreat

But even the dietetic method of treatment, cautious though it was, was a novelty and offended those physicians retaining the attitudes of prewar days. After publication of the temporarily influential paper on the Hammersmith experience with the Bull regimen for patients with "crush syndrome," the *British Medical Journal* carried a letter from H. A. Harris, an Oxford University professor. He made, perhaps for the last time in public, the case for the ancient, alternative, expectant, Hippocratic method of disease management, dominant in the holistic medical views of the 1920s:

Crush injuries are not new. . . . The treatment is careful nursing and non-interference, rather than physiological and biochemical assay. The cases from the [Hammersmith] Postgraduate Medical School suggest a syndrome which might be called the "continuous interference syndrome." Not only had the patients been subjected to continuous readings of pulse, systolic and diastolic blood pressure, estimations of haemoglobin, oscillometric readings of leg volumes on already injured right and left legs, electrocardiographic examination, and even [bladder] catheterisation, which itself may give rise to shock. The repeated examinations for so-called blood chemistry and urine chemistry give a picture of the extent to which rest was not allowed to figure in the treatment.[38]

But the professor's confidence in the healing power of nature had its limits, especially in a war.

War in Korea

In the Korean War of the early 1950s, doubts were emerging about the non-dialysis management of renal failure in the badly injured troops. In World War II, evacuation of the wounded was slow, infection was common, and in the mortally wounded, any renal failure, if noted, went untreated. Biochemical blood tests were in their infancy and thus were rarely obtained and seldom repeated, and the true extent of renal failure was thus unclear.

In the Korean War, combat injuries were managed differently. The wounded were resuscitated, transfused, given antibiotics, and promptly evacuated by helicopter. Routine and regular blood testing of the increasing numbers of immediate survivors showed that acute renal failure was common. The kidney failure in these severe trauma cases was quite different from the milder civilian incidents successfully managed by the "conservative" method. In 1950, after Colonel William Stone had pointed out the apparently new prominence of acute renal failure in the wounded survivors, a center dedicated to its treatment was established in 1952 at Wonju, attached to the 11th Evacuation Hospital. Acute renal failure was now separated from the other general effects of trauma as a condition that could possibly be treatable. It was a major paradigm shift.

Far from the purview of skeptical senior medical staff in the hospitals back home, young army doctors in the war units began using an early dialysis machine of the Kolff-Brigham type. Even in the difficult setting of a combat zone, the machine's usefulness was impressive, and the careful collection of medical data showed a trend. With dialysis, there was a significant improvement in overall survival rate.[39]

Hemodialysis treatment was thus established through wartime experience and success. Improved artificial kidney machines soon became more widely available for use in civilian hospitals, first in Boston, then regular use in Britain at Leeds, with conservative London following slowly thereafter.[40]

Blood vessel surgery also improved greatly as military surgeons began practicing new techniques. Human reconstructive vascular surgery hardly existed until this time, notably because vascular disease was not yet a prominent clinical challenge. In World War II, a famous U.S. Army study by Michael DeBakey showed that in the major arterial limb injuries dealt with at the battle front, direct repair was attempted in only 5 percent of cases; the large limb arteries were simply tied off nearer the heart. This approach was surprisingly trouble-free in young men, with only occasional consequential amputations.

By the time of the Korean War, however, many factors made it possible to perform successful direct reconstructive vascular surgery. The availability of stored homograft vessels provided a range of options, and surgeons had many opportunities to practice immediate repair of the vessels. The myth that late rupture would follow direct suturing was put aside, and the new techniques gained in Korea were carried over into civilian practice, where surgeons encountered increasing numbers of traumatic injuries and a rise in vascular disease. The confidence gained in vascular surgery was also a major stimulus to experimental and clinical organ transplantation.

Human Kidney Transplants of the Early 1950s

By 1950, laboratory scientists had increased their understanding of tissue transplantation mechanisms, but no usable method of preventing rejection in clinical practice had emerged. The brief prolongation of homograft survival using steroids or radiation was judged not to be of any clinical value.

As the decade began, however, surgeons were exhibiting signs of impatience, and, with willful empiricism, some surgical units independently decided to proceed with human kidney transplantation attempts. These pioneering kidney transplants, now seen as the obvious and celebrated first step in the development of organ transplantation, were bold ventures at the time and were seen by many, both inside and outside the profession, as distasteful human experiments without hope of benefit.[41] Moreover, some leaders of opinion considered these operations contrary to the spirit of "scientific surgery," thus suggesting once again that clinicians should await new understandings handed down from the lab in the accepted one-way flow of enlightenment. To deviate from this path would, it was said, diminish the new authority and status of surgery and attach a humiliating label of empiricism. Dempster, the Hammersmith surgical researcher, was expressing a widely held opinion when he wrote at the time that "it is unwise to carry out such procedures [kidney transplantation] without any scientific knowledge of the fundamental processes involved. . . . It is quite out of the question that kidneys should be homotransplanted in man just in case a permanent survival might be obtained. We feel that little knowledge is to be gained at this stage by homotransplanting human kidneys. . . . From the immunological and histological point of view, there can be no doubt that the human kidney can provide little or no information which could not more extensively be derived from animal experiments."[42]

Some were even harsher in their private judgments, but it turned out that human beings do have quite unique responses to organ grafts. *Homo sapiens* proved again to be the "odd mouse out."

The "unmodified" human kidney transplants of the early 1950s were labeled as such because no attempt was made to suppress the immune response. Most of these operations took place in Paris and Boston. There was also a small series of less well-known Soviet human kidney transplants carried out in the late 1940s by Yu. Yu. Voronoy, the pioneer transplanter of the 1930s. Although these transplants were not therapeutic successes, they did yield valuable information until 1955, after which time these unmodified transplants ceased.

Voronoy's Later Cases

Voronoy, the pioneer transplanter of the 1930s, had, by 1949, attempted five more human kidney grafts. By that time, Voronoy was director of the Department of Experimental Surgery in the Ukrainian Institute of Experimental Biology in Kiev. The institute's administrator was O. A. Bogomolets, whose "antireticular" serum, an alleged stimulator of healing, had political support and widespread use in the Soviet Union but notoriety elsewhere. Voronoy's scientific articles of the 1930s had been ahead of their time and advanced in their analysis, but his publication of 1949 is disappointing.[43] Instead of building on his earlier attempt with the world's first human-to-human kidney transplant, Voronoy had to fit his new study into the paradigm of attitudes acceptable under Soviet philosophy. Instead of exercising his earlier perceptive awareness, he had to follow the teachings of Vladimir P. Filatov (1875–1956), the academician and Stalin Prize winner. Filatov had made the remarkable claim that prolonged storage of tissues prior to grafting was required and gave better graft survival via "biogenic stimulators" that increased the cell's vitality and were produced in the tissues after encountering unfavorable, but not lethal, internal and external environmental conditions.[44] Filatov had official support, and the government set up laboratories to produce these allegedly stimulatory substances. All tissue transplantation activity had to follow the Filatov paradigm and deliberately store tissue prior to transplantation.[45]

In this troubled period of Soviet biology, scientists working under the system's constraints also had to relate medical theory to the earlier work of Ivan Pavlov, famous for his studies of the nervous system and the "conditioned reflex" and considered a hero by Soviet authorities. Some researchers began to suggest that reflexes could cause kidney failure. In Soviet labs, even immunological responses were to be incorporated into conditioned reflex arcs via the central nervous system. This "neuroimmunology" prospered for a while in the Soviet Union and was taken seriously as psychoneuroimmunology by left-leaning European biologists in the 1950s.[46] The result of the Filatov-Pavlov stance in kidney transplantation was a complex hybrid proposal that biogenic stimulation after deliberately delayed insertion of the graft would produce a "disinhibitory reflex," which would annul the central, nerve-mediated curb which was said to be destroying the patient's diseased organ.[47]

This improbable official theory explains much about the human transplant cases Voronoy reported in 1949. He had to use kidneys transplanted after long periods of storage between one and twenty days after removal from the donor, but no convincing benefit was claimed. But there was one genuine and interesting innovation mentioned in Voronoy's 1949 paper: the renewed use of the surgical stapling machine for joining the kidney graft vessels—the same device Demikhov had been using in his experimental heart transplants.[48]

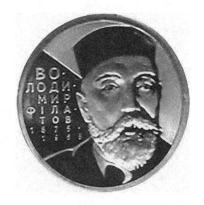

Vladimir (or Volodymyr) Petrovich Filatov, whose image here graces a Ukrainian coin, pioneered human corneal grafting in 1931 at his innovative unit in Odessa.

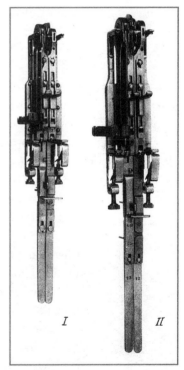

I   *II*

These pioneering Soviet stapling machines were developed for stitching blood vessels, and Yuri Voronoy used the device in his human kidney transplants in the late 1940s. From *Annals of the New York Academy of Sciences* 87 (May 1960): 539.

Richard Lawler's Bold Initiative

In 1950, Richard Lawler (1896–1982) attempted a human kidney transplant in Chicago. Although often seen as an isolated and maverick effort, it had an important influence at the time since others watched the event closely prior to making their own attempts. On June 17, 1950, at Chicago's Presbyterian Hospital, Lawler removed a polycystic left kidney from a forty-four-year-old patient who was not yet in terminal renal failure but had pain and infection. Having carried out the necessary kidney removal, Lawler then transplanted a blood-type-matched cadaver donor kidney into the left renal bed using the stumps of the host renal vessels. The operation was filmed, and large numbers of hospital staff were present. The media reported on the event, and the *New York Times* and *Newsweek* published supportive editorials one week later. The transplanted kidney gave some evidence of function, namely a larger output of urine, and the transplant was viable as judged by radiology. It was said to have a normal appearance when explored shortly after for a ureter problem. Later, the graft's function proved to be doubtful, and several months later, the kidney appeared shrunken. The patient's own right kidney function sustained life for four more years.

While the public response was supportive, there was prompt professional criticism of Lawler, and he was "excluded from polite company" in the medical community. The American Urological Association issued a negative verdict on kidney transplantation and on Lawler's conduct. His colleague Patrick McNulty, the urologist involved, was asked to appear before the AUA public relations committee, and the association called for a moratorium on kidney transplantation until the immunological problems had been solved.[49]

In contrast to this professional disdain, others who had been ready to proceed with kidney transplantation were heartened by Lawler's initiative. Lawler's bold venture encouraged surgeons in Paris and Boston to start attempting kidney transplants, since Lawler's technical side of connecting the kidney had gone well. The French surgeon René Küss later acknowledged the influence: "Lawler had an extraordinary impact. . . . It gave us reason to believe that transplant surgery was possible in human beings. . . . His results and conclusions were not entirely convincing, but we used Lawler's success as an excuse to begin kidney transplants in man."[50]

Details of Lawler's historic effort appeared in the French newspaper *France-Soir,* and terminally ill patients and relatives of patients started requesting the operation in Paris.[51] One other lesson learned by those watching in Boston was to avoid publicity and to delay professional publication and clinical presentations until well after the surgery. There were

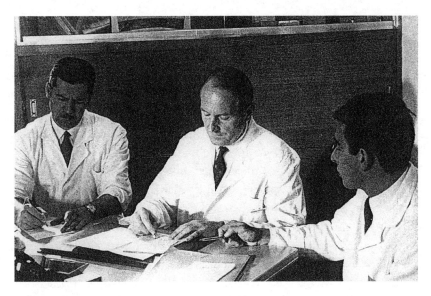

René Küss, urologist and pioneer Paris kidney transplanter. Image courtesy of René Küss.

few such concerns in Paris, and French public opinion did prove to be very supportive. The Paris transplanters gave fairly well-received presentations at scientific meetings and published their cases quickly. The Boston transplanters delayed reporting for some years.

Paris Transplants

In France, the nine kidney transplants of the early 1950s were performed by three teams in two hospitals in Paris—the Centre Medico-Chirurgical Foch and the Hôpital Necker.[52] The eminent surgical teams included Oeconomos, Dubost, and Auvert at Necker, René Küss at Foch, and M. Servelle, who reported one case elsewhere.[53] The physicians involved were Jean Hamburger (1909–1992) at Necker and Marcel Legrain at Foch.[54] Organizationally, Hamburger, the physician, brought in the surgeons to assist him at Necker, while at Foch the surgeons were the activists. The rivalry between these two groups in Paris was well known but is poorly documented.

Servelle and Charles Dubost did the first French transplants, using the kidneys from a guillotined prisoner in early January 1951. In spite of the opportunities offered by this distasteful situation, up to two hours elapsed between death and the removal of the donor kidneys, since the procedure had to be carried out in unsuitable surroundings. Dubost had proposed this source of kidneys, and Küss later recalled his unease at being involved—"c'était une atmosphère extrêmement pénible [fraught]." When removed, the two kidneys went to two different surgical teams in two different hospitals, using favorable blood type matches. The French surgeons placed their transplanted kidney in the pelvis close to the bladder, the position later used routinely by kidney transplant surgeons. In the Boston cases, soon to follow, the kidney was instead placed superficially in the thigh, as Voronoy had done. No urine output was obtained in either case in Paris, perhaps surprisingly, and these transplanted kidneys, when studied after death, showed little evidence of rejection.

Both cases were promptly reported to a Paris medical society in mid-January. The Küss team proceeded with the first of its six cases, doing the surgery on January 20 and publishing the details in the French medical journals that year. In Paris, lay comment was supportive, but an unpleasant anonymous attack by a Paris medical insider reached the newspapers, doubtless reflecting some professional distaste at the time. It described how a "pitiable young woman became the needless victim of a needless experiment . . . which ended in a grave, sacrificed on the altar of the surgeon's ambitions. When will our colleagues give up this game of experimenting on human beings? And when will they realize that dying, too, can be a mercy?"[55]

First Living Kidney Donor

On December 26, 1952, surgeons in Paris performed the first transplant using a kidney donated by a close relative of the patient.[56] The recipient was a sixteen-year-old carpenter injured in a fall from scaffolding. When

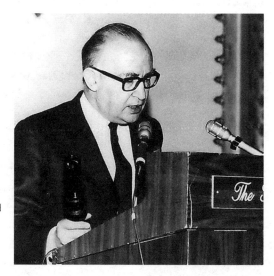

In the early 1950s, Jean Hamburger, a Paris nephrologist, developed an improved model of the artificial kidney and also encouraged human and experimental kidney transplants.

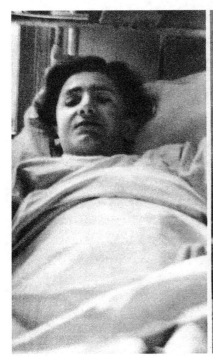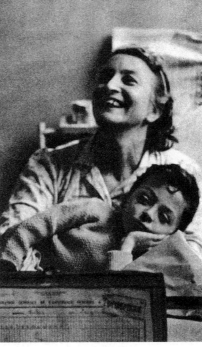

In Paris in 1953, Marius Renard (*left*) was the first patient to receive a living-related kidney transplant, from his mother (*right*). Image courtesy of *Paris Match*.

his badly damaged kidney was removed, the medical team quickly discovered that it had been his only kidney. As he rapidly deteriorated, the boy's mother proposed that she would donate a kidney, and Jean Hamburger agreed to organize the transplant. Unlike all earlier attempts, the kidney functioned immediately, and the recipient's uremia was quickly relieved. The local and international media followed the events closely.[57] On the twenty-second day the graft abruptly ceased functioning because of rejection, and with renal failure returning, the patient died shortly after. However, French public interest was intense, and public opinion was favorable.

Kidney Transplants in Boston

The Boston cases started three months later and were carried out at the Peter Bent Brigham Hospital, where there was a culture of innovation in the small, close-knit collaborative academic group with a range of clinical and laboratory skills. The chief of surgery, Francis D. Moore, is credited with directing the effort, and the renal physicians had the artificial kidney available.[58] Associated with them was an energetic young surgeon named

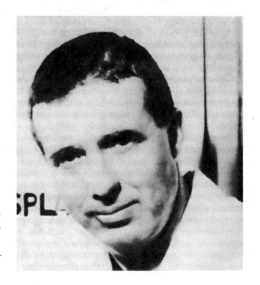

David Hume trained at Harvard and carried out the pioneering Peter Bent Brigham Hospital kidney transplants in the early 1950s. He moved to the Medical School of Virginia at Richmond in 1956. Image courtesy of *Transplantation Proceedings*, from vol. 6, supplement 1 (1974).

David Hume (1917–1973).[59] Hume had made himself available for the repeated surgical insertion of tubing into the patient's arteries and veins necessary at that time for use of the dialysis machine. For each dialysis, new vessel sites had to be found, and thus the number of treatments each patient could receive was limited.

The hospital had a modified Kolff machine on site, and Merrill's experience with it meant the referral of many patients with renal failure to Brigham and considerable understanding of the problems of acute and chronic renal failure, particularly in regard to fluid and electrolyte balance resulted.[60] In the kidney transplants attempted at Brigham, the modified Kolff machine was used not only to prepare patients for surgery but also to support some patients after transplant while waiting in hope for the donor kidney to begin functioning.

At Brigham, Hume had already experimented with an unusual use of a kidney graft in an attempt to treat acute renal failure. In 1947, he used a human homograft kidney in a patient with postpartum kidney failure, stitching the kidney to the arm blood vessels at the elbow under local anesthetic, as had the pioneering xenograft surgeons in the early part of the century. The other trainee surgeons involved were Charles Hufnagel and Ernest Landsteiner, who was the son of Karl Landsteiner and the chief resident in urology. The young men were apprehensive about the senior staff's reaction to such experimental therapy, and, in addition, as Hufnagel diplomatically recalled later, there was the not-unfamiliar situation that "because the patient's condition appeared extremely critical, there was some administrative objection to bringing the patient to the operating theater." The procedure was accordingly carried out not in the operating theater but in a side room of a ward at midnight, famously with the aid of two "goose-neck" lamps. The cadaver kidney was donated after the death of a patient in the hospital (the husband of a member of staff), and the kidney did function immediately and continued to do so for two days, with some clinical improvement in the patient's condition. The kidney output declined on the third day, the furtive project was terminated, and the organ detached without the senior staff being involved. The patient's acute renal failure resolved three days later, and the role of the homograft in this survival is not clear. The patient died of hepatitis a few months later.[61]

In 1951, four years later, at the invitation of Thorn and Merrill, Hume commenced a series of human kidney transplants.[62] The first patient in the Boston area treated by kidney transplantation in this series was also the first to be treated by the artificial kidney in preparation for a transplant. The patient did not have the operation at Boston but in the nearby town of Springfield. The thirty-seven-year-old patient had been diagnosed with chronic renal failure and sent to Brigham for dialysis. Then, by coincidence, a patient at the Springfield hospital was found to require removal of a normal kidney because of a cancer at the lower end of the ureter, and the transplant operation using this "free" kidney was carried out there by James V. Scola. The kidney functioned for a short time only.

Thereafter, the patients Merrill chose for transplantation were in chronic renal failure. One grim situation was that some had presented with apparently acute reversible failure and were successfully started on dialysis but then proved to have chronic renal damage instead. All involved knew that these patients were doomed, since dialysis could not continue when all arteries and veins suitable for dialysis had been used.

Six of the Boston transplants took place in the five-month period from March to July 1951, following the busy January-February transplant activity in Paris. The remaining three Boston cases came later, between 1952 and 1953. The publication describing the work did not appear until 1955, and none of the data was presented formally at surgical meetings, as a result of concern over peer disapproval or adverse media publicity.

These transplants were carefully planned. Six out of nine patients had had pretransplant dialysis. The donor kidneys were obtained from patients who had died during risky heart surgery or from children who had a kidney removed as a part of the Matson procedure, an operation for hydrocephalus introduced in Boston by the surgeon Don Matson.[63] Donor kidneys were flushed briefly with saline but not cooled. The Boston team had considered using kidneys taken, as in Paris, from executed criminals but decided not to do so. Most of these transplants had blood type compatibility, but in two cases there was a serious incompatibility.

The kidneys were all placed in the upper thigh using the main vessels to the leg—the Unger/Voronoy position—rather than the pelvic position favored in Paris. Using this site, the kidney could be covered, with difficulty, by a skin flap, and the ureter was brought out onto the skin. In this way, blood flow could be observed and any urine produced could be collected unmixed with any residual output from the patient's own kidneys.

All transplant patients were given short courses of ACTH, as had one Paris case, on the basis of the spectacular but unconfirmed claim by M. James Whitelaw in January 1951 for prolongation of skin grafts in this way. Some patients also received large doses of cortisone for a short time, from George Thorn's early Brigham supply. All patients were also given testosterone, a hormone then thought to improve kidney function and protect the organ against damage.

One technical matter clearly reveals the particular mindset of the day. Hume awkwardly enclosed one of the kidney grafts in a plastic bag, which was a muddled response to his misunderstanding, shared by Dempster, of Loeb's homograft experiments when slices were placed under the rat kidney capsule. Hume may have believed that he could avoid rejection by preventing invasion by thigh tissue cells. He paid surprisingly close attention to the histological study of the capsule of the rejected kidneys, as did Dempster. Hume found no signs of a local rejection mechanism via the capsule, and he was thus able to join Dempster in the fashionable denigration of Leo Loeb.

The results of these nine early Boston kidney transplants were generally poor. Five of the transplanted organs failed to function at all, but the other four showed some function for periods ranging from five weeks to five and a half months. The technical side of the surgeries went very well, even in one case that involved the use of multiple donor arteries and ureters. Rejection was the inevitable outcome, but loss was not as rapid as expected, and there was that one remarkable success. The longest survivor was a twenty-six-year-old South American physician, and his was the last case reported in the series. The kidney in that case, although slow to regain function, survived for five months and twenty-five days, at which point the patient died from rapid onset renal failure and hypertension.

David Hume described this series of patients in a remarkable paper published in 1955. Even his review of the literature can be admired, not only for the 139 references quoted but also for its quality, since he had been the first to unearth the obscure report of Voronoy's pioneer human kidney transplant in the Soviet Union and he had cited the recent French literature. Hume also had noticed the forgotten work of James Bumgardner Murphy at the Rockefeller Institute, which emphasized the role of the lymphocyte in graft loss. Hume used the word *rejection* to describe graft loss throughout the paper, being perhaps the first to use this word consistently in its later technical sense. Many of his tentative conclusions from his small and varied group of grafts show impressive intuition and foresight. Among them was his correct hunch that, since one of his patients had kidney failure from polyarteritis, which then affected the graft blood vessels, the return of the original kidney disease might be a problem to consider in future transplant work. He also noticed that even with kidney survival of modest duration, the donor renal arteries developed atheroma and rapid narrowing; he mentioned changes that were later termed "chronic rejection." He concluded that, after all, blood typing might be important in kidney transplantation, since the most rapid rejection found occurred when a type B donor kidney went to a type O recipient.[64] Hume even suggested, far ahead of his time, that pretransplant blood transfusion might be beneficial to kidney survival, and the Brigham team established that removal of the host's own diseased kidneys might be necessary if there was intractable hypertension after transplantation. Not the least of his conclusions was that human transplantation differed from the experience in animal models, not only on the immunological side but also in terms of management and complications. His empirical venture had sprinted ahead of theory and showed, not for the first or last time in transplantation, that theory had shortcomings.

The Brigham pathologist Gustav Dammin contributed to Hume's historic paper. Dammin described a "round cell" lymphocyte infiltrate of variable intensity in the rejected kidneys. Dempster's and Simonsen's verdict on the microscopic appearances in their experimental kidney homografts was that a vigorous and mysterious internal reaction was responsible for the death of the organ. Dammin and Hume declined to follow this lead, and Prof. L. Michon's report on the microscopy of the lost kidney in the living-related donor case in Paris had also avoided this complexity. The two teams instead concluded that a cellular infiltrate was coming from the host, reflecting the immunologists' changing views. Acceptance of the lymphocyte's role was reemerging.

When David Hume left Brigham in 1956, the kidney transplantation work in Boston continued under Joseph Murray, the plastic and head and neck surgeon. There were perhaps six more human cases, never reported, carried out at about this time, and the team gained further experience by performing experimental dog kidney transplantation. In 1954, Murray's group had the opportunity to carry out the first of its historic kidney transplants between twins.

Other patients in the United States, Canada, and Britain received kidney transplants without immunosuppression around this time. Britain's only case was at St. Mary's Hospital, London, in 1955.[65] It is likely that similar transplants were carried out elsewhere but not reported because the operations caused controversy at the institutions involved. In Paris and Boston, the attitudes of the local staff were crucial in allowing the surgeons to proceed.

Gordon Murray in Canada

At Toronto, three human kidney transplants were carried out in 1951–1952, but little is known about them, though they were reported briefly in 1954 before the publication of the paper about the Boston transplants. The surgeon involved was the gifted Gordon Murray (1894–1986), best known as the pioneer of the clinical use of heparin. Frederick Banting and Charles Best had isolated the blood-thinning substance in Canada, and Murray had been first to use it, at Toronto General Hospital in 1935.[66] About this time, he also devised new methods of dealing with poorly united bone fractures, including bone grafting. By 1946, he was also the Canadian pioneer of heart surgery, including use of hypothermia, and was the first to deal with heart valve disease by grafting preserved human valves. In 1947, he constructed his own artificial kidney and used it in Toronto patients at a time when the Boston kidney machine was just being developed.

In the early 1950s, Murray made a study of kidney transplantation in the dog, and, like others, found that, individually, antihistamines, cortisone, irradiation, or pretransplant injections of antigen were ineffective in prolonging the life of a graft. Murray's publications show that he realized early that donor kidneys should be cooled, doubtless drawing on his heart surgery experience and the advice of Wilfred Bigelow, also working in Toronto. In addition, Murray found that, contrary to the accepted view, careful low-pressure irrigation of the donor kidney with a heparinized saline (known as "Markowitz's modification of Locke's solution") was not harmful but helpful, and he attempted preservation of donor kidneys by perfusion. Of his four human kidney transplants in the early 1950s at about the time of the Paris and Boston ventures, he remarked that these attempts were made "in spite of the heavy odds against the possibility of survivals and the vast amount of work to support the futility of the work."[67]

Despite Murray's many contributions, this inventive man has not achieved the place in the history of surgery he deserves. The reasons for this neglect are that Murray wrote little, and when he did, his accounts were regrettably telegraphic. They gave little detail about his methods, which he regarded as uninteresting, nor did he elaborate on his results, which he regarded as self-evident. He funded his own laboratory, did not encourage visitors, sought no collaborators, and did not attend scientific conferences. Later, he ensured at least short-term neglect of his contributions by dabbling in simplistic immunotherapy of cancer in the late 1950s, and he was forced into early retirement after embarrassing his friends and his hospital by publicly claiming to have cured paraplegia by excising and suturing the damage in the spinal cord.[68]

Transplant Activity Elsewhere

The broader surgical world took little interest in these early attempts at organ transplantation, an era of surgery that now seems important in retrospect. The first invited lecture on transplantation to a surgical society since Carrel's visionary contribution in 1914 came when Blair Rogers addressed the American College of Surgeons in 1949. In Britain, Michael Woodruff used his experimental transplant work as the basis for his prestigious Hunterian Lecture at the Royal College of Surgeons of England in 1952. At the annual meeting of the American Association of Surgeons in 1955, Lloyd MacLean, from Minneapolis and then working with Robert Good, gave a paper on experimental transplantation. MacLean urged the surgical audience to be "aroused by these immunological challenges, and by virtue of greater interest bring sooner to successful practice, clinical, homovital organ grafting. Such an accomplishment represents a maturation of surgery that is a bright vista to contemplate." The historian of the association records that no questions or discussion on this bright vista followed, and the speaker was merely thanked for these fine words. No further papers were presented on transplantation to this major academic surgical society until 1958, when the first clinical transplant account of the Boston transplants between twins was reported. Even then, no further papers were given to the association on this subject until 1960. Organ transplantation was not yet respectable.[69]

These innovators in clinical transplantation in the 1950s had this rather unusual and isolated interest, and they always had other surgical projects, some of which were moving at a faster rate. This isolation of transplant innovators was aided by the geographical and institutional separation of those involved. Boston and Paris had their pioneer kidney transplant surgeons, but no immunology laboratories in those metropolitan areas were yet interested in the subject. London had talent in fundamental transplantation immunology, but the surgical community in that city was uninterested or even hostile to human transplant surgery. New York had neither organ transplanters nor interested immunologists but still had the group of involved plastic surgeons, who still did their best, with diminishing influence, to encourage the skeptical surgical world.

The Hiatus

By 1954, despite the hesitant start in Boston, Paris, Toronto, and elsewhere, clinical kidney transplantation came to a halt, its practitioners having learned some valuable lessons. Experimental organ transplantation also failed to thrive or explore any new initiatives, though some useful findings went unnoticed, notably that steroids and nitrogen mustard might be a useful combination.[70] There was a similar hint from the work from a distinguished group in Paris on the power of the same combination.[71]

One reason for the clinical hesitation was that, as many had hoped, a strong lead did come from the laboratory. In 1953, Medawar achieved the long-sought goal of obtaining prolonged graft survival in small animal transplantation work using a method that prevented rejection completely, easily, reliably, and specifically. Such was the power of this "tolerance" strategy that investigation of the modest effects of cortisone, antimetabolites, and radiation was put aside. Although the original form of tolerance induction was unsuitable for immediate use in human organ grafting, it gave confidence and hope for a way forward. After a delay, a modified form of tolerance was ready for human use by the late 1950s.

11 Transplantation Tolerance and Beyond

URING THE EARLY 1950S, while human and experimental organ transplant attempts were under way, in the laboratory steady progress was being made toward understanding graft rejection, and the advance of great significance resulted. In 1949, Peter Medawar met Hugh P. Donald, an Edinburgh veterinarian, at a scientific conference in Stockholm, and he asked for Medawar's help in solving a familiar problem: distinguishing at an early stage between identical and nonidentical twin cattle—that is, between mono- and dizygote twins. Dizygote, or non-identical twins, when one was male and the other female, could look very similar, since the female twin had been masculinized during gestation. This female twin or "freemartin" will produce no milk and thus is of no economic value. Medawar told Donald that the results of a skin graft from one twin to the other would distinguish between these two types of twin, since he was confident that only the identical twins would accept grafts exchanged between them.

Later Medawar recalled the events and his advice: "Let him only assemble a collection of twin pairs of doubtful classification and we would exchange skin grafts between them. If the skin grafts survived the twins could be classified as monozygotic [identical]; if not, not. In the relaxed and matey atmosphere of international congresses one sometimes enters upon commitments that one later regrets; being busy at home I was not overjoyed when Hugh Donald wrote to me a month or two after the congress and reminded me of my promise to carry out skin grafting in twin cattle."[1]

Reluctantly, but under this obligation and knowing that surgery and skin grafting in such animals was technically difficult, Medawar and his group started the research at Cold Norton Farm in Staffordshire, near their Birmingham laboratory, where Donald had the necessary animals for study. The skin grafting was carried out on the animal's ear, using local anesthetic. As expected, the identical twins accepted each other's

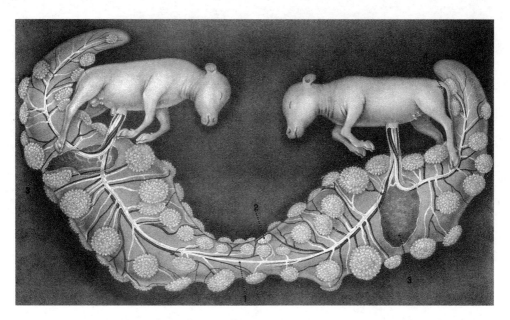

F. R. Lillie explained the phenomenon of the freemartin cattle twin as the result of shared circulation due to the fusion of the placentas from two separate pregnancies, one in each uterine limb. From F. R. Lillie, "The Theory of the Freemartin," *Science* 43 (1916): 611–13.

grafts. To the researchers' surprise however, they found that grafts exchanged between mature nonidentical twin cattle, even those of a different sex, were also accepted. The finding broke the very paradigm that had been established with such difficulty by Medawar and his school—that grafts between different adult individuals are always rejected. The team's other projects, including some difficult pigment spread experiments and studies of the interesting but modest immunosuppressive properties of steroids, were not going well. The cattle puzzle was certainly a diversion.

Ray Owen's Observations

Donald was told of the skin graft findings, and he then informed Medawar that there was a more than useful lead from earlier work on the freemartin cattle by Ray D. Owen, a veterinarian then working in Wisconsin, the dairy farming heartland of the United States. Owen's research work was supported by grants from the Guernsey Association because freemartin cattle were a financial loss to the industry. Owen had studied one family of quintuplet freemartin cattle and showed that they shared each other's blood types, a condition that he called "mosaicism."[2] All looked different and were genetically diverse, but each animal's red blood cell population had some red cells from the other four.

Owen had gone further and had solved the puzzle of these changes by unearthing a 1916 study by Chicago veterinarian Frank R. Lillie that showed the curious anatomy of the twin cattle placentas: "Development begins separately in each horn of the uterus. The rapidly elongating embryo sacs meet and fuse in the body of the uterus. The blood vessels from each side then anastomose in the connecting part of the chorion . . . so that either fetus can be injected from the other. . . . If one is male and the other female, the reproductive system of the female is largely suppressed. . . . This [freemartin state] is unquestionably to be interpreted as a case of hormonal action."[3]

This arcane matter had been well known in the field of reproductive endocrinology, but Owen was first to detect the provocative blood type mixture, and it is one of many "experiments of Nature" that continued to advance immunological knowledge.[4] He not only proposed blood typing as a useful early test for looking for the freemartin state but also remarked that "speculation on the immunology would be fruitful." He did make moves in 1951 to encourage study of the effect of experimentally injecting foreign cells into the rat fetus, and, though his graduate student did show production of artificial "erythrocyte mosaicism," this line of research was not formally published nor pursued.[5]

Macfarlane Burnet's Interest

Owen had reported his original findings on the freemartin cattle in 1946, and Macfarlane Burnet (1899–1985), when writing the second edition of his textbook *The Production of Antibodies* (1949), had noticed Owen's paper and, as a result, made the general suggestion that the fetus would recognize as "self" all tissue, notably protein antigens, encountered in prenatal life. Burnet had written that "if in embryonic life, expendable cells from a genetically distinct race are implanted and established, no antibody response should develop against the foreign cell antigen when the animal takes on independent existence."[6]

Medawar, working on the puzzle of their cattle skin grafts, realized that the unexpected graft survival was the result of the fetal cross-circulation. He recalled that "light dawned when we read Burnet and Fenner's *The Production of Antibodies* (1949) and learned of the work on twin cattle of R. D. Owen—work which, along with Traub's investigation of lymphocytic choriomeningitis in mice, formed the principal empirical basis of Burnet's audacious theory of the biology of self-recognition, from which the notion of acquired tolerance was a natural inference. We first used the word 'tolerance' in writing up the work for publication in the journal *Heredity*."[7] In fact, they had used the related word *tolerant* slightly earlier, in 1951.[8]

Burnet realized that some embryologists had routinely inserted tissue from one embryo into another and produced hybrid adults, and Herbert Eastlick at Washington State University had raised chickens with variegated plumage using this strategy. In 1952, William Longmire and Jack Cannon had noted a related phenomenon in that a proportion of newly hatched chicks could accept a third wing homograft indefinitely.[9]

The important addition by Medawar's group was that although persistence into adulthood of tissue introduced early in life had been noticed, no other group proceeded to retest the adult animal later with any second graft of tissue from an identical source. This crucial difference in emphasis undoubtedly derived directly from Medawar's unusual clinical background. Blood type chimerism or persistence of fetal grafts alone did not interest him; strategies for obtaining prolonged survival of grafts in adults did. He had been personally involved in the challenge of human homografting, dating from the problem of RAF pilots' burns and his involvement thereafter in patient care at the Glasgow Burns Unit. A new kind of "second set" testing came naturally to him, and this time he used it to detect the absence of an immune response rather than faster rejection.

University College Research

In 1951, Medawar and Rupert Billingham (1921–2002) moved back to University College London, and a graduate student, Leslie Brent (born 1925), joined them. In the laboratory, Medawar's team attempted to replicate the twin cattle situation using chickens in an interesting revival and extension of J. B. Murphy's method of studying fetal immune responses. Hens' eggs seemed to constitute the simplest available model because during incubation the eggs could easily be opened to display the yolk sac and then sealed again. The group injected cells into the eggs, a few of which ultimately hatched, and the chicks later accepted grafts.

The experiments proved to be more easily carried out with inbred mice, however. Medawar had preferred to work with outbred stock, attempting to keep close to human relevance.[10] Perhaps reluctantly, he ceased that practice since tolerance work required grafting adult mice with tissue identical to the cells introduced into the fetus. Moreover, understanding of mouse transplantation genetics was rapidly advancing. The inbred strains alone offered the possibility to do simple, repeatable transfers and transplantation of identical donor cells and tissues to groups of identical recipients. Such experiments could be replicated over lengthy periods of time and repeated in other labs.[11]

Grafting in Inbred Mice

Medawar continued to say unkindly that Loeb had found that inbred animals rejected grafts from each other. In reality, however, the transplant world was in Loeb's debt for highlighting the reliability that could be obtained with inbred animals. Each lab began regularly checking stocks for uniformity by using the skin graft test Loeb had introduced. Medawar used white A strain mouse skin grafted onto darker CBA hosts supplied by Peter Gorer in London, who in turn had used J. B. S. Haldane's University College lines brought from Bar Harbor.[12]

The skin graft work was surprisingly simple, since mice were quite easily grafted with small patches of thick tail skin. Groups of ten or twelve identical animals were given identical tail skin grafts from the other strain. The time to skin graft loss within the group was remarkably constant, with no outlying results, and little observer error, thus allowing very precise experimental comparison of different groups. These rejection times with small standard deviations became, as Medawar proudly claimed, "one of the most precise and repeatable observations in biology," and although differences between groups were usually self-evident, statistical analysis of the survival curves permitted confident statements when there were subtle differences between groups.[13] This approach provided the measure of sophistication that had previously been lacking in experimental transplantation, and the once poorly regarded business of skin grafting finally gained respectability in academia and neutralized the claims that immunological precision was to be found only in reductionist in vitro models.

Neonatal Tolerance in Mice

In a famous study in which Billingham, Brent, and Medawar extended their findings in cattle and chickens, they injected cells from adult donor white A strain mice into CBA fetuses in the uterus. When adult, the now "tolerant" CBA mice permanently accepted A strain skin grafts. The results were reported in brief in their classic paper of 1953.[14] Later, this approach was greatly simplified after the researchers realized that the donor cell injection was still effective when given immediately after birth and that the cells were as effective when introduced into the peritoneal cavity as when injected intravenously.[15]

But Medawar's group did not rush into print. He and his colleagues published the tolerance work in brief in 1953, and the detailed papers only emerged in 1956. They described the findings at the 1954 transplantation conference in New York, and Blair Rogers recalled years later that their presentation of the data, perhaps surprisingly, did not arouse any excite-

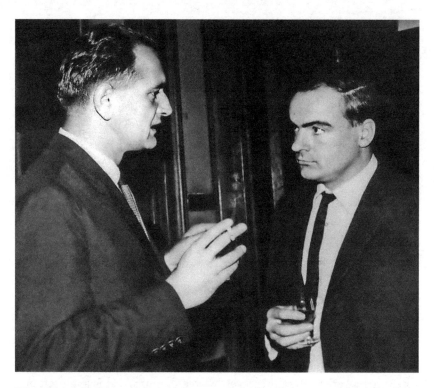

Milan Hašek (*left*), shown with N. A. Mitchison, worked at the Charles University in Prague from the 1950s, and his fetal parabiosis experiments showed tolerance induction. Image courtesy of the Novartis Foundation.

ment. Even George Snell, also attending the meeting, did not think that the paper was of much significance.[16] Nor had Ray Owen pursued his findings any further. But in coming years, after this delay, the phenomenon of tolerance was to be a dominant issue in twentieth-century immunology, and hopes for creating human tolerance of foreign tissue became the elusive Holy Grail of clinical transplantation. It was these experiments and concepts that earned Medawar a Nobel Prize in 1960, one shared with Macfarlane Burnet.[17]

Milan Hašek's Experiments

Milan Hašek (1925–1985) of Prague had made a similar observation in 1953. At first, Hašek was keen to fit his work into the Soviet Lamarckian/Lysenko biological paradigm of the day, then at odds with conventional Western genetics. His first paper, on neonatal injection of adult tissue, held out hope for permanent genetic alteration. It starts: "The method of so-called vegetative hybridization developed for plants by Mitchurin and

Lysenko is one of the methods providing excellent proofs which disprove the genetic theory of hereditary."[18]

Lysenko had claimed to have altered plant lines permanently by environmental change, and Hašek's initial hope was not only that chimerism would modify the animal but that the genome would also change and thus chimerism would be passed on to future generations.[19] But Hašek's injection of embryos with adult tissue in an attempt to alter their genetic structure had simply taken him into tolerance work, which led to close contacts with biologists in the West. He visited London, and two of his group worked with Snell at Bar Harbor each year. Although supported and encouraged by his friendship in the West with left-leaning Morten Simonsen, Hašek soon turned against the official flawed Soviet biology. Doing so left him in an uncomfortable position in his own country, and his discomfort worsened after the Soviet invasion in response to the "Prague Spring" of 1968. He was demoted, and many of his group, including Jan Klein, left for the West.[20]

Cellular Immunity

While this work on tolerance was in progress, the hunt for the elusive antibody postulated to play a part in graft rejection continued but was finally put aside in the light of new findings. In a slow revolution, compelling evidence emerged to support and resurrect the older Murphy/Loeb view that lymphoid cells, not antibodies, were indeed the agents causing graft destruction. At this time, Medawar exchanged letters with the surgeon Blair Rogers in New York on their shared research interests, and, in 1951, Medawar wrote to him regarding the discouraging hunt for the antibody:

I wish you [Blair Rogers] every possible success in your hunt for antibodies and it will be a great weight off my mind when I get a cable from you reporting success! We are discouraged here. Under Coombs guidance (he is probably the best straight immunologist in England now) we have done some extremely careful conglutination and anti-globulin tests. . . . We have also done tests in which donor tracheal epithelium and phagocytes have been cultivated in immune serum and the tracheal epithelium goes on beating and phagocytosis is unimpaired. . . . My ex-pupil Avrion Mitchison in Oxford says he is now almost sure he can secure passive transfer of immunity by leucocytes from peritoneal exudates. His work is still in progress; it is done with scrupulous care.[21]

By late 1952, Mitchison's proposals for the major role of cells and "cell-mediated immunity" to homografts began its entry into received wisdom.

Mitchison's Contribution

Nicolas Avrion Mitchison (born 1928) was an undergraduate student studying under Medawar at Oxford, and although he remained there when his mentor moved to the chair of zoology in Birmingham, he assisted with the awkward cattle skin grafting experiments conducted there. Mitchison began his cellular transfer work in 1951, spent a year working with Tracy Sonneborn in Indiana, and published the important results of his work in 1953.

Mitchison also took advantage of the powerful tool offered by the inbred strains of mice, which permitted successful cellular transfers from one animal to another within an inbred strain. The first surprise was that lymphoid cells proved to be more robust than had been thought and were largely unharmed by the manipulations required to make cell suspensions outside the body. Secondly, contrary to the old assumptions, upon injection into the peritoneum of mice of the same strain, the cells from the lymphoid suspension migrated promptly throughout the body and resumed their usual activities. The long-held view that the featureless lymphocyte was an idle wanderer in the blood and an indolent bystander in connective tissue was wrong.

Mitchison immunized one group of mice using tumor grafts (as a form of normal tissue) and took lymphoid cells from the mice. Normal mice of the same strain injected with these lymphoid cells rejected the same tumor graft more promptly. Mitchison could not transfer immunity with immune serum. He boldly proposed that a cellular mechanism was the main agent providing immunity to tumor and tissue grafts.[22]

Fine Discrimination

Helping this reemergence of cell-mediated immunity was Philip Gell (1914–2001) in London, who had been asked by the Ministry of Supply to look at the high incidence of contact dermatitis in factories making the explosive trinitrobenzene. Gell noticed that the skin reaction was delayed, appearing ten to fourteen days after exposure, unlike most allergic reactions. It was a new form of delayed sensitivity, one suggesting that skin proteins were changed by this simple chemical and that a cellular immune response could detect and then react against this tiny change in body protein. Although reluctant to add to the complexity of immunological discourse "for reasons of economy," Gell did support the idea that "wandering cells carry a special kind of antibody."[23] Mitchison pointed out that this cell-bound antibody system had finer discrimination than that of conventional antibodies and that "the homograft reaction is concerned with antigenic differences of a much slighter nature than in classical immunological studies."[24]

When Mitchison visited Bar Harbor, he continued this work in Snell's laboratory and again emphasized that serum alone could not transfer homograft sensitivity. He reported to the 1954 transplantation conference in New York that "several reasons can be found for supposing that the serum antibodies are less important than might be supposed. . . . In further experiments, we have been able to show that detectable titers of serum antibody are neither necessary nor sufficient for homograft breakdown."

Medawar also came around to this view, but, reluctant to dismiss the role of antibodies, he also proposed that fixed, not free, antibodies were responsible for cellular immunity.

This cautious but incomplete acceptance of the existence of another system continued to restore the lymphocyte to a central role. It was an important change in understanding, one that others supported. When new "privileged sites," which lacked lymphatic drainage, were created in the animal body, visiting lymphocytes could not exit, and the resulting "immune ignorance" meant that homografts placed there could survive well.[25] In particular, a study by G. H. Algire from the National Cancer Institute at Bethesda was important in changing attitudes on the topic and in elevating the status of the lymphocyte.[26] In conducting his studies, Algire placed tissue homografts in a millipore chamber, whose perforations allowed fluids but not cells to pass in and out. Trapeznikov had used this model in his anthrax parchment pouch experiments in the "lost era" of immunology during the 1890s. Homografts inside Algire's barrier were exposed to antibodies but not to cells, and the grafts survived nicely, even in sensitized animals. A major paradigm change was occurring.[27]

The Paradigm Change

The proposed existence of cell-mediated immunity greatly simplified the spectrum of immunological responses. It immediately explained the puzzle of some special cases, notably the survival of corneal homografts, which have no blood vessels and are thus not in contact with lymphocytes. It explained that the so-called "missing antibody" in some diseases characterized by lymphocytic infiltration, ranging from contact dermatitis to tuberculosis, was indeed missing. It recalled James Bumgardner Murphy's finding of graft survival in "privileged sites" not reached by cells, such as the brain. The hamster cheek pouch was soon added to this list.[28] Leo Loeb's view that the fetus was a protected homograft was also revisited. The new view acknowledged that Murphy and Loeb were right and that the massive lymphocyte infiltrate in rejecting grafts meant something. This concept gave a provocative new explanation for the so-called autoimmune diseases, long known to be associated with marked lymphoid infiltration.

At this point, Loeb's 1930s insights on the lymphocyte should have been recognized, but instead the old animus to his allegedly abstruse contributions continued. Though a convert to the Murphy/Loeb view, Medawar still wrote unkindly of Loeb's work: "It was full of fine talk about individuality and differentials and the like, but it did not lend itself to experimental testing, and so may confidently be classified as so much nature-philosophy."[29] Loeb had, however, documented his experimental testing fully and carefully in his original papers. Medawar's group even received credit for "Loeb's Test," since a book on experimental transplantation by Rupert Billingham was soon credited with the grafting method of quality control for inbred mice.[30] The geneticist C. C. Little's bizarre polemic attack on Loeb in 1926 was found and unfairly quoted again against Loeb.[31]

The marginalizing of Loeb had yet another unfortunate effect, since the excellent lymphocyte-oriented work of the "lost era," on which Loeb built, was uncoupled from any continuity with this revival in the role of the lymphocyte in the 1950s. The boom in transplantation cellular immunology of the 1950s was seen as entirely new and without any earlier lineage, a judgment that, if it were true, would be unique in the annals of science.

New Paradigm's Slow Growth

The new thinking about the lymphocyte's role was isolated for a while, and conventional immunology circles were slow to accommodate the revolution. Cellular immunity was still in a world apart, and, until about 1960, it did not feature in the serology-dominated immunology journals, notably the *Journal of Immunology*. In 1956, William C. Boyd's standard text, *Fundamentals of Immunology*, had only one vague reference to the lymphocyte, stating that, "in the absence of more definite knowledge of lymphocyte function, a rational account of the lymphocyte in pathological conditions is impossible."[32] Joseph Yoffey's standard textbook on the lymphocyte and the lymphatic system also failed to assist in this matter. Also slow to catch up were the pragmatic surgeons in their search for practical methods of prolonging kidney grafts. Clinicians like Joseph Murray still assumed that antibodies caused homograft rejection.[33] It did not matter. Successful empirical innovators could ignore the theory; it was results that counted.

In the laboratory, the insights from the new cellular immunology meant continuing progress in understanding not only the mechanisms of graft rejection but also much else. Many talented research workers were entering the field, attracted by the intellectual challenge and the feeling that the bland little lymphocyte, all brain and no muscle, and much more mobile and powerful than it cared to reveal earlier, might have some further secrets to reveal. The new cellular immunologists also knew that the tissue rejection mechanism and its "exquisite specificity" (Mitchison's phrase) clearly had some form of fundamental biological role, as Loeb had taught, through its ability to recognize any tissue that did not match that of the host. Biologists like Bill Hildemann (1927–1983) traced the cellular transplantation response further and further down the phylogenetic tree.[34] A few invertebrates among the annelid worms and tunicates like sea squirts could also show graft rejection; since they failed to make antibodies, the dark thought arose that antibody formation was the junior evolutionary partner.[35] Later, with fine irony, the humble hydra species, which Abraham Trembley had used in his classical grafting experiments in the eighteenth century, were shown in 1970 to be intolerant, after all, of lasting unions with bits taken from others. Trembley was lucky in his short-term observations in his experiments in 1744.

Cell Studies

From the success of the cell transfer experiments came a new interest in methods of studying isolated lymphoid cells. Mitchison-type transfer and in vitro methods helped expand this field. The robust lymphocyte was soon to show great stamina and vitality in the test tube, now often the economical, disposable tubes provided by the plastics revolution. Concerns that study of parts separated from the living body would show effects not found in the body, that is, findings not seen in the intact animal, were put aside.

This reductionist biology was also aided by the emergence of better growth media for cell cultures. New solutions used for short-term cell suspensions were improvements on the traditional Ringer's, Hartmann's, and Locke's salines favored from the earlier part of the century. New variants like Hank's, Eagle's, and RPMI-type solutions allowed sustained vitality of dissociated cells. Elegant layered density gradients allowed separation of cell types, notably lymphocytes, and the use of unsorted lymphoid cells ceased.[36] Newly available isotopes could label cells for cell-killing tests or could track cells' movement through the body.

Long-term Preservation

To these in vitro techniques was added the important ability to freeze, store, and revive cells. This capability further revolutionized the study of the lymphocyte, since it allowed particular cells to be put aside and restudied or used at will. Red blood cells, lacking a nucleus, had been easily stored, but the serendipitous discovery of a method of freezing and reviving nucleated cells came from a group at the National Institute for Medical Research at Mill Hill in London. Allan Parkes (1900–1990), Chris Polge (1926–2006), and Audrey Smith were attempting to freeze and revive animal sperm, a goal with considerable commercial significance in the animal breeding world. They described their unexpected and striking success in a paper published in *Nature* in 1949. The trick was to use "the action of glycerol and related compounds, to which our attention was directed by a chance observation"—that the reagent bottles had been mixed up. The accidental use of Meyer's albumin, only used in the lab for mounting histological specimens, preserved the sperm, and it was the glycerol component of the solution that was crucial for cryopreservation.[37]

Using increasingly simple freezing schedules, the team regularly obtained successful results, and, by 1954, long-term storage of viable corneas was possible.[38] More successful variants on the method, notably the use of agents such as dimethylsulfoxide (DMSO), emerged and eventually cryopreservation became a remarkably simple matter. By 1970, early-stage embryos could be preserved, but attempts at long-term subzero preservation of complex tissues and organs like the kidney failed.

Genetics of Graft Rejection

Since the late 1930s, Peter Gorer in London had been studying experimental transplantation, and, unlike those studying normal tissue grafts, he had already found host antibodies against tumor grafts. George Snell in Bar Harbor had been working with complex mouse breeding experiments to try to unravel tissue incompatibility. It was only in the mid-1950s, however, that the general significance of their work for practical transplantation was realized and Gorer's antibodies noticed, paradoxically at a time when the role of cell-mediated immunity was accepted anew.

Peter Alfred Gorer (1907–1961) had begun his scientific research at University College London in 1936, when he blood-typed the inbred mice Haldane had brought back to the department from the Bar Harbor lab.[39] Gorer identified three red cell antigens, which he numbered simply as I, II and III. Antigen II was not restricted to the mouse red blood cells but was also found on most of the other cells of the body, including white cells.

Gorer used a sarcoma tumor that had arisen in an A strain mouse bearing antigen II, and the tumor grew in some, but not all other inbred strains, and there was a pattern of growth or loss. The animals in which the tumor grew also had antigen II; it failed to grow in mice lacking antigen II. The widespread antigen II seemed unlikely to give rise to the "host susceptibility to cancer" concept that had earlier beguiled others like C. C. Little. Gorer accordingly shifted the emphasis to determining

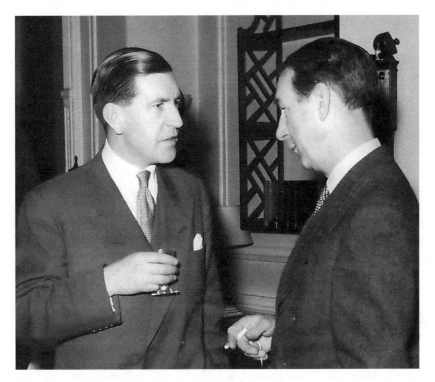

Peter Gorer (*right*) found an antigen controlling the outcome of tumor transplantation in mice, and in the Department of Pathology at Guy's Hospital, London, he and his pupils developed an early understanding of histocompatibility testing. Image courtesy of the Novartis Foundation.

why the tumor would be lost in some cases rather than why it persisted in others, concluding that the tumor's failure was explained by a reaction against antigen II.

Moreover, Gorer found that when the tumor cells from the antigen II mouse failed to grow and were rejected, the host produced an antibody against antigen II. This was the first such "allo-antibody" to be detected, though Gorer was careful not to claim that this antibody was responsible for graft loss. Medawar commented much later that:

Gorer was now in a position to reformulate the genetical theory of tumour transplantation along immunological lines. His predecessors had been inclined to speak of genetic factors the possession of which conferred susceptibility to the growth of foreign tumours. Gorer saw that . . . it would be more in keeping with immunological theory if the possession by the tumour of Antigen II were said to excite resistance in mice that lacked it. . . . Although in later years he kept his mind open to the possibility that malignant tissue might be antigenically distinguishable from normal tissue, there was no reason to doubt that the rules governing the transplantation of normal and malignant tissues were essentially the same.[40]

Gorer's research was interrupted by an increase in his routine clinical work as a pathologist during the war, but he visited Snell at the Jackson Laboratory in Bar Harbor in 1946.[41] The two discovered that they were in broad agreement about the role of the tissue antigens in tumor rejection.[42] While Gorer used serological methods, Snell had used complex backcross experiments to make progress with the genetics of tissue transplantation in mice. This research benefited from the fortuitous association of the obvious fused tail trait with the region that controlled graft loss—what Snell called the "H region." The two investigators merged their independent genetic terminology—Gorer's "Antigen II" and Snell's "H" to designate "H2" as the region on the mouse chromosome responsible for the cell surface antigenic differences and thus graft loss. Because the mouse red cells were easily studied and bore these important antigens (unlike the red cells in some other animals), the mouse was the animal of choice in such work. Together Snell and Gorer discarded the assumption that the genes involved were dominant or recessive, having realized that there were many alleles with independent action and a graded influence on graft outcome.

Gorer, after his visit to the lab in Maine, returned to London and continued his work as a pathologist at Guy's Hospital, London. In 1948, he and Snell collaborated on an important publication that recorded their joint understanding and terminology of the genetics of graft rejection, and in the title they used the word *histocompatibility* for the first time.[43] This term had echoes of the earlier emphasis on tumor graft survival, even susceptibility, rather than normal tissue rejection. But the word *histocompatibility* did at least reflect the later clinical need to match donor and recipient to enhance the likelihood of graft survival.[44] Snell, who had spent time in St. Louis, had admired Leo Loeb since that time and had loyally used Loeb's terminology for graft types, but the arcane usage, notably Loeb's "homoiotransplant," fell from favor and the older term "homograft" took its place.

Enhancement Found

In 1946, Snell repeated an observation from the "lost era" that was to haunt transplantation immunology thereafter. When mice immunized with transplanted tumors were treated with sera against the tumor, he expected more rapid rejection but found instead that such sera could prolong the graft, a phenomenon he called "enhancement" of the graft's survival—that is, antibody-mediated protection of grafts from rejection.[45] This experiment raised hopes and concerns. There was the more than interesting possibility that human organ grafts might survive through use

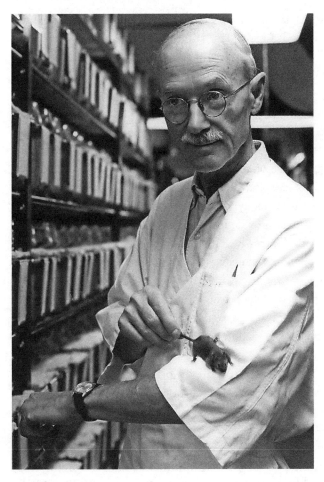

George Snell pioneered the study of transplantation genetics in mice using backcross and other breeding techniques. Image courtesy of the Jackson Laboratory Archives, Bar Harbor, Maine.

of such enhancing sera (a hope never fulfilled) but also the fear that any attempts at immunotherapy of human tumors might result in more rapid growth (also never observed). Enhancement was indeed obtained in some special experimental transplant models later, but this was not of general application.

The Missing Antibody

Snell continued with closer and closer inbreeding of mice, which had the useful commercial by-product of producing "congenic" mice differing by only one histocompatibility antigen. Gorer in London meanwhile concentrated on improving methodology for the detection of antibodies appearing after tumor transplantation. Medawar, who had abandoned the hunt for the "missing antibody," had, surprisingly, not met Gorer, such was isolation of the small number of transplant researchers at the time. Not until Medawar returned to London in 1951 did the two meet. Gorer supported a humoral view of transplant rejection in the 1950s and continued a scholarly jousting campaign with the new proponents of cell-mediated rejection, namely Mitchison and Medawar.[46]

Although members of Medawar's group were now enthusiastically exploring the significance of cellular mechanisms, they cooperated with Gorer's team at Guy's Hospital. Bernard Amos, working with Gorer, first detected the "missing antibody" in mouse homograft experiments using skin-grafted animals provided by Medawar's colleagues Rupert Billingham and Elizabeth Sparrow.[47] This finding deepened the debate in the 1950s on the role of the previously elusive antibody. In 1957–1958, Paul Terasaki of UCLA was a visiting worker in Medawar's laboratory, where he started his distinguished lifelong work on transplantation antibodies. For the rest of his career, Terasaki enjoyed revealing to cellular-leaning transplanters that with each advance in serological technique, additional subtle, unsuspected antibodies were found in graft rejection. His listeners responded by pointing out that even antibody formation required the help of the T-cells responsible for cell-mediated immunity.

The Lymphocyte Studied

Gorer had sensed that, to extend the serology of transplantation beyond the mouse and toward "tissue groups" in humans, he had to move from studying the helpful but unusual mouse red cell and seek to identify the antigens on other available cells. The hope was to study the lymphocyte, and eventually the human lymphocyte. Gorer attracted talented postgraduate students, and the group gathered for this research included the later pioneers of human tissue-typing, namely Bernard Amos (1923–2003), Richard Batchelor (born 1931), and Edward Boyse (1924–2007); it was Amos who, in 1953, first devised a successful method of studying suspensions of white cells.[48] Further improvements allowed the difficult early tests and erratic results to be replaced, and Gorer's lab soon reported the first direct lymphocyte killing test.[49]

Gorer's shift to studying the mouse leukocyte as the serological target cell opened the way for human studies. He was not deterred by the huge number of antigens emerging in animal studies. He had found strong and weak antigens, and perhaps not all needed detection: "It is therefore possible that we might greatly prolong the life of human homografts if we could match them for a relatively small number of antigens. It would very seldom be possible to obtain compatibility for all of a very large number of antigens." He suggested perceptively that antibodies would be found after any human organ transplant, predicting that such antibodies could then be used to type the transplant donor and recipient. Thinking even further ahead, he warned that these antibodies could present some possible dangers after human organ transplantation. His fear was that blood transfusion or a pregnancy after a successful organ transplant might encounter dangerous antibodies: "It will be seen that if homografts are to be used in clinical practice, the question of an antibody response is not entirely academic. One must be able to type people so as to minimise the risks (i.e. of future blood transfusion and pregnancy) in recipients."[50]

Ironically, events took a different turn. Unknown to Gorer, pregnancy and transfusion had already produced these antibodies and would provide the first sera to be used for tissue typing. His plea for close matching at the time of transplantation, if only to minimize sensitization, is still sound.

Gorer did not live to participate in the exciting early days of tissue typing, which developed along the lines he anticipated and in which his methods and his pupils played a major role. He died in 1961, and Snell was awarded a Nobel Prize in 1980, at the age of seventy-seven, an award that Gorer, had he lived, would certainly have shared.

By the early 1960s, most researchers were in agreement about the relative roles of the two aspects of the immune response. The power and specificity of the cell-mediated rejection component, particularly in first grafts and weak genetic combinations, meant that antibodies were relegated to a secondary role. In second grafts, very strong combinations, or xenografting, the humoral component was judged to have greater importance.

These rapid advances in basic and applied immunology continued in the mid-1950s, at a time when, paradoxically, clinical attempts at organ homografting had ceased after the attempts in Boston and Paris. Although the lymphocyte was now considered to have a role in immunological reactions, there was little understanding of its detailed behavior. The usual teaching on its function had since early in the century acknowledged one striking feature, namely, that the cell emerged in huge numbers from the thoracic duct to connect with the bloodstream. The simplest interpretation was that the cell had an extremely short life, and since the thoracic output predominantly consisted of small lymphocytes, many researchers concluded in despair that the small version was an effete "end cell," a former lymphocyte of some sort.

Howard Florey, as noted earlier, had a long-standing attraction to this puzzle, but, in the late 1930s, his first coordinated attempt to study the cell, with the Medawars on the team, had come to nothing. Thereafter, he was fond of quoting Arnold Rich's view on the lymphocyte: "The complete ignorance of the function of this cell is one of the most humiliating and disgraceful gaps in all medical knowledge." In the 1950s, Florey once more revived his Oxford department's interest in this cell. He suggested to James "Jim" Gowans (born 1924) in his department that "if he could find out where the lymphocyte travelled to, then they might find out what it did."[51] Tracing the movement of this cell had once been difficult, but by this time it was possible to track it using isotopes. In 1954, Ottesen in Copenhagen had labeled the lymphocyte and proved that it was very long-lived cell, not a short-lived one, and this finding deepened the mystery of the huge output from the thoracic duct.[52] Aided once again by new technology, in this case fine-bore, nonwettable plastic tubing, Gowans established long-term thoracic duct fistula drainage in rats.

Tracing the Cell

Gowans showed that the huge output of cells from the thoracic duct declined after a few days but that the output could be restored by reinfusion of the same cells into the general circulation. Using an isotope to label lymphocytes, he showed in 1959 that these labeled cells, given intravenously, would appear promptly in the thoracic duct.[53] He had solved the puzzle of the huge output from the thoracic duct, proposing that the small lymphocyte was a recirculating cell, moving from blood to lymph and back again. It was not until 1964 that Gowans's view was accepted, since it proved difficult to find the cell in the act of crossing over.[54]

The recirculation findings had profound influence and increased the interest in the lymphocyte. The discovery suggested that lymphocytes could visit transplanted tissue and the draining lymph nodes and then spread as sensitized cells, retaining memory thereafter. But lymphoid cells came in all sizes and occupied many different organs and tissues, including the mysterious thymus. The neutral and functional phrase "immunologically competent cell" was widely used for a while to reflect the powerful potential of the lymphoid cell group, usefully replacing classifications based on the size or location of the cell.

Graft-versus-Host Response

Major assistance in understanding the function of the lymphocyte arose at this time, it is sometimes forgotten, from study of the graft-versus-host response. Its use came at a time when lymphocytes were still not easily studied outside the body. The only way of exploring lymphocyte behavior

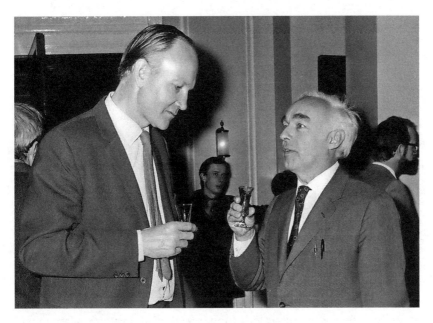

James Gowans (*left*), shown with R. E. Billingham (*right*), demonstrated at Oxford the recirculation and immunological competence of the lymphocyte. Image courtesy of the Novartis Foundation.

at the time was by cell transfer, a method that, though cumbersome, has the attraction of revealing behavior in the intact animal. It is a strategy free of reductionist criticism.

The idea that lymphoid cells in the *graft* might attack the *host* (GvH) had been suggested more than tentatively, as mentioned earlier, by Morten Simonsen and Jim Dempster early in the 1950s. Simonsen still found the general idea to be of interest, and he began to look for this possible GvH reaction by injecting lymphocytes into hosts of various kinds. He started with the convenient chicken embryo model, unaware of James Bumgardner Murphy's earlier use of it and Murphy's important findings. Simonsen immediately noticed Murphy's long-forgotten finding of marked enlargement of the chicken embryo spleen when foreign lymphoid cells were added.[55] Simonsen, now aware that the lymphocyte could migrate, realized that his introduced lymphocytes (which were not rejected by the embryo) had migrated and attacked the host, notably the embryo's spleen, with vigor. Simonsen soon realized Murphy's priority and gave a gracious acknowledgment to his prescience.

Simonsen developed his idea by using the newly available inbred strains of animals, and he began studying the GvH response in the adult animal, injecting various types of lymphocyte into hybrids made from two parental inbred strains; these animals could not react against injected parental strain cells. But the injected parental cells recognized half of the hybrid host antigens, which increased spleen weights. This phenomenon proved to be remarkably reproducible, and he could quantify the immunological response. It was the first powerful tool with which to investigate the powers of the various "immunologically competent cells," since the injected cell type, origin, and numbers could be controlled. His rat spleen assay method was published and used from 1957, and the simpler rat popliteal thigh lymph node assay followed later, in 1970.[56]

Other GvH Situations

Around this time, three other research groups had made independent and puzzling observations that turned out to be explicable by this GvH mechanism. Medawar and Brent had noticed in their early experiments that many of the CBA animals made tolerant by neonatal injection of A strain lymphoid cells eventually became ill. This chronic malaise involved a failure to thrive, with hair loss, lung infection, and spleen enlargement, a syndrome they descriptively termed "runt disease." They at first understandably blamed the infection commonly found in animal houses from time to time. Later they realized that "runting" was simply a GvH reaction, caused by the persisting, tolerizing injected lymphoid cells reacting against the recipient tissues. Thereafter, for further tolerance studies, they also used Simonsen's strategy of injecting adult CBA/A hybrid cells to induce tolerance, neatly avoiding the GvH.

Another team, D. W. H. Barnes and J. F. Loutit at the Medical Research Council Radiobiology Research Unit at Harwell, had a similar experience. They were seeking ways to protect against lethal irradiation. Experimenting with homograft bone marrow as a protectant, they noticed what they called "secondary disease" in their surviving bone marrow recipient animals, again noticing an enlarged spleen. Initially, they also blamed infection, but the situation was once again recognized as a GvH response caused by the lymphocytes transferred in the foreign marrow. In the United States, Delta Uphoff made a similar observation on radiation chimeras studied at the National Cancer Institute.[57]

Mid-1950s Attitudes

By this time in the mid-1950s, the growing group of transplantation immunologists had established the primacy of cell-mediated mechanisms and the existence of GvH, and there were hopes for tissue matching. To add to this, Medawar's group had demonstrated a highly successful specific and safe way of preventing graft loss by inducing tolerance. But the surgeons did pause and wait. Medawar, as always, had human organ transplantation as a goal, and, in 1954, he was increasingly confident it could be achieved: "I now feel certain that the clinical homograft problem is soluble; workers all over the world are discovering gaps in the immunological defences that were unheard of even five years ago, and there seems no reason to doubt that if homograft problems continue to be the subject of systematic and careful research, the gaps can be made a great deal wider yet."[58]

The main defensive gap, almost an open door, seemed to invite the use of tolerance induction, rather than continuing efforts to prolong graft survival by the other means. Still, it was difficult to see how tolerance could be put into clinical practice. To mimic the animal model in its simplest form required placing tissue from the future donor into a fetus or newborn child. Making children tolerant of parental tissue as insurance for serious disease later was a possible scheme, and Michael Woodruff had moved in this direction and injected prematurely born children in this way. Upon hearing of the GvH danger, he quickly terminated this project before doing any harm—or achieving any tolerance.[59] But the elegance and specificity of tolerance induction continued to offer an exciting challenge, and the mechanism attracted the attention of more and more immunologists. It was also a topic favored by those funding basic biological studies.

Early Transplantation Conferences

The scattered group of transplantation enthusiasts had no organizational structure until the 1950s. In 1950, Medawar hosted a small meeting in Birmingham for scientists and clinicians interested in transplantation, and among the attendees were Simonsen, Coombs the immunologist, and the surgeons Woodruff and Archibald McIndoe. Better known was the first American transplantation conference, organized by E. J. Eichwald (born 1913) of New York. This group gathered at Arden House on the Harriman Campus of Columbia University, New York, in 1952. The meeting was simply called the Tissue Transplantation Conference, and its proceedings were published the following year.[60] Support for the meeting came from the American Cancer Society and the National Institutes of Health, and Eichwald later gave long service as an editor of the transplantation journals.[61] The 1952 conference, held at a time when transatlantic travel was still by sea, provided travel funding for two European speakers—Medawar from Britain and Pieter Gaillard from Leiden.[62]

At that historic meeting in 1952, papers were given by Longmire, George Gey, Snell, Eichwald, and Theodore Hauschka, and extra material

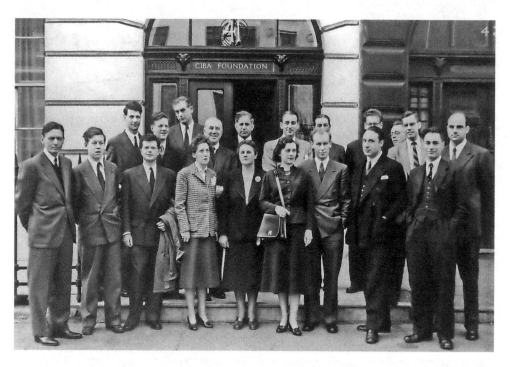

Some of the participants at the CIBA symposium, Transplantation of Normal Tissues, in London, 1954. Image courtesy of the Novartis Foundation.

was presented in discussion by Gaillard, Hume, Herbert Conway, Algire, Richmond Prehn, Medawar, and Nathan Kaliss. An attempt was made during the meeting to standardize the anarchic nomenclature of transplantation, as noted earlier. Interestingly, there was barely any mention at the meeting of the now important series of human kidney transplants from 1950 to 1953, except for a brief comment by Hume in the discussion; the matter was sensitive.

In 1953, a conference was held at the CIBA Foundation in London, with Medawar's help, on the topic "The Preservation and Transplantation of Normal Tissues."[63] The foundation continued to take a close interest in immunological topics and host other important invited-speaker conferences.[64]

The historic New York meeting that gave rise to the later transplantation conferences had a different origin, one closely linked to the still continuing interest in transplantation by American plastic surgeons. John Converse, as noted earlier, had been attached to the U.S. Army in Europe, and upon his return to New York, he brought in other plastic surgeons, notably Blair Rogers and Lyndon Peer, to share his interest. Converse's wartime work spurred the group's interest in skin grafting. In the early 1950s, he persuaded the New York Academy of Sciences, of which he was a council member, to host a conference on tissue transplantation, and it took place in 1954, two years after Eichwald's meeting. Such was the sentiment of the day that, Converse recalled later, "it was difficult to attract any respectable immunologists."[65]

Casting around for help with the organization for the meeting, a colleague, Sherwood Laurence, then in charge of the student health service at Bellevue Hospital, suggested that Felix Rapaport (1929–2001), a hospital intern convalescing from hepatitis, had available free time and would be suitable as the organizer. After the conference, Rapaport and Laurence joined Converse's research group, as America's first transplantation immunologists. They had a major influence thereafter.[66]

This New York Academy of Sciences meeting of 1954 was held in the Barbizon Plaza Hotel, New York, and was called the First Tissue Homotransplantation Conference.[67] The sessions that attracted papers at these early conferences involved special cases and privileged sites and the hunt for the missing transplantation antibody. Several attendees unconvincingly claimed to have found the antibody. Cellular mechanisms were not yet on the agenda in that year of 1954, and the only speaker to raise the matter cautiously was Marion Sulzberger, a New York dermatologist; in the discussion that followed, Avrion Mitchison supported him.

Following the success of this meeting, a regular biennial series resulted.[68] Up to 1956, the main theme was still the search for the antibody responsible for rejection (now allegedly cell-bound). Blair Rogers made considerable efforts to include papers from surgeons in the out-of-favor Soviet Union, but difficulties continued, and, in 1960, Anastasy Lapchinsky, though expected as a speaker, was unable to attend, and his interesting paper on Soviet transplantation, which described the use of stapling devices and organ perfusion machines, was instead read by Blair Rogers. Lapchinsky's other transmitted contribution to the conference—on dog limb transplantation—was less well received.[69]

The meeting format remained the same until the early 1960s.[70] During this early period, the plastic surgeons Converse and Rogers had continued as cochairs of the meetings. But, poignantly, the world of clinical transplantation was steadily moving away from the realm of plastic surgery. Skin grafting of human patients and laboratory animals had been the basis of all early transplantation hopes and observations, but now transplantation of other tissues and vascularized organ grafts were gaining prominence.[71] Added to this was the irony that skin proved to be more vigorously rejected than most internal organs.

As transplantation specialists began to gather for meetings, new publications appeared to report their work. A lively but short-lived journal called *Transplantation Bulletin*, edited by Eichwald, appeared in 1953; it was the first periodical devoted to transplantation studies. It had short articles, current affairs, and reviews, together with massive scholarly, historical bibliographies of the literature relevant to each aspect of transplantation. In 1958, the *Bulletin* was incorporated unhappily into *Plastic and Reconstructive Surgery* as a supplement, and, four years later, this arrangement ceased. Soon after, new and lasting niche transplantation journals began to appear.

Corneal Grafting Begins

While these important early events in transplantation immunology were unfolding, one type of human grafting was becoming routine in the early 1950s. Because the cornea has no blood circulation, no white cells reached the graft, and thus, in straightforward cases, rejection did not occur. With no immunological hurdle to overcome and technical mastery achieved, the corneal grafter's main challenge was to obtain donor tissue. This entry of corneal transplantation into accepted clinical practice had important, albeit forgotten, effects on the development of organ transplantation. Those pioneering this new service of corneal grafting were the first to grapple with supply and legal issues. At the time, the transplant-minded British surgeon Michael Woodruff noticed that progress was being made in corneal grafting, notably in the drive for donors, and that eye surgeons were successfully obtaining changes in the ancient and outdated British laws on tissue donation. Woodruff, like others, hoped organ transplantation would eventually become routine, and he commented that "all interested in homotransplantation must be deeply grateful to the ophthalmic surgeons for bringing this matter before the public and government."[72]

In 1877, Arthur von Hippel (1841–1916) devised a clockwork trephine, an implement that permitted extreme precision in cutting and fitting corneal grafts. The first successful human corneal homograft was reported by the Vienna-trained ophthalmologist Eduard Zirm (1863–1944) in 1905, in the university town of Olomouc, one hundred miles east of Prague.[73] Zirm presented his patient at the prestigious Vienna Medical Society in 1906, and at this time the same society also heard about experimental kidney transplant attempts in eastern Europe.

The continuous era of corneal grafting started in the 1930s, when Vladimir Filatov established a routine service in Ukraine, with Moscow following shortly afterward.[74] Filatov had sufficient cadaveric eye donations to perform his work, because the collectivist Soviet system either successfully encouraged such donation or allowed routine removal without any legal formalities, as was normal practice with cadaveric blood. Filatov's unit grew in size to become the impressive, one-hundred-bed Ukrainian Experimental Institute for Eye Diseases, founded in 1936. Although specialty hospitals were not entirely a novelty in medical care, the institute's multidisciplinary structure and linkage of research facilities to a clinical service was new, and the institute was widely admired internationally at the time.

Elsewhere, however, the lack of corneal donation posed serious supply problems for transplant surgery. The eye surgeons in Europe and the United States, though aware of the surgical possibilities and ready to develop corneal grafting service, met public resistance to donating tissue after death. Those New York surgeons who were interested in this operation in the 1930s had to improvise and use various sources:

There was a constant struggle to find donor material most of which came from therapeutic enucleations—eyes with suspected intraocular tumors, traumatized eyes ... and cadaver eyes which were usually derivatives of "private deaths." That term euphemistically referred to the occasional opportunity that corneal surgeons had to gain private access to the dead body of a patient or family friend, in order to remove the eyes before the undertaker removed the body. There was no paper work. . . .

For the early corneal surgeons, therefore, the supply line for keratoplasty called for considerable discretion and resourcefulness. One solution that was practiced by Townley Paton was the use of donor material from executed prisoners. Paton lived in New York City just 30 miles south of the notorious Sing-Sing Prison. . . .

There is no record of the frequency of Paton's visits to Sing-Sing, although there is a family recollection that the trip was made rather often in the early 1940s.[75]

In Britain, the Welsh surgeon Tudor Thomas (1893–1976) attempted to set up a cadaveric eye donation service in the late 1930s. The effort failed, and he was thus limited to using the corneas occasionally available from eyes surgically removed from patients for various reasons. He appealed to colleagues for assistance in obtaining corneas, and a surgeon working near London recalled a donation from 1936: "[I] removed the eye in Reading at about 9 o'clock in the morning, had a porter standing outside the theatre, and having packed the eye carefully in a jar in cotton wool and saline surrounded by ice, it was taken straight to the Great Western station and handed to the guard of the train going to Cardiff. Mr Tudor Thomas collected it from the guard at the Cardiff station and took it to his theatre, where he performed the graft later on in the afternoon."[76]

But these were only occasional events. Tudor Thomas's assessment was that public attitudes did not favor donation, and he was gloomy about obtaining regular donations: "It is difficult to contemplate the establishment in this country of a scheme requiring elaborate organization and intense publicity."[77]

Changing Attitudes

Remarkably, attitudes to postmortem corneal donation changed. In the 1940s, the clinical demand in Britain and the United States for corneal grafting increased, mostly as a result of wartime injuries, especially facial burns, which had also encouraged study of skin grafting. The war effort seemed to bring a new collectivist cohesion to society, and eye donation to assist blinded veterans could now be presented as an altruistic, worthy service to the community.

In the United States, Townley Paton and Ramon Castroviejo became actively involved in efforts to promote donation, as did Louis Paufique, Philippe Sourdille, and G. Offret in France and Albert Franchescetti in Italy. The surgical activist in Britain who helped bring about local change was Benjamin W. Rycroft (1902–1967), at Queen Victoria Hospital, in East Grinstead, and he acknowledged that, before the war, "the country was not yet informed or ready."

Rycroft started corneal grafting at Queen Victoria Hospital in 1947. Like the plastic surgeons there, he dealt with the delayed legacy of the war, notably deformities of the face and eyes. Rycroft also inherited the political skills of McIndoe, his wartime predecessor, in negotiating with bureaucratic military departments and reluctant governments.

The legal difficulty in starting a formal program for the donation of corneas after death was that the matter was covered by the Anatomy Act of 1832. The oldest British law relevant to the practice of medicine, it dated to the excesses of the grave robbers of the nineteenth century. The Anatomy Act prohibited dissection or removal of tissue from a corpse unless the person had gifted their body to medical science, usually a medical school, or if the body was unclaimed. The body parts had to be returned for burial later. The wording of the act not only did not meet the needs of corneal grafting but actively precluded it. Lord Justice Davies looked back later at the status of the Anatomy Act, which "required that the body [parts] be decently interred after dissection and it therefore had nothing to do with retention of tissue or organs for any purpose. Nevertheless, the grafting of the cornea from the dead to the living had become a frequently performed operation for several years. There are times when the bold medico makes the cautious lawyer gasp."[78]

But the surgeons of the 1950s were in no legal danger. Those tending the war wounded, like Harold Gillies, Archibald McIndoe, and Benjamin Rycroft, had particularly heroic status and were unassailable.

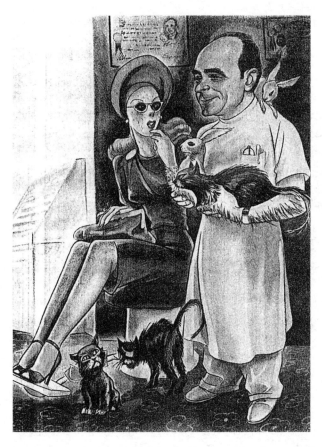

Ramon Castroviejo, the Spanish-born New York corneal graft pioneer, whose science was never far from his clinical work. From Mark J. Mannis and Avi A. Mannis, *Corneal Transplantation: A History in Profiles* (Oostende, Belgium: J. P. Wayenbourgh, 1999).

Public Campaigns

In the United States, the wartime pressure for dealing with corneal injuries had not been so great, but there was a need, and activation of public support for donation started. The ophthalmologist Townley Paton (1901–1984) harnessed the formidable energies and social connections of the New York philanthropist Aida de Acosta Breckinridge, who was afflicted with glaucoma. She also supported John Marquis Converse's plastic surgery for disfigured veterans.[79] The result was the appearance in 1945 in New York of the Eye-Bank for Sight Restoration, Inc., supported by an advisory council of thirty persons drawn from the great and good of the nation, including five former U.S. presidents' wives. The legal side was assisted locally by an amendment to the New York State autopsy law, which allowed the next of kin to authorize removal of eyes after death. The attitude of the media was favorable, and support from the *Reader's Digest* was important. Townley Paton fronted the Eye-Bank's publicity, but his emergence as a public icon was criticized by his colleagues.

The new charity served thirty-two local hospitals, and, by 1950, it had obtained and placed twelve hundred corneal grafts. By 1956, most major U.S. cities had similar corneal donation schemes, assisted now by tissue storage improvements, and the efforts were usually funded by charitable organizations such as the Lions International or the American Legion. These developments eventually led in 1961 to the Eye Bank Association of America, which organized the corneal grafting service, supported research, maintained standards, and monitored quality control.

In Britain, Rycroft mounted a campaign to make the public aware of the possibility of corneal donation after death, to change the nineteenth-century law, and to give corneal donation not only respectability but also nobility. In his energetic campaign, he sought support from the media and was soon helped by interested tabloid journalists. The result was Britain's Corneal Grafting Act (1952), which allowed for the prompt removal of eyes from recently deceased persons if they had proposed such a gift during their lifetime.[80] The law made no mention of asking the next of kin to make the donation. Remarkably, the act also had what current terminology identifies as an "opt-out" arrangement, which allowed surgeons to proceed with the removal of eyes if there were "no known objections by the deceased," but this clause in the law was ignored. Rycroft organized national publicity for his donor drive and put pressure on the Ministry of Health to help him expand the service.[81] It was the first time central government had been asked to become involved in such a matter. Rycroft deliberately encouraged would-be donors to contact the ministry directly for details of the nonexistent national government scheme. This met a cool reception. The minister of health even declined to set a good example by arranging to donate his eyes after death and also stated that any data collection on the numbers of grafts carried out nationally was the responsibility of voluntary bodies, such as the Royal National Institute for the Blind, not government.

The response from the public was more enthusiastic, helped by a program on corneal grafting in the British Broadcasting Corporation's series *Your Life in Their Hands,* which for the first time showed surgeons at work. Celebrities and would-be celebrities hastened to make it known that they would donate their eyes for corneal grafting after death. A surplus of donated eyes was soon available, and there were requests from other countries for corneas, notably in the Middle East and Far East, where citizens, rich and poor, had major eye problems but where laws and customs forbade such tissue removal. These profitable opportunities were not always turned down by the surgeons involved.

Papal Support

In 1956, a conference on corneal grafting at Rome was addressed by Pope Pius XII. As was the routine at medical conferences in that city, the pope was asked by the local organizers to send a message, and he and his advisors often used his address as an opportunity to deal with any current ethical issue. At this time, hopes for use of animal corneas had arisen, and, in his address, the pope ruled that use of animal tissue for grafting was acceptable, provided no genetic or psychological damage was done. This interest and input on a medical matter from organized religion presaged the rise of advice from lay medical ethicists later. Generally, the pontiff's statements thereafter were liberal and helpful to organ transplantation, as his views were based on advice from Italy's distinguished and innovative transplant surgeons.

Kidney Transplantation between Twins

After the Boston and Paris kidney human homografting attempts of the early 1950s, there was a surgical hiatus in such ventures until 1958. In the interim, however, there was a major event. Toward the end of 1954, an unusual patient was admitted to the Brigham Hospital in Boston. He was a young man in end-stage renal failure, but his daily bedside visitor was his identical twin, and the twin was entirely well. The possibility of transplanting a kidney from the healthy twin to his sick brother arose. The medical team was confident it could be done, and they were competent in dealing with the purely surgical aspects of kidney transplantation. The challenge in this case was purely surgical.

David Hume was no longer at Boston, and Joseph Murray (born 1919) had taken his place. He had trained as a plastic surgeon and was a surgical resident with James Barrett Brown and Bradford Cannon during World War II.[82] Murray had therefore emerged from the influential American plastic surgery/transplant milieu. The choice of a plastic surgeon to take charge of the Harvard Medical School Research Laboratories, with its interest in kidney transplantation, seems odd in retrospect but was not unusual at that time, and he continued with his Boston plastic surgical practice. Murray was to have a major role in Boston and in international transplantation until the late 1960s, and he later earned a Nobel Prize for this work.[83]

Murray knew about twins. He was well aware of reports in the plastic surgical literature from the 1930s onward demonstrating the success of skin grafts exchanged between identical twins. His surgical mentor, James Barrett Brown in St. Louis, had published the definitive paper on this topic, bringing order to the disorder of the times. But Brown's work had been an immunological experiment rather than treatment for clinical need, and the first use of twin tissue for therapy was by Converse in 1947, when he found that a burned patient had an identical twin who willingly donated skin.[84]

The Boston twin with kidney failure was twenty-three, and after dialysis his condition improved somewhat. The twins were shown to be identical by an exchange of skin grafts, and the donor's health was carefully checked. There remained the ethical problem of performing nontherapeutic surgery on a healthy person. This dilemma was resolved, as it often was later, by the donor's clear wishes, though he sought reassurances about his future health and health care. The plan proved newsworthy after an unwelcome leak, and the Boston media followed the preparations for surgery with interest.[85] Murray and other team members had some private professional pressure put on them not to proceed. But the ill twin had declined and become disoriented, agitated, and violent and suffered convulsions. This was not the "death with dignity" described by those who were soon to oppose the introduction of dialysis and transplantation.

The operation proceeded, and Brigham's urologist, Hartwell Harrison, later described it:

The operation was rehearsed in the department of pathology on a cadaver on December 21. On December 23, 1954, the operation was done exactly as planned. Excellent communication was maintained between operating teams in the two adjacent rooms by the Moseley Professor of Surgery at Harvard, Francis D. Moore. When all was ready in the recipient room for anastomosis of the vessels, Murray gave a signal and Harrison clamped the [donor] renal artery close to the aorta. The artery was severed, the kidney was allowed to empty itself of blood and then the renal vein was clamped and divided. The ureter had previously been separated. The kidney was delivered in a sterile basin to Murray in the next room. Immediately anastomosis of the vessels was begun and finished expeditiously. No attempt was made to cool or perfuse the kidney. Harrison then joined the team operating on the recipient for the purpose of exposing the bladder, opening it, and transplanting the ureter. . . . A polythene catheter was left in the ureter going to the renal pelvis and emerging with a cystostomy tube from the superior end of the incision of the bladder. This avoided the use of an indwelling urethral catheter and permitted separate collection of urine from the transplanted kidney as well as allowing separate function studies on the transplanted kidney.[86]

This operation used the Paris pelvic position for the transplant, not the leg placement used in the earlier Boston cases. Other junior surgical staff involved in the management of the twins at this time were distinguished later in transplantation matters, and among them was E. Donnall

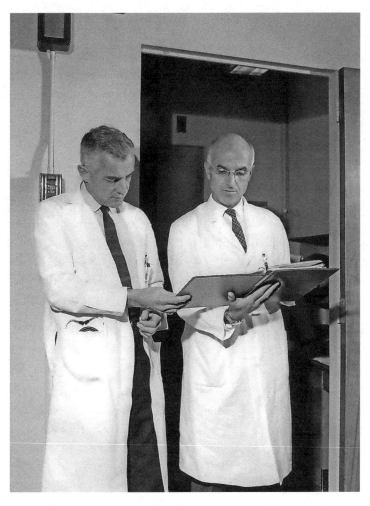

The Boston surgeon Joseph Murray (*right*), shown with physician John Merrill (*left*), cooperated on many aspects of renal replacement therapy, including the twin and homograft kidney transplants at the Peter Bent Brigham Hospital in Boston from 1954 onward. Image courtesy of Joseph Murray.

Thomas, who acted as an attending physician for the twins and was later the pioneer of bone marrow grafting.

The donated kidney started to function within a few days, and it steadily restored the patient to clinical and biochemical normality. The expected complication of high blood pressure appeared, and to deal with this, the patient's own kidneys were removed later. Thereafter, his health was excellent for many years. His twin brother, who donated the kidney, remained in good health.

After this first transplant success in twins, doctors from afar began referring similar cases to the Boston transplant team.[87] Similar operations were carried out elsewhere, notably one case in Montreal, another in Paris, and one in Oregon, often proceeding only after local controversy. By 1976, the Boston team had performed transplants on twenty-nine pairs of twins. All donors had remained healthy after the operation, and all involved were reassured when life insurance companies, whose rules are always a sensitive index of short- and long-term disability, agreed to insure kidney donors at the usual rate (though not the recipients).

During the Boston experience with twins, the team encountered many complications and surprises, which crop up during any radically new therapy. One of pleasantest circumstances involved an ill patient who, like all patients with renal failure, was infertile, and received a kidney from her twin in 1956. Later that year, she realized that she was pregnant.[88] This unexpected triumph of transplantation caused concern because of the pelvic position of the kidney, and an elective Caesarean section was thus recommended. Later, it was found that a normal delivery was routinely possible in transplant recipients, and these happy events were later collated in the Philadelphia Pregnancy Registry.

Long-term Results

These kidney grafts between twins were the first to result in long-term kidney replacement by transplantation for patients in chronic renal failure. The experience added to the insights gained in the early 1950s and gave vital information for the homograft (i.e., allograft) era to come. A number of questions had arisen about the potential outcomes, and the answers were clear. The biochemical effects of uremia could be completely reversed by a single kidney transplant. In addition, the kidney and ureter, though transplanted to a strange situation and deprived of both their nerve supply and lymphatics, functioned normally in the long term. Finally, the bladder, perhaps collapsed and inactive for some time, was ready to spring into action again.

Some other important practical lessons were learned. Donor kidneys supplied by two or more arteries from the aorta, rather than one, were more regularly encountered than the anatomy books suggested. To anticipate this anomaly, doctors undertook full radiology of the relevant blood vessels in the donor, albeit reluctantly. Apart from technical problems, notably a number of immediate urine leaks, the only discouraging feature of the transplants was that many of the donor kidneys ultimately developed the same disease that had destroyed the recipient's own kidneys. Four out of eight of the recipients in the Boston twin series died later of such recurrence. Eventually, this particular problem was largely solved in a curious way. The drugs that became available after 1960 to prevent rejection in homograft kidney transplants also prevented return of some common kidney diseases.

Legal Hurdles

The twin transplants also raised the problem of obtaining legal consent for this unique operation. The Boston success meant that twins were being considered in increasing numbers for transplantation, and operating on a normal person for donation was now accepted. But these referrals also included potential donors who were not yet twenty-one, the age of consent. The Boston doctors first asked a court to consider the matter and obtained a decision on June 12, 1957. The ruling was that the transplant operation could proceed, since the parents and young donor were both willing. The legal opinion went further than expected, since it concluded that the distress that the donor would experience upon the death of the untreated, ill twin outweighed the risks of the operation. This type of judgment also came into play later in cases elsewhere. But the situation was less clear when the twins were younger teenagers, or when the donor's health was not perfect, or when learning difficulties existed.

The kidney transplants between twins were a highly successful form of therapy, and the success increased the morale of those involved in transplantation in Boston and elsewhere. The publicity surrounding the cases was intense and favorable, though some in the medical profession were less positive. The purely surgical technique of donor kidney removal and then transplantation to the pelvis was now well established and changed little thereafter.

A Way Forward

By the late 1950s, there was support from laboratory studies that the rejection mechanism could be overcome, possibly through use of tolerance induction. It is sometimes said that Medawarian tolerance merely gave "hope without help" to the transplanters. Hope was indeed given, but the help was also there, if carefully sought historically. For the next few years, human kidney homografting work proceeded in a logical way from the hope that graft tolerance could be achieved.

These protocols for achieving tolerance derived not from the Medawarian paradigm of injecting cells early in life but from a variant on tolerance uncovered by others during attempts at mitigating radiation injury. Radiobiologists had found that they could replace the marrow and blood cells in adult animals using foreign cells, and this "adult tolerance" had an interest well beyond the narrow needs of radiation protection.

12 Hopes for Radiation Tolerance

THE FIRST HESITANT STEPS that marked the start of the modern, continuous period of human organ transplantation were taken in 1958, when attempts were made to thwart organ graft rejection in humans. The strategy used came from radiobiology—the study of the effects of lethal radiation and its treatment using bone marrow infusion. An infusion of an animal's own bone marrow allowed it to survive the effects of radiation, but a surprise was that "foreign" marrow cells from donors would also be effective. After recovering, the test animals had marrow of donor origin and would accept grafts from this donor indefinitely.[1] This heroic lethal radiation/marrow infusion method of "adult tolerance" induction was attempted in two cases in human transplantation, but it emerged that sublethal irradiation alone could be an effective immunosuppressant. Within a short time, the clinical strategy for organ grafting shifted away from finding tolerance and moved toward the less sophisticated, nonspecific forms of immunosuppression.

Radiation and Tolerance

In the 1950s, studies of the biological effects of radiation resumed as part of essential cold war research. Moderate nonlethal doses were known from the early part of the twentieth century to cause diminished antibody production. Other studies during this "lost era" of transplantation immunology showed that radiation increased the susceptibility of animals to disease, notably tuberculosis, and that radiation could prolong the life of tumor grafts. Jim Dempster, having experimented with radiation in dog kidney grafting, found no benefit. This discouraged others from reviving use of this modality, and researchers thus failed to discover the useful immunosuppression provided by moderate doses of radiation, as observed later in mice and rats—and humans.

Post–World War II attention instead centered on the lethal results of high-dose irradiation and protection from it. The use of atomic weapons at the end of the war, and fears of their use in the cold war period that followed, produced an intense interest in the immediate effects of atomic explosions and the delayed biological damage from the consequent fallout. A number of research laboratories were well funded for such studies.[2] Surprisingly, some were allowed freedom to publish their studies, even in this sensitive area.

The U.S. Navy Radiological Defense Laboratory at Hunters Point in San Francisco and the Oak Ridge National Laboratory in Tennessee were the centers for this American research, and the Radiobiology Unit at Harwell was the equivalent in Britain.[3] In the Netherlands, there was distinguished work done at the Medical and Biological Laboratory of the Defense Research Organization at Rijswijk. A useful by-product of this research and development was the preparation and sale of radioactive isotopes, not only for therapy and new imaging techniques but also for investigative medical research.[4] This powerful new technical innovation had a major impact on the methodology of biological and clinical research, including immunology, notably assisting, at last, in tracing the movements of the mysterious lymphocyte.

Radiation Protection

Studies of Japanese civilians who survived the initial wartime nuclear blasts showed that their bone marrow function was depressed, their blood levels of white cells, platelets, and eventually red cells were reduced, and infections developed.[5] The cold war threat of nuclear conflict necessitated a search for methods of treating or mitigating radiation effects, particularly as "limited" nuclear wars were still thought to be possible and disasters at the growing number of nuclear installations had to be contemplated. Although there were some claims for a protective action of cysteine or estrogens, these and other pharmacological strategies proved of little use when given after high doses of radiation.

The first hope for effective treatments came in 1949, with experiments confirming the finding in the 1930s that, if an animal's spleen or marrow was shielded during administration of a lethal dose of radiation, then the animal survived.[6] In America, Leon O. Jacobsen of the Argonne National Laboratory near Chicago, a classified research institute that developed nuclear reactors, studied this striking empirical finding and looked for the factor emerging from the protected spleen that seemed to restore the hematopoietic system. He showed that the effect was a speedy one, since even if the shielded spleen was removed a few hours after radiation, its brief earlier presence had still provided protection for the animal. Since the researchers of the day were still caught in the pre-Gowans mindset that lymphoid cells, in this case the spleen cells, were neither mobile nor capable of returning to earlier forms, the necessarily tunnel-vision analysis was that a "humoral factor" came from the spleen and stimulated the depressed, irradiated native marrow. Jacobsen wrote that "it seems unlikely that cell migration from the shielded or transplanted tissue and subsequent proliferation of these cells can account for the reconstitution of hematopoietic tissue."[7]

This faulty assumption led to further error. Injecting the lab animals with bone marrow cells also produced the protective effect, but, ignoring the exciting alternative possibility of cellular migration and colonization, researchers looked for an alleged potent marrow-stimulating factor. Such was the supposed reasonableness of the theory that they soon reported having isolated this factor.[8] Leonard Cole's research group at Hunters Point carefully described this "nucleoprotein" and offered short-lived hopes for a useful, chemical, storable radioprotectant. Given by injection, the protective extract was also isolated from bone marrow taken from all kinds of donor—identical, homograft, or even xenograft. This finding seemed to strengthen the humoral case.

A flurry of experimental activity followed from 1954 to 1957, with the analysis still trapped in the humoral marrow protection idée fixe, but the humoral paradigm was being strained to the limit, and collapse was imminent. It was Britain's Harwell group, notably John Loutit (1910–1992), who from 1952 cautiously raised the unlikely, alternative cellular explanation of the protection given by shielding experiments or marrow infusion, namely that the donor cells settled and functioned.[9] This new view gained credibility when Avrion Mitchison and Jim Gowans's work showed the mobility and versatility of the lymphocyte.

Grafting after Marrow Infusion

In 1955, Joan M. Main and Richmond T. Prehn, part of a new group at the National Cancer Institute interested in immunology, were studying large doses of irradiation and confirmed that donor bone marrow infusion from the same or different mouse strains would protect the recipient animal from the lethal effects of high-dose radiation. Thinking that the radiation might have suppressed immunity for an extended period, they tested with skin grafts and made a simple, crucial observation: only skin grafts from the marrow donor strain of mice would survive; all other grafts were rejected promptly.[10] Graft survival thus could not be attributed to the earlier radiation but to the marrow donor.

By this slightly circuitous route, the researchers had discovered a way of obtaining safe, profound immunosuppression that was donor specific, as in "Medawarian" tolerance. They named this effect "adult tolerance," in contrast to the strategy for obtaining tolerance in the newborn.[11] These workers had also realized that the findings were "consistent with the cellular repopulation theory of radiation protection" and that the new marrow and blood cells were of donor origin and not the result of host cell revival by the stimulant postulated earlier.

Chimerism Revealed

The year 1956 was the annus mirabilis of radiation protection and marrow replacement studies, and the humoral versus cellular debate resembled the Loeb/Medawar choices at this time on the antibody/lymphocyte choices in the mechanisms of rejection. It is even reminiscent of the much earlier Ehrlich/Metchnikoff debate. Researchers quickly accepted the cellular explanation of marrow replacement and quietly dropped the hunt for a humoral factor. In that year, six papers from the centers active in this field all directly showed the marrow repopulation by cells of donor origin (chimerism) and thus that the survivors were hybrids. In this "year of chimerism," ingenious ways of identifying engrafted donor marrow quickly emerged.[12]

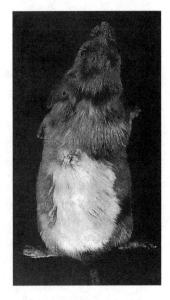

A mouse treated by lethal irradiation and bone marrow replacement showing survival of skin taken from the marrow donor. From J. M. Main and R. T. Prehn, "Successful Skin Homografts after High Dose X-radiation and Homologous Bone Marrow," *Journal of the National Cancer Institute* 15 (1955): 1023–30.

The most notable contributions came from Cole's group (now accepting the "new testament"), from the Netherlands, and from Harwell.[13] It was Mitchison who first used the term "radiation-chimera," and this classical term was quickly preferred, with a little help from Medawar and Loutit.[14] Late that year at Harwell, C. E. Ford, in his famous study, shifted course from his work on chromosomal radiation damage to show that the revived marrow of the irradiated mice had the characteristic cellular marker present in the cells of the donor strain—namely the donor's easily detected T_6 chromosomal translocation.[15]

This work was also important because medical teams realized that bone marrow transplantation was now a technically feasible measure for treating blood diseases.[16]

Graft versus Host

All those who were experimenting with radiation and "foreign" bone marrow rescue noticed later onset of disease and poor survival of their animals, in spite of successful marrow engraftment. John J. Trentin and Delta Uphoff in the United States and Loutit in Britain first reported this effect, calling it "secondary disease." Morten Simonsen and Medawar's group, as previously noted, had already noticed "runting" illness and enlarged spleens after foreign lymphocyte injections. Synchronous scientific enlightenment arrived in 1957. All these studies—radiation and nonirradiation—had been touching the same elephant; the various effects were manifestations of the graft-versus-host response in which donor (foreign) lymphocytes attack the host.

What had started out as a hunt for radiation protection had produced a strategy for inducing specific transplantation tolerance in adults. This newfound strategy raised hopes for human organ transplant success. The earlier neonatal "Medawarian" strategy for achieving tolerance for human transplantation seemed unrealistic and also hazardous. The clinical world took note of the new radiation/marrow Main-Prehn strategy, as it was now called, and the Boston clinical transplant group saw in this adult tolerance strategy a possible way forward for organ transplantation: by giving lethal irradiation to the recipient plus bone marrow rescue followed by an organ transplant compatible with the marrow. In Boston, this regimen was used first in experimental organ transplantation, then briefly in human patients.

Another Boston clinician had noticed other extended possibilities for marrow grafting beyond radiation protection or transplantation. As described later, Edward Donnall Thomas soon started his celebrated work on marrow grafting, hoping to deal with blood cell malignancies.

Boston Kidney Studies

In Boston, the nephrologist John Merrill had been involved earlier in David Hume's 1953 series of "unmodified" human kidney transplants, namely grafting without immunosuppression, and shortly after 1956, the "year of chimerism," Merrill assisted Joseph W. Ferrebee (1908–2001), a Brigham Hospital physician, in writing a review on the future of homografting, and they highlighted the possibilities offered by inducing chimerism via donor marrow infusion.[17] The main constraint of such a plan was that the transplant operation had to be planned around the time of the irradiation and thus could not be scheduled to coincide with the unpredictable availability of a cadaveric organ. Living-related donor kidneys or a "free" kidney removed in elective surgery were the only choices. And there was one other unknown—the strong possibility of graft-versus-host disease from the donated marrow.

Merrill traveled in Europe in 1957, the year after publication of the important chimerism papers. He sought and developed links at this time with transplantation immunologists like Medawar and the British radio-biologists at Harwell, picking up the methods on the use of radiation and techniques for bone marrow harvesting and administration. He even published a paper with the Harwell radiobiologists, and Loutit recalled later that "John Merrill did get about. We discussed various problems, or the one problem from a variety of angles. He went to Paris and amongst those with whom he had discussions was Pierre Grabar and somehow or other a publication arose from the various visits. I guess he was around in the summer of 1957."[18]

Merrill also visited his old "renal replacement" friends in Paris, now increasingly skilled in hemodialysis, thus keeping up the personal clinical ties between Boston and Paris.

The Radiation Cases

Back in Boston, Merrill and the Brigham Hospital group, which included Ferrebee and Donnall Thomas, tried the radiobiologist's chimerism protocol in dog kidney transplantation and obtained considerable experimental experience with it. But the results were poor and mortality high. There was one exception, and it came when Thomas and Ferrebee moved to the Mary Imogene Bassett Hospital in Cooperstown, New York, and attempted further similar experimental dog kidney transplantation with John Mannick, later to succeed Moore at the Brigham. This mysterious long-term success in which the kidney survived seventy-three days gave encouragement at a discouraging time.[19]

However, it was decided to proceed in Boston with transplantation of some patients in renal failure using this Main-Prehn strategy, and this was first attempted in 1958. It was assisted that year by some very helpful technical information about likely human dosage, obtained by a hematologist in Paris. He had to deal with some heavily irradiated people surviving from a nuclear reactor disaster.

The Nuclear Incident

In Paris, Georges Mathé (born 1922), who had trained with Loutit, found himself in the unexpected situation of having to carry out pioneer, emergency human bone marrow transplantation. In 1958, six Yugoslavian physicists who had been involved in a nuclear reactor accident were sent to Mathé in Paris for treatment of their marrow suppression. One who had received about 400 rad did not require treatment other than isolation and barrier nursing. The clinical situation and blood findings were ominous in those who had received 700 rad, and Mathé treated them with bone marrow from unrelated donors. Initially, these donor cells were established, but in the four men who survived, spontaneous recovery of their own marrow occurred later and chimerism disappeared.[20] However, even the short-term technical success gave some encouragement for kidney transplanters contemplating use of lethal human irradiation plus bone marrow. Mathé's estimate of the dosage and effects in these cases was important, and the transplanters in Paris and Boston sought and heeded his advice that 400 rad was about the limit for nonlethal human irradiation. Any more would require marrow rescue.

The first kidney transplant operation on a human patient using significant immunosuppression was carried out in Boston in March 1958. The recipient was pretreated with radiation and marrow given from an unrelated donor.[21] The Boston patient did not have chronic kidney disease, but, in a surgical disaster, her only kidney, congenitally misplaced in the pelvis, had been removed when it was mistakenly thought to be a chronic appendix abscess. She was admitted to the Peter Bent Brigham Hospital in Boston for treatment on the artificial kidney and improved considerably, but, at that time, long-term treatment by dialysis was not possible, and repeated dialysis could only be given up to a limit.

Kidney transplantation was proposed for this doomed patient, and in preparation, she was given 600 rad of radiation. Marrow from a patient about to have removal of a kidney during a Matson operation for hydrocephalus was used. In this procedure, a tube was led from the patient's brain and placed in a ureter after removing the kidney, thus draining the excess brain fluid into the bladder. The hope was that the marrow would induce tolerance in the transplanted patient, who also received additional marrow from other donors to provide a broad range of effects. Donnall Thomas and Robert Schwartz prepared the marrow.[22] The possibility of graft-versus-host disease was accepted.[23]

The kidney graft functioned immediately, but marrow function continued to be depressed, with little evidence of donor marrow engraftment. The patient died of uncontrollable hemorrhage, sepsis, and intestinal ulceration thirty-two days after irradiation. The only feature of this case to offer hope was that at postmortem the kidney transplant had been a technical success and showed no signs of rejection.

The second and last attempt using this adult tolerance protocol came in the case of a twelve-year-old boy who was flown from Sweden to Boston in July 1958. His one kidney had been injured and had to be removed. His mother was willing to donate one of her kidneys, and the boy received radiation followed by marrow from the mother, but when he quickly developed marrow suppression and serious coagulation defects, the transplant was postponed. He died shortly afterward.

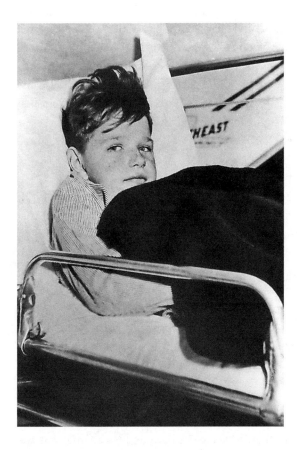

The pioneering Boston kidney transplant and dialysis group brought in cases from afar for treatment. This boy lost his only kidney as the result of an accident, and, after dialysis in Sweden by Nils Alwall, he was flown to Boston in 1959, where a transplant from his mother was proposed. Image courtesy of Joseph Murray.

Experience from these two cases suggested the need for a change in the dosage levels of both radiation and marrow, but in what direction was not clear. Even proceeding further was a fraught issue, since at the normally supportive Brigham there was hospital criticism of the two attempts.[24] The Brigham group chose to lower the x-ray dose to safer, sublethal levels and omit the marrow transfer, but they were still seeking and hoping for tolerance of another kind. Merrill suggested that the kidney itself was effectively a large dose of antigen, and this, with the modest irradiation plus the naturally lowered immunity of patients in the chronic uremic state, might result in tolerance. He wrote that "we reasoned that the kidney might [then] be transplanted at a time when the lymphopoietic system was temporarily incapable of responding to foreign antigen. It is in this fashion that tolerance is produced in the embryo. . . . A small dose of radiation might allow the recipient bone marrow to become tolerant . . . without the necessity for transplantation of marrow."[25]

From May 1958 to April 1962, five patients received transplants in Boston using these smaller, safer, divided doses of irradiation and no marrow transfer. Surgeons in Paris soon followed suit using the same low-dose strategy. Some success followed. The grafting seemed to offer some form of tolerance, or the host "adapted" to the graft in a way not seen in the lab. Clinical attitudes were drifting away from the idea of using the imported, sophisticated methods of the laboratory and moving instead toward new empirical surgical strategies.

The Lower Dose Cases

The transplanters in Boston and Paris increased their experience with the use of smaller doses of radiation used alone, without marrow transfer. This protocol was immediately rewarded by two remarkable successes, one in each city. The Boston case was in 1959, when a twenty-three-year-old patient with chronic renal failure presented with a healthy twin and was considered for transplantation. But investigation showed that the twins were in fact nonidentical.

The Boston team employed the now accepted highest nonlethal dose of irradiation for transplantation—450 rad—in two sessions separated by seven days and then performed the transplant.[26] Despite a stormy postoperative period, the donor kidney worked well.[27] The patient, J. M. Riteris, was well for many years and took an academic philosophy post in Indianapolis. He gave a personal testimony at the Fourth Congress of the Transplantation Society in San Francisco in 1972 and for a while was the world's longest survivor after kidney transplantation over a genetic barrier. He died in 1979, of unrelated causes.[28]

In Paris, the low-dose radiation approach had attractions, and kidney grafting restarted. In June 1959, some months after the success in Boston, one patient transplanted by the Hamburger team at the Hôpital Necker obtained similar long-term survival.[29] The wife of the patient had heard of the Boston nonidentical twin case success and had written to Merrill, who, replying in French, suggested that they consult Jean Hamburger in Paris.[30] The twin donor in this case again was nonidentical, and the recipient received low-dose irradiation without marrow transfer.[31] Merrill traveled to Paris to observe and advise during this time. Of great interest was that in the third week after the transplant a temporary rejection crisis occurred, and although no therapy was known or given, kidney function spontaneously improved. This *"crise fonctionnelle réversible"* was the first use of the word *crisis* for the rejection episodes to be familiar later. When rejection started again in August 1960, the Paris team knew by then, through a visit by Roy Calne, that the anticancer drug 6-mercaptopurine might be of use, and administering it was met with success.

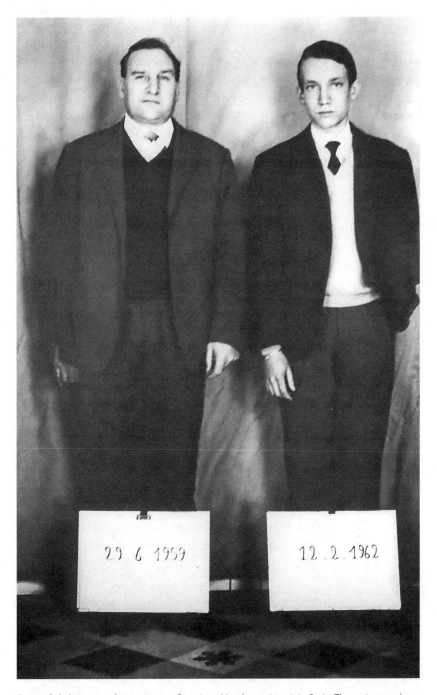

29 6 1959   12 . 2 . 1962

Two early kidney transplant successes from Jean Hamburger's unit in Paris. The patient on the left received low-dose irradiation and a kidney from his nonidentical twin in 1959. In 1962, the patient on the right was the first to receive a kidney selected from the extended family using early tissue-typing methods. Image courtesy of Jean Hamburger.

These isolated successes hinted at some features of human transplantation immunology that were confirmed later. First, human results differed from those with dogs, since radiation failed to prolong dog kidney grafts. Second, even if episodes of rejection did occur, kidney function could return. Third, if a human organ survives for an initial period as a result of short-term immunosuppression, like that provided by irradiation, then the graft seemed to induce tolerance or adapt to the host.[32] Such features were not found or even suspected in experimental animal transplantation.

These immunological puzzles, observed only in human transplantation, were later to beguile the transplant community and were reanalyzed after each development in immunological understanding and technique. In addition, the occasional long-term, unexpected kidney transplant successes gave hints at some unknown factors that, once identified, would give routine success. The most likely factor at the time was genetic closeness of the donor and recipient, which raised hopes for support from future tissue matching methods. In Paris, associated with Hamburger's hospital, Jean Dausset had already made some progress in identifying tissue antigens, and he was making the first effort at tissue matching. In one of the pioneer low-dose radiation cases, a choice was made between a number of possible family donors by using Dausset's early methods to detect the best match.

Encouraged by these two cases of long-term success in human kidney grafting, the two Paris transplant units subsequently did twenty-five transplants using low-dose irradiation. In 1960, they had their first success with an unrelated donor—a brother-in-law. But the overall results were poor in both Paris and Boston, and interest shifted instead to hopes for chemical immunosuppression. Moreover, since radiation had to be planned, use of cadaveric donors was not feasible, so in most cases a close relative had donated the kidney, thus affecting two patients rather than one.[33]

The Results

This radiation-only phase of organ transplantation sustained hopes for the future and gave valuable experience in transplant management.[34] René Küss wrote later that the experience had provided "gains from the progress made in donor and recipient preparation, [the need for] a very short ischaemia time for the transplant organ, the experience acquired in postoperative intensive care, infection prophylaxis by placing the patient in a sterile room and the curative treatment of haemorrhagic complications."[35]

In Boston and Paris, the transplant teams now concluded that the results did not justify use of kidneys from living-related donors, in spite of the advantages of a planned operation and immediate graft function. But

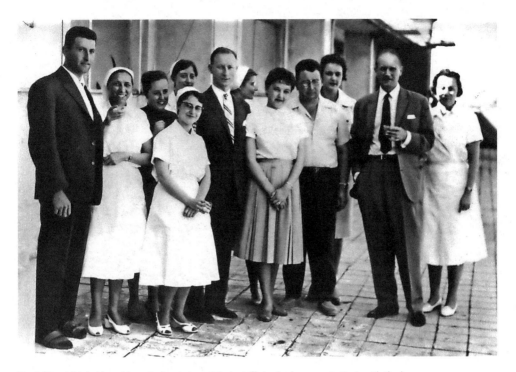

René Küss (*right*), Marcel Legrain (*center*), and their staff also had success in Paris with the low-dose, radiation-only regimen. The patient (*center*) received a kidney transplant in 1959 from her brother-in-law using this nonlethal irradiation and was the first nonrelated living donor success. Image courtesy of Marcel Legrain.

other sources of usable kidneys were declining. The Matson operation, which offered a "free" kidney, was out of favor, and cardiac surgery was increasingly successful.

The Innovators

Around this time, most of the rest of the surgical world had serious reservations about organ grafting, not only because of the poor results and the challenging ethics of donation from living donors but also from a deep-seated view that it was wrong to try to thwart one of nature's fundamental mechanisms. Only at the innovative centers in Boston and Paris were there senior surgeons interested in kidney transplantation, plus supportive internists managing dialysis facilities and other noninvolved staff who were generally tolerant of the attempts. Elsewhere there was a cautious, even hostile attitude to transplantation on the part of most internists.[36] Thus, referrals to surgeons for transplantation were rare. In this pioneer series of transplants, many cases came directly to the surgeons, following

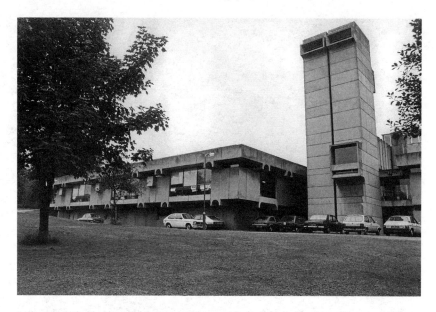

In the 1960s, the problem of infection and the need for isolation led to the construction of custom-built transplant units. The Edinburgh unit, supported by the Nuffield Foundation, opened in 1968. Image courtesy of Sir Michael Woodruff.

traumatic kidney damage, the removal of a single kidney, or even as self-referral following press reports of transplant attempts when doomed patients and their families felt they had nothing to lose. Not until the mid-1960s did internists in general start to consider this risky surgical option for their patients.

Although the kidney transplanters had now abandoned the bone marrow/lethal radiation approach, simplifying it to low-dose radiation only, the Boston laboratory experience in the more heroic protocol was put to good use in a direction whose significance was not obvious until later. E. Donnall Thomas, the chief medical resident at Brigham Hospital from 1951 to 1953 and then a hematologist there until 1955, started kidney transplantation studies in chimeric dogs while working with Ferrebee at Cooperstown. Thomas traveled back and forth between Cooperstown and Boston and was still involved in many of the Brigham transplants, including the lethal radiation/bone marrow cases. He realized that radiation offered a way of wiping out and replacing the blood cells of patients with hematological malignancy, and so he began studying bone marrow transplantation, not as a means toward tolerance but as an end in itself. One year after the discouraging Boston experience with the radiation/marrow attempts, in 1959, like the Boston kidney team years earlier, Thomas encountered an ill patient with leukemia who had a healthy twin who was willing to be a marrow donor. After irradiating the patient, Thomas successfully transplanted marrow harvested from the twin brother. This mimicry of the kidney transplant success in twins was rewarded with short-term success, but the patient's leukemia returned later. Nevertheless, a remarkable period of enthusiasm for clinical bone marrow transplantation followed. The numbers of marrow transplants attempted in this manner greatly exceeded the number of organ transplants of the time.[37]

Kidney Transplant Attitudes

The mood of those involved in this period of transplantation efforts can be seen in the published discussions from Milan Hašek's Mechanisms of Tolerance conference, held at Liblice near Prague in 1961. Attempts with low-dose radiation were continuing at the time, and the first hopeful findings on chemical immunosuppression had appeared. But the conference participants' view of the way forward was far from clear; some still hoped for induction of tolerance.

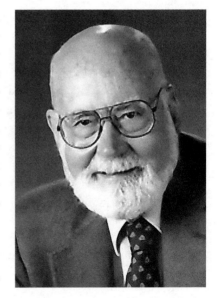

E. Donnall Thomas, the Nobel Prize–winning pioneer of bone marrow transplantation, started his life's work while he was serving as an internist and hematologist and dealing with the Boston kidney transplants. Image courtesy of Donnall Thomas.

In the closing discussion of the conference, Peter Medawar asked those present to imagine that they were dying from kidney failure and, rather than accept their fate, they had to choose a treatment. Simonsen spoke up first and "requested" a living-related kidney transplant with tolerance induced by small regular doses of x-rays plus spleen or marrow from the same donor. A local surgeon named Nakić wished to have the same but pointed out the risk of graft-versus-host disease. Leslie Brent preferred bone marrow rather than spleen with his radiation but added that he also wanted immunosuppression after the transplant by a course of a-methopterin (methotrexate) administered by Paul Russell, the Boston surgeon. Russell, present at the conference, wanted the same regimen for himself. Nathan Kaliss said that 6-mercaptopurine could be used instead of radiation and requested it be followed by a massive, tolerogenic dose of connective tissue rather than marrow or lymphoid cells, in the hope of avoiding graft-versus-host disease. E. J. Eichwald disloyally said he would send a telegram to Willem Kolff at Cleveland and hope there might be an available slot for treatment with the artificial kidney.

By 1960, the prospects for using radiation in human kidney transplantation seemed poor. But there was new interest coming from a new direction—chemical immunosuppression. One other matter was soon unpleasantly clear: if tolerance could not be induced for human organ transplantation with a short, sharp, single sophisticated, specific, tolerogenic intervention, and nonspecific immunosuppression was instead the way forward, then the surgeons faced a different kind of future. It would require balancing kidney and patient survival and prolonged encounters with a daunting array of purely clinical and potentially fatal complications. These included coagulation disorders, hemorrhage, common and exotic infections, delayed healing, and much else. These problems were notably absent in inbred brown mice made tolerant of skin grafts from white mice.

13 The Emergence of Chemical Immunosuppression

IN THE EARLY 1960s, the approach to organ transplantation changed, allowing attempts with radiation to be put aside in favor of progress by other means. Immunosuppressive drugs appeared, and they proved to be more controllable and more effective than irradiation, and the surgeon's assumptions changed from hoping for "one-shot" tolerance to accepting the use of long-term, continuous medication. Soon after this shift, in the mid-1960s, rapid developments in tissue typing showed promise for close and beneficial matching of the recipient and donor, either within the family or with a deceased donor organ. There was also at this time rapid growth in basic immunological knowledge, which continued to raise hopes for fuller understanding and control of transplantation immune responses. Many believed that more sophisticated methods of tolerance induction or specific immunosuppression would appear, that the modest but growing success of chemical immunosuppression, with all its risks, was only a temporary phase, and that a final, immunological solution would certainly appear.

The word *immunosuppression* entered clinical discourse in the early 1960s to denote depression of immunological responses by drugs, radiation, or other agents.[1] Ways of reducing antibody responses had been studied quite closely in the earlier "lost era" and were then forgotten. But when new anticancer drugs emerged in the 1940s, marrow depression was one of their features, along with an associated susceptibility to infection. There was soon a modest interest in the fact that these oncological agents could reduce immune responses. These studies throughout the 1950s went largely unnoticed by the transplant community, then preoccupied with the lure of human tolerance induction and the related hopes for irradiation use.

In cancer therapy, the first drug of value in the modern era was nitrogen mustard, the unpleasant poison first used in 1915 in World War I and held in reserve during World War II. This agent was at the beginning of a path that led to trials of 6-mercaptopurine, and thence to azathioprine and the first successes in organ transplantation.[2]

Nitrogen Mustard

In World War I, mustard gas was directed downwind to cause fatal damage to the lungs of enemy combatants. Survivors of these attacks showed a reduced white cell count and a susceptibility to infection. In the laboratory, experiments by E. B. Krumbhaar and others showed that this poisonous gas could reduce antibody production. After the war there were serious accidents involving stocks of the gas, notably an explosion at the gas munitions dump at Breloh in 1919. The site's medical officer carefully described the medical effects of this exposure, and his book was found and restudied with interest in the 1940s.[3]

Mustard gas was occasionally used by the military in the interwar period, and during World War II, stocks were kept in reserve near the front lines for retaliatory use. The toxicity of mustard gas in humans was again established in 1943, when the U.S. naval vessel *John Harvey*, backing up the invasion of Italy with a cargo that included five hundred tons of the poison, plus munitions, was hit and exploded in the harbor of Bari during a German air raid. About seven hundred sailors and one thousand Italian civilians died, many from the immediate and delayed effects of the gas.

The U.S. Medical Corps studied the casualties, and tissues from forty dead sailors were sent to the chemical weapons research and development centers at Edgewood Arsenal in America and Porton Down in Britain.[4] The effect of the gas on bone marrow and the finding of reduced white cell counts were again prominent, and the American Office of Scientific Research and Development and the military renewed their study of the poison.[5] Cornelius "Dusty" Rhoads, the controversial chief of the Biological Branch of the U.S. Army Chemical Warfare Service, then started research on the action of mustard gas derivatives. Alfred Gilman and Thomas Dougherty at Yale University were brought into the study, and they reasoned that the poison's potent action on active marrow cells might also be of use in dealing with rapidly dividing malignant cells. Using nitrogen mustard and its derivatives, notably tris-nitrogen mustard, they were the first to show that such substances were indeed active against mouse lymphoma tumors.

This wartime work was secret, as were the first tentative trials of the derivative drug at Yale in 1942. Louis S. Goodman and Gus Lindskog, then assistant professor of cardiothoracic surgery and later head of the department, tested the drug on human cancer patients.[6] The ban on publication of secret wartime work was removed in 1946, by which time the promising effect of nitrogen mustard on various malignancies had been confirmed.

Cancer Chemotherapy

At this time, the only effective therapeutic remedies in clinical medicine were a few ancient favorites. In the practice of internal medicine, traditionalist physicians laid more emphasis on holistic adjustment of lifestyle. Nitrogen mustard's reputation was as a poison, and the idea of giving such a toxic substance by mouth or, worse still, intravenously, met reflex resistance from patients and physicians alike. Gilman later recalled that, "as a result of the impact of the sulphonamides, medicine was beginning to emerge from a period of therapeutic nihilism, . . . [but] in the minds of most physicians the administration of drugs, other than an analgesic, in the treatment of malignancy was the act of a charlatan."[7]

Such therapeutic adventures were in any case thought to be doomed, since it was reasoned that any powerful agent would equally attack the tumor and the patient's normal tissues. The task was seen as almost as hard as finding some agent that will dissolve away the left ear and yet leave the right ear unharmed, so slight was the difference.

However, in the development of cancer chemotherapy, much new ground was being broken. Although the nitrogen mustard derivatives were difficult to use, the first impressions were favorable, and a beneficial effect on human leukemia was soon established. It was the first of the alkylating agents, and similar anticancer drugs were to appear in the 1950s.[8] One of the new drugs that appeared in the wake of this new confidence was the antimetabolite 6-mercaptopurine (6-MP), which was to be important later in transplantation. Introduced in 1953, it was given only in short courses, and proposals for more continuous chemotherapy were reflexively opposed at first.

Immunosuppression Studied

Until the late 1950s, the interest in these drugs was only in reference to human and experimental malignancy, and any effect on immunity was a side issue. Only one new study of the effect of these drugs on antibody formation was made, and this careful 1947 Edgewood Arsenal study of moderate doses of mustard gas in the goat (an animal favored in biological warfare studies) showed a marked lowering of antibody production. In addition, the Edgewood research group proposed a simple new scheme, later accepted as self-evident, that irradiation, mustard gas, and benzene all acted through the common path of marrow suppression.

A small number of similar studies followed, confirming that antibody production could be reduced in this way. It is curious that in the early 1950s none of these drugs was considered for human or experimental animal kidney transplant work, with one exception.[9] The explanation is that transplanters focused their hopes on "one-shot" methods of obtaining permanent graft survival. This mindset muted any thoughts on the use of continuous, nonspecific, toxic, chemical immunosuppression. There had likewise been opposition to continuous therapy with cortisone, in any ailment, when it first became available.

6-Mercaptopurine Use

In 1959, at the time when strategies using radiation were being explored for human kidney transplantation, Robert S. Schwartz and William Dameshek, at the New England Center Hospital and Tufts University School of Medicine in Boston, were attempting bone marrow transplantation in human patients with blood malignancies. Like the Brigham Hospital kidney transplanters and Donnall Thomas, they were using lethal radiation to destroy the patient's own defective marrow and blood cells, then providing marrow donation from a relative. Like the surgeons, they found that total body irradiation was difficult to use, and they were also discouraged by early deaths from its use. Casting about for an alternative, they turned to using large doses of anticancer drugs, instead of radiation, to destroy the patient's bone marrow prior to grafting donated marrow.

Schwartz and Dameshek showed experimentally that the Burroughs Wellcome lab's 6-mercaptopurine (6-MP) was a promising agent with a more predictable effect than radiation. As part of their studies, they found that 6-MP reduced the antibody response of rabbits.[10] They then found that other agents, notably methotrexate, and, ironically, azathioprine, were less effective. In 1959, Schwartz and Dameshek went further and reported that a short course of 6-MP, plus suitably timed dosing of antigen, could induce long-lasting failure to respond to this antigen. They had induced tolerance chemically, exactly the hoped-for strategy in transplantation at this time.

It was this tolerogenic capability, not just the immunosuppression effect, of 6-MP that caught the attention of some, and when Schwartz and Dameshek published their report in the prestigious general science journal *Nature*, the title of their work included this claim.[11] Less dramatic at the time was the additional information Schwartz and Dameshek reported to the Seventh European Congress of Haematology in London in

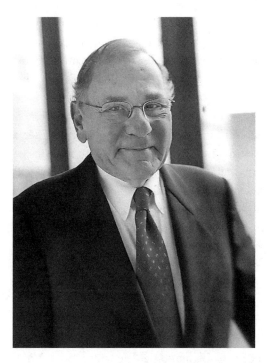

In 1960, Robert Schwartz abandoned the use of lethal radiation for marrow transplantation in favor of 6-mercaptopurine. The drug also reduced antibody formation. Image courtesy of Robert Schwartz.

September 1959, namely that 6-MP, given continuously, modestly prolonged the life of skin grafts in rabbits to about twenty days. This figure should not have disappointed them, but it did. It was the first report of the "continuous chemical therapy" approach to tissue grafting.

Interestingly, Schwartz and Dameshek sought to downplay any hopes for clinical use, particularly continuous use, fearing that, by analogy with microorganisms, "antibody-forming cells might develop resistance to the drug." They added that, in any case, "toxicity in man and its limited effects preclude immediate application to the problems of tissue transplantation in humans."[12]

Kendrick Porter and Roy Calne

The Boston paper on 6-MP in *Nature* was not unexpected news to Kendrick "Ken" Porter, professor of pathology at St. Mary's Hospital London. He had recently returned from working in Boston, where, with Schwartz, he had been involved in the radiation/bone marrow studies and had published, with Joseph Murray, on cryopreservation of marrow cells using glycerol.[13] Back in London, he was not inclined to use irradiation in marrow grafting and like the others, was looking instead at the anticancer drugs as possible marrow "space-makers" to allow success with marrow grafts, even though the results of this strategy until then had been discouraging.[14]

About the same time, Roy Y. Calne (born 1930), a young trainee surgeon at the Royal Free Hospital in London who had spent some time in research in the Anatomy Department at Oxford, had been attracted to the challenge of clinical transplantation.[15] While continuing to train in London, he was also keen to start experiments on kidney grafting. In the conservative world of London surgery, Calne was lucky to have one senior supporter, John Hopewell, a urological surgeon at the Royal Free Hospital who had started to treat patients with an artificial kidney at that hospital in the late 1950s. Hopewell made the introductions necessary for support of Calne's interest, and, with the encouragement of David Slome, the energetic professor of physiology at the Royal College of Surgeons, Calne first attempted to do rat kidney grafts using Payr-type stents to link the vessels. This effort did not go well, and Slome then arranged for Calne to have facilities for dog kidney transplantation at the college's Buckston Browne Research Farm, then under Slome's direction. The staff there had considerable experience in such work, since William "Jim" Dempster, the Hammersmith surgeon, had worked there on his long series of similar experiments on the mechanism of dog kidney transplant rejection. As described earlier, Dempster had found no way of prolonging the survival of the grafts. Calne did the experiments again, since clinical transplant use of radiation offered some hope. He found that, as Dempster had previously reported, even the lethal 900-rad dose of radiation did not affect the outcome of dog kidney transplantation.[16]

At this point, Calne sought Porter's advice, and Porter told him about the 6-MP studies just published by Schwartz and Dameshek. With this information, Calne began using 6-MP in the hitherto fruitless and discouraging dog kidney transplant work at Buckston Browne.

The 6-MP Effect

The administration of 6-MP gave the first positive results in the prolonged dog kidney graft studies of the 1950s. Use of this agent significantly prolonged survival of some of the grafts. In February 1960, Calne published his results in the *Lancet*.[17] Contrary to the mood of the times, he raised the possibility that the action of 6-MP might be simpler than was thought. Skeptical, as always, about invoking a complex immunological mechanism, he placed tolerance second in his analysis, stating that the encouraging results could be "explained either by a non-specific toxic effect on the immune system, or by a true specific production of immune tolerance [i.e. by the graft as antigen]."[18] He made the bold, and entirely correct, claims that not only could use of the drug have advantages over total body irradiation but, in addition, its action might have more effect on cellular immune reactions than on antibody responses. This was an important possibility, since many believed that adequate immunosuppression would inevitably entail lethal infection.

One discouragement for Calne at the time was an unhelpful and patronizing response from Dempster, also published in the *Lancet*. Dempster's earlier pessimism continued, and he repeated the view that "any measure which can suppress the homograft rejection process must also render the host an immunological cripple."[19] But Calne did receive encouragement from Charles Zukoski (1926–1983) of Richmond, Virginia, who was working in David Hume's department in the medical college there, where Hume was now vigorously engaged in transplant studies. Zukoski wrote to Calne after reading his paper in the *Lancet* and told Calne that he too had found 6-MP to inhibit cellular immune reactions.[20]

Calne received an invitation to visit one of the Paris units, where René Küss listened attentively to Calne's findings and soon employed the drug in reversing a late rejection episode in the recipient successfully grafted in 1959; the patient had received a kidney after single-shot low-dose irradiation as the only initial immunosuppression.[21]

Further Developments

At this time, Calne and his mentor Hopewell felt sufficiently encouraged by the early results from the dog experiments to attempt three human kidney transplants using 6-MP as the immunosuppressant—one case in 1959 and two in 1960. Cadaver donor kidneys were used in two cases and a living-related donation in the third. All of the patients died without showing any function of the kidney, though one of the deaths was from rapid reactivation of preexisting tuberculosis.[22] Publication of these cases was delayed until 1964, since the principals were well aware that not only the results but also the attempted transplants met with disapproval. In retrospect, these cases were among the historic first attempts at transplantation with a purely chemical immunosuppressive regimen.

At this point, in 1960, with Medawar's help, Calne obtained a Harkness Fellowship to work in Boston with Joseph Murray, and Calne proposed to carry out further dog transplant work using 6-MP.[23] Keen to try any newly available variants, Calne, on his way to Boston, visited the Burroughs Wellcome Research Laboratories at Tuckahoe, New York, where

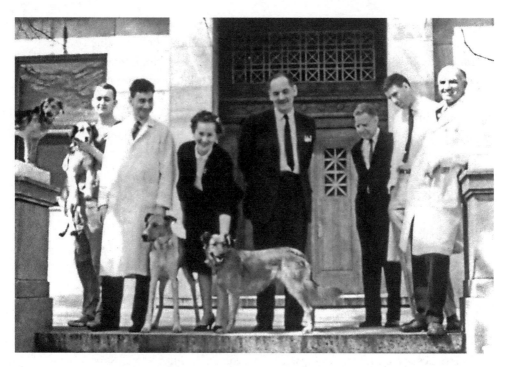

Roy Calne (*left*), Joseph Murray (*right*), Gertrude Elion and George Hitchings of Burroughs Wellcome (*center*), and Donald Searle, medical director of Burroughs Wellcome (*rear*), present the dogs that received the first successful long-term kidney transplants, achieved with the use of azathioprine, on the steps of the Harvard Medical School. Image courtesy of Joseph Murray.

George Hitchings (1905–1998) and Gertrude "Trudy" Elion (1918–1999) provided him with a supply of the required chemicals, as they had previously done for Schwartz and Dameshek.[24] Among these chemicals was the compound BW57-322 (later known as azathioprine/Imuran).

As soon as Calne arrived in Boston, Murray proposed that he instead get involved in their traditional radiation work, but when Murray left on vacation, Calne managed to introduce his chemical studies.[25] The dog kidney transplant work proceeded rapidly, and Calne and Murray soon showed that azathioprine was more successful as an immunosuppressant drug than 6-MP.[26] As they gained experience in using azathioprine, they obtained increasing periods of kidney graft survival in some dogs, as well as fewer complications.[27] At the Brigham Hospital in Boston, Calne and Murray presented a healthy dog with a successful kidney transplant at a historic hospital clinical meeting. As before, the occasional success gave encouragement. Calne and Murray briefly tried azathioprine in empirical combination with other agents in the transplant laboratory but without success.

Use of Azathioprine in Humans

Azathioprine was not available for human use until 1961, and in the waiting period of 1960–1961, 6-MP was used in a number of human kidney transplants, including two in Boston, to add to Calne's three earlier Royal Free Hospital cases. Occasional use of the radiation-only strategy continued until 1962, as it did in Paris, but in all the Boston cases results were poor, and no lasting human kidney transplant function was obtained with 6-MP. Even when azathioprine was available for use in humans, even with added azaserine or actinomycin C, the results were no better. By 1962, only one patient out of eight had survived beyond three months.[28] David Hume, having returned to transplantation studies, had a slightly better experience at Richmond using immunosuppression with azathioprine plus local radiation to the kidney.[29] In Edinburgh, Michael Woodruff, who started with a successful transplant between twins in 1960, now had a single survivor using chemical immunosuppression, and this living-related, father-to-son transplant was carried out in 1962 using azathioprine obtained via Boston. The graft was to last for twenty years and by then was one of the two longest survivals in the world. But with the high death rate among transplant patients in the early 1960s, whether the primary treatment was with irradiation or drugs, infection was the dominant factor, and the survival of the kidney itself may have been better than these figures suggest. Doomed patients did not return to dialysis, and some kidneys at the time of the patient's death showed little sign of rejection. In retrospect, the azathioprine dose was high and toxic, but there was no alternative.[30] The feeling grew that azathioprine, in spite of some experimental successes in dog work, was after all, only too similar to radiation in having an unacceptably difficult and narrow range of therapeutic action.

In the 1962–1963 period, few new human kidney transplant cases were attempted, and this hesitation arose from the poor results, scarcity of donor organs, and a growing reluctance to use living-related donors. Roy Calne was quite pessimistic in early 1963:

Clinical application of renal transplantation between individuals other than identical twins has been attempted and occasionally has proved to be moderately successful.

A surgeon proposing to remove a healthy kidney from a living donor takes upon himself a large share of moral responsibility. It is a tribute to human nature how often relatives and friends of a dying uremic patient will offer to donate one of their own healthy kidneys, if there is even an infinitesimal chance of the transplant being successful.

With the exception of twins, the present position of experimental renal transplantation would not in general justify clinical transplantation from a live donor.[31]

At other times the roles were reversed, with surgeons seeking a related donor. In such cases, they entered the complex dynamics of human families, encountering donors who were willing but medically unsuitable, as well as suitable donors who were unwilling. These matters added to the growing bioethics agenda of the day.

The Combined Regimen

The route by which steroids gained a crucial role in transplantation came from attempts to delay loss of grafts that had started to reject. In 1960, Willard Goodwin at UCLA had noticed prompt reversal of human kidney rejection after using a relatively large daily dose of prednisone in a patient managed with a nitrogen mustard regimen. Goodwin had one other success with this protocol but no others, and when he ceased kidney transplantation in 1961 after a run of dismal results, the strategy was forgotten when he described this experience briefly in 1962.[32] He did not report the interesting use of steroids until early 1963.[33] Meanwhile, early the previous year, Thomas Starzl, with his colleague Tom Marchioro (1929–1995), had found steroids of benefit in dealing with rejection in dogs on azathioprine, particularly in liver grafts. As Starzl knew, liver rejection in dogs was less powerful and showed occasional spontaneous reversal.[34] Goodwin visited Starzl at the Denver VA Hospital in May of that year, and Starzl soon found that the massive steroid dosage regimen was successful in treating human transplant rejection.[35] He reported this important finding late in 1963, after having difficulty getting his papers on the subject accepted.[36] From this publication the term "rejection crisis" came into general use.

Starzl also considered that "it might seem reasonable to administer these agents prophylactically from the time of transplantation." This approach meant supplementing the azathioprine therapy with steroids from the start, with further large doses of steroid for rejection episodes. Starzl later pointed out that this crucial development was an empirical one, with the role of animal models being secondary:

In occasional dogs, a protracted life proved possible after renal transplantation with the use of steroids, 6-mercaptopurine or azathioprine as the sole immunosuppressive treatment. In man similar successes were occasionally achieved solely with 6-mecaptopurine or azathioprine. Thus both the animal data and the initial clinical experience discouraged further trials. The most important development which made immunosuppression practical was the discovery of the way in which azathioprine and prednisone could be advantageously used together. There was essentially no preceding laboratory data to indicate that the benefits with this now universally accepted combination of agents would be as great as proved to be the case.[37]

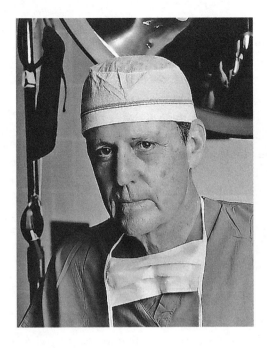

In 1963, Thomas Earl Starzl introduced the "combined therapy," namely the addition of steroids to azathioprine from the outset in kidney transplantation, which led to regular success in kidney transplantation. His pioneering liver transplants, also carried out in 1963 at the Denver Veterans Administration Hospital, resumed in 1967 with the use of antilymphocyte serum. He moved to Pittsburgh in the 1980s and, with Roy Calne, established liver transplantation as a routine service.

Using this new combined regimen, Starzl was obtaining very promising results in a rapid-fire series of patients.

National Research Council Meeting

In September 1963, twenty-five doctors involved in transplantation worldwide were invited to meet at the National Research Council (NRC) in Washington, DC, and to consider the status of kidney transplantation.[38] Their expenses were met by the pharmaceutical companies Burroughs Wellcome, which sold azathioprine, and Parke Davis & Company, which marketed cortisone and, if not impressed by the potential the transplantation market might hold for their two existing, inexpensive products, they were impressed by the quality of those involved in the endeavor. Few transplant centers were not represented. In total, experience with 244 living-related and 68 cadaver kidney transplants were reported.[39] Easily the largest series was the 67 cases from Boston's Brigham Hospital dating from the late 1950s, followed by Starzl's 27 cases carried out over a much shorter period of time after his arrival in Denver in 1962. Hamburger reported on 20 patients, and Küss, also from Paris, described 16 transplants. Hume, having recently restarted transplants in Richmond, contributed 20 cases.[40] Lower numbers were reported by Goodwin from Los Angeles (13), Ralph Shackman from London's Hammersmith Hospital (12), Woodruff in Edinburgh (11), Willem Kolff at Cleveland (9), Paul Russell from Boston's Massachusetts General (6), and smaller numbers from other groups. Woodruff had the longest individual survivals at this time.

Other centers not represented but mentioned as being active were headed by Guy Alexandre in Belgium, Priscilla Kincaid-Smith in Melbourne, and Anthony Walsh in Dublin. Some who were not in the informal network, like Gordon Murray in Toronto, were perhaps not invited or did not respond. It is likely that scattered single, nonreported kidney transplants were carried out elsewhere with discouraging outcomes.

Overall transplant results up to that year had been poor, and many expected that the NRC meeting would be a reflective and gloomy one, but there was good news. The attention was on Starzl's results with his new combined steroid/azathioprine regimen. He had a late invitation, through Goodwin's suggestion, and he reported excellent results from Denver: twenty of his recent twenty-seven kidney transplant patients had survived for noteworthy periods of time. Goodwin forewarned Starzl that the Denver results might not be believed, so he brought his patients' large wall charts, the first single-sheet data charts of the kind that were later in common use. The group admired the chart format and carefully scrutinized the data.[41] The meeting participants returned to their own units and followed Starzl's lead.

Group Experience

The group review of these early efforts at human kidney transplantation revealed important practical details. It suggested that blood group mismatching could, after all, cause immediate kidney loss, and there was a shift toward using the blood-typing rules of transfusion in organ grafting.[42] While there was still some unfounded nervousness about cooling or flushing the donor kidneys, Starzl and Calne advised the meeting attendees that flushing and thoroughly cooling the donor organ was helpful.[43] Cooling had finally achieved acceptance.[44] And it was clear that patient mortality was not always from kidney rejection. Half the early deaths were from surgical complications or infection. There was a tense dispute on the use of living donors, with many speaking against their further use and promoting cadaveric sources instead.

A few transplant centers, including those in Denver and Cleveland, had full dialysis support for transplantation, but centers elsewhere, including Boston, were less fortunate. Keith Reemtsma (1925–2000), the transplant pioneer at Tulane, had no dialysis facilities available to him in New Orleans, nor did the Belgian surgeon Guy Alexandre (born 1934), who had trained in transplantation at Boston in the early 1960s. On his return home, no artificial kidney was available in Belgium at that time.

Among meeting attendees, opinion was split on the need for radiology of the kidney vessels in assessing a living donor, but there was agreement that bilateral kidney removal for serious hypertension before or after transplantation was sometimes essential.[45] The meeting featured no discussion of early tissue-typing methods or brain death issues as related to donation, which would later become important.

Joseph Murray's Analysis

Before the NRC meeting, Murray had asked the invited participants for information and then prepared an analysis to present at the event. When the proceedings of the meeting were published, he added a careful introduction and summary. As a result of the conference, the International Human Kidney Transplant Registry, the first cooperative clinical venture of its kind, was set up in Boston to collect data and watch yearly trends, although in the end only a few active transplant centers contributed.[46] Murray took responsibility for the registry but credited Medawar with the idea.[47] Although this registry seems an obvious idea in retrospect, such sharing was an innovative concept at the time. Reemtsma perceptively noted this change in clinical scientific behavior: "In the past, scientists have considered their work as personal property, to be presented when and how they choose. We have an opportunity [in human kidney transplantation] to revise drastically both our methodology and record-keeping and our philosophy of data-sharing. By the use of biomedical computers, data collected from world-wide sources as work progresses could be made available to all investigators."[48]

This openness was laudable and served as a template that was to be routine in many later clinical endeavors. Murray did point out that in any rapid growth phase of innovative medicine, the recent results were usually better than those of previous years and that some centers were more successful than others. Pooling all cases could dilute the year-on-year success and conceal what could be attained by the new treatments in the best cases.[49] However, the pooling of outcome figures was a form of audit whose time had come. Such data were useful in many ways and later would assist in the choice between transplantation and regular dialysis for

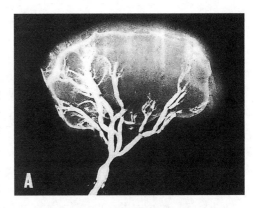

By the mid-1960s, it was apparent that ABO blood-type matching had significant impact on human kidney transplantation. This image shows a type A kidney that had to be removed shortly after grafting into a type O recipient; angiography revealed the intrarenal vascular disaster. From Thomas Starzl, *Experience in Kidney Transplantation* (Philadelphia: Saunders, 1964).

kidney failure. Having factual data on transplant outcome was soon to be important to health care planners and governments wanting to know the usual results in the hands of those offering a routine service.

With this caveat on the value of pooled data, Joseph Murray regularly enlarged and extended this valuable analysis of kidney graft survival, an enterprise later taken over by the American College of Surgeons and the National Institutes of Health when the numbers of kidney transplants increased rapidly. The registry continued to produce valuable data until it was overwhelmed by the numbers of transplants carried out worldwide, and local collection of data took over. Of these local data registries, the most authoritative was to be the European Dialysis and Transplant Association (EDTA), formed in 1964, which in 1965 started its unique collection of survival data for both dialysis and kidney transplant patients.[50]

One initially puzzling aspect of the early registry reports is that kidney survival is not described, and the only outcome recorded after transplantation was the patient's death or survival. In 1963, kidney survival and patient survival were not considered separately. Rejection followed by death, or complications without rejection leading to death, were added together. Not until the late 1960s was it routinely possible to return to regular dialysis following loss of a transplant, and only then did kidney and patient survival become different lines on the registry graphs.

Organ Supply and Demand

With an awareness that future donation might not be mainly from living donors, the transplant community made the first estimates of future supply for cadaveric organ donation versus demand. A thoughtful contribution on this matter came from Nathan P. Couch at Peter Bent Brigham Hospital.[51] His assumptions are interesting: he believed that kidney and liver transplantation would eventually become routine and would use cadaveric rather than living donors. His view was that transplantation would be restricted to recipients between the ages of four and sixty. He used data from *Vital Statistics of the United States 1963* showing a death rate from major kidney disease at 114 per million (a figure that did not require serious modification later), with 40 per million dying in the "transplantable" group. In looking at the pool of potential donors, he assumed these would be patients dying suddenly from brain lesions, notably subarachnoid hemorrhage. Interestingly, he ruled out donations from those dying from head injuries after accidents. Although these types of injuries were common enough, in this preventilation era such pre–critical care patients usually died with multisystem complications and infection. His calculations showed that there were 32 deaths per million in the acute brain disease group, and with each donor giving two kidneys, the potential supply was adequate. Couch knew that few hospitals had been involved with transplantation to that time and all would have to help in the future if organ donation was to expand. Couch added that a full supply of donor livers for those with liver failure was also mathematically possible. It was indeed a time of optimism.

But increasing the cadaveric donor supply presented difficulties. In Boston, Murray described the routine at the time, a reminder now of the rushed, undignified, and often unpleasant early days of obtaining the needed cadaveric kidneys. The orderly world of intensive care and assisted ventilation of the critically ill was still to come. Kidney removal had to follow death in the ward, or emergency rooms, and the organ had to be implanted quickly into patients with fluid or electrolyte problems and suboptimal anesthetic preparation. The likely recipients with kidney failure were not on dialysis or on a waiting list but were simply those with a suitable blood group who were in the hospital at the time. Murray wrote that "suitable cadaveric kidneys are not frequently available for several reasons: a potential donor must be free from infection and have normal renal function; legal permission must be obtained immediately from the medical examiner in cases of acute trauma or from the family if the examiner waives jurisdiction; a potential recipient must be constantly available in the hospital; and finally, the operating teams and theatre must be ready. Only two or three hours can elapse from the death of the donor to revascularization in the new host."[52]

When Roy Calne returned to London from Boston, there was a coolness toward his work, and his proposals to obtain cadaver kidneys in his hospital offended some: "We hit a serious snag: the nurse superintendent of the operating theatres would not permit dead bodies to be brought into her operating theatres. So we had to remove the kidneys in the open ward. Looking back on the procedure it must have resembled a horror film."[53]

Nevertheless, the pioneer transplant units at this time looked to cadaveric donation as the future source of organs. Donors were sought only in the hospitals pioneering transplantation, and none were initially obtained elsewhere, not only because of the need for speedy grafting but also because other hospitals were uninterested in participating in such efforts. Exchange of kidneys with the other scattered and distant transplant units was not considered.[54]

Clinical Optimism

Shortly after the 1963 National Research Council meeting, twenty-five new kidney transplant programs began at centers across the United States. One of the first of these was in San Francisco and under the direction of John

Najarian (born 1927). Transplantation had been only part of the work of the surgical departments involved thus far, but identifiable specialist transplant units began to emerge as patient numbers increased. Starzl's new combined immunosuppression regimen was a vital innovation. An initially large but incrementally reduced steroid dose was used after transplant, and the now smaller azathioprine dose could be adjusted daily according to the patient's white cell count in hopes of avoiding infection and other consequences of marrow depression. After some weeks, the doses of the two drugs could be cautiously reduced to levels that would have been ineffective at the time of transplantation. This was the drug combination that was to be generally successful and unrivalled for almost twenty years.[55]

It was soon obvious that the first three months after transplant were crucial and that, thereafter, acute rejection was less likely. The word *tolerance* was used at this time to explain any long-lasting grafts, in a somewhat general sense, but use of the term also conveyed the hope that specific immunological tolerance might have been achieved, for which there was evidence later. Most writers preferred the neutral terms *adaptation* or *accommodation* for the undoubted decline of rejection episodes with time.[56] Surgeons were fascinated to discover that some patients with long-surviving grafts had privately concluded that their medication need not be taken fastidiously and that temporary or permanent stoppage of their immunosuppression did not always lead to rejection. This was a phenomenon not seen in animal transplant work, and the interesting news was proudly given back to the labs. The puzzle of this helpful adaptation continued to be unsolved for decades.[57]

Into the Unknown

Clinical surprises, both pleasant and unpleasant, emerged from the growing number of successful kidney transplants carried out in the first half of the 1960s. Infection with common organisms was frequent, but as surgeons gained experience, fewer patients died of early sepsis than in the pioneering early 1960s and management of the technical surgical problems improved. As more patients survived the early, hazardous weeks, they entered into an uncharted area of clinical care. They were found to be prone to exotic infections, notably those controlled by cell-mediated immunity, such as pneumocystis, nocardia, candidiasis, and aspergillosis. Less exotic old-fashioned killers, like reactivated tuberculosis, were encountered routinely, and normally mild viruses such as herpes, chickenpox, and cytomegalovirus could be lethal.[58] These challenges, often appearing rapidly and aggressively, taxed the talents of the staff involved and required improvisation in these novel areas of clinical management.[59]

Rolla B. Hill's laboratory group commented on their Denver experience: "The transplant recipient has joined the growing legion of patients whose therapist treads a thin, barely observable line: too little therapy, and the patient succumbs to his biological abnormality; and too much and a new constellation of unrelated but equally ominous pathological processes arises. To find and stay on the narrow middle road requires alert individualization of dose and a considerable delicacy of response to changes in the patient's condition."[60]

With longer graft survival, novel surgical complications affecting the ureter and artery emerged, notably renal artery stenosis, which caused narrowing near the junction of host and graft renal arteries.[61] The expected side effects of the large doses of steroids were common—poor wound healing, diabetes, pancreatitis, gastrointestinal hemorrhage, muscle loss, and the classic "moon face" and "buffalo hump."

Functional Assessment

By later standards, however, radiological assessment of the transplanted kidney in the 1960s was primitive, being restricted to traditional intravenous urography. This imaging was certainly helpful in showing obstruction of the ureter in functioning transplants but was of little assistance in monitoring a nonfunctioning kidney. Angiography of the kidney was possible and could show blood flow and assist in assessing nonfunction but could not be repeated frequently. Sophisticated imaging of transplanted organs and interventional adjustments were still to come.[62] David Hume hesitantly began to employ biopsy of the transplanted kidney in 1963 but soon abandoned that practice because of the danger to the organ. It was cautiously reintroduced in 1968 by the Melbourne team, which added a twelve-hour histological processing regimen as an aid to diagnosis of rejection.[63] Regular biopsy soon became routine.

Delayed Effects

In transplanted kidneys, the expected return of the original disease, notably glomerulonephritis, was helpfully delayed by the immunosuppression. However, an unusual form of bone disease—avascular necrosis—emerged regularly in the increasing number of survivors and was eventually linked to the large initial steroid dosage.[64] Hyperparathyroidism could worsen after transplantation and was cured by surgical removal of most of the glandular tissue.[65] Units with the longest surviving grafts, notably in Denver, first found and defined the prevalence of mild "chronic rejection" of otherwise successful kidney grafts.[66]

Patient Eligibility

With a greater range of patients being considered for transplantation, they inevitably had significant related illnesses, notably diabetes, vascular disease, and previous malignancy. As transplanters gained experience, they honed the criteria for transplantation. Some diseases, oxalosis, for example, showed prompt recurrence in the transplanted kidney, and transplantation for later patients with the condition was reluctantly ruled out.

At first, there was a narrow age range criterion for transplantation, and it excluded young children; they were also not considered suitable for regular dialysis. The post-graft phase was judged to be too much of an ordeal for the young, and the exposure to growth-inhibiting steroids was thought undesirable. But as the transplant results improved and management became simpler, children were reconsidered for grafting. The first bold pediatric kidney transplants were carried out in Denver and Richmond beginning in 1962.[67] These pioneering efforts were highly successful, and a major series was reported later from Minneapolis.[68] The surprise was that immunosuppression in the young was tolerated better than in adults, though skeletal and hormonal maturation was usually delayed.

In this early period of transplantation, diabetic patients with kidney failure were not eligible for kidney grafting. The argument was that, because diabetes was a multisystem disease, it was pointless to replace the kidney, since complications and comorbidity would continue and be dominant. It was also expected that the grafted kidney would promptly suffer diabetic damage and that immunosuppressant steroids would worsen the diabetes. The assumption that diabetics were unsuitable for kidney transplantation was first set aside in the Minneapolis unit, and kidney survival figures were good, with patient survival less so.[69]

Two other pleasant surprises emerged. The first, reported by Hume in Richmond, was that a second kidney transplant might succeed in a patient after the first graft had been rejected. Regrafting had been avoided, since accelerated "second set" rejection was a hallowed part of transplant lore and was thought to be unavoidable. The second welcome event was that pregnancy was possible after non-twin kidney transplants. In spite of an early scare that azathioprine caused birth defects, there was relief when further experience showed that immunosuppression drugs had no harmful effects on the fetus.[70]

Transplantation and Tumors

Less welcome was the first case of a malignant secondary deposit in a kidney taken from a donor known to have a lung carcinoma. John B. Dossetor (born 1925), a Canadian nephrologist, reported the first such instance in 1963, and by 1965 there were two more cases.[71] This contradicted the conventional wisdom that common solid tumors rarely shed cancerous cells to the kidney. As a result, a new view emerged that there was early diffuse, occult spread of common malignancies. In affected recipients, removal of the transplant with its tumor deposits, plus cessation of immunosuppression, successfully controlled some of these transferred malignancies. Shortly afterward, a number of kidney recipients had other types of de novo tumors, ones not carried over as metastases in the graft. When three cases of reticulum cell sarcoma had appeared by 1968 in Denver, it became clear that these cancers were transplant related, and similar single cases were soon reported in Edinburgh, Auckland, and Minneapolis.[72] There was even concern at the time, ultimately unwarranted, that malignancies would limit the transplant service. Further research soon established that the tumors were mainly lymphomas, plus superficial skin carcinomas, rather than a general increase in malignancy. Cessation of immunosuppression usually resulted in remission of the lymphomas, and, happily, in only half of the cases was withdrawal of immunosuppression followed by rejection of the kidney.[73] These events firmly encouraged the idea that cell-mediated immunity might hold back early tumor cell growth. This "surveillance" was to be a favorite concept for a while, seemingly answering the puzzle first posed by Leo Loeb: that cellular immunity was surely "designed for" some vital role within the body, other than to reject transplants.

An international register of post-transplant tumors—the Denver Transplant Tumor Register—was established in 1969. Israel "Sol" Penn (1930–1999) led the registry's effort to record and study such tumors and advise on the many individual clinical challenges presented. The registry eventually moved to Cincinnati and was renamed in his honor.[74]

Other Organs Considered

Encouraged by the growing success with kidneys, surgeons soon began to attempt transplants of other human organs, including the liver, lung, intestine, and pancreas. Although these early operations are now considered the "firsts" for each organ and were generally well conducted and based on experimental experience, they were controversial at the time because the grafts all failed, promptly and unpleasantly in most cases. Few of the surgeons involved continued to try at that time, and only in scattered surgical units did hopes for such organ transplants persist. These various moratoria after initial attempts were self-imposed, though often heeding local professional concern. There were as yet no national regulatory bodies or local ethical committees to be consulted before any important clinical innovation. Grafting of some of these organs did not resume until the advent of cyclosporine for immunosuppression.

Liver Transplantation

After the power of the azathioprine/steroid combination became apparent in 1963, Thomas Starzl, working in Colorado, attempted the first human liver transplants. Starzl had been preparing the ground carefully for some time.[75] Others also had an interest in transplanting the liver, and Jack Cannon (born 1919), working in William Longmire's unit in Los Angeles, was probably first to attempt experimental liver transplantation.[76] The first full reports of experimental liver transplantation came from C. Stuart Welch (1909–1980) of Albany Medical College, New York, who described auxiliary hepatic homografts in dogs in 1955.[77] From 1955 onward, Starzl had taken the possibility of human liver transplantation seriously and gained considerable experience and routine technical success in dogs. He started work in the Department of Surgery in Miami, headed by one of Welch's protégés, and after Starzl moved to Chicago in 1958, he regularly succeeded in autotransplantation, namely removing an animal's liver and then returning it, with full function, to the same animal. He shared the kidney transplanters' interest in immunosuppression with radiation at that time but found that it did not prolong liver graft survival in dogs. Francis Moore in Boston also had gained experience with dog liver replacement.[78]

When Starzl moved to Denver in late 1961 as head of the academic surgical department in the Veterans Administration Hospital, he had intended to set up a liver transplant unit. Sensing that the time was not right, a view shared by his hospital colleagues, he instead commenced a successful kidney transplantation program. With the success of his combined regimen and growing experience in the complexities of immunosuppression and organ transplantation management, in 1963 he attempted human liver transplantation. He carefully discussed his plans with other hospital staff and even with key legal and political figures in the state.

In spite of Starzl's considerable experience with experimental liver grafting, these historic human operations posed additional formidable difficulties that proved insurmountable. The first five human liver transplant patients all died within six to twenty-three days of grafting, including one operative death from uncontrolled bleeding. He did no further liver transplants at this time while carefully taking stock.[79] Shortly afterward, others had similarly discouraging experiences and desisted at an even earlier stage. Moore in Boston and J. Demirleau in France, both of whom had considerable experimental experience, stopped after attempting one human case each. The comments on the Paris case, presented at the Académie de Chirurgie in February 1964, guardedly mentioned Demirleau's "grand courage moral et physique" but raised "l'aspect éthique de la transplantation du foie."

These early forays into human liver transplantation, although disappointing, did offer some lessons. The major issue was the massive blood loss from a general ooze that occurred after removal of the patient's own liver and prior to insertion of the graft.[80] Postmortem study showed that rejection of the liver was not prominent and that some function had been obtained, but ischemic damage to the graft in the period between donor death and organ insertion was a major factor. Based on the experimental transplants with dogs, surgeons had used a venous bypass (later shown to be unnecessary for humans), which led to blood clots in the lungs. The delay from donor death to transplant and consequent damage could be accepted in cadaveric kidney transplantation, because immediate function was not needed and dialysis might be available, but for the liver no similar support was available and any organ damage was fatal. Aware of this problem, Starzl attempted general cooling of any cadaveric donors after death and prior to removal of the liver, the only strategy available at the time.

Early Lung Transplants

In this period of optimism about human grafting, single lungs were transplanted in approximately twenty patients with terminal lung disease. Experimental lung grafting had been pioneered by Alexis Carrel and Charles Guthrie in 1905, but no more reports of lung transplantation had appeared until the considerable experience reported by Vladimir P. Demikhov in the Soviet Union in the late 1940s.[81] Thereafter, experimentalists, notably Wilford B. Neptune at the Hahnemann Medical College in Philadelphia, went through the familiar evolution of establishing a standard experimental surgical technique, obtaining autotransplant success, then showing that dog-to-dog grafts rejected routinely.

The first human lung transplant attempt was in June 1963 by James D. Hardy (1919–2003) at the University of Mississippi Medical Center in Jackson. The recipient was a prisoner serving a life sentence for murder, and he died eighteen days after the operation.[82] All of the other patients receiving lung transplants elsewhere, including one in Edinburgh in 1968, died after a short time, as did those receiving the first double-lung or heart-lung grafts, pioneered by Clarence Lillehei (1918–1999).[83] The major surgical problems of single lung transplantation proved to be necrosis, air leakage, and stenosis at the junction of the donor and recipient bronchus. Thereafter, lung transplantation was abandoned but later revived, in the early 1980s.

Pancreas Transplantation

Early attempts at pancreas gland transplantation in the 1960s had the usual evolution—technical experience gained first with animal models, then tentative human attempts with poor results, followed by a self-imposed moratorium. For the diabetic patients, the alternative of remaining on insulin treatment was safer, at least in the short term, and only a few diabetics with poor blood sugar control were considered for grafting. In 1966, William Kelly and Dick Lillehei at the University of Minnesota carried out the first vascularized human cadaveric pancreas graft, plus a kidney from the same donor, in a patient with diabetic kidney disease. Six further attempts followed at this time in this unit.[84] The problems encountered were usually not immunological but surgical, since the pancreas graft had to drain its other digestive secretions into the bowel or urinary bladder, and any enzyme leaks were disastrous. Single pancreas implantation operations declined and kidney-with-pancreas grafting was preferred for a while. The early results were poor, with only a single one-year survivor.[85] A register of the small number of transplants of the time was set up in 1966, but it was not until 1978, with the use of cyclosporine, that there was a resurgence of interest. David Sutherland was the activist, working at Minnesota.

Pancreatic Islet Grafting

The alternative to the considerable surgical challenge of whole organ pancreatic transplantation was the attractive and apparently simple and accessible strategy of implanting the insulin-secreting islets of the pancreas, free of the surrounding enzyme-producing tissue. There had been many earlier, uncritical attempts and enthusiastic claims in the gland-graft era using implantation of fragments of whole pancreas.

With successful immunosuppression using azathioprine and steroids emerging in 1963, a number of groups started work on islet transplantation in the mid-1960s. The necessary first step—the separation of pancreatic islets in quantity—proved to be difficult. The work of Paul E. Lacy at St. Louis, which allowed a fair yield of islets from a whole gland, spurred progress in 1967.[86] But careful studies, helped by the ability to measure the levels of the relevant hormones in the blood, showed that islet transplants were destroyed by an usually powerful rejection mechanism.[87] Clinical interest waned, but the goal remained.

Other Organ Transplants

Now forgotten are the reports of a small number of human spleen transplants. The attraction was the reasonable hope (not fulfilled) that such grafts would help in the treatment of hemophilia and agammaglobulinemia. Although the spleen graft was technically easy, no survival of the spleen was obtained nor any therapeutic effect obtained.[88] In any case, a serious graft-versus-host response might have prevented success.

A surgical "first" at this time of hope was carried out in February 1964 at the Clínica Guayaquil, Ecuador, on a soldier who lost a hand after a grenade accident. The prolonged operation using a hand from a cadaveric donor was apparently technically successful, and the immunosuppression was monitored with the help of advice via telephone from Richard Wilson of the Peter Bent Brigham Hospital in Boston. Wilson then traveled to Ecuador and, after assessing the situation, transferred the patient to Boston, but twenty-one days after the transplant, rejection forced removal of the hand.

In 1964, two intestinal transplants were attempted in infants by Ralph A. Deterling (1917–1992), a distinguished vascular surgeon at the Boston Floating Hospital, a long-established innovative pediatric unit associated with Tufts–New England Medical Center. The results, however, were not reported at the time.

Xenograft Organs

With the confidence gained from Starzl's successful combined immunosuppression regimen, kidney transplanters now looked confidently beyond human sources to consider animals as donors. Using monkey organs for human transplantation held appeal because of their size and blood types shared with humans. "A period of collective madness" was a rueful verdict later, but the temporary enthusiasm for these xenografts is explicable by the circumstances of the times. The rapid progress after 1963 suggested that newer methods of immunosuppression would appear shortly and that routine success with homografts would follow. It was a time of considerable progress in basic immunology, and, with further progress expected in the near term, xenograft organ survival would presumably be achieved. The other factor was that opinion was still turning away from use of living-related donors. That trend coexisted with increasing numbers of patients being considered for transplantation and the resulting awareness of a shortage of cadaveric donor organs, helping the notion that grafts from animals would meet the need. Such grafts would be available for planned human operations and would function immediately.

In Minneapolis in February 1963, C. R. Hitchcock had grafted a ba-

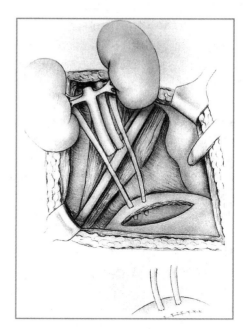

An "*en bloc*" technique was used when, in the 1960s, surgeons grafted monkey kidneys to human patients. In the technique, both kidneys and the large vessels were grafted, as was used later, when children's kidneys were transplanted to adult recipients. Image courtesy of Keith Reemtsma.

boon kidney to the thigh of a human patient, and the kidney functioned well for three days before arterial thrombosis occurred. Shortly thereafter, chimpanzee kidneys (which have A and O type blood) were used in six cases by Reemtsma, and, in Denver, Starzl did six human kidney transplants using baboon donors (which possess A, B, and O antigens) and then stopped to assess the series.[89] These xenografts showed spectacular postoperative urine outputs and did not fail immediately; one chimpanzee kidney functioned for six months, and the patient returned to work.[90] But rejection episodes in the xenografts continued to be severe, closely spaced, and eventually irreversible.

During the short period when these monkey kidney grafts functioned well, the news spread and surgeons in other nations enthusiastically made plans to start xenografting. Roy Calne traveled from Britain to New Orleans to study the experience there, and on his return he enlisted the aid of the London Zoo. Edinburgh's Michael Woodruff also visited American transplant centers in 1964, and he told the Medical Research Council that he was impressed with the "astonishing progress." When the MRC funded his proposed use of monkey donor organs, the proposals were enthusiastically supported in the press.[91] When reports of the discouraging longer-term results in America became public, these international plans were dropped. The media also took an interest when James D. Hardy used a baboon heart in the first attempt at human heart transplantation, with immediate failure.[92] Hardy faced professional criticism, most notably at a transplantation meeting in New York two weeks later. George Hitchings also sounded an ominous warning at about this time: "Publication in the lay press is responsible for much of the enthusiasm in the field of transplantation. The lay press lives from day to day. . . . Reporters are nice people, but should be shunned like lepers during the early phase of clinical investigation."[93]

Legal Issues

The transplanters' activities also risked legal disapproval. The urgent donor organ removal and informal permission arrangements raised some questions that others noticed. Most nations had brought to bear various "Tissue Acts" to regularize the removal of material for use in tissue banks and corneal grafting. These legal measures usually allowed the "person lawfully in charge of the body" to give permission for tissue donation, after "all reasonable inquiry." But use of cadaveric donor organs proceeded at a different tempo. In Britain, one judge, Lord Davies, soon had to remind doctors that there was a person legally in charge of a dead body and that that person was to be consulted, and he reflected on who would make inquiries as to organ donation and when such inquiries were to be made: "Medicine and Law serve the community best when they walk in step. If they proceed at different speeds, trouble is apt to arise. Unfortunately law is often a laggard and at times medicine gains the lead by long and rapid strides. Doctors are then startled to learn that their projects may land them in Court for breaking what they condemn as myopic and arthritic laws. The reason is not far to seek. 'Law' it has been said 'does not search out as do science and medicine; it reacts to social needs and demands.'"[94]

The law relevant to early tissue grafts, if not myopic, had been overtaken by the new need for rapid cadaveric organ donation at a time when the public did not think about future organ donation after death. The deficiencies and omissions in the law were becoming increasingly apparent, but serious legal entanglement was avoided—barely.[95]

But the public was supportive, and the transplanters could now give out good news. Some units actively sought good public relations.[96] Patients who had resumed important work or gone on to worldly or sporting success gave particularly valuable testimonies.

The Language of Transplantation

One sign of the change of pace at this time was that the nomenclature of clinical and basic transplantation immunology was tidied up. The activist in this matter was the tenacious Peter Gorer, and he had first advocated the changes in 1960 at Milan Hašek's "tolerance" conference at Liblice. Gorer had gained so much respect from his tissue-typing contributions that he persuaded all involved that a vocabulary overhaul was required, and his aim was to bring the language of transplantation into line with serology and classical languages. His most noteworthy proposal was to abandon the word *homograft* and other older terms. Gorer wrote that "this situation [i.e., the terminology] reaches its full flowering with that dismal trio isologous, homologous and heterologous. . . . I have asked several classical scholars for their advice and the term I like best is 'allogenic.'"[97]

Gorer also suggested the change from *heterograft* to *xenograft,* a word that had desirable classical roots. Although there was some grumbling, Gorer continued to push the matter, gaining supporters over the next four years, including George Snell.[98] Snell was preparing a new edition of *The Biology of the Laboratory Mouse,* and, determined to tidy up the nomenclature, he asked experts in the field for their views. His advisory group, which may or may not have included surgeons, voted to dump the term *homograft* and substitute *allograft,* but the vote was only 9 to 6. At the last minute, he canvassed five of his panel, proposing *xenograft* instead of *heterograft,* and the vote was 4 to 1 in support of the change.[99]

Because of the narrow verdict, the older term *homograft* persisted in the journals and was regarded with affection by the pioneers, particularly so by the transplant surgeons and by many in America. By the end of the 1960s, though, a new generation of transplanters had emerged who had no loyalty to the older words. Newcomers found that *homograft* was rather old-fashioned and dated, and *allograft* increasingly became the standard term.[100]

The word *immunosuppression* had quickly found widespread acceptance as a method of continuous, reversible medication. The term *rejection* had been in use for some time to describe the final loss of a graft, and the neologism *rejection crisis,* which had first been used as the French *crise,* was popularized by Starzl, and the phrase suitably suggested possible survival from such a threat.[101] Left untouched were the rather militaristic and even xenophobic metaphors in transplantation immunology, notably *attack, defense, invasion,* and *foreign bodies. Harvesting* of organs seemed insensitive, but *tolerance* and cellular *cooperation* had more kindly nuances. The success of regular dialysis also encouraged attempts to move away from the melancholy phrase "terminal renal failure," but no substitute found favor, with some using the scarcely more cheerful "chronic renal failure" or the depressing "end-stage renal failure."[102] The phrase "cadaveric donor" lasted for a surprising length of time, since there seemed no alternative, but was replaced in about 2000 by the less gruesome "deceased donor."

A New Journal

At this time, the journal *Transplantation* appeared, acknowledging a new need, and it was the first of many specialized journals to serve the transplant community. The only niche publication prior to this time was the increasingly neglected supplement, "Transplantation," carried in *Plastic and Reconstructive Surgery* as an evolutionary relic of the considerable and commendable efforts of the American plastic surgeons in nurturing transplantation studies in the 1950s and earlier. But times had changed. Medawar's "Introduction" to the slim first issue of *Transplantation* in January 1963 hailed the new publication as timely and stated that it "would be met with a sigh of relief by the editors of orthodox journals who have looked fearfully on the rising tide of manuscripts written in the private language of transplantation research."

The new journal, with E. J. Eichwald again serving as an editor, had original articles, an abstracts section, and frequent bibliographies on specific areas of research. It carried the regular scholarly reports and data analysis from the Kidney Transplant Registry run by Murray in Boston. The journal expanded rapidly, reporting in brief on the papers given at relevant conferences, and it had no competition in the area until *Transplantation Proceedings* appeared in 1969. This second journal carried the reports of the activities of the new Transplantation Society, which had emerged in 1966. The earlier transplantation gatherings had been of small groups of invited well-informed experts, and the shift in structure to larger meetings, open to all, was not to the liking of some.[103]

Mid-decade Hesitation

After hopes in the early 1960s that a routinely successful kidney transplantation service was at hand and that success with other organs would follow, there was a pause in mid-decade. Results were not improving rapidly, and regular cadaveric donation was slow to emerge. Hopes for using grafts from monkeys were dashed. But the alternative method of treating end-stage renal failure by regular hemodialysis was now developing rapidly, and it offered a safer, though less complete or satisfying, way of restoring lost kidney function. Patients and their doctors now had a choice.

14 Support from Hemodialysis and Immunology in the 1960s

I N 1960, the medical community made significant progress toward a full understanding of cell-mediated immunity. Most notably, researchers uncovered the central role of the thymus and defined the two types of lymphocyte and their links with cell-mediated immunity. Also in 1960, Peter Medawar was awarded a Nobel Prize for his work on tolerance, a signal that transplantation immunology had come of age. And 1960 was also the year in which regular dialysis was first used to sustain patients in end-stage renal failure. Dialysis and kidney transplantation were to be closely linked thereafter.

Regular Dialysis

Beginning in the mid-1950s, the use of the kidney machine to deal with acute renal failure slowly started gaining acceptance and dialysis techniques steadily improved. But to keep patients with end-stage renal failure alive in the long term with such treatment seemed inconceivable.[1] Not only was the concept considered "unnatural" in some quarters, but there were also practical constraints. For each dialysis treatment in the 1950s, separate surgical procedures were needed to connect the patient's circulation to the machine.

In 1960, there occurred a simple change in the method of this "access" to the circulation for dialysis, which was immediately successful. This advance came from creative tinkering with bits of the new plastic tubing widely used for covering telephone cables. Regular dialysis was possible, and this new treatment not only immediately opened up many clinical challenges but also changed the practice of medicine, provoking a new public debate on a range of issues. This new form of treatment developed exactly as hopes grew from 1960 to 1963 for successful kidney transplantation. This was perhaps simply a historical coincidence, but it certainly seemed at the time that treatment of end-stage renal failure was a venture whose time had come.

In 1960, Belding Scribner (1921–2004), a nephrologist in Seattle, Washington, devised a method for gaining permanent access to arteries and veins for the purposes of regular hemodialysis. Scribner developed a simple shunt using a length of electrical cable.[2] The cable was sheathed in the newly available, nonwettable, heat-malleable Teflon, and, removing the cable, he was left with a hollow tube. He thinned down the two ends to give narrow tips, bent the tube into a loop, and inserted and tied one narrow tip into an artery in the forearm and the other into a nearby vein.[3] With the loop led outside of the skin, this gave an external conduit for blood flow, and a junction inserted into the loop created an opening for connection to the machine. Blood flowed nicely through the device without clotting, aided by the dispensation of the low viscosity of the anemic end-stage renal failure patients' blood, plus their subtle clotting defect.

The shunt continued to work remarkably well. Tentatively, Scribner started to carry out repeated dialysis treatments in a patient with end-stage renal failure.[4] It was reasonable to expect that the treatment would simply postpone the inevitable and result in a lingering death with unpleasant and intractable complications. To Scribner's surprise, the treatment went smoothly from the start, and when a shunt firmly clotted or became infected, a new site could be found.

Scribner reported his clinical experience,

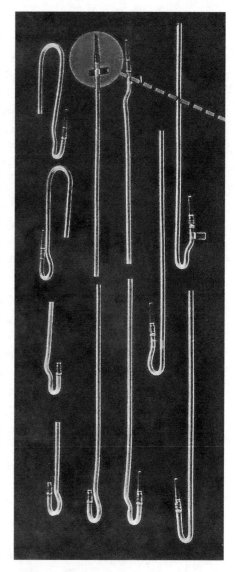

Belding Scribner developed a shunt that provided permanent access to arteries and veins, to allow repeated hemodialysis. Available commercially, in many variant forms, the shunt could be placed at the wrist or at the ankle.

only ten weeks into the treatment of his first case, to the American Society for Artificial Internal Organs meeting in Chicago in May 1960, and he took to the meeting ten of his simple shunt-making kits for others to use. Because of interest in the device, he was allowed to substitute this presentation for a paper previously accepted and already on the printed program.[5] In Scribner's unit, four patients started on regular dialysis in the first year, the first living for eleven years thereafter, and the second had eight years on dialysis and lived for a further nineteen after a transplant. Four more patients were taken on in the second year, including a young London doctor, Robin Eady.[6] Apart from Scribner's technical success, he could show that the expected nutritional problems and neurological damage predicted by skeptics had not appeared. Although new challenges emerged from this venture into the unknown, the physicians promptly devised new solutions.

Scribner's shunt and method were quickly used elsewhere, with similarly good results. It was the only "access" method used in the first six years of regular dialysis, but, in 1966, another strategy emerged when Michael Brescia and James Cimino in New York, looking for alternatives to the shunt, created a deliberate arteriovenous fistula between a superficial vein and the radial artery at the wrist.[7] This use of the wrist fistula, and variants on it, later became the standard strategy for access to the circulation for regular hemodialysis. Thereafter, the shunt retained some niche uses, notably in acute renal failure, until use of percutaneous dialysis lines emerged.

When the availability of hemodialysis, the so-called "endless," and expensive, treatment emerged in Seattle, it produced a local resource crisis. Encouraged by Scribner, the debate became public.[8] Indeed, the origins of modern bioethics are often dated to this episode.[9]

Ethical Debate over Regular Dialysis

Historically, new medical therapy is often expensive, controversial, uncertain in outcome, or hazardous. As a result, skeptical doctors and cautious patients are slow to accept new approaches. Patients with advanced illness may get the treatment first, and thus the first results of a novel treatment may be poorer than when given later to healthier patients.[10] Accordingly, though in short supply, new treatment modalities usually enter only slowly and uncertainly into common practice.

Scribner realized that his new treatment was not following this usual pattern of heroic but hazardous innovation. Regular dialysis was surprisingly safe, and many patients were immediately candidates for this life-saving, long-term, expensive, and labor-intensive treatment. The immediate problem was that his patients could not pay the costs, and no money was available from Scribner's hospital, insurance, or from research funding. Instead, he sought help from local charitable groups, and, supported by the John A. Hartford Foundation (which had also provided financial support for the pioneering transplants in Boston), an artificial kidney center opened in Seattle in 1962. Still, only a few patients in the local community could be treated, and the prospect emerged that some eligibility criteria would be needed to determine which patients could receive dialysis.

Selecting Patients for Dialysis

Scribner took the unusual approach of deliberately setting up a structured mechanism for choosing which patients would receive the life-saving treatment. To remove the burden of the decision from his own shoulders, an Advisory and Policy Committee of doctors made a preliminary selection of clinically suitable patients. Then came a novelty, when a second, anonymous committee, with lay members, made a final choice. The members of this second committee, it became known, included a bank president, a labor leader, a minister of religion, two physicians, a housewife, and a lawyer. The medical committee's criteria were that the patients should be under forty years of age, emotionally stable, not suffering from high blood pressure or other comorbidity, and be part of a supportive family unit. Less clear were the attitudes of the lay committee regarding selection.

The use of these committees, particularly the lay involvement, was unique, and when revealed, it attracted wide interest. This committee marked the first such lay input in medical decision making or regulation, and such involvement was later to become common when ethical matters arose. The choice of who would live or die naturally intrigued commentators curious to know the criteria used. Of the medical committee, it was pointed out that their own professional work ethic might count against those without it—"the dilettante student or the non-productive heir." A more obvious target for the commentators was the possibility of conservative attitudes within the second committee. An observer commented dryly at this time that in Seattle the lay members might rule out treatment of the "creative non-conformists, who rub the bourgeoisie the wrong way but who historically have contributed so much to the making of America. The Pacific North-West [i.e., Seattle] is no place for a Henry David Thoreau with bad kidneys."[11]

Interest Spreads

The pioneering kidney transplants of the early 1950s and 1960s were newsworthy in the short term, but regular dialysis with the artificial kidney provoked a sustained public debate, centering on the Seattle method of choosing those to be treated. An article on Scribner's work in Seattle by the journalist Shana Alexander appeared in *Life* magazine on November 9, 1962, ensuring national interest. In addition to harrowing descriptions of individual cases of end-stage kidney failure, the article gave details of the criteria for selection of dialysis patients and included a discreet, shadowy picture of the assembled lay committee.

This public examination of how a limited resource like dialysis treatment was allotted to patients piqued interest in other parts of the medical community. In academia, a sophisticated philosophical and legal discussion on the allocation of scarce life-saving resources also emerged, and the subject also attracted detailed, scholarly attention that yielded articles in legal journals, notably the *Columbia Law Review* and the *Harvard Law Review*. Previously, only arcane theoretical life-and-death choices had been studied rather than the practical application of life-and-death decision making.[12] The world's major religions, the usual arbiters on matters moral, had no obvious theological stance on this niche issue of renal dialysis, and they merely watched from the sidelines. The way was open for emergence of a new cadre of lay bioethicists, particularly as these ethical problems seemed to be increasing in number.[13] These bioethicists wryly noticed that earlier writers, like Aldous Huxley in *Brave New World*, had assumed that high technology would eliminate such questions and create an amoral society. The reality was that the reverse seemed to be happening, particularly in medicine.[14]

Patient Selection Criteria

A number of well-defined ethical issues emerged when it was obvious that demand for regular dialysis treatment outstripped supply in the early 1960s. At last, a real "doctors' dilemma" had emerged, one succinctly dramatized by George Bernard Shaw in his play, *The Doctor's Dilemma:* "Well, Mr Saviour of Lives: which is it to be? That honest decent man Blenkinsop, or that rotten blackguard of an artist, eh?" Shaw's famous options arose from a new immunological treatment, one known to him from his visits to Almroth Wright's Vaccine Department in London. Wright had told Shaw of the possible shortage of his powerful new vaccine and that it would be necessary to judge whose lives to save. That situation was never reached.

The debate on allocation of dialysis in the 1960s was not an academic exchange about hypothetical vaccine shortages, though it did recall the scenarios popular with philosophers, namely, who to discard when an overcrowded sledge is being overtaken by wolves or who to put overboard when an overcrowded life raft is sinking.[15] The ethical and legal problems raised by these scarce medical resources were real, and new dilemmas were to emerge. The neophyte ethicists' contributions were made at first in plain language, but technical terms soon professionalized their discourse.

However, most renal units in the United States at this time did not use Scribner's high-profile selection method when they began offering regular, long-term dialysis. Instead, they simply muddled through when choosing patients for treatment.[16] A "first-come, first-served" principle for those meeting reasonable clinical criteria seemed to work in practice. Commentators remarked that this random acceptance "mimicked fate," a concept probably more acceptable than the decision of anonymous committees.

Death with Dignity

Adding to the debate on how to allocate treatment such as long-term dialysis was a second issue: the quality of life on regular dialysis. A further question was whether life should be prolonged in this way at all. Irvine Page (1901–1991), the distinguished physician-editor of the generalist journal *Modern Medicine,* spoke out on the issue in 1963. In a number of editorials, he attacked the growth of hemodialysis treatment. His own hospital, the Cleveland Clinic, had a transplant unit and a dialysis service run by Willem Kolff, and the two men were not close. Page asked, rather disingenuously,

Who would look on a loved one with equanimity, knowing that his life is wholly dependent on the functioning of some mechanical aid? Is this right in a world so full of simple need? It is a nightmare world in which a segment of our (least fit) population is kept alive hooked up to ingenious machines. Is death to be looked upon as evil? Cannot man have confidence in the orderliness of nature—that death like birth, will be painless, and is not to be feared? In our desperate attempts to prolong life, we are, I think, losing sight of these simple ideas. . . . Life cannot be replaced by the artificial. Death cannot be averted by a substitute.[17]

Page thus raised the specter of the dialyzers as insensitive latter-day Dr. Frankensteins, going beyond the normal limits of medical science.[18] In the years that followed, Page was less temperate, singling out Kolff again for his disapproval.[19] Patients surviving on dialysis were depicted as frail, chronically ill, and prone to suicide.[20] But supporters of dialysis pointed out that the type of death suffered by untreated end-stage renal failure patients was far from dignified, with nausea, vomiting, psychoses, convulsions, and blindness. To neutralize the negative perceptions of the quality of life of the dialysis patients, it became common for their doctors to present pictures or film of their best patients or to have them testify at clinical meetings.

In 1964, J. R. Elkinton, the Quaker editor of the respected *Annals of Internal Medicine,* joined Page's campaign against regular dialysis treatment. Elkinton's criticism of transplantation and dialysis was less ad hominem and came from the simpler, older holistic approach of noninterventionist medicine. Like Page, he quoted with approval the Osler/Hippocratic view, expressed in the famous words of Sir Francis Bacon, that the "office of medicine is but to tune this curious harp of a man's body and reduce it to harmony."[21] He thus praised the body's self-righting mechanisms, as aided by advice from a learned physician on diet, exercise, and change of climate. This "airs, waters, and places" approach to disease and therapy, so popular in the 1920s and 1930s, was itself dying with dignity as a result of the rapid advances in medicine in the 1960s. But even the modernizers among the physicians balked at the prospect of using an artificial kidney and that a learned physician might need to be familiar with machines and their gadgetry.

Cardiac Resuscitation

An additional ethical concern in the 1960s relating to "death with dignity" arose with the introduction of another high-technology intervention, one that heralded momentous events to come later. By the early 1960s, attempts at resuscitation of patients were becoming routine in hospitals, and sometimes these efforts after sudden collapse and cardiac arrest in the hospital setting were successful. These heroic, undignified, and far from private efforts in the wards were entirely directed at restarting the heart, without any attention to supporting respiration.

In 1961, an editorial in the *Medical Tribune,* published in the United States, commented on concerns about this type of medical intervention: "From time to time we are criticized for the overly dramatic and desperate treatment of moribund patients—for surrounding the poor soul with infusions, oxygen, pressor amines, residents and attendings [doctors] that the relatives can barely have a glimpse of him amid a forest of equipment. . . . A plea is made for the dignity of a patient's last hours when he ought to be allowed to die in peace."[22]

Missing from the *Medical Tribune* editor's list was intubation of the trachea and assisting ventilation thereafter. However, the early form of resuscitation he describes was increasingly attempted even in the last moments of those expected to die. This "imperative to resuscitate" involved these undignified and largely unsuccessful scenes at the bedside, which might include a final direct attempt, after the heart stopped, with cardiac massage, after opening the chest in the ward. These unpleasant scenes were eventually reduced to being used only after sudden collapse, but it was temporarily a lively addition to the ethicist's agenda. By the mid-1960s, the medical community realized that seriously ill patients with a chance of survival should instead have a different form of support, namely assisted respiration, which was increasingly used. Such patients were moved, with less drama, to a new type of unit: intensive care.

Funding Dialysis

Regular dialysis would require substantial funds, from what was increasingly recognized in the developed world to be finite health care budgets. Some doctors thought that the considerable publicity generated by the new renal replacement services distorted the debate on funding. The debate also alerted government officials in America that voters might soon demand federal action to make the expensive regular dialysis treatment more generally available, since the costs were prohibitive for most individuals and unattractive to insurance companies.

Internationally, the response of individual countries to the challenge of the new treatment corresponded to budgets, the type of health care system in place, and the expectations of patients. In the United States, a few found that their insurance companies would pay part of the cost. Communities attempted to provide support to the small number of patients needing the treatment, and fund-raising for this purpose proved popular. Then, in a surprising move, in 1963 the Veterans Administration proposed setting up thirty dialysis centers. Shortly thereafter, the U.S. Public Health Service also approved some funding from its end-stage disease programs, notably from its Kidney Disease Control Program (KDCP), and its Crippled Children Program funded the treatment of children with renal failure. A federal grant in 1964 funded a dialysis center in Seattle, and twelve more such grants followed in 1965, but all of these grants were based on "step funding," which meant that support would decline each year, thus appeasing congressional conservatives by encouraging the development of other sources of funding, which never emerged. The possibility of home dialysis was also investigated as a cheaper alternative to hospital dialysis.

In 1965, the U.S. government established Medicare to provide health care coverage for senior citizens and those with certain disabilities. Two years later, the confidential Gottschalk Report, submitted to the Bureau of the Budget, stated that transplantation and regular dialysis were not experimental treatments but established therapies and recommended a national treatment service for renal replacement.[23] This prestigious report, chaired by a distinguished nephrologist, encountered a shrewd awareness at the government level of the magnitude of the open-ended financial commitment required by the report's main conclusion that dialysis and transplantation were "sufficiently well advanced today to warrant launching a national program." The report, though eventually published, had only limited circulation in government circles and was then shelved, but not forgotten.

Although the Gottschalk Report is usually remembered only for its early proposals to support regular dialysis treatment, it also envisaged a national kidney transplant service. Some of its proposals were accepted, and some low-key national transplantation initiatives soon emerged. One reason for those moves was that the Public Health Service had noticed that successful transplantation was emerging as a cheaper option to dialysis treatment, and, in 1969, its KDCP not only gave some support to transplant units but also funded seven cadaveric procurement agency contracts.

After the Gottschalk Report's quick relegation to obscurity, there was continuous pressure to obtain federal funding for dialysis via repeated bills and continuous lobbying from professional groups and consumer organizations At last, in 1972, the Social Security amendments, Section 2991, and Public Law No. 92-603 did extend Medicare coverage to those with end-stage renal disease or their families if they received Social Security disability payments. The legislation followed only after complex political maneuvering, since many in Washington regarded the debate on dialysis as a "stalking horse" and a forerunner of a larger one thought to be imminent, namely on universal health insurance for Americans. In spite of high-level political opposition, not only on the question of cost but also the principle involved, Congress agreed for the first and, to date, the last time to extend Medicare coverage for a specific disease. As Francis Moore, the Boston surgeon, crisply observed, "The United States seemed to be approaching a socialized health service via the urinary tract." The legislation was assisted by a dramatic demonstration of dialysis by a patient, Shep Glazer, on the floor of Congress. The cost of regular dialysis to treat those under fifty-five with no systemic disease (e.g., diabetes) was expected to level off at one billion dollars in ten years' time, but, as critics had anticipated, this figure was exceeded within three years.[24] In the wake of this legislation came the first federal government oversight of medical treatment in the United States, since regular dialysis was paid for by government funds. However, these arrangements did not include features that would benefit the government, namely doctors paid by the government and the ability for the government to make bulk purchases, control costs, and utilize central planning with sensible geographical placement of units of viable size.

There was soon to be a major international renal failure/industrial complex comprising the suppliers of dialysis machines and consumables plus the network of hospital and freestanding dialysis units. In some health care systems, profitable dialysis units were often accused of being cool toward kidney transplantation, since it took away business.

Dialysis Funding in Britain

In Britain, further government support for dialysis was also increasingly sought.[25] Fund-raising for purchase of kidney machines, a visible and worthy project, became a favorite charity. This sort of community effort pressured the hard-pressed government into providing the less obvious, but necessary, support for running these machines. The health minister released precious "top-sliced funds" from his Special Medical Developments Fund to set up ten hemodialysis units in Britain. He wished only to "prime the pump" and urged local health authorities to take over the expensive units thereafter, similar to the "step-funding" plan in America, though these local authorities were also paid by the Ministry of Health. His advisors noted gloomily that, as usual, the existence of the treatment seemed to increase the incidence of even an old and familiar disease. The minister's civil servants were relieved when expert advice indicated that only 10 percent of new end-stage renal failure cases would be suitable for treatment.[26]

Hepatitis Appears

By the mid-1960s, the first ominous cases of hepatitis B appeared in the new renal units, and soon the disease appeared in endemic and epidemic form in the units. Medical and nursing staff dealing with dialysis patients were also affected, and many of the nephrologists and pioneer transplanters, including Roy Calne in London, Thomas Starzl in Denver, John Najarian in Minneapolis, Allan Birch in Boston, and Georges Mathé in Paris, had a brush with this disease. In some units, there were patient and staff deaths from the disease, among them Starzl's chief research technician in Colorado. In Britain, the Edinburgh outbreak claimed eleven lives, including three staff, and it was the worst of twelve outbreaks in Britain.[27] Contact with the renal patients' blood was quickly shown to be responsible.

This viral infection outbreak reached a peak in 1966, and, during this time, there was some hostility shown to the renal units within larger hospitals and at administrative levels. Britain's chief medical officer, keen to contain the funding going to regular dialysis, cynically wrote that if the hepatitis outbreak continued, they would not need to stop priming the pump; it would stop itself.[28] The cases continued, but in less dramatic outbreaks, and the appearance of the initially expensive hepatitis B vaccine, developed in Edinburgh, resolved the clinical and professional difficulty. There was at first an interesting ethical mini-debate on who should get the expensive vaccine. Its use virtually eliminated the epidemic aspect of the disease.

Professional Attitudes

Regular dialysis treatment also changed professional attitudes and relationships. Practitioners of "modern uremia therapy" were at odds again with the senior nephrologists of the "salt and water school" who had earlier lost the debate on the value of the emergency dialysis treatment of acute renal failure. To the traditionalists, the empiricism and monotony of regular dialysis was an additional intellectual affront, and when hepatitis appeared, the expensive units were additionally viewed as dangerous and it was privately considered by some to be a fitting nemesis for the dialyzers' hubris. The University of Minnesota School of Medicine declined to house a new regional dialysis center, and, in Boston, staff left the prestigious Brigham Hospital to set up a freestanding dialysis service. Eli Friedman, one of America's first nephrologists and an early proponent of regular dialysis, recalled that "New York's medical establishment was resistant to acceptance of maintenance hemodialysis as legitimate. . . . Columbia University, New York Hospital, New York Medical College and New York University virtually excluded modern uremia therapy as important components of their Department of Medicine. For at least a decade, the [dialysis] team at New York Hospital were denied faculty appointments in the Department of Medicine."[29]

Younger staff at these conservative New York academic institutions often encountered patients suitable for regular dialysis and diverted any such deserving cases to Friedman's unit at Downstate Medical Center in Brooklyn. In London, at St. George's Hospital, senior staff were similarly hostile, and junior staff spirited away doomed patients to the new dialysis units in nearby hospitals.

Immunology in the Early 1960s

This period of progress in clinical transplantation and the emergence of regular dialysis also coincided with an equally distinguished growth spurt in immunology in general and transplantation immunology in particular. The roles of the thymus and bursa were recognized, as were the two kinds of lymphocyte, and when it was found that the lymphocyte could be made to perform in vitro, immunology shifted increasingly away from "whole animal" studies to a reductionist approach.[30] Thereafter, this previously poorly regarded cell attracted wide attention, and outside the immunology field it was increasingly used as a model for understanding the fundamental biology of the cell, particularly the cell membrane.[31]

Fundamental Advances—Mitogens

Methods of studying, storing, and handling the lymphocyte had been improving as a result of the emergence of better culture media and successful long-term storage. But the revelation that the lymphocyte could be activated in vitro encouraged studies of the formerly enigmatic cell. The potential of the lymphocyte to expand into an active "blast" form outside the body was discovered accidentally by Peter C. Nowell in Philadelphia in 1960. He was looking at methods of separating lymphocytes from red cells in a density gradient, and, studying the cells two days later, instead of immediately, he noticed that the lymphocytes had

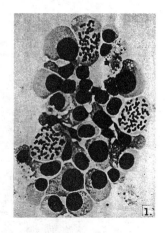

Peter Nowell noted cell division and large mononuclear cells in four-day cultures of lymphocytes after phytohemagglutinin was added. From P. C. Nowell, "Phytohemagglutinin: An Initiator of Mitoses in Cultures of Normal Human Leucocytes," *Cancer Research* 20 (1960): 462–66.

transformed into large, pre-mitotic lymphoblast forms. Analysis showed that the stimulant proved to be the agent used to clump the red cells—the plant lectin phytohemagglutinin, obtained from the bean *Phaseolus vulgaris*.[32]

Events moved quickly when the same effect could be shown when lymphocytes taken from tuberculin-positive humans were exposed to tuberculin in vitro. This revealed the potential of the cell to react outside the body to specific antigens. This discovery led to a huge array of tests of lymphocyte function. Further research showed that, after stimulation of these cells, the culture fluid was found to have soluble factors of interest, the first being MIF (migration inhibition factor), noted in 1961. This factor prevented out-migration of macrophages, which measured the intensity of cell-mediated immunity (still called "delayed hypersensitivity" at the time).[33] Many important similar "lymphokines" were to be identified later.

A further triumph in the study of the lymphocyte in culture came in 1964, when Fritz Bach and Barbara Bain in New York managed to obtain lymphoblast transformation in vitro when mixing cells of different individuals, mimicking the host response to a graft. This method was soon used in the first tests of human compatibility in relation to transplantation, as described later.[34]

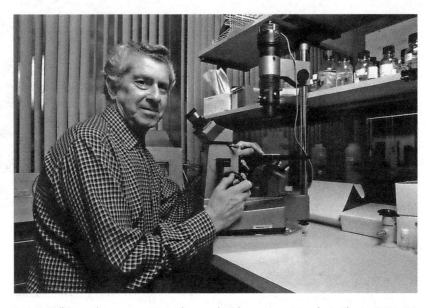

Jacques Miller's work on an experimental mouse lymphoma virus at London's Chester Beatty Research Institute led in 1960 to the demonstration of the immunological functions of the thymus gland. Image courtesy of Jacques Miller.

Thymus Function

In 1961, researchers had a major insight into immunological function when they discovered that the thymus gland, often regarded, in spite of its size, as inactive or vestigial, instead had a central role in immunological responses. Generations of anatomists, with one exception, had studied the thymus and its cells without profit, and generations of experimentalists had removed the thymus gland from a huge range of species without apparent detriment to the animal. Humoralist explanations came from some who claimed that extracts of the thymus had potencies of various kinds or even that the thymus was an endocrine gland whose unknown product was "something to do with growth."

Another episode of classical serendipity also occurred in 1961, when Jacques F. A. P. Miller (born 1931) discovered that removal of the thymus gland from mice at birth would eliminate cell-mediated immunity. Miller had been working at the Chester Beatty Research Institute in London on an experimental mouse lymphoma virus that replicated first in the thymus, and he was doing earlier and earlier thymectomies. After mastering the tricky technique of thymectomy on the animal's first day of life, a period not considered important, he noticed that the animals deprived of the thymus lacked vitality later. He then found that these mice did not reject skin grafts.[35] Rapid confirmation, analysis, and extension of the discovery followed, and the once mysterious thymus was quickly elevated to the position of central controller of cell-mediated immune mechanisms. It emerged that Robert Good (1922–2003) had done similar experiments, and a lasting, unresolved dispute over priority arose.[36]

The Bursa's Role

To add to these insights on thymus function, researchers realized that years earlier, Bruce Glick (1927–2009), working at Ohio State University, had already filled in the other half of the immunological puzzle. As the result of yet another serendipitous event in 1956, he had shown that early removal of the chicken's bursa of Fabricius, the pelvic cloacal lymphoid organ, could prevent antibody formation.[37] The journal *Science* had rejected the paper "as lacking general interest," and instead it was humbly published in the small circulation niche journal *Poultry Science*. When the study was ultimately pointed out to Robert Good, he and others realized that a new, simpler understanding of the immunological system was emerging—that the thymus controlled cell-mediated immunity and that the bursa or its equivalent controlled antibody formation.

This understanding also offered insights into the various human immunological disorders, notably the so-called "experiments of nature," that is, the defects responsible for some congenital human immunological diseases.[38] Some patients had defects of cellular immunity, and some had poor antibody production.[39] But there seemed to be overlap. The remaining puzzle was resolved in 1966, when, in yet another serendipitous event, one cheerfully acknowledged, Henry Claman found that, while a limited range of antibodies could be made in animals deprived of their thymus, if thymus cells were added, they would "help" these animals with only bursa-derived cells make the other antibodies.[40] The two types of cells were christened T (thymus-derived) and B (bursa-derived) by Ivan Roitt in 1969. By 1969, Martin Raff had demonstrated the presence of a surface marker on mouse T-cells that made them identifiable in tissues and organs, and the dynamics of the T- and B-cells were soon displayed.[41] Numerous subsets of the T- and B-lymphocyte were also described. Robert Good recalled the achievement of the period: "All of the experimental research of at least two decades fell clearly and agreeably into alignment. The scientific meetings at which these findings were presented and discussed were filled with joy, excitement and anticipation."[42] There was even one authenticated "Eureka" incident, when the pediatrician Angelo DiGeorge (1921–2009), while listening to a presentation on the thymus at a conference in 1965, realized its significance to one of his patients. Hurrying to the microphone, he announced that his puzzling patient must have absence of the thymus, thus correctly identifying the congenital deficiency and achieving eponymous fame as the discoverer of DiGeorge syndrome.[43]

Laboratory-Clinic Linkage

Assessing the role these important immunological discoveries played in advancing clinical organ transplantation in the 1960s (indeed, the role of basic transplantation science at any time) is of interest. In the mid-1950s, clinicians had looked for help from the laboratory, and the advice and guidance from distinguished scientists on using tolerance and radiation chimeras offered a way forward. Using these laboratory strategies, surgeons embarked on human kidney transplant attempts in the late 1950s. In the 1960s, the new understanding of the role of the thymus, and the rapid rise in methods of study of lymphocyte activity, might suggest that these laboratory insights also assisted the rise of clinical organ transplantation at this time.

But a one-way enlightenment model does not fit the events of the 1960s. Instead, it was the surgeons' new use of azathioprine, borrowed from oncology, plus widely available steroids that constituted the first successful immunosuppressive regimen in clinical organ transplantation. Moreover, many novel findings can be credited to the clinical observations of the pioneer surgeons—the reversible rejection crises, the blood typing effect, graft adaptation, and even the occasional inexplicably successful graft, which hinted at favorable immunological factors unknown from experimental work. This growing success with human kidney transplantation, and the way it was achieved, came as a surprise to many scientists. Paul Terasaki recalled that "large numbers of live-related kidney transplants were performed in rapid succession . . . and took the scientific community by surprise, for the scientific background for such a monumental step simply had not been laid."[44]

Some scientists were still critical that the clinicians had moved forward with transplantation without the "homograft problem" first being solved in the laboratory. With immunology advancing rapidly in the early 1960s, researchers believed that they might soon be able to offer new tools for use by the impatient surgeons. Their focus was generally on their hope for obtaining tolerance methods that would be applicable in clinical transplantation; this was the leitmotif of the immunologists. The scientists also loftily criticized the lack of any sophisticated immunological studies or monitoring by surgeons during the early efforts with kidney transplants. "Measurements are at the heart of good science," the scientists reminded the surgeons.[45]

Although there were these critics about, the surgeons and scientists continued to seek and foster professional and personal links. Medawar in particular was not critical of the surgeons' bold actions. His earlier involvement in clinical work in Glasgow and his own preference for whole-animal surgical models made him an honorary and honored member of the surgical world. He generously conceded "that the success of renal homografts in clinical practice, however meager it may yet be, is very much greater than people working in laboratories had dared to hope."[46]

Surgical empiricism was defended from within. Keith Reemstma, the Tulane University transplant surgeon, added a wry analysis of the timeless resistance to clinical innovation: "I do not doubt that the first cave man who trepanned a skull was assailed for trying an unproved operation, for proceeding without conclusive animal experiments, for forsaking the medical regimen of powdered owl feathers, for getting too much publicity, for siphoning off public funds for his work and denying support to the tiger tooth necklace project, for interfering in the plans of the Great Spirit, and of course, prolonging the lives of the unfit individuals and thereby placing in jeopardy the future of the Cro-Magnon race."[47]

Joseph Murray also gave a stout advocacy of this clinical empiricism in his welcome to those gathered for the NRC conference in Washington in September 1963: "The clinician is eager to grasp at any potential technique and may apply hypotheses prematurely. While the non-clinical investigator may be useful as a curb to rash clinical action, he also may retard clinical progress by overly rigid experimental restrictions. . . . Clinicians will never succeed in organ transplantation if they wait for the solution of problems derived from lower animals to be extrapolated to man. There are even variations of immunological patterns between different strains of the same species. . . . No test system has universal applicability."[48]

Joseph Murray's view of the limitations of animal models is of interest. Mice are not sensitive to steroids, unlike guinea pigs, and dogs are hypersensitive to this agent. Irradiation in dogs has little effect as an immunosuppressant and has a narrow band of usefulness, but radiation proved effective in supporting transplantation in rabbits, mice, and humans. Guinea pigs show significant "delayed hypersensitivity" reactions, but rats do not; graft-versus-host reactions vary by species, and some mice show an "alternative path" sensitization. Animals that are not inbred, humans being a prime example, are difficult to tolerize, but inbred lines of laboratory animals can present numerous anomalies and oddities, including spontaneous acceptance of organ homografts. Liver transplantation in pigs proved to make such animals tolerant to future kidney grafts, and though dogs need a venous shunt during liver replacement, humans fortunately do not. Later, cyclosporine proved to be toxic to human kidneys, a result not seen in preliminary animal testing.

Surgeons and scientists, though separated by differing traditions and agendas, had considerable personal and organizational links at a number of levels—local, national, and international. Other influences, too subtle to appear in the scientific papers of the time, were at work. It was a unique experience for surgeons to be associated so closely with a highly sophisticated branch of fundamental biology, one that was staffed by scientists of eminence. There was always the hope that a new solution might emerge from the vitality of basic research, and each of the new immunological insights of the 1960s and the steady stream of new immunological tests, watched with awe, seemed to give new hope for the addition of further tools.

On their side, scientists also desired to maintain links with the clinicians. The 1960s were a time when governments, medical research organizations, and charities looked toward support of applied research of practical worth, seeking Baconian innovations "of use as well as light." The grand surgical endeavor of transplantation was beginning to show results, and the related basic science could easily be shown to be supportable on grounds of utility. The transplantation immunologists, when seeking funds, were understandably keen to demonstrate that they were engaged in a joint effort with the clinic toward a desirable goal. It was not necessary to mention that the transplant-related biological mechanisms, the study of which required funding, were of more fundamental significance than simply causing organ graft rejection. Basic research served both agendas.[49]

New Pills

One source of innovation, dominant in other clinical endeavors, was notably absent from the world of clinical transplantation in the mid-1960s. Transplant surgeons at this time were not looking to the pharmaceutical industry for new products, and none were offered. Pharmaceutical companies still considered the market for immunosuppressive drugs to be too small for a major investment in research and development. Transplanters and laboratory scientists were on their own and expected to develop their own immunosuppressive methods from their base in unworldly academia. Thus far, their choices had ranged from the sophisticated solution offered by tolerance induction to the use of familiar, economical medications already on the shelf. The transplanters still assumed that future pharmacological solutions would come from their own efforts.

But the successful combination of azathioprine and steroids that had emerged in 1963 was not quickly improved upon, and the results were leveling off by the mid-1960s. There was also disappointment at the failures with other organs and with the xenograft attempts. At this time, two developments showed promise for rapid progress anew. One was maturation of useful tissue-typing methods and the resulting promise of helpful matching. The second was the emergence of a new powerful biological immunosuppressant—antilymphocyte serum. And it came from a surgical research laboratory.

15 Progress in the Mid-1960s

THE TECHNICAL SIDE of kidney transplantation was now well established, and there was growing confidence with the surgical management. Policy shifted to encourage the use of cadaveric organs, thus removing the concerns associated with living-related donation. The only source of kidneys for transplantation so far had been from patients dying in those hospitals interested in transplantation, but as the results improved, more doctors and more hospitals were prepared to consider helping with donation.

Experience with both living and cadaveric grafts yielded one very important observation about the comparative results. Although cadaver grafts could do well, living-related kidney donation within the family provided better overall results than did cadaver kidneys. The freshness of the donor organ from a living relative and the less hurried aspect of the dual operation contributed to the more positive results, but the beneficial effect of a family donation was clearly due to favorable genetic factors.

This finding encouraged the use of tests for human tissue compatibility, the hope being to improve the results of cadaveric transplantation, and by matching, bring the results up to the level of living donor grafts. Few patients might have a fully matched sibling donor, but all might get a fully matched cadaver donor kidney. Testing would also assist in choosing a donor within the family. The occasional excellent cadaveric graft outcome without use of matching raised hopes that the genetic system controlling human transplantation might not show much complexity. This was not to be the case.[1]

Tissue Individuality

In Karl Landsteiner's broad-ranging analysis, included in his Nobel Prize lecture of 1931, he predicted that serological methods, akin to blood typing, would eventually aid tissue grafting.[2] But the failure of blood type match-

314

ing to influence human skin graft outcome, noted in the 1930s, may have suggested that seeking further tests of tissue matching might be futile. Landsteiner himself turned away from the study of blood types and moved instead in the 1920s into reductionist realms, finding that the study of the chemistry of antigen and antibody interaction was more inviting.

The first investigations of tissue compatibility were by Peter Gorer and George Snell, as described earlier, and these studies in mice developed steadily and inconspicuously from the 1940s and were mature by the 1950s. But similar methods for detecting human transplant antigens did not emerge until the mid-1960s. Prior to that time, the surgical pioneers had for a while been casting about for some method of judging closeness of human identity, an important matter when live donors were being considered. These interim "whole person" methods, now forgotten, deserve a review.

Early Matching Methods

The first tissue-matching strategies were various cumbersome forms of direct testing in vivo. Only live donors and their prospective recipients could be studied in this way, the goal being to choose the best donor within a willing family. Three main approaches emerged, and all three simply judged the recipient's reaction to the future donor's tissues.[3] These ingenious methods not only revealed genetic differences but also gave a useful estimate of host reactivity, later largely ignored, which was known to be variable in chronic renal failure patients. A low-reactivity patient could have a good result even with a poorly matched kidney.

The first tissue-matching method was the most direct one: grafting skin from the donor or donors to the recipient and noting the survival times, thus estimating outcome. London's Hammersmith Hospital surgeons described this "prelusive" skin grafting, and they used this method to study forty-three patients prior to transplantation, giving small doses of azathioprine to the patient to delay the pace of rejection and thus assist quantification. The method seemed of value when a choice of donor was available.[4]

A further approach to testing came from Peter Medawar's group: their "normal lymphocyte transfer test," which they studied in outbred guinea pigs.[5] Lymphocytes from one animal were injected into the skin of another. The reaction taking place within a few days was shown to be a brief graft-versus-host reaction; a host-versus-graft component followed some days later, and it could be quantified. This method was used by Paul Russell at Boston's Massachusetts General Hospital prior to twelve human kidney transplants. A variant was J. Wayne Streilein's "irradiated hamster test" in which lymphocytes from the human donor and recipient were mixed and injected subcutaneously into hamsters made nonreactive by irradiation. A visible two-way reaction, which could also be measured, occurred, and this method also showed promise. The third suggestion, coming from Felix Rapaport (1929–2001), was the "third man test" in which a normal volunteer was grafted with skin from the proposed recipient of a kidney graft. The sensitized volunteer was then grafted with skin from all possible family donors, looking for the accelerated rejection indicating that the recipient and donor shared the same antigens. Studies at Boston using the same approach were carried out in normal human volunteers, but preliminary sensitization was by lymphocytes, rather than skin, followed by skin grafting from possible donors.[6]

These methods, though reasoned and well intentioned, had a number of defects, scientific and ethical. Skin grafts from a human donor to recipient might sensitize the patient to a future kidney graft from this or other donors and accelerate rejection. Another problem was the later realization that any transfer of cells and tissue between recipients and donors or, worse still, third parties, might not only sensitize the patient but also transfer disease, notably hepatitis B, then on the increase in dialysis units.

Testing for these indicators of compatibility was slow relative to the urgent pace of cadaveric transplantation; such methods were also not easily employed for "typing" the increasing numbers of patients kept alive on regular dialysis while waiting for a cadaveric transplant. The routine use of such direct tests of compatibility for intrafamily grafting, after a short period of experimental popularity, was overtaken in the mid-1960s by the rise of serological tissue-typing methods that had been slowly developing over fifteen years.

Jean Dausset in Paris

The first understanding of the human histocompatibility system can be dated to 1952 and Jean Dausset's pioneering work, for which he was later awarded a Nobel Prize. A number of clinical hematologists entered this new field of tissue typing, becoming the latest discipline to join the developing, patchwork structure of transplantation immunology.[7]

In 1952, Dausset (1916–2009) studied a curious antibody in the blood of a patient with aplastic anemia who had required multiple transfusions. This antibody could destroy white blood cells taken from some but not all healthy people.[8] Dausset explained his observation by invoking other mechanisms known at the time, concluding that an auto-antibody was damaging the patient's own cells.[9] In other cases, a similar antibody appeared, with the autoimmune explanation being awkwardly applied to the data. Dausset soon accepted the need for a paradigm shift and concluded that the antibody was acquired from the white blood cells in the

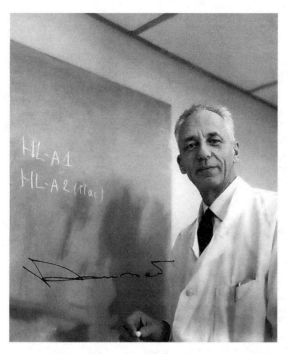

Jean Dausset, pioneer of tissue-typing methods, described the first human tissue "group" in 1958. In 1983, he shared a Nobel Prize with Baruj Benacerraf and George Snell. Image courtesy of Jean Dausset.

many blood transfusions these patients received. His most potent white cell antibody was tested on a variety of cells, and using the initials of those donating cells destroyed by the serum, in 1954 the shared tissue antigen thus identified was called "MAC."[10]

Three years later, Rose Payne (1909–1999), a California hematologist, came to similar conclusions. She had also found these antibodies in multiply transfused patients and noted that patients who had had a febrile episode at the time of blood transfusion but who showed no evidence of destruction of red cells were those who later had the interesting antibodies, having reacted to the transfused white cells.[11] She extended Dausset's analysis when she noted that women had such antibodies more often than did men, and she then realized that previous pregnancies were responsible. Independently, Jon van Rood (born 1926) in the Netherlands had also found that women who had been pregnant often had antibodies directed against their baby's cells.[12] The survival of the baby in the presence of apparently damaging antibodies during pregnancies deepened the mystery of the role of the antibody and revived the view that the fetus was indeed a graft and one mysteriously surviving in spite of a reaction against it.

These hematologists knew of the comparable but more advanced studies by Gorer and Snell on mouse red cell antigens, and thus these new human tissue typers had many leads to follow.[13] But at this time in the late 1950s, organ transplantation was not an active topic; any human studies were not of immediate value, and they thus appeared only very slowly. Only by the mid-1960s was there a need for methodology to use in testing humans for transplantation. In a surprise development, human matching promptly uncovered human genetic susceptibility to some diseases, a scientific adventure that continues.[14]

Typing Methods

The tissue typers initially used a fickle agglutination test to look for clumping of white cells. Serum samples from multiply transfused patients were studied first and inevitably gave wide reactions, but van Rood managed, first with data punched on machine-readable Hollerith cards and then with a computer analysis, to sort out these patterns.[15] There was temporary enthusiasm for obtaining more specific sera by injecting white cells into human volunteers, a strategy abandoned after concerns, ethical and practical, were raised. Sera from multiparous women proved to be more specific, and more persistent, and later some helpful post–kidney transplant antibodies were also available. High-quality specific sera were sought, greatly prized, and shared among the pioneer labs. There were hopes that the tissue types might not be much more complex than the blood types. This was not the case.

Matching and Graft Survival

In Paris, Jean Dausset worked at the Hôpital Necker, where Jean Hamburger's transplant team in the early 1960s had begun using low-dose radiation immunosuppression. In 1962, Dausset used his early tissue-typing sera for the first time to assess the likelihood of success when there was a choice of donor for a proposed living-donor kidney transplant. A first cousin of the patient had volunteered, and the simple testing of the time showed that the cousins shared antigens. This matching effort yielded a successful transplant outcome.

But studies to establish any general benefit of typing faced difficulties in the early 1960s. The number of kidney transplants being attempted was small. Storage of white cells for later analysis was not yet routine, and factors other than rejection had a major influence on the outcome. Deaths from infection complicated any effect of tissue matching, yet there were high hopes that tissue matching could play a dominant role in transplant successes. Since kidney transplantation seemed unlikely to provide the vital data in the near future, some scientists again turned to experimental skin grafting for the answer.

Felix Rapaport had continued the skin homografting research work started in the 1940s by Blair Rogers and other research-minded plastic surgeons in New York. From 1956 Rapaport had been carrying out experimental skin grafts on volunteers sought among the blood donors at his hospital, and he used microscopy of the blood vessels in the graft, rather than inspection, to give a better assessment of the rapid rejection found in normal humans. Anxious to confirm Medawar's acquired immunity theory, he transferred second grafts from the same donors, and these new sets of tissue could show a "second set" or "white graft" response with a reduced survival time. When using a second graft from a different donor, he sometimes found a rapid, second set response. This testing offered a way of revealing any shared antigens.[16]

When Dausset encountered the French-speaking Rapaport at a meeting in 1962, they decided to merge their skills.[17] Rapaport had the human surgical test system and Dausset had an increasingly sophisticated bank of sera to type Rapaport's volunteers. The New York surgical team's ambitious series of human skin graft experiments, eventually totaling nine hundred, extended from 1963 to 1977. These grafts were carried out in New York at first, but, when concerns about human experimentation emerged in America, the surgical work moved to Paris, resuming at Dausset's laboratory.[18] The considerable expense of the work was met by a New York philanthropist. Other groups, led by van Rood, Ruggero Ceppellini, and Richard Batchelor, also started human skin grafting to investigate the role of tissue typing, but demonstrating the expected link with graft outcome was proving difficult. Nevertheless, the researchers agreed that these studies were the way forward, and, in 1960, when scientist Paul Terasaki wished to start tissue typing, he was advised to "get into skin grafting, that's where the action is"—advice he did not take—and instead kidney transplants for him to study soon emerged locally at UCLA.

Tissue Typing and Kidney Transplantation

Terasaki, who was to be a dominant force in this tissue-typing endeavor thereafter, had started work in William Longmire's transplant-oriented surgical department at UCLA, and his talents were soon recognized. In 1958, Longmire encouraged Terasaki to go to Medawar's laboratory in London for a period of study.[19] Members of Medawar's group were by then prominent converts to, and notable advocates of, the primacy of cellular rejection mechanisms. However, they did not discourage Terasaki from taking up the unfashionable study of the transplantation antibodies, particularly since Gorer's nearby laboratory had at last demonstrated the presence of such antibodies after mouse skin graft rejection.[20] Terasaki met with Bernard Amos (1923–2003) and Edward Boyse (1923–2007), in Gorer's group, who were devising better methods for detecting such mouse antibodies. Terasaki visited Paris at this time and saw Dausset's work on human tissue typing.

On his return to Los Angeles, Terasaki worked toward improved human typing methods, and after unsatisfactory experience with traditional tests, he improved on Gorer's dye exclusion method.[21] By 1964, Terasaki had gathered from a number of centers early data on the role of typing in human kidney transplant outcomes. He was not a hematologist nor was he involved in the blood transfusion service, so he initially had limited access to sera. The immunosuppressed kidney transplant recipients were awkward to study, since their blood lymphocyte levels were low. Terasaki then successfully developed a micro-method of his test in 1964, largely through necessity. Using plates with tiny wells instead of the usual test tubes, Terasaki could conserve cells, sera, and reagents, and the plates were read with an inverting microscope using a coating of oil to prevent drying of the reagents. Terasaki made these plates plus sera available to other interested laboratories, and his work soon garnered substantial support from the transplantation funds of the National Institute of Allergy and Infectious Diseases in the United States. His method soon became the worldwide standard.[22]

Gorer died in London in 1961, and his pupils Edward Boyse and Bernard Amos moved to the United States, where they established important tissue-typing laboratories. Richard Batchelor was now unexpectedly in charge of Gorer's laboratory, and he successfully moved the unit's interest from the mouse to human studies, just as kidney transplantation was starting in Britain.

Retrospective Transplant Assessment

The first assessments of the role of tissue typing in organ transplantation were carried out by studying the early cases in the scattered kidney transplant centers. The expected difficulties soon arose. No stored cells existed, which meant that none had survived from any earlier cadaveric donor. Also, since no patients had returned to dialysis after loss of a kidney graft, no idea of their match could be obtained. The only patient/donor pairs for which cells were available for study were those who had successfully been transplanted with a living donor's kidney. Since graft failures could not be studied, the project was inevitably biased.

However, these retrospective studies provided some useful data to occupy researchers while they waited for data from a reasonable number of recent transplants in which tissue typing had been done.[23] Van Rood looked at as many living donor cases as possible at this time, pooling the data from Boston, Denver, Edinburgh, Brussels (Charles Toussait's cases), Louvain (Guy Alexandre's cases), and Minneapolis (William Kelly's cases), and the analysis did provide the hoped-for evidence of better kidney survival with better matches.[24] Rapaport and Amos made a study of David Hume's successful family donation cases at Duke University. Tissue typing appeared to relate to successful kidney transplant outcome.[25]

By 1968, a few cadaveric graft outcomes could be studied for the first time, because Ken Porter at St. Mary's Hospital in London, who had published earlier on bone marrow cell storage, had introduced systematic retention of donor lymphocytes, particularly from cadaveric donors, using the new glycerol preservation methods.[26] Porter had the first collection of this kind, and van Rood made early retrospective use of the St. Mary's stored material for the first "prospective" (though retrospective) investigation of cadaveric graft outcome, and the analysis was again favorable.[27]

Prospective Studies

Typing and outcome data for transplants involving cadaveric donation slowly emerged. Good correlation was reported in separate studies by Terasaki, Peter Morris, van Rood, and Batchelor. Meanwhile, in Denver, there was a unique situation, since Starzl had embarked on an unusual living-unrelated kidney donor program, using volunteers from among the inmates at Canon State Prison. He tissue-typed the inmate donors to obtain matches for his patients. Of the 108 prisoners that he and Terasaki typed, many had all of the four antigens then identified, and fourteen provided a well-matched kidney. Starzl concluded that by choosing the best match for his patients from among the prisoners, he increased the one-year survival of unrelated kidney transplants from 33 to 55 percent.[28]

There remained, however, the puzzling observations, particularly in cadaveric transplantation, that long-term graft survival could occur in spite of major incompatibility and, conversely, that complete matching did not guarantee success. Further experience in

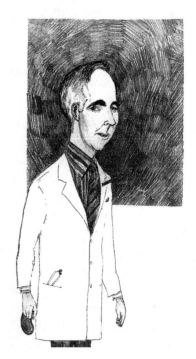

Sir Peter Morris pioneered kidney transplantation in Melbourne and then in Oxford. He reported early on the role of tissue typing, and later, with Alan Ting, he showed the importance of the HLA-D system in human kidney grafting. Sketch by the late E. G. Lee. Image courtesy of Oxford University Transplant Unit.

cadaveric kidney transplantation provided increasing amounts of data, yet the overall tissue-typing influence was still not clear cut and certainly a major, self-evident benefit of typing in cadaveric grafting was not emerging.[29] But typing and matching results were often incomplete, and there was always hope that as the number of newly identified antigens grew or when the importance and different strengths of the various antigens were identified, predictions would be more accurate.

A further hint that there were more antigens to be uncovered came when researchers compared the outcomes of cadaver and living-related kidney grafts that had similar levels of tissue matching. The researchers expected to find no difference in the outcomes, but they found instead that the living-related graft survival was clearly better than that of the apparently similarly matched cadaveric kidneys. This result meant there were missing antigens and unknown loci, and it was clear where they were inherited en bloc within families nestling close to the loci identified so far. The hopes that close cadaveric matching would quickly eliminate the need for family donation had not been fulfilled. These findings caused the transplant community to hesitate in the late 1960s when it was on the verge of changing policy to reduce the use of living-related donors.

Genetics

Genetic research finally revealed that an individual's four antigens, as detected by serology studies, came from four genes, with two on each copy of the chromosome 6 pair. The two genes were transmitted close together and were called the "haplotype" by Ceppellini in 1967. One haplotype came from the mother and one from the father. In a large family, the offspring could have only four possible combinations of these two haplotype blocks: one quarter would have identical haplotypes, one quarter would have completely mismatched ones, and half would be half matches. The children would always be a half match with a parent. As data on the outcomes of kidney transplantation in these living-related cases emerged, the results very neatly tied in with the three levels of matching. These findings were a remarkable vindication of the much-maligned report by Leo Loeb in the 1930s, when he picked up the same three levels of homograft survival in these proportions in his simple slice graft experiments between siblings in outbred rat families.

Using even the limited range of sera testing available, surgeons could study a family in search of a full match and thus avoid transplanting a completely mismatched kidney. Whether to go ahead with a half match was problematic at this time.

Role of Antibodies

One dimension of this major serological effort provided immediate benefits in human organ grafting and was to be of lasting importance. Peter Morris (born 1934), working in Melbourne, showed that antibodies useful for tissue typing could also result from kidney transplant rejection, and many of these antibodies soon assisted the tissue typers. However, these preexisting antibodies were also soon found to explain why some grafts failed immediately.[30] In 1966, Flemming Kissmeyer-Nielsen in Åarhus, Denmark, reported two cases of immediate graft failure similar to a major blood group mismatch but in which no ABO blood-type mismatch existed, and he identified a preexisting antibody as the cause.[31] Terasaki had also noticed this hazard earlier, and, by 1967, he had collected seven such incidents, of which five were the result of antibodies from previous pregnancies.[32] By 1969, these "positive cross-matches," when identified before transplantation, were clearly shown to risk a hyperacute loss of the kidney, and pretesting for these antibodies soon became not only desirable but obligatory. This cross-match delayed the insertion of a donor kidney, and this extra wait caused difficulties: it increased the pressure to find organ preservation methods.

Typing Workshops

In the early 1960s, the laboratory methods used by the pioneer tissue typers differed greatly, as did the nomenclature. The need to seek uniformity in methods, and to collect data, led to a meeting at Duke University in 1964, another initiative taken by Ernst Eichwald, now chair of the Committee on Transplantation of the National Research Council. Bernard Amos was the local organizer.[33]

This first tissue-typing meeting was not particularly successful, yet it did serve as a hesitant and important start to what was ultimately a successful and remarkable series of cooperative international workshops. Those invited to the Duke University meeting brought their own reagents and sera and attempted to type the same batch of cells with their very disparate methods. However, when Ruggero Ceppellini collected the data, all he could do was to announce the few agreements and play down the many inconsistencies. The Duke meeting at least defined the major questions to be addressed, and those present resolved to meet again in the Netherlands the following year.

When they gathered at Leiden, sixteen teams again used their most interesting sera against the white blood cells or platelets from a panel of forty-five local blood donors. Richard Batchelor recalled:

It has to be remembered that 1965 was several years before the micromethods of Paul Terasaki had been developed and adopted. Virtually all of us were using approximately 10–15 microlitres of sera per test and corresponding amounts of target white cells before reading . . . [The] supernatant was removed by Pasteur pipettes, dye added and mixed and cells transferred for counting. . . . The conclusions were both statistically significant and very exciting. They showed that different labs were able to identify the same antigens in many instances, the extent of polymorphism was large, and that it was imperative to agree on a standard terminology.[34]

The most commonly encountered human leukocyte antigen (later called HLA-2) was Dausset's MAC, also known in these anarchic times as Shulman's P1GrLy, Payne and Bodmer's LA2, Terasaki's "Group 2," and van Rood's 8a. This apparent act of "touching the same elephant" gave justifiable hopes for a grand simplification.

Many problems remained unresolved, and, by the third workshop, in Turin in 1967, the hoped-for uniformity was close. At this meeting, to denote the entire system, the term HL-A was chosen, as a compromise, thus incorporating the terms Hu-1 of Dausset and Bodmer's LA, though later the term was widely believed to mean Human Lymphocyte/Leukocyte Antigens. The hyphen in HL-A was soon dropped, and the two regions within the newly termed HLA were named HLA-A and HLA-B. The whole chromosomal region was later renamed the human Major Histocompatibility Complex (MHC), although this term understandably tended to perpetuate the assumptions that the mechanism's function was primarily concerned with transplantation. From 1965 onward, the National Research Council regularly published the results of the workshop in its Histocompatibility Testing series, and, after each workshop, an expert committee met to agree on the terminology of the growing number of newly found tissue antigens.

Between these meetings there was a regular exchange of useful HLA typing sera, and, as storage methods evolved, cells could also be transported and shared in this way. This international cooperation was remarkable in bringing in all the major investigators, and no major laboratory declined to join the joint enterprise. The international effort mirrored the innovative data sharing by the kidney transplanters.

Sharing Kidneys

In the 1960s, the dream of using tissue typing to produce better outcomes in cadaveric renal transplantation had an inevitable corollary: that, when a cadaver kidney was obtained and typed in one center, the widest possible search should be conducted for the best match among already typed potential recipients. But transporting kidneys took time, and, until the mid-

1960s, time was short. At the 1964 NRC conference in Washington, it was clear that the old antipathy to the flushing and cooling of donor kidneys was fading and there was now a quiet revolution in attitudes toward kidney preservation. Simple cooling was found to prolong organ survival for about six hours—just enough for rapid dispatch to another nearby center.

With more "cold time" thus available, kidney sharing brought many benefits, and formal sharing schemes started to emerge. After blood type matching, the new sharing schemes could provide not only good tissue matches and avoid positive cross-matches but also enable recipients with rarer blood types to receive a donor organ. For patients in urgent need, a scheme could provide a kidney graft quickly from the greater resources of any sharing organization. In addition, the tissue typing provided an objective way of choosing between patients from the pool of those waiting. This absolved and removed the doctors from the difficult choice in judging between the patients waiting for a kidney, and it preempted any allegations of allocation bias by local doctors. But this scheme rested in its entirety on the assumption that tissue typing mattered in routine cases.

The sharing schemes also meant that considerable amounts of data could be collected, which raised hopes for resolving the controversy over the role of tissue typing, since clinical data on outcomes were sent back to the typing labs. This abundance of data also encouraged analysis of other factors of influence, notably the efficacy of preservation of organs, the role of original disease, age, previous blood transfusions, and much else.

Sharing Schemes

The first sharing schemes were local, informal cooperatives in the small number of major cities with pioneer transplant units. Paul Terasaki started an organ-sharing group in Los Angeles in 1967, and this group, which had an innovative donor procurement team who traveled and served a wide region, reported its first audit in early 1969.[35] The Northern California Transplant Bank and the Boston Interhospital Organ Bank both started in 1968. In 1969, Bernard Amos and David Hume at Duke University provided a tissue-typing service and organized a major sharing scheme for their region. The Southeastern Organ Procurement Foundation initially worked with eight Virginia hospitals, plus the university hospitals at Duke, Emory, Johns Hopkins, and the Medical College of Virginia. In 1975, this group expanded, and, when incorporated as a foundation, it took initiatives to encourage donation in all hospitals in the area. The success of the scheme led to an extension of its service area. The Richmond scheme later served as the template for the national UNOS organization—the United Network for Organ Sharing—and Richmond was chosen as the UNOS headquarters.

In Paris, two hospitals had been involved in kidney transplantation from the outset. In 1967, René Küss and Jacques Poisson organized Paris Transplant, and the city started sharing kidneys, and other organs later, based initially on blood group matching, then on tissue typing. The Paris group kept a degree of independence thereafter, but after joining the Rhône-Méditerranée scheme in 1969, the enlarged organization was renamed France Transplant. In 1967, van Rood, in the Netherlands, suggested amalgamating kidney-sharing organizations in his part of Europe, in order to obtain the best tissue match in an extended geographical area. The result was the Eurotransplant organization, which initially included patients in the Netherlands, Belgium, and northwestern Germany and later covered an even wider area. It was the first scheme to have a sufficiently large number of patients on the waiting list to obtain the optimally close HLA matching. Similar large sharing schemes soon evolved elsewhere, notably Scandiatransplant, which, by the mid-1970s, had seven hundred patients awaiting transplants. In Britain, informal sharing was run from the London Hospital, starting in 1969; in February 1972, the Department of Health and Social Security established the National Organ Matching and Distribution Service (NOMDS) at Bristol, after the National Tissue Typing Reference Laboratory was established there in 1969. It was renamed the United Kingdom Transplant Service (UKTS), later shortened to UKT, and served Ireland as well.[36]

Speedy Sharing

For the sharing and transporting of kidneys, the major constraint was still the limited time available after donation and before transplantation of the organ. Most kidneys had been used locally until the late 1960s, and a 1968 survey by the National Kidney Registry in the United States reported that most transplants were under way between two and four hours after donation—an astonishing figure. This meant that, after doctors removed a donated organ, they still turned first to renal failure patients then in the same hospital, and preparation of such patients for surgery and anesthesia would not be ideal. By the late 1960s, more time was available and the chosen recipient could be summoned from home. The maximum of six hours of "cold time" allowed more distant sharing of kidneys, and rapid communication and speedy transport of the organ meant regular success in long-distance donation and transplantation. In the Netherlands, an army helicopter was placed at van Rood's disposal for Eurotransplant work, and other countries provided similar assistance. Although difficult to believe now, the highly desired fully matched kidneys were flown between European nations and implanted within six hours. The internal British sharing scheme used police transport or the St. John Air Ambulance Wing, an organization set up by volunteer pilots in 1972, and both had free use of landing facilities at military airfields, where police escort cars met each flight. These early "mercy flights" captured the public's imagination, and the movement of organs proved newsworthy, though the flights were risky. Later, when surgical teams flew out to distant hospitals for donations, they had some brushes with death.[37]

Organ Perfusion and Preservation

As described earlier, physiologists had been keen to study perfusion of isolated organs to unravel some features of their function. The workable "heart-lung" machines of the 1880s had provided stable short-term survival to allow useful metabolic studies, and the first report of perfusion of the kidney was in 1915, by Alfred Newton Richards and O. H. Plant at the University of Pennsylvania. Later, in the 1930s, as described earlier, Alexis Carrel, supported by Charles

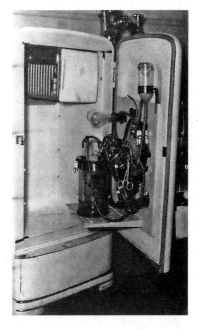

In 1960, Soviet surgeon Anastasy Lapchinsky described his machine for cold perfusion of organs for transplantation in a paper presented at the meeting of the New York Academy of Sciences. From *Annals of the New York Academy of Sciences* 87 (1960): 541.

Lindbergh's engineering skills, reported development of a closed, sterile perfusion device and had apparent success, claiming thirty days of survival of the thyroid gland but not the kidney.[38] The matter was put aside, but, with the new success of organ transplantation in the 1960s and the need to transport organs to obtain the best match in the sharing schemes, attention naturally turned again to attaining longer-term preservation by perfusion.[39]

Perfusion Reemerges

In the mid-1960s, the revived Carrel continuous perfusion approach seemed to offer the most promise for obtaining the long periods of preservation needed for widespread organ sharing. If the donated organ could be preserved for a period of time, the medical team would have more time for careful cross-matching and tissue typing and for summoning and preparing recipients for surgery. Moreover, perfusion using a pump, rather than simply holding the cooled kidney in a storage container, was thought initially to be more "natural." It was also hoped that organs damaged prior to removal would benefit from this perfusion period, which also gave the medical team time to assess the kidney for damage. In 1961, Francis Moore in Boston proposed a simple glucose oxidation isotope test to judge the vitality of a donated organ. Other methods followed and offered hopes of excluding organs that might already be irreversibly damaged at the time of donation and thus have poor or absent function when transplanted. No single test found wide acceptance, however.[40] Increasing the period between organ retrieval and transplantation also meant that there might be time to apply tolerance induction schemes which might emerge, still a goal hoped for by some.

The leader in this area of kidney preservation was Folkert O. Belzer (1930–1995), and, starting in the Department of Surgery in the University of California Medical Center at San Francisco, he patiently studied all promising leads that appeared over decades.[41] His evolving designs of perfusion machines were widely adopted and were manufactured commercially.[42] His early pumps used perfusion with a plasma-based solution and pulsating flow, again mimicking the natural process, also a temporary trend in the design of cardiac surgery bypass pumps at the time. To these kidney perfusion machines was added the other surgical fashion of the day: high-pressure oxygenation of the perfusion fluid.[43]

Considerable research effort went into such work. By 1967, Belzer's approach had achieved seventy-two-hour preservation of dog kidneys.[44] Mobile perfusion teams, traveling in vans with the perfusion apparatus, were impressive in action and captured the public imagination. Particularly newsworthy was any international transfer of a kidney, and the moving of a machine plus kidney from San Francisco to Leiden on Christmas Day in 1971 was a major story. Denver surgeon Larry Brettschneider, who devised an improved perfusion machine in Starzl's department, had a remarkable, brief professional lionization.[45] In Denmark, Kissmeyer-Nielsen, the tissue typer, was becoming a well-known public figure and announced that worldwide sharing was the goal and with complete matching would result in 100 percent graft survival.

Intracellular Fluids

In 1966, a British group working in Newcastle reported that a new fluid based on *intracellular* electrolyte levels (high potassium and low sodium), rather than the high sodium and low potassium of blood, offered better preservation for cooled organs.[46] This approach was another borrowing from the world of cardiac surgery; in 1955, Denis Melrose had shown that potassium-rich solutions not only arrested the heart and eased the surgeon's task but also protected the heart.[47]

Research revealed that, for organ transplants, a simple flush with this type of potassium-rich fluid, followed by chilled storage, offered better tissue preservation than had previous perfusion methods. Lars-Erik Gelin in Sweden and Geoffrey Collins, in Terasaki's laboratory, took this idea further.[48] By 1969, Collins had produced an improved "intracellular" preservative solution, with little extras like magnesium, glucose, mannitol, phenoxybenzamine, procaine, and heparin.[49] The success of the intracellular fluids signaled the decline in the widespread use of the perfusion machines, but not without controversy. Terasaki recalled that "pulsatile perfusion was so well entrenched that very few surgeons were willing to consider a method as primitive as cold storage. The objection in the Los Angeles area was that our little cardboard box with ice would be offensive to the operating room personnel who were accustomed to the Belzer ambulance with its impressive machine, paraphernalia and perfusion technologists. . . . In our desperation to have the cold storage method accepted, dog kidneys were sent by ordinary air freight to Dr. Collins who went round the world implanting kidneys in London, Tel Aviv and Sydney."[50]

Soon the Collins solution and various derivatives, like the Euro-Collins solution, became standard. Later, the University of Wisconsin solution was a further improvement and was widely used after 1987.[51] The perfusion machines were not forgotten, however, since many believed that they ought to be used. There was renewed interest in the machines later on, after claims that, after all, they revitalized substandard donor organs.

Experimental Grafting, Large and Small

The mid-1960s was a time of increasing confidence with experimental liver and heart transplantation in larger animals, work that steadily paved the way for human grafting. The traditional outbred dog kidney transplant model was still employed to test new strategies in organ transplantation, but in the development of heart and liver grafting, large animals, notably pigs, were increasingly used. As always, experimental work on new species offered surprises. Roy Calne's pig studies, carried out with the assistance of the Agricultural Research Institute of Animal Physiology at Babraham, immediately revealed that outbred pig liver transplants might be surprisingly successful.[52] In addition, these grafts could induce unexpected "tolerance" of a future kidney graft.[53] The resulting familiarity with pig breeding, husbandry, surgery, and genetics had longer term importance because, when human xenograft organ replacement became a possibility in the 1990s, these large pigs, with their human-sized organs, became a more likely source of future human xenografts instead of chimps or baboons.

At the other end of the scale, the development of microvascular surgical methods in the 1960s opened up the study of organ transplants in small laboratory animals. Rat organ transplantation was achieved by joining the tiny vessels, and with a sophisticated immunological understanding of the inbred rat strains already in place, useful insights were possible, and, as ever, there were further surprises.

This new interest in microvascular methods arose in the 1960s, when neurosurgeons began using the operating microscopes already necessary for some ear, nose, and throat procedures.[54] After tiny needles and sutures became available for eye surgery, the first use of these ultrafine sutures in vascular surgery was reported by the neurosurgeon Julius Jacobsen of the University of Vermont, who used 7/0 needles experimentally in 1960 to repair vessels two millimeters in diameter.[55] These micromethods found immediate application in plastic surgery for digit and limb reimplantation and for movable "island flap" work in which areas of skin with their attached small blood vessels were removed and grafted elsewhere on the body.

The first attempts at organ grafting in small animals had been in 1957, when Sun Lee had finished his basic surgical training at the University of Pittsburgh and Bernard Fisher encouraged him to look into using rats for experimental organ transplantation. Fine sutures were not yet available, but, in 1958, after persevering and designing new vascular clamps, Sun Lee obtained his first success with joining the portal vein and vena cava in the rat, using 7/0 sutures, and his improved method was published in 1961.[56] With even finer sutures available in 1964, his method was extended to transplant the rat heart.[57] Progress continued, with transplanting of the rat liver in 1966, kidneys in 1967, pancreas in 1968, and lung, testis, and small intestine in 1971.[58] Eventually, tiny 11/0 sutures were available, and, by 1999, vascularized thymus gland transplants in the mouse were achieved.

The attractions of these small animal transplant models were considerable. Highly sophisticated knowledge of the transplantation genetics of small inbred animals was available, and small animal work allowed a greater output of data. Small animals, being more economical to purchase and house, spared the use of larger animals at a time when animal experimentation was increasingly under public scrutiny and subject to criticism. But, as always, there was the reservation that, although

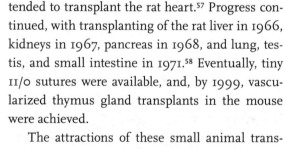
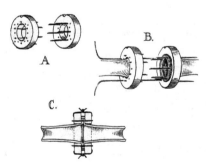

Micro-methods of joining small animal blood vessels first emerged in 1960. Success with microsurgery led not only to new models of organ transplantation but also to innovative plastic surgery. From J. H. Jacobsen and E. L. Suarez, "Microsurgery in the Anastomosis of Small Vessels," *Surgical Forum* 11 (1960): 243–45.

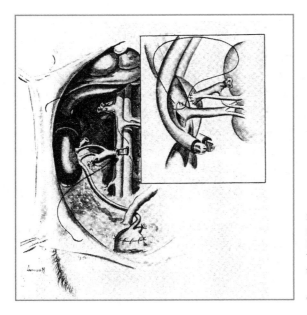

Sun Lee's illustration of rat kidney transplantation. From S. Lee, "An Improved Technique of Renal Transplantation in the Rat," *Surgery* 61 (1967): 771–73. Image courtesy of *Surgery*.

immunological insights certainly emerged, the relevance to the outbred human situation was problematic.

These rat studies did immediately yield novel findings. Some rats showed spontaneous acceptance of mismatched kidney transplants from other inbred strains.[59] But the most exciting finding was of an "enhancement" mechanism, already well known in tumor transplant work but never seen in decades of skin graft work in small animals. Giving immune sera against an organ graft plus this graft could, instead of shortening graft survival, prolong survival. It offered, like tolerance, a powerful specific suppression of the immune response, with all the associated attractions for clinical work. This finding revived the possibility of achieving human graft survival by sophisticated immunological means.[60] Careful plans were made to use this type of enhancing antibody in human transplant patients, but their use did not result in success.[61]

Antilymphocyte Serum

In the optimistic mid-1960s, in addition to the considerable promise offered by the introduction of tissue-typing methods, hopes for rapid progress in clinical transplantation were further raised by the emergence of a new immunosuppressive agent. For a while it promised to be the final, or near final, solution to tissue transplantation.

Antilymphocyte serum appeared at a useful time. In 1966, the rapid progress in kidney transplantation that had begun in 1963 had slowed. The Kidney Transplant Registry confirmed this slowdown, recording a commendable 65–70 percent one-year kidney survival rate for living-related kidney transplants, but also pointed out a "certain stability" in the results. Many other attempts had been made to improve outcome. Other immunosuppressive drugs, including methotrexate, azaserine, and actinomycin C, had been tried briefly and then discarded. Other strategies were investigated, notably selective forms of irradiation beamed at only the central lymphoid organs or the transplanted kidney or by irradiating the patient's blood as it passed through an external shunt. Combining surgical removal of the thymus or spleen with immunosuppression efforts proved to be of no benefit, nor did removal of both spleen and thymus help, particularly since such surgery also had its risks. There were initial hopes for the use of human thoracic duct drainage to deplete lymphoctyes, a tactic introduced by Joseph Murray and Nicholas Tilney in Boston.[62] None of these strategies found a permanent place later in the management of kidney transplantation, but antilymphocyte serum (ALS) and its descendants were to find a lasting role.

Antisera that killed cells had been made and used in the "lost era" of transplantation immunity. Elie Metchnikoff had tried this approach, and Alwin Pappenheimer, working in New York in 1917, as discussed earlier, had made and tested a very effective serum against leukocytes. In 1937, W. B. Chew and John Lawrence in New York also followed this approach and made a serum for guinea pig studies. In Britain in 1941, Alan Cruickshank, working at Oxford and later in Aberdeen, had prepared an active anti–rat leukocyte serum as part of Howard Florey's failed but determined attempt to understand the lymphocyte.[63] Shortly thereafter, in the Soviet Union, Alexander Bogomolets (born circa 1881) made an antireticular serum using multiple spleen cell immunizations and absorptions, but its healing properties could not be confirmed in the West.[64] The lymphocyte killing or inactivation strategy was revived by the surgeon Michael Woodruff while in an academic surgical post in Aberdeen from 1948–1952, and there Cruickshank told him of the neglected Oxford work. Later, after moving to Edinburgh, Woodruff worked steadily from the 1950s on antibodies raised against lymphocytes, improving the methods and refining the crude serum until he had a potent ALS to use against rat cells.[65] By 1964, Woodruff could prolong experimental rat skin grafts with his ALS. Byron Waksman at this time also devised an effective protocol for making a similar cytotoxic serum.[66]

Others, notably Anthony Monaco (born 1932) in Boston, followed Woodruff's lead and soon confirmed the immunosuppressive action of such sera

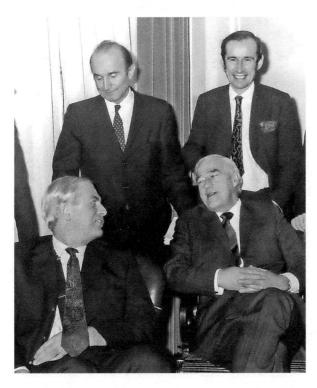

Michael Woodruff (*bottom right*) seen here with Peter Medawar (*bottom left*) and Georges Mathé (*top left*), made many contributions to transplantation, including the development and study of antilymphocyte serum. Image courtesy of the Novartis Foundation.

in small animal work.[67] Medawar, ever watchful for useful clinical strategies, put some young surgical visiting research workers onto the project. This group produced and studied a nontoxic, antithymocyte serum (ATS) for use in mice, and it markedly prolonged skin grafts.[68]

The excitement arose from the observation that the action of ATS/ALS seemed restricted to a marked effect on cell-mediated immunity, via elimination of circulating T-cells, while leaving antibody formation largely intact. Allografts and xenografts in mice (which Medawar still loyally termed "heterografts" in 1968) were accepted indefinitely.[69] Immunological memory could be wiped out, and, if adult thymectomy was performed in addition to provision of ALS, a profound, longer lasting effect resulted. Even tolerance could be induced in adult mice after pretreatment with the agent, which once again resurrected clinical hopes for this strategy. There were also short-lived hopes that, by inducing tolerance to ALS itself—as to any other protein—an attenuated, safe, and economical action would result. In short, ALS seemed to be the answer to the challenge of the times.

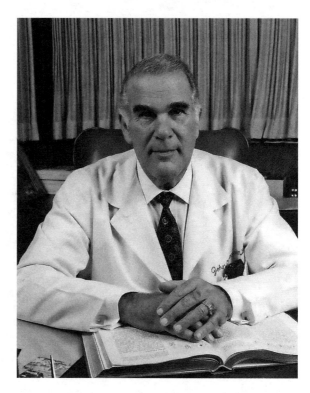

John S. Najarian at the University of Minnesota extended kidney transplantation to children and diabetic patients and made early use of human antilymphocyte serum.

The News Spreads

News about ALS spread rapidly and was a dominant topic at the 1967 conference on tissue transplantation held in Santa Barbara.[70] Starzl made his own ALS and started human trials.[71] John Najarian, working in Minneapolis, inventively used a line of cultured human lymphoblasts as his unchanging antigen for making a horse serum, refining it to antilymphocyte globulin (ALG) alone, that is, the globulin fraction.[72] Improved kidney transplant results were reported from ALS use in these units and elsewhere, notably from Ross Sheil in Australia. ALS was immediately used in treating marrow cell suspensions prior to infusion for bone marrow transplantation, since it usefully removed the troublesome lymphocytes causing graft-versus-host damage.

Much effort went into varying the protocols used in making the antilymphocyte serum. There were choices between the many sources of lymphoid cell to be used and the antibody-producer animals (rabbit, pig, or horse), plus various immunization regimens, as well as the choice between the globulin fraction or the whole serum. These combinations led to a flurry of catchy acronyms, including RAMLS, PAMLS, and HAGLS. Batches tended to be variable in effectiveness, so tests of potency were sought. Prolongation of skin grafts was the obvious quality control test in small animals, and for testing ALS, the best in vitro method to emerge was to use the serum's capacity to block T-cell "rosetting," a test announced by Jean-François Bach in Paris. However, most makers of human ALS preferred the direct test—monkey skin grafts—a method that also detected any residual toxicity. This expensive service was provided by Hans Balner of the Primate Center at the Rijswijk Radiobiological Institute in the Netherlands.[73]

Pharmaceutical Company Interest

After the development of the new sera, pharmaceutical companies took an interest for the first time in the history of clinical transplantation, and they moved quickly to develop the new immunosuppressive agent. High development costs and other difficulties slowed the process, however. Production finally commenced, notably by the Upjohn Company in Kalamazoo, Burroughs Wellcome in Britain, and Behringwerke AG in West Germany, joined later by the Fresenius and Merieux companies. In Britain, a worthy Medical Research Council committee, chaired by Woodruff, advised Burroughs Wellcome on manufacturing methods, and the council planned to purchase the ALG and proceed to a controlled clinical trial. Deliberations started in late 1967, but plans were immediately stalled by reports from the United States that ALS used in humans could on occasion cause platelet damage, anaphylaxis, and kidney damage. The new Committee on Safety of Drugs ("Drugs" changed to "Medicines" in 1971), set up in Britain in 1963, became involved, and its concerns on side effects further delayed the MRC study and use of this novel agent. The regular use of homemade ALS in America by Starzl and Najarian was announced and reported to the committee, but the rest of the cautious MRC committee members were unmoved when the surgical members urged that use of ALS should proceed.[74]

Clinical and Research Uses of ALS

Only short courses of ALS were recommended for human patients because of the usual risk of sensitization from a foreign protein, and the globulin was painful when injected either under the skin or directly into muscle. It proved fairly safe to use intravenously but could cause kidney lesions after prolonged use. Soon the consensus was that the spectacular success in small animal transplantation could not be obtained in human patients, particularly as humans could not be given a dose as large as the equivalent of the animal's dose. By the mid-1970s, clinicians considered ALS merely helpful rather than essential, and it found more favor in North America than in Europe.

ALS use remained an important tool in laboratory work. Monoclonal versions later largely supplanted the polyvalent sera, and the monoclonal antibodies to lymphocyte subsets gained niche therapeutic uses and became a vital routine research tool in the study of immune responses.

Liver Transplantation Resumes

After ALS emerged, Starzl achieved favorable results with it in human kidney transplantation, and these results led him to restart liver transplantation in 1967 in Denver. Roy Calne in Cambridge followed shortly afterward, and thereafter they supported each other for some years against a skeptical surgical world.[75] In spite of Starzl's adverse experience with human liver transplants in the early 1960s, he had not abandoned the goal, notably because his early failures were mostly technical rather than immunological. Meanwhile, Calne had moved from London to the chair of surgery at Cambridge, and, joining up with Roger Williams's liver unit at King's College Hospital London, he started liver transplantation, though Calne had little enthusiasm for ALS.

Both men obtained encouraging early results with their new liver graft cases.[76] Experience with the technique, better donor organs, better coagulation control, and better management of conventional immunosuppression all played a part, and, in the late 1960s, some long-term survivals of patients with liver transplants were reported. Others in America, including David Hume in Richmond and Joseph Fortner in New York, started liver transplantation but encountered serious difficulties similar to those seen earlier. In 1968, two liver transplant units opened in continental Europe—at Groningen in the Netherlands and Hanover in West Germany. The three European centers started to share donated livers via Eurotransplant, aiming to obtain at least ABO blood group compatibility. The development of ALS/ALG was also an encouragement for further pancreas transplants, and Carl-Gustav Groth in Sweden and Jean-Michel Dubernard in Lyon began attempts, as did the Mayo Clinic.

Renal Replacement

In the mid-1960s, in large urban hospitals, patients began to have a choice between regular dialysis treatment and kidney transplantation. The existence of such a choice varied from country to country, and city to city, and even from hospital to hospital according to attitudes and the skills available. In most regular dialysis units, the staff were proud and protective of their small but growing number of surviving patients in whom they had invested so much effort. Although kidney transplantation was becoming more common, these doctors might not even consider referring these precious, successfully dialyzed patients to the transplant surgeons. They judged the hazards of grafting to be too great, and although life on dialysis was not ideal, the patient was at least alive. There was also a mindset that a patient should have one chance with one therapy, and not receive both, and at this time there was no return to dialysis after loss of a kidney graft. Some support for this apparently heartless policy was the finding that survival was poor on dialysis after the debilitating struggle with a failing transplant.

In London, dialysis treatment was well established at the Middlesex and the Royal Free hospitals. In 1967, J. D. N. Nabarro, of the Middlesex Hospital, wrote that "renal transplantation remains a hazardous procedure, and I am still a little hesitant about recommending it. Chronic haemodialysis seems at the present time to be the most encouraging approach." As late as 1972, physicians of the London Hospital, in planning for the next five years, concluded, "We feel that the present indications for transplantation are those of failure of haemodialysis on medical, social or psychological grounds."[77]

The patients receiving transplants at this time were a mixed group, including those judged unsuitable for dialysis or doing poorly with dialysis, or those with a suitable, willing living donor. In hospitals where both dialysis and transplantation facilities and skills existed, the professional relations between the nephrologists and surgeons involved varied. In some places, purely surgical transplant units were emerging, with physician input, while elsewhere the physicians took on the management of the transplants and simply embedded helpful surgeons on the team to do the technical work. In Denver, Joseph Holmes, the chief of nephrology, started a new dialysis service, with all the incumbent difficulties, but it was linked to Starzl's transplant efforts. Holmes, "approaching sixty, . . . became the oldest member of the transplant team. Chronically fatigued by overwork and lung disease which he 'treated' by constantly smoking cigarettes, he fought to hold back the tide of desperate patients who flocked to Colorado General Hospital. Not far behind them came an avalanche of remonstrances from administrators who complained that his dialysis unit was consuming 10 percent of the entire hospital budget, which was true. Unanswered mail surrounded him in his tiny office."[78]

But an important change, not least for the patients, was in allowing a return to dialysis after loss of a kidney transplant, and this came about very slowly and not until the late 1960s. By 1972, the Renal Transplant Registry in Boston announced a novelty in their annual report: transplant failure no longer meant death. New format graphs were presented—one for kidney survival and one for patient survival. The authors indicated that "this report differs in some ways from the structure and format of previous reports. Statistics are given on both patient survival and on duration of function of the transplant. Thus a given patient may be alive with dialysis after his graft has ceased functioning. Interpretation of the data will be more accurate when this fact is kept in mind."[79]

Another change resulted from the new strategy. As regular dialysis became routinely available for those with failed transplants, the surgical priority after transplantation became the life of the patient rather than heroic attempts to sustain the life of the graft, notably with more profound immunosuppression. When the surgical team judged the graft to be doomed, they no longer resorted to the "no-lose" measures, and an orderly, safe return to dialysis became the strategy. The pioneers graciously accepted the fact that this move took some months off their graft survival times, figures that were important to them in the pioneer days.

Legal Issues

As confidence with kidney transplantation rose and a routine service began to evolve, the demand for donor kidneys increased and further efforts to seek wider donation began. The legal issues involved in organ donation now increased in number and complexity. Some countries had no relevant legislation at all. In France, for example, since 1947 a limited number of hospitals had been allowed to remove tissues and do postmortems, without legal formalities, "in the interests of science," and this practice seemed to legalize routine cadaveric organ removal. Some countries had ancient restrictions on tissue removal, usually in places where there had been scandals over the use of bodies, such as the excesses of nineteenth-century anatomists and resurrectionists in Britain. But even when legal frameworks existed, the law had assumed that any gifts were for anatomy schools, tissue banks, or corneal donation and donation was not urgent.

In the mid-1960s, most countries moved toward a necessary clarification of the relevant laws. In the United States, lawmakers used the Commissioners on Uniform State Laws to consult widely, seeking to replace the patchwork of variable state laws on donation of tissues after death. After five years, in 1968, the commissioners introduced the Uniform Anatomical Gift Act as a model for legislation by individual states. According to the policy's language, a gift could be made during life through a will or on a card designed to be carried on the person and that would override the demands of relatives after death. It allowed for donation to proceed in the absence of any known wishes during life and if no relatives attended. It had one other dispensation that favored transplantation: it protected anyone involved in removal or transplantation of organs from the threat of civil proceedings, provided they acted in good faith.

In Britain, discussion about reforming the Human Tissue Act (1961) started in the mid-1960s, with the goal of modifying it in the light of a changing world, together with consideration of measures to encourage organ donation. These new discussions also attempted to deal with the ancient, unresolved issue of ownership of a dead body. Modification and clarification of the law were proceeding well until 1968, when there was the major setback. The year 1968 proved to be a turbulent one in the world of transplantation.

16 Brain Death and the "Year of the Heart"

A MAJOR CHANGE in hospital practice occurred in the mid-1960s when gravely ill or injured patients could receive respiratory support on a ventilator. This shift transformed resuscitation into a focused, successful strategy. Intubation and ventilation of patients, followed by care in the orderly calm of the new intensive care units, constituted an increasingly standard procedure if recovery was deemed possible.

The pioneers of intensive care were encouraged by outcomes in the Denmark polio epidemic of 1953, when respiratory support for a period of time allowed some patients to survive. Traditional anesthetic practice taught that prolonged anesthesia was dangerous, but, with more adventurous surgery being attempted, it became commonplace to continue ventilation postoperatively, rather than to assume that the patient's breathing would resume promptly. This ventilation proved beneficial rather than harmful, and the "long-is-bad" anesthesia paradigm was discarded.[1] New ventilators were more sophisticated, and, with backup from the frequent biochemical and blood gas measurements that had just been introduced, longer and longer periods of safe ventilation and nutritional support could be achieved.

New Units

Resuscitated patients were initially left in the wards where they had been receiving treatment, but soon it was deemed more sensible to place these patients in one location. The first such specialized units appeared in 1958, notably the Uppsala University Hospital Respiratory Care Unit. At Baltimore that year Peter Safar (1924–2003) established such a unit, naming it "intensive care." Later, these areas were often called "critical care" or "intensive therapy" units. The growing use of these new units is seen in data from Boston's Massachusetts General Hospital's Respiratory Care Unit, established in 1961. The number of cases that facility managed in this way quickly rose from about one hundred to six hundred by 1966, but the survival rate was only 50 percent in this early period.

In the early years of ventilation, respiratory support continued in critical care units until recovery or when the heart finally failed, and, in this pioneer era, the period of time until "cardiac death" could be quite short. But with experience in management of such cases, hospitals increasingly faced a new situation: there were patients who showed no spontaneous breathing but survived purely as a result of this essential ventilation and other increasingly skilled supportive measures. The ICU staff were increasingly faced with the decision of how long to continue treatment, and it was at the Massachusetts General Hospital where an orderly solution was first sought to deal with what was increasingly admitted to be occasions of "pointless ventilation."

By the mid-1960s, the situation was quite common, and it was distressing both to families and to the staff involved. Practical and ethical concerns about this situation were discussed at local and national professional meetings, and they became part of the fast-growing agenda of the new field of medical ethics.[2] Support for terminating pointless ventilation came readily from outside the medical profession, notably from advocates of "death with dignity." For those seeking the input of religious leaders, useful ethical guidance had already been given in an earlier pronouncement by Pope Pius XII in 1957. Speaking by invitation on the matter of resuscitation to the International Congress of Anesthesiologists in Rome, he stated that "ordinary means only" should be used to keep patients alive and that any added "extraordinary treatment" was not a moral obligation. He stated that death was the time when the soul departed from the body, and he also argued that the soul could have left at the time of resuscitation from an otherwise fatal incident.[3]

Questions on Death

There had never been a legal concern about the definition of death until this period in which the use of new medical machinery blurred the line between life and death. Up to this time, death was confirmed when a doctor certified life extinct, and the time of death recorded was the moment when the heart stopped. But prolonged survival on a ventilator raised new questions. The legal issue had come up first, indirectly, in an Arkansas case involving the determination of, for inheritance purposes, which of two accident victims had died first.[4] In that case, only the more seriously injured wife was ventilated, and she survived her husband for some days. A claim was made that she died first, at the time of resuscitation, but the judge concluded that anyone still breathing, even on a machine, could not be dead. The case was taken to higher courts, but the Supreme Court was uninterested, since the definition of death was "so settled." The Supreme Court went further, delivering a sharp warning that attempting to debate the definition of death might open the way for tasteless legal advocacy.

But the question of defining death would not go away. The "settled principles" were being unsettled.

One of the first to attempt a redefinition of death was Robert Schwab (1903–1972), the senior neurologist at Boston's Massachusetts General Hospital. The hospital's critical care unit had consulted Schwab with increasing frequency to assess brain function in comatose, unresponsive, ventilated patients, and, as early as 1963, he had drawn up a "triad of grave prognostic signs," as he called them, and then studied the outcomes. His three "grave signs" were as follows: no brain electrical activity (the "flat" or "isoelectric" electroencephalogram), no eye pupil reflex, and no response to noxious stimuli. His study of outcomes included postmortem examination of the brain, which always demonstrated irreversible damage, and this careful study gave him confidence in the significance of his triad of signs.

Schwab was accordingly prepared to make a diagnosis of death of the brain when others understandably hesitated, feeling they were on uncertain ground. In 1964, three years before the historic meeting of the Harvard Ad Hoc Committee which first formally considered brain death, a colleague noted Schwab's leadership: "[He] had accepted responsibility with the support of his colleagues for death pronouncements by EEG some 15 times during the past two and one-half years. The experience has proved eminently satisfactory to all concerned, diminishing grief and anxiety for the family of the victim in a state of limbo, also relieving the travail and expense of skilled personnel, special equipment and service."[5]

The Organ Donation Factor

There was considerable uneasiness about terminating respiratory support. Among the many expressing reservations were surgeons like James D. Hardy, who, though interested in the future of transplantation, in 1964 was troubled about withdrawing ventilation in general surgical patients: "In fairly rapid succession three young men were admitted with fatal head lesions. . . . Each of these patients died after variable periods of mechanical pulmonary ventilation, a fact that raised a disturbing moral problem: when, if ever, would a physician be justified in switching off the ventilator in a patient whose voluntary respiratory effort had long ceased, to permit the hypoxia that would be followed by cardiac arrest. We were not able to conclude that we would be willing to do this."[6]

Still, the number of occasions when those in charge of the case terminated ventilation was growing. At this point, the suitability of a patient's organs for donation was only rarely an issue, if considered at all, since there were few transplant units in the mid-1960s and many large urban hospitals had not started kidney transplantation. But if donation was possible, events moved swiftly after the ventilator was switched off and cardiac death that followed soon after was certified. This routine emerged in the mid-1960s, sometimes assisting the small number of kidney transplants of the time, and some deterioration of the kidneys was accepted, as always. Removing organs before stopping ventilation in brain-dead patients was unthinkable at the time.[7]

In 1966, Michael Woodruff organized a historic CIBA Foundation meeting in London: "Ethics in Medicine."[8] Woodruff invited the distinguished jurist Lord Kilbrandon, a colleague on the board of the Edinburgh Royal Infirmary, to assist with the conference, which was also attended by transplant surgeons Roy Calne and Tom Starzl. There they heard, apparently for the first time, of the removal of organs from a brain-dead donor before the removal of ventilator support, and these surgeons responded with surprise, caution, and reserve.[9] Calne believed that "if a patient has a heart beat he could not be regarded as a cadaver." Starzl went further: "I doubt if any of the members of our transplantation team could accept a person as being dead as long as there was a heart beat. . . . Would any physician be willing to remove an unpaired vital organ before circulation had stopped?"[10]

Attitudes began to change, however. By the mid-1960s, Norman Shumway at Stanford had reluctantly concluded that although surgeons could briefly delay removing donor kidneys after a patient's heart stopped beating, there could be no delay when a heart was to be transplanted. At the Santa Barbara conference in 1967, the year before his first human heart transplants, Shumway made this point again but acknowledged that the public was not ready for the idea of organ donation before cardiac function had ceased: "It is indeed unfortunate, that the traditional definition of death is cessation of the heart beat. . . . There is an untapped source of potential heart donors in the Intensive Care Unit of every hospital. . . . These are patients who are essentially dead. Accordingly, research must continue in the area of cadaver heart resuscitation and storage while medical and social policy slowly make room for the concept of heart beating donation for heart transplantation."[11]

By the mid-1960s, increasing numbers of transplanters did come to accept the future possibility of this so-called "heart-beating" donation and raised the matter carefully with local critical care staff and neurologists.

But the matter was thrust on the public suddenly in 1968, not slowly, as Shumway had hoped. And the public reacted adversely, as had the surgeons at the CIBA conference in 1966.[12]

The Harvard Committee

On September 29, 1967, Henry K. Beecher (1904–1976), Harvard University's long-serving Henry Isaiah Dorr Professor of Research in Anesthesia, sent out a historic letter calling a meeting of the medical faculty's Standing Committee on Human Studies. Beecher, who had already stirred controversy by alerting his American colleagues and the American public to issues regarding human experimentation, now wished to discuss the issues arising from "pointless ventilation." Beecher was well aware of the growing problem in his Massachusetts General Hospital intensive care unit and wished to pursue the matter further. No pressure for the meeting came from local transplant surgeons, but, perhaps unfortunately, the surgeon Joseph Murray from the Brigham Hospital transplant unit was already a member of the Standing Committee and was thus automatically involved.

This committee was a prototype of the "ethical committee" that was later to be a familiar part of hospital life. The chair had fallen to Beecher because of his spirited stance on earlier, broader issues. His continuing interest in medical ethics meant that he had contacts throughout the various faculties at Harvard, including that of the Divinity School.

About 1967, Beecher had come to consider that making patients respirator dependent was almost a medical experiment, one that violated the principle outlined in his 1967 lecture, "The Right to Be Left Alone: The Right to Die," although this dimension faded from the "brain-death" debate as it matured. Others on the committee, notably William Curran, professor of public health, shared Beecher's interest in bioethics. But the committee member with the greatest practical input was Robert Schwab, now confident that his "triad of grave signs" was helpful in determining when death of the brain had occurred.

Committee Deliberations

At the meeting of the committee on October 19, 1967, Beecher gave a presentation on ethical problems that arise when an individual is "hopelessly unconscious."[13] Beecher had prudently made sure that the dean of Harvard Medical School was aware of this proposed discussion on a difficult matter. He wrote to Dean Robert H. Ebert that "the developments in resuscitative therapy have led to many desperate efforts to save the dying patient. Sometimes all that is left is a decerebrated individual. These individ-

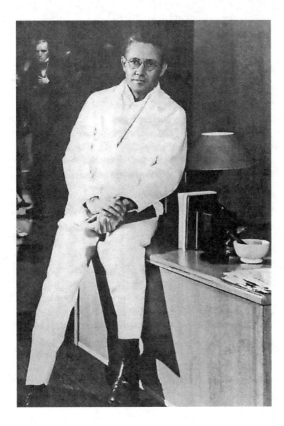

Henry K. Beecher, Dorr Professor of Research in Anesthesia at Harvard Medical School, was the activist in setting up in 1967 the famous Harvard faculty Ad Hoc Committee that suggested a set of criteria for the diagnosis of brain death in ventilated patients. Image courtesy of the National Library of Medicine.

uals are increasing in number all over the land and there are a number of problems which should be faced up to."[14]

Ebert suggested that a subcommittee be set up, and he appointed Beecher as its chairman. Some members of Beecher's subcommittee were obvious choices, notably Curran and Schwab. The surgeon Murray was also added, and he wrote to Beecher after the committee meeting. Murray, referring to their discussion, mentioned a "second question": "The first problem requires merely a definition of death. No longer is cessation of heart beat or respiration applicable. . . . Brain death is the essential requirement and the faculty of the Harvard Medical School is in a suitable position to make a statement. The second question regarding organs for donation is really simple. Once the patient is dead the legal mechanism then applies. . . . All that is required is proper permission from either the patient [i.e., permission given earlier in life] or from the next of kin."[15]

Murray was supporting brain death as a new clinical standard for a declaration of death. He was also simply pointing out that if brain death was accepted as a legal criterion for death, organs could, as always, be removed after the declaration of death, without legal entanglement. He was not urging use of heart-beating donation, and Murray's own view on this at the time is not clear: he never spoke in support of such donation.[16]

While Beecher was working on getting members for a new subcommittee that the dean had recommended, the world received the dramatic news of Christiaan Barnard's heart transplant attempts.

The Committee at Work

By January 1968, Beecher had his subcommittee, famously called by its new title—the Ad Hoc Committee on Brain Death—and it had wide-ranging cross-faculty membership. It seems this famous committee never met, with members simply considering and responding to various drafts of the policy document Beecher produced; the document went through five revisions. When Beecher had initiated discussions on the problem of "pointless ventilation," the matter was seen, reasonably, as a clinical challenge to which Harvard academics could contribute ethical insights. But as the controversial events surrounding heart transplant attempts unfolded, the issue of brain death was already in the public domain. Although the Ad Hoc Committee had been set in place before the flurry of heart transplants, one view, almost a conspiracy theory, was that it seemed remarkably convenient that the criterion of brain death should emerge at such a useful moment for some transplant surgeons. Raymond Adams, one of the committee members, did address this possible criticism, which he pointed out to Beecher during the exchange of drafts. One of the policy drafts may have pointed out the obvious: that organ donation could benefit from criteria that permitted cessation of ventilation. With loss of brain function as the criterion for death, the usually rushed process of organ removal could be avoided, since removing ventilation and cardiac death could be planned for a certain time. Adams's comment on the drafted text was, "I object to using the need of donor organs as a valid argument for redefining cerebral death." Dean Ebert also noticed this undesirable apparent linkage and told Beecher that one paragraph was "unfortunate, for it suggests that you wish to redefine death in order to make viable organs more readily available to persons requiring transplants."[17]

Beecher revised the document yet again to meet these concerns. Because of the sensitivity of the matter, Harvard's president, Nathan Pusey, was also asked to read it, and he approved the final wording, which was entirely about brain death, with a passing remark about critical care units as a source of donors.

The Report's Publication

The report of the Harvard Ad Hoc Committee on Brain Death was published in the *Journal of the American Medical Association* on August 5,
1968. Much had happened in the ten months since Beecher's initiative,
and the heart transplantation controversies had profoundly changed the
biomedical ethical landscape. The *JAMA* editorial leadership was uneasy
about the report. The editor and the association thought it proper to follow
the Ad Hoc Committee's report with a statement on the status of transplantation from the American Medical Association's Judicial Council.
This perhaps deliberately adjacent, seriously worded statement, "Ethical
Guidelines for Organ Transplantation," contained, in code, a rebuke for
the excesses of the heart transplanters. It hardly mentioned the historic
Harvard report on the preceding pages.[18] This silence was significant: it
was one way of attempting to undo the already widespread perception that
the needs of organ donation had stimulated the arrival of the brain-death
criterion.[19]

In normal circumstances, this much-needed new definition of death
might have encouraged a slow but orderly change in medical practice. But
the times were not normal: Barnard's transplantation of a human heart,
performed just after the Harvard committee had been launched, had
changed everything.

Heart Transplants

In early December 1967 in Cape Town, Christiaan Barnard performed the
first human heart transplant, and public interest was immediate, massive,
and sustained.[20] Barnard (1922–2001), a South African cardiac surgeon,
had postgraduate surgical experience in the United States, and, beginning in 1965, he carried out kidney preservation studies at Groote Schuur
Hospital in South Africa.[21] He then visited North American surgical departments again, including a short spell with David Hume at the Medical College of Virginia, where he gained experience in kidney transplantation and witnessed Richard Lower's experimental heart transplants.[22] He
spent time at the Denver and Minnesota units, and, in visiting Shumway,
he knew of the long-standing experimental heart graft project at Stanford and the use of an atrial cuff to simplify the connections.[23] Surgeons
elsewhere had considerable experience with experimental heart transplant work, notably Donald Longmore in London, who told the Ministry
of Health that he was ready to perform human heart transplants but was
dissuaded by his hospital.[24] All these groups had held back from human
attempts, since the experience with dog heart transplants at the time was
not encouraging.[25] The lessons of the dismal failure of Hardy's solitary

human xenograft heart transplant in Mississippi in 1964 were not forgotten.[26] The awesome responsibility of the preliminary removal of the patient's heart, which to some was the seat of the soul, weighed heavily even on those with experimental experience.

Barnard's own hospital had an excellent cardiac clinic, and he had been the first to do open heart surgery in South Africa.[27] His first step upon returning from his second stint in the United States was to perform his nation's first kidney transplant. He had no direct personal experience in experimental heart transplantation, and thus his human heart graft in late 1967 was a bold step.[28] It was an attempt that might have been expected to fail and attract criticism. Instead, the reverse was the case.

Immediate Effect

Instead of prompt failure, the patient's graft was working well in the days following surgery. The graft worked long enough to answer the crucial question of the time: could a human donor heart, removed from its considerable nerve supply and lacking what some proposed to be a mysterious synergy with its familiar lungs, produce immediate, normal cardiac function? The answer was yes. This technical triumph released others who had built up the necessary experimental experience, and some who had not, from their many inhibitions and concerns, and a remarkable number of such human heart transplants immediately followed. Three days after Barnard's first operation, Adrian Kantrowitz (1918–2008), a pediatric surgeon at the Maimonides Medical Center in New York, was the first American surgeon to attempt the procedure. He had a long and distinguished record of innovation in heart valve and pacemaker use and had begun making and using auxiliary artificial heart devices in 1966 without any publicity. He also had vast experience in experimental heart transplantation over five years, and, with some doomed young patients already under consideration for such surgery, he proceeded to do a human heart transplant, but the patient died shortly afterward.[29]

Barnard's first heart transplant patient died eighteen days after the operation, as a result of problems with the immunosuppression regimen, rather than rejection. Barnard then carried out a second heart transplantation, and, remarkably, this graft, for a dentist named Philip Blaiberg, sustained reasonable quality of life for two years.[30] Barnard, his patient, and their hospital did not discourage publicity, and the South African government, isolated at that time and attracting international censure for its racial policies, was also delighted to have this sudden gift of a place in medical history.[31] A special issue of the *South African Medical Journal* was rushed into print.

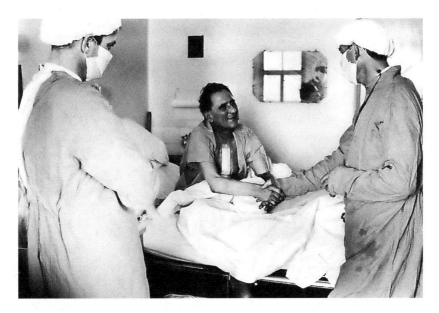

Louis Washkansky and his surgeon, Christiaan Barnard, at the Groote Schuur Hospital shortly after he underwent the world's first human heart transplant operation. Image courtesy of D. K. C. Cooper.

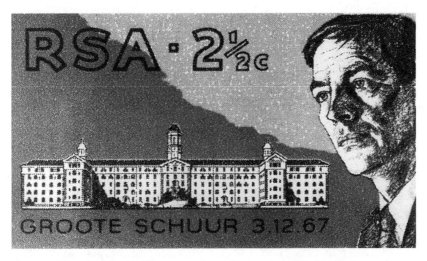

Christiaan Barnard achieved celebrity status after performing the world's first heart transplant in December 1967. The South African government issued a postage stamp honoring him in July 1969.

Barnard's successful heart transplants caused an international sensation, and in the short run, his success won approval.[32] Barnard traveled the world but was noticeably absent from the surgical and scientific meetings where such experience is normally shared. He had a high profile among the general public, however, appearing in the media as a handsome young man offering polished, optimistic comments. He also assisted American physicians' organizations that sought his support after they encountered public opposition regarding medical and ethical issues. In 1968, U.S. senator Walter Mondale had responded to widespread public concern over the ethical, social, and legal implications of high technology medicine and had proposed a commission to oversee such matters. The Senate called Barnard to testify, and, at the height of his fame, he took a thoroughly libertarian stance at the hearings. With a burst of bravado, he warned that the senator's proposed commission would threaten American surgical research: "If I am in competition with my colleagues in this country [America] which I am not . . . then I would welcome this Commission, because it would put the [American] doctors so far behind me, and hamper the group of doctors so much, that I will go so far ahead that they will never catch up with me."[33] Mondale's bill did not progress at that time, but a less intrusive version was incorporated into other legislation in 1974.

Poor Results

Among the heart transplants carried out worldwide between the historic first in South Africa and May 1968, only Barnard's second case had a significant survival. Even with his experimental experience, Norman Shumway's two heart transplant attempts in January and February 1968 sustained life for only fifteen and three days, respectively. Kantrowitz's second heart transplant patient lived for only eight and a half hours. There were also failed attempts in experienced cardiac surgery units in Paris. Other cases in the "Year of the Heart," as it might be called, followed in places not known for transplant innovation or notable cardiac surgery. Barnard's audacity had suggested there was no need for previous experimental heart transplant experience. National pride often seemed at stake, and since South Africa had managed to show the way, surgeons throughout the world decided there was no need to wait for studies from the usual leaders in Europe and North America. Immediate death was the result of most of the first, and often only, heart transplants carried out in Bombay, São Paulo, Buenos Aires, Prague, Sapporo, Caracas, Madrid, Leningrad, Ankara, Istanbul, and Warsaw. There were also failed attempts in better-known cardiac surgery units, including those in Paris, Montreal, and Sydney.

Six months after Barnard's first case, two major figures at famous American units both started heart transplantation: Denton Cooley (born 1920) and his local rival Michael DeBakey (1908–2008), both working at cardiac surgery centers in Houston.[34] Cooley quickly carried out a series of seventeen transplants with initial success, and his public status soon rivaled Barnard's. Cooley's unit expanded, but problems appeared and soon there were only two survivors of twenty-one transplanted patients.[35] Six months later the unit contracted and closed in late 1968, with dying but hopeful patients still camped in motels around the hospital.[36] At the Montreal Heart Institute, seven out of nine patients survived for six months, but all died thereafter, and the surgeon, Pierre Grondin, agreed under pressure from colleagues to cease trying.

Many of these cardiac units that tried heart transplants with little success were not linked to experienced kidney transplant units, and they also lacked the immunological research support that had traditionally been part of the pioneer kidney transplant units.[37] Another factor was that heart surgery units were accustomed to a rapid turnaround, with patients quickly returning home to distant towns for further management and follow-up by their own physicians. The "cut well, stitch well, get well, home well" cardiac surgery philosophy encountered difficulties taking on the continuous postoperative surveillance needed in organ transplantation.

Public Attitudes Change

By May 1968, public support for heart transplants had begun a dramatic decline. The increasing number of deaths, the hints of competition between the heart units, the intrusive publicity, and the obvious national rivalries and chauvinism were increasingly considered to be distasteful. In addition, there was adverse publicity surrounding the circumstances of donation, one example being when a brain-dead donor was flown by private jet from Massachusetts to Texas and the subsequent transplant was unsuccessful. In April 1968, Cooley used a controversial new artificial heart in a human patient as a temporary support and made a dramatic public appeal for a donor heart. Investigations and local professional censure followed this episode, and the director of the National Heart Institute at Bethesda also delivered a firm rebuke to these cardiac surgeons.[38] A less obvious feature was that some famous transplantation centers had decided to wait and watch in silence. Francis D. Moore in Boston, who had done so much to foster kidney transplantation from its early days, broke ranks and issued a rebuke to all involved in heart transplantation.[39]

In London, heart transplantation efforts got under way with the formation of the Joint Cardiac Transplant Committee in May 1968. Its mem-

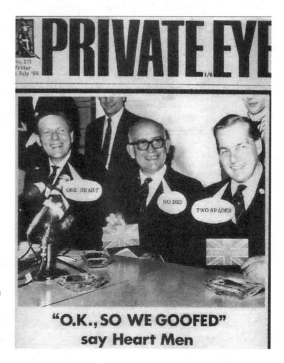

This satirical magazine's version of the British heart transplant press conference reflected growing public concern in mid-1968 over such attempts.

"O.K., SO WE GOOFED" say Heart Men

bership linked three hospitals and planned to avoid "the element of competition and secrecy which has grown up," but events soon discredited the committee's efforts.[40] In the first transplant case under the committee's aegis, a brain-dead donor was moved across London with attendant publicity, since the media had been alerted, and the names of the patient and donor emerged. The next day, the hospital organized a news conference, the first given by any British hospital, which featured triumphal detail, a background of Union Jack flags, and the surgeons sporting a team tie. After the death of this first London patient, the *Observer* and the *Times* in London condemned the operation, and the *New Scientist* called for a halt to such "human experiments." The transplant received less than enthusiastic support from Britain's medical journals; the *Lancet* called the news conference "a fatuous spectacle." Career controversialists waded in, one concluding that the transplants were "a step backwards towards final degradation of our Christian way of life." Britain's *Sunday Telegraph* called for a halt to the "gruesome medical Olympic Games."

Further Concerns

The heavy media coverage of the London heart transplant revealed to the public for the first time precise details about how heart donations took place there and elsewhere. In some cases, the heart donation occurred shortly after the ventilator was switched off. Barnard and Kantrowitz had waited for the donor heart to stop beating but then started cardiac massage and restarted ventilation to maintain heart vitality, which the London surgeons had also done. In Shumway's third case, a private California neurosurgeon certified a brain-dead patient as dead while still ventilated, marking the first heart-beating donation for heart transplantation.[41] Although this practice was to be routine decades later, the idea repelled the unprepared public, abruptly stirring up ancient, latent fears of burial while alive.[42] At Stanford in 1968, the local district attorney and coroner both warned Shumway that they might investigate his donor procedures, and he survived a legal case against him in 1974. In May 1968, in Richmond, Virginia, after a heart was removed from a brain-dead "unclaimed" person, family members later emerged and alleged that their relative had been murdered by the ventilator "switch-off" and the organ removal operation, which was not a heart-beating donation.[43] In August 1968, in Japan, the heart surgeon Juro Wada was indicted for the murder of a brain-dead heart donor. The charges were eventually dropped, but the episode cast a long shadow, and two decades had elapsed before heart transplantation could be considered again in Japan. Not until 1998 could the legal status of brain death be discussed calmly again in that country.

Meanwhile, kidney transplant surgeons watched the increasingly unpleasant public reaction with dismay, since public and professional hostility was spilling over into their noncontroversial service, which had no need of heart-beating donation.[44] Organ donation rates had fallen. Many hospitals were declining to consider donation, and, if asked, families were refusing permission for donation. Even in the calm, well-established niche world of corneal grafting, eye donation also declined at this time.

Legal Events

Brain death was now a sensitive public issue, but brain death was a universally accepted standard in the world of critical care units. It was in routine use as the criterion for terminating ventilation in the CCUs of all major hospitals, but, in the public eye, it still seemed linked to the needs of organ transplantation, small though they were. A further effect was that governments, medical organizations, and justice departments that needed to regularize laws and procedures regarding brain death now were reluctant to get involved, even though the issue had nothing to do with transplantation. What did have relevance to transplantation was the long-awaited and noncontroversial Uniform Anatomical Gift Act, which appeared across the United States in 1968. Although drawn up to assist tissue donation, in the febrile atmosphere of that year, it omitted any reference to the diagnosis of death. A briefing accompanying the draft act stated carefully that "no attempt is made to define the uncertain point in time when life terminates.... The answer depends upon many variables, differing from case to case.[45]

The Uniform Determination of Death Act finally passed in legislatures across the United States in 1980, when public opinion was fully ready, and Britain's Law Lords in 1981 brought in similar closure when they legally equated brain death with death.[46] Until then, most intensivists had no legal backing for their well-established use of the brain-death criteria.

Other Stumbling Blocks

In Britain, the "Year of the Heart" also halted some other initiatives already under way to assist transplantation. The minister of health, like the Commission on Uniform State Laws in the United States, had moved toward much-needed legal changes by revising the outdated Human Tissue Act. The minister had already asked a committee to advise him on the Human Tissue Act and held an invitation-only conference in March 1968 to finalize matters.[47] The meeting was regarded with public suspicion, however, and the normally serious-minded *New Statesman* described the conference as "a gathering of mini-sages behind closed doors as part of the notorious Chris Barnard show." The minister's advisory committee, now called the Advisory Group on Transplant Problems, prudently took its time, aware of the adverse shift in public opinion, and it transmitted a fairly bland report to the minister one year later, in May 1969. The report covered wider matters and was clear that press intrusion must cease, donors were not to be identified, and dying organ donors should not be moved to transplant units for organ removal.[48] As in the United States, the British report avoided discussion of brain death, though the advisory committee, in a timid aside, opined that "determination of death is a clinical matter; useful criteria are the absence of vital functions, including particularly circulation and breathing."[49] The advisory committee decided that its report required approval by Prime Minister Harold Wilson.[50] The prime minister then judged that the timing was not right for its release, and its publication was delayed further.[51]

The broader transplant community, far from having sought the brain-death criteria and urged the change on a reluctant world, were themselves hesitant. At a meeting of the Transplantation Society in The Hague in 1970, there was a tense reaction to a draft document drawn up by the society's committee that cautiously recognized brain death rather than cardiac death as an acceptable standard. The members supported this proposal by only a 2-to-1 margin. It was clear that there were still misgivings about brain death, even within the transplant community. Transplant units were few, and only kidney grafting was being attempted routinely. The kidney was a robust organ, and when removed after cardiac death, dialysis would support the recipient patient until the organ resumed function. The kidney transplant community generally declined to raise the sensitive matter of using heart-beating donations when called by critical care staff, and when donation was possible, it followed cardiac death that resulted from withdrawal of ventilation.[52] Most CCUs, though using the brain-death criterion in their own clinical management, waited for about ten years until the different needs of heart and liver transplantation were clearer. A slow change in attitudes then brought about routine heart-beating, multi-organ donation.

The "Year of the Heart" Ends

The long "Year of the Heart" ended in the spring of 1969, after one hundred operations by sixty-four teams in twenty-two countries over fifteen months, attended by very poor results, constant media interest, and public unease. The peak of this enthusiasm had been the month of November 1968, and of the one hundred cases, only twenty-four patients lived beyond six months. With these poor results, challenging complications, lack of donors, and continuing professional and lay criticism, the enthusiasm of most of the heart transplanters waned. The world of transplantation had received a setback. Bad early results had not been unusual in the early days of other organ grafting. If experienced and respected groups had made a start with a careful appraisal of a limited series of heart transplantation work, as had been the case earlier, the history of transplantation might have been different.

Pondering the Future

In the United States, the National Heart Institute's Ad Hoc Task Force on Cardiac Replacement was asked to take stock of the events of the "Year of the Heart." The institute undertook this investigation because, although it controlled huge research and development funds and was seemingly a freestanding organization, its budget was influenced by Congress; thus, public opinion mattered. The stern report, issued in October 1969, concluded that cardiac transplantation had moved too precipitously from animal experimental work to human transplants. The report called for more research into transplantation immunology and determined that only cardiac units linked with ongoing transplant immunology research would be eligible for research grants. The report also found that some funds for nontransplant research and development had been diverted to human cardiac transplantation, an internal bookkeeping practice that was common at the time. Grants that had been transferred in this fashion were terminated, with a rebuke. To prevent further maverick enthusiasm, only focused funding from the National Heart Institute was to be used for such human cardiac transplant work. It was a centrally imposed moratorium, one unique in American clinical culture.

The effect was that Lower, at Richmond, continued to receive support for a while, but then only Shumway at Stanford had long-term funding for this form of cardiac surgery. Placing this grant at Stanford nearly failed, since both the American College of Cardiologists and Shumway's local hospital trustees called for a national moratorium. He first had probationary funding, and then, impressing the National Heart Institute not only with his careful study of his early cases but also his ability to keep a low profile, his unit received full funding.

Other national institutions and governments had watched with disquiet the transplantation developments during 1968. In Britain, local surgeons had traditionally been free to explore new avenues, and the costs were met locally by the National Health Service after professional discussion and advocacy. But this freedom was about to be curtailed. George Godber, Britain's chief medical officer, later described disingenuously how he managed to get the desired moratorium on heart transplantation:

In consultation we agreed to call together the small number of surgeons, cardiologists and clinical physiologists then working in this field to consider whether it would be best to continue work in human patients or to await the outcome of further work in animals. We agreed unanimously a letter of advice offered by the whole group which I was to send to the small number of medical staffs working in this field. It was of course informal and not simply the Chief Medical Officer's view or the Department's. It was well received and by consensus, further human transplants were delayed until more research had been done. . . . Of course, someone leaked the letter but it was accepted as a reasonable conclusion by informed people—in no sense an instruction.[53]

In reality, the clinical transplanters were not waiting and hoping for new insights from basic research. The lessons from kidney transplantation earlier in the decade had taught them otherwise, and surgical empiricism would doubtless again be dominant. But the "back-to-the-lab" mantra had to be voiced by all. Instead, the transplant world was quietly waiting for empirical innovation. They were waiting for Norman Shumway to obtain regularly good results in human cases, and this he was to do.

The clinical experience gained in this spate of heart transplants, though patchy and scattered, had been significant and would be available whenever the operation might resume. Experience had shown that tissue matching did not significantly affect outcome, nor did the graft need its former nerve supply. Hyperacute rejection was not a problem. Minor imbalance of size

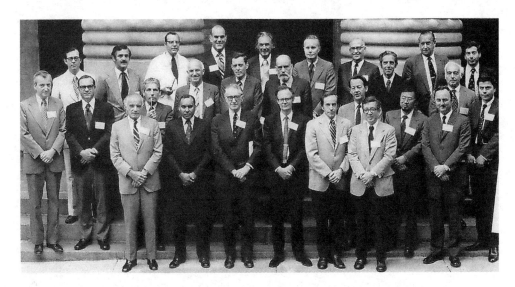

The pioneers of clinical transplantation in the 1960s assembled at a meeting in honor of David Hume. From *Transplantation Proceedings*, December 1974, supplement.

did not matter, but one crucial factor probably explained many of the immediate deaths in the best units. If lung damage was present in the patient from years of heart failure, a donor heart might not overcome the lung resistance and the graft could thus fail within hours of insertion. New tests for graft rejection were sought at this time, and the electrocardiogram and cardiac enzyme studies were prime candidates in that search.

Legacy of the "Year of the Heart"

The legacy of the year 1968 was considerable. Transplantation now had powerful critics outside the medical profession, and many within. Some humility on the part of the transplant community was expected. Central governments and funding agencies had been involved, and they had seen the need to place moratoria on further transplants. Governments were also displeased to have had to shelve measures intended to help organ transplantation. The high cost of transplant operations led some health economists to advocate transferring funds to preventative programs instead, and research bodies lent an ear to the "back-to-the-lab" advocates and the pleas of immunologists that funds should go to them rather than to heedless surgical empirics.

The surgical profession had lost standing in the public's eye. Formerly, surgeons could do no wrong, but now there were questions. The public and the media could be hostile, and publishers were not slow to realize that tales of irresponsible surgery and science would sell. A string of transplant-related novels appeared beginning in 1969, and some centered on dubious transplant practices, gothic horror plots, and unscrupulous organ donation rackets.[54] Few of these novels sold well. But one of them, almost the last to emerge from this genre, seriously affected public opinion for a while. *Coma,* written by a Boston doctor, was a best seller and a successful film in 1977. The plot involved a medical racket in which organs were sold from patients deliberately made brain-dead by unscrupulous anesthetists.[55]

Outlook for the Future

These events left the clinical transplantation community rather demoralized. It was a self-inflicted, and possibly avoidable, setback, and events might have taken a different course in the hands of others. But there was still a sense that the pioneering work in kidney transplantation would be applicable to other organs. The keynote speakers at the Transplantation Society meeting in late 1968, when discussing the future, no longer assumed that kidney grafts alone were being considered, as in the past. Although attempts with other organs were still in the hands of a few, this work gave a new texture to the transplanters' discourse, namely, that there were new vistas possible beyond kidney replacement. Sir Peter Medawar was asked to address the conference on the topic of "The Future of Transplantation." As a distinguished laboratory worker who had done so much to foster clinical organ grafting, he might reasonably have been judgmental in his reaction to that year's events. But instead, and loyally using the word *we,* he cheered the conference with his vision that the difficulties of the year would be put behind them and that development of human organ replacement would move forward: "The transplantation of the heart has been the instrument of a great catharsis. From the press and the pulpit and the judge's bench we have had a stream of advice and comment and warning and exhortation. But I think the Society ought to express collectively the view that the transplantation of organs will one day be assimilated into ordinary clinical practice. . . . There is no need to be deeply philosophical about it. It will come about for the simple and sufficient reason that people are so constituted that they would rather be alive than dead."[56] Events were to prove him right: even heart transplantation was to become respectable, in time.

But in the short term, there were also some domestic clinical discouragements. The advances in tissue typing had, unexpectedly, not brought routine success with cadaveric grafting, and human antilymphocyte serum had not fulfilled its initial promise. Moreover, the results of kidney transplantation were not improving. The effect was that the early 1970s was a period of hesitation, and of stocktaking.

17 The Plateau of the Early 1970s

I N T H E E A R L Y 1970 S, there was a hesitation in the development of organ transplantation. The results of kidney transplantation had been encouraging in the late 1960s, but thereafter the pace of improvement stalled.[1] The numbers of kidney transplants also leveled off after 1972, and the results then got mysteriously worse. After the major promise of anti-lymphocyte serum had faded, the hunt for new drugs ensued, and there was but brief enthusiasm for each new agent tried.[2] The hopes for a dominant role of tissue typing in cadaveric kidney transplantation declined, and the matter became problematic. The development of liver transplantation, which had restarted in 1967, reached a plateau, with Starzl's outcome at one year fixed for some time at 35 percent survival. Heart transplantation was restricted to Shumway's low-key attempts, which were edging slowly toward clinical and political respectability. Transplants of lung, small bowel, and pancreas were rarely attempted. The best news in the transplant world was growing confidence in the technique of human bone marrow replacement.[3] One new development was that kidney transplantation was beginning to spread beyond the developed nations and there it met new challenges.

Even in the world of immunology there was a hesitation after the buoyant 1960s, with little novelty emerging. The doyen of the new cellular immunology, Niels Jerne, later a Nobel Prize winner, famously stated that "the end of immunology is in sight."[4] Some transplant pioneers believed that, although organ transplantation was not finished, there was an impasse. Some moved enthusiastically into other fields, notably cancer immunology and cancer immunotherapy, the promise of which proved to be short lived. To add to the uncertainty of these unsettled times, there were some incidents of scientific misconduct in transplantation research in the early 1970s.

Taking Stock

At the Transplantation Society meeting at The Hague in 1970, the society issued a declaration summarizing the place of organ transplantation in the clinical world. Only kidney transplantation was considered to be a routine service, and grafting of other tissues and organs, notably the heart and bone marrow, "deserved careful clinical trial by experienced teams." This was a coded warning, if one was needed, to prevent any repeat of events in the "Year of the Heart." Thomas Starzl's verdict on transplantation at the time was that "surgeons interested in the extrarenal organs brooded in their self-made dungeons, smuggling messages to each other or communicating by secret signals, tapped on their academic walls. There were very few who continued to try."[5]

Outside of transplant circles, few considered that even kidney transplantation was a treatment generally available. In the cautious world of life insurance, transplantation continued to be viewed with fiscal disdain. In 1973, Richard Simmons in Minneapolis polled seventy-seven major insurance companies in North America, and 90 percent responded that no life insurance could be offered at any premium to those with a kidney graft. Only 12 percent of the companies surveyed would consider life insurance even for a recipient of a kidney from a twin donor.

Bone Marrow Grafting

The first experimental attempts with marrow grafts in the mid-1950s had been intended to protect animals and hence human patients after radiation injury. The technique was an apparently simple one, but it presented an immunological challenge not faced by the surgical transplanters, namely, that the effects of carrying over even small numbers of foreign lymphocytes with the marrow caused an immediate and troublesome graft-versus-host reaction (GvH). Organ transplantation had been largely free of this particular complication, at least in its overt form.[6]

The Boston-trained physician/hematologist E. Donnall Thomas had been involved in the early use of radiation plus "tolerogenic" bone marrow in the Boston human kidney transplants, and, in 1955, he began studying marrow transplantation as a separate, independent project. Over many years, his persistence, and that of others, solved the many discouraging challenges in this field. Thomas moved to Cooperstown in 1955 but maintained his Boston links, and in 1959, as described earlier, he had treated a human patient with leukemia using a twin as the marrow donor, although the leukemia returned later. Thomas moved to Seattle in 1963 and persevered with radiation to destroy the host marrow. But it was the improvements in tissue typing that proved essential in establishing bone

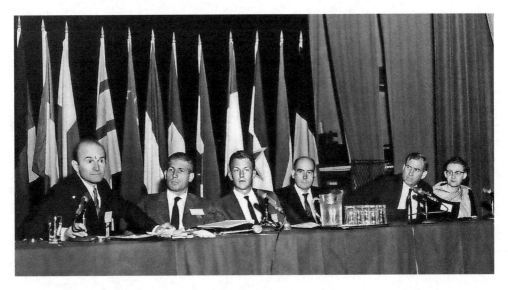

Many of the pioneers in bone marrow research attended a conference on the subject in Paris in 1971. Pictured (*from left to right*) are Georges Mathé, Dirk van Bekkum, Donnall Thomas, Charles Congdon, and Delta Uphoff. Image courtesy of Donnall Thomas.

marrow grafting. In 1968, the first clinical successes with marrow transplants were reported in patients with rare congenital immunological deficits.[7] But treating common blood malignancies was the real goal of marrow transplantation.

New Methods Using Marrow Grafts

Further improvements aided progress in treating blood cancers. The first was the use of strategies to separate out the cells responsible for GvH reactions from the remaining marrow cells to be injected. Dirk van Bekkum began using these pioneering methods in 1968.[8] For the recipient, total body irradiation was used up until 1968 to "make space" for the donor marrow, but George Santos at Baltimore introduced an improvement by using cyclophosphamide; this drug regimen could be controlled more easily than radiation.[9] Donnall Thomas's work greatly benefited from the arrival of antilymphocyte serum, and GvH in the marrow recipients, when it occurred, was treatable.[10] There followed some success in treating blood malignancies using marrow donors within the family, and Thomas soon had some cases without recurrence after four to nine years.

The ultimate goal was the use of unrelated marrow donors, and, in late 1968, Thomas and Robert Good started human bone marrow transplantation using unrelated tissue-typed bone marrow.

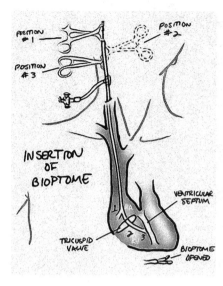

Routine intracardiac biopsy was devised in Norman Shumway's unit at Stanford in 1973, and the procedure greatly aided in the diagnosis of rejection in heart transplants. Image courtesy of the CTS Net, Mayo Clinic.

Slow Progress

In the "extrarenal" situations—liver, pancreas, lung, and heart—only a few surgeons continued to attempt transplants.[11] After his unpromising start in January 1968, Norman Shumway in California alone managed to obtain funds to continue heart transplantation, and results in his unit improved slowly, aided by better quality donor organs, care with recipient selection, and growing confidence with clinical management.[12] By 1972, his results had reached a 40 percent one-year survival rate. In the next year, results again improved, with major support from a new device inserted into a neck vein and passed into the heart and used for routine, repeatable intracardiac biopsy of the heart muscle, thus allowing for regular rejection testing.[13] In 1973, there was one important acknowledgment that heart transplantation would shortly be generally acceptable. Shumway's local Blue Cross insurer, which administered Medicare funds, surprisingly started paying for heart transplantation; the important criterion that the procedure was no longer experimental had thus been met locally. It was a significant milestone, one that others seeking success with liver and other organs had still to reach.

Elsewhere, in Europe, the only heart transplant unit to resume work was in France, where Daniel Guilmet decided to restart his heart transplant work in 1973, after one failed attempt in the "Year of the Heart." He raised private funds for the transplant effort and defied the authorities to stop him, but poor results again terminated the work. The unofficial heart transplantation moratorium in Britain remained in place for some years. Elsewhere, some centers started cautiously again, and, in 1973, with interest growing and results improving, the International Society of Heart Transplantation emerged. A registry of cases had been proposed in 1968 but had been abandoned after the reverses of that year. In 1973, the society drew up a small registry of new transplants.

Blood Transfusion Paradox

But in the early 1970s, the results of kidney transplantation reached a plateau, and then, in some units, the one-year survival got worse. Not all units were affected, and at first it was thought that this was the result of less fit patients being treated or that the newer units did not possess the skills of the pioneers. The explanation, when found, seemed unreasonable at first and was resisted, but there soon was no doubt that the otherwise laudable plan of reducing the number of blood transfusions given to the always-anemic dialysis patients was responsible.[14] This policy had been adopted to prevent the appearance of the undesirable antibodies. This paradox had no known immunological explanation.[15] The finding caused some academic excitement, since it seemed to be a form of specific tolerance, one induced by the physicians.

A new paradigm appeared, and there was a return to cautious empirical blood transfusion, and, as hoped, the results of graft survival did improve, but still without understanding of the mechanism involved. Deliberate blood transfusion continued until the cyclosporine era, and the practice soon included the almost unthinkable deliberate blood transfusion from a future living-related donor to the recipient. This controversial strategy, which apparently risked sensitization of the patient, was successfully introduced by Oscar Salvatierra in 1978.[16] But before the mechanism of this effect could be unraveled, the better results using cyclosporine made the slightly risky transfusion strategy unnecessary.

Verdict on Tissue Typing

At this time in the early 1970s, clinicians were slowly admitting the failure of close tissue typing to ensure excellent results in cadaveric renal transplants. Although some groups, notably in Paris and Leiden, still reported encouraging experience using HLA in predicting graft outcome, the tipping point came at The Hague meeting of the Transplantation Society in 1970.

Paul Terasaki's extensive tissue-typing service in California allowed him to study outcomes, and at The Hague he bravely announced that in a large follow-up study of these cadaveric kidney grafts, there was little or no benefit from pretransplant tissue matching.[17] This result was unexpected, and concerned tissue typers made haste to disagree with this verdict. Possible explanations were offered, notably that not all tissue antigens had yet been identified and that Terasaki's series included only a small number of fully matched patients. The puzzling discovery did not affect the manifest benefit of typing within families to choose the most suitable donor. It also did not diminish the value of typing in bone marrow transplantation, platelet transfusion, or the crucial pretransplant cross-match, and all agreed that close matching would certainly reduce future sensitization in the recipient patient. Tissue typing was thus still secure as a service, but Terasaki's results were still a troubling blow.

The unwelcome message Terasaki delivered in The Hague seemed to threaten the whole edifice, and some took the stance that the messenger had to be shot. Members of the U.S. National Institutes of Health who had attended the meeting in The Hague agreed that Terasaki's histocompatibility studies had no future. After an emergency site visit, the NIH promptly withdrew Terasaki's four-hundred-thousand-dollar grant, leading to the closure of most of his laboratory.[18] Terasaki's unit scraped by in the short term largely by making and selling his own sixty–well tissue–typing trays, called "Terasaki Plates" to this day. These trays, sold for fifteen dollars each, were soon considered to be better than the free, government-supplied typing trays from the NIH Serum Bank. Terasaki retained his honored place as a dominant figure in applied histocompatibility and transplantation studies, and the government later restored funding for his work.

More Typing Methods

Tissue matching did increase in sophistication, and it took a new direction in the mid-1970s. This change in direction may be traced to basic cellular immunological studies by Fritz H. Bach (born 1934) and Barbara Bain, who both reported in 1964 that mixing two sets of lymphocytes would cause the cells to become large blast forms, as in the action of the newly described mitogens like PHA.[19] The response of one set of cells alone could be studied by preventing the reaction of the other set by radiation or mitomycin C. This "one-way" mixed lymphocyte culture (MLC) test initially seemed to be a useful and simple in vitro model of transplantation, that is, of host lymphocytes reacting against donor antigens carried on these donor lymphocytes.[20]

Bach's cellular response was immediately compared to the HLA differences between the cells. At first it seemed, as expected, that within a family, the MLC response was proportionate to the HLA antigen differences. Cells from fully mismatched siblings reacted strongly when mixed while fully matched siblings' cells did not. But cells from fully HLA-matched *unrelated* persons did stimulate each other to become large blast forms. The puzzle of the better survival of related as compared with unrelated grafts at the same level of HLA match was now explained. Something else was the stimulus for the MLC response; it was not HLA but an important genetic area that was close to HLA.[21] The new locus was called HLA-D or DR or Class II, and it was soon found to affect cadaveric graft outcome.

HLA-D Typing

Sera for DR antigens did soon emerge, but, in the interim, target cells had to be used for typing. Fortunately, there was only a single locus DR on each chromosome pair, and the number of DR antigens there was small. This meant that if cells with two identical antigens could be found, they could be used as stimulatory "typing cells," since they effectively possessed only one antigen. To find these homozygous cells quickly, researchers hunted for them among isolated populations with little outside genetic influence. The Inuit of northern Canada found themselves of interest to immunologists, as did some closed religious communities in North America and the headhunters of Borneo. In Europe, the cousin marriage registers of the Catholic Church were an obvious, but possibly confidential database, and although access to such records in France was denied, in Italy and the Netherlands the Catholic Church's records were opened up to the transplant scientists.[22]

At first, only this homozygous cell stimulation method was possible, but the tissue typers moved quickly to develop routine serological testing. Peter Morris and Alan Ting first reported the added value of matching for the DR system in organ transplantation in 1978, and thereafter it was used in addition to HLA-A and HLA-B tests.[23] DR typing again raised hopes for complete prediction of outcome in cadaveric kidney transplantation, although this goal again proved elusive. However, each advance in typing meant an advance for bone marrow grafts between unrelated persons.

More Immunological Insights

This period was characterized by the clinical introduction of the use of the many in vitro tests which had appeared in the immunological labs in the 1960s. Proud of these insights, the immunologists had teased the surgeons, accusing them of measuring nothing, and this challenge was now responded to with gusto. With a plethora of tests available which apparently offered hope of assessing transplantation outcome, or monitoring rejection, or judging appropriate levels of immunosuppression, the surgeons made haste to attempt to avoid the "empiric" label. These tests simply mixed donor tissue of some kind with the host's responding lymphocytes. Although prodigious amounts of experimental work were done, the complexity of the intact human response was never reproduced in the test tube.

There were hopes that routine levels of migration inhibition factor (MIF) would help.[24] Clinicians were already using MLC and cell-mediated lympholysis (CML) tests, which mimicked graft destruction, and T- and B-subset cell counts plus lymphocyte mitogen transformation tests, colony inhibition, and cytokine production measurements were also available to surgeons.[25] If advanced laboratory facilities were available to clinicians, a battery of these new tests could be used in post-transplant management. There was then a period of enthusiasm for intensive and expensive "immunological monitoring." Interest faded when no single indispensable test or even a group of in vitro tests was found to relate usefully to ongoing clinical events, notably in regularly anticipating rejection and thus allowing clinicians to make a preemptive strike to stave off a rejection crisis. The hunt was abandoned when the use of cyclosporine reduced the daily threat of rejection.

Basic immunology made one huge, practical contribution to transplant management at this time. In 1975, Georges Köhler and César Milstein managed to fuse antibody-forming cells with tumor cells, thus producing robust cell lines that made specific antibodies.[26] These "monoclonal" antibodies revolutionized not only the scientific study of antibodies but also produced powerful reagents for day-to-day use in research, diagnosis, therapy, and tissue typing.[27] In clinical transplantation, monoclonal antibodies also signaled the availability of new, pure, antilymphocyte sera directed against the various new subsets of lymphocytes, thus raising new hopes for clinical immunosuppression. Benedict "Ben" Cosimi was the first to report favorable experience in dealing with human graft rejection using the monoclonal OKT3, prepared by E. L. Reinherz and S. F. Schlossman and active against CD3 lymphocytes.[28]

Also in the mid-1970s came a long-awaited insight into the "real" role of histocompatibility and cellular recognition when Peter Doherty and Rolf Zinkernagel made their Nobel Prize–winning observation of "restriction," namely that T-cells could only kill virally infected cells which carried the same histocompatibility antigens as these T-cells. The major histocompatibility complex (MHC) seemed to control a membrane region to which cell constituents were constantly moved for study by outside T-cells.[29] This finding at last explained the puzzle, first highlighted and then partly explained by Leo Loeb, that dead allograft cells do not provoke an immune response.

Also at this time, more findings emerged to remind the medical community that tissue typing had wider significance beyond tissue transplantation. The first noteworthy finding was the report of an association of particular tissue-typing antigens with disease. In 1973, Donald Kuban and Terasaki noticed a relationship between the presence of HLA antigen B13 and the skin disease psoriasis, and in the following year D. P. Singal showed more such disease links.[30] Many similar findings appeared quickly, of which the most notable was the association between ankylosing spondylitis and antigen B27. Thereafter, a large range of diseases, especially autoimmune diseases, showed tantalizing associations, weak or strong, with HLA, as part of the ever-widening linkage of disease and genetic susceptibility.

Improved Transplant Management

The search for better methods of immunosuppression continued in the early 1970s, and some showed promise. The pharmaceutical industry still had little interest in transplantation, and it was to older ideas and familiar drugs already on the market that surgical attention turned. The anticancer agent cyclophosphamide made a brief return to favor in kidney transplantation in 1971 as a possible substitute for azathioprine.[31] There were also short trials of cyproheptadine (an antihistamine), the antihelminthic drug niridazole, and macrophage blockers such as silica and carrageenan. Pretransplant thoracic duct drainage also had new supporters.[32] Total lymphoid irradiation (TLI), that is, radiation restricted to the lymphoid organs, which had been used safely in the treatment of the lymphoid malignancy Hodgkin's disease, also had a new vogue.[33] Support emerged for pretreatment of the cadaveric donor to remove mobile "passenger" cells like mobile lymphocytes with the hope of making the graft less antigenic.[34] None of these measures found a routine place in graft management. The most important and permanent improvement was that lower doses of steroids were found to be as effective as the higher dose assumed from earliest days to be necessary in the post-transplant regimen. These lower doses lessened many of the dangers and reduced the side effects prominent in the early post-transplant period.[35]

Surgical Management

Day-to-day surgical care for transplant patients steadily improved. Early detection and early treatment of infection was still crucial, and it was a time of the helpful arrival of newer antibiotics in the penicillin and cephalosporin groups. Fungal infections, particularly in those patients receiving antilymphocyte sera of the various kinds, were prominent and promptly addressed. Treatable *Pneumocystis carinii* lung infections were recognized.[36] A major advance came when the usually benign cytomegalovirus infection was found to be a more common post-transplant event than previously suspected. This virus was transferred in the donated organ, and detection of previous infection in the donor permitted prophylaxis or early diagnosis and treatment of infection in the recipient.[37]

Renal biopsy had had a controversial entry into management of transplants in 1968, but the Melbourne transplanters eventually persuaded other units around the world that routine use of the improved Vim-Silverman biopsy needle was safe and helpful in assessing kidney graft function.[38]

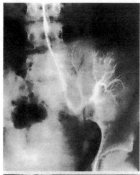

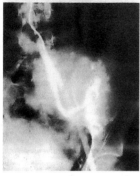

Angiography of the transplanted kidney could reveal renal artery stenosis as a cause of post-transplant hypertension. From D. Carr, R. O. Quin, D. N. H. Hamilton, et al., "Transluminal Dilatation of Transplant Renal Artery Stenosis," *British Medical Journal* 2 (1980): 196–98.

Radiological Assistance

Imaging of the transplanted kidney had, until the early 1970s, been restricted to conventional examination via intravenous pyelography (IVP) of grafts that were functioning well. Such radiological imaging merely showed dye in the ureter and renal pelvis and at best a faint shadow of the kidney. Even the traditional retrograde studies of the ureter by inserting a fine catheter from the bladder upwards were usually impossible because of the awkwardly situated and fragile new entrance of the transplanted ureter in the dome of the bladder. Angiography of the kidney blood vessels with injected contrast media, although displaying the arterial supply in detail, was not suitable for repeated use, and it revealed little about the quality of function other than that there was flow in the renal artery—or not. Angiography still had a niche role in showing renal artery stenosis, a short narrowing of this vessel, which posed an unpleasant surgical challenge until alternative methods for dealing with it emerged using balloon catheter dilatation from within.[39] When isotope scanning became available, it was frequently used to study the post-transplant kidney.[40] These scans with isotopes excreted by the kidney offered noninvasive reassurance that blood flow existed, or did not, particularly during any period before the graft functioned. Scans could be repeated, and serial comparisons helped transplanters diagnose rejection.

But it was the rise of ultrasound in the 1970s—simple, economical, safe, and repeatable—which was to emerge in a key role in transplant management and was to supplement and then largely replace isotope scanning. One surprise seen regularly on the new ultrasound scans was the accumulation of lymph adjacent to transplanted kidneys, and these areas could be aspirated by needle by the increasingly confident "interventional" sonographers.[41] Ultrasound could also detect complications arising in the ureter, which often could be dealt with without open surgery.[42]

Kidney Transplantation Funding

The funding of transplantation varied according to the type of health care system involved. In the United States, growing alarm at the costs of regular dialysis meant that the government encouraged kidney transplantation, enacting Medicare amendments from 1970 onward. Under the new

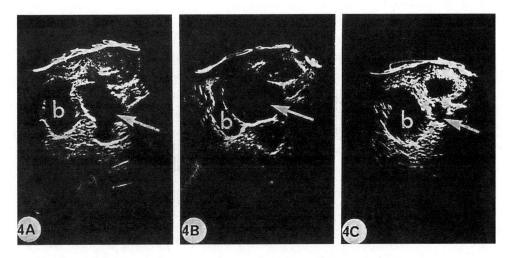

Ultrasound played an increasing role in imaging the transplanted kidney and aided the steady improvement in management from the mid-1970s. Its earliest success was in detecting and draining lymph collections around the graft. From P. Morley, E. Barnet, P. R. F. Bell, et al., "Ultrasound in the Diagnosis of Fluid Collections Following Renal Transplantation," *Clinical Radiology* 126 (1975): 199–207.

guidelines, the health care program paid not only for the transplant operation and twelve months' care and medication but also for organ procurement agencies. This government transplant funding carried with it increasing oversight and audit, and, allied to this activity, certification of individual units followed. The first stipulation came in 1973, and was an interesting "volume" condition, of the kind to be routine later, namely that only units carrying out fifty kidney transplants per year would get unconditional Medicare certification; the remaining units would be watched. Protests were made, particularly by states like Georgia, with small transplant units, and reflex opposition also came from libertarian medical politicians who opposed any ceiling and disputed that greater volume necessarily meant greater quality. The threshold for automatic Medicare certification was eventually lowered to fifteen grafts per year, thus leaving kidney transplantation in the United States well funded, but largely unregulated, for some time.[43] But central funding could give some distortions.[44] Payments for regular dialysis were still generous, and this flow of funds still provided a predictable and profitable income for private nephrologists caring for even a small number of regular dialysis patients. Such units sought and retained these valuable patients (a practice flippantly called "cattle rustling"), and the system discouraged referral for transplantation. Lower-cost home dialysis failed to flourish in spite of considerable U.S. government encouragement, financial and otherwise.

Other countries did not have the same type of funding concerns. In Britain, the centrally funded National Health Service and its salaried staff encouraged the emergence of a joint transplant/dialysis service. By 1972, both were accepted as established modalities of treatment and these were to be integrated as a single renal replacement therapy. Transplantation and home dialysis were encouraged because of lower costs.[45] A dilemma for patients and doctors was, as ever, that dialysis often gave better patient survival, but the quality of life with a successful transplant was better.

As transplant patient survival improved during the 1970s, and with dialysis after a failed transplant now an unquestioned routine, patients increasingly opted for the hope of a "no-lose" transplant. In most countries in the early 1970s, the average age for kidney graft recipients was about twenty-five, with only occasional recipients over the age of fifty. A new trend emerged, however, with older, younger, and higher risk patients being treated by dialysis. The criteria for patients receiving transplant approval were also broadening. Those with heart disease, diabetes, or previous malignancy in particular were no longer automatically excluded from consideration.[46] With these changes, the estimates of future numbers requiring renal replacement proved to be seriously flawed.

Donor Drives

In the United States, the Special Services Administration in 1973 brought the existing organ sharing agencies under a single regulatory umbrella, and, by the mid-1980s, there were about forty organ sharing agencies, funded by reimbursement through Medicare. The Uniform Anatomical Gift Act had encouraged donation and donor cards. As the number of donations rose, and the work involved in donation grew, a new position emerged in the transplant units worldwide to share the organizational work with the surgeons: the transplant coordinator.[47] Their activities aided in the procurement of organs, organized the procedures surrounding surgical donation, and took on liaison activities with the local and national sharing schemes. They could also be responsible for public and professional education and contacts with the families involved.

Many governments also took some initiatives to increase donation rates, notably issuing kidney donor cards indicating a person's willingness to donate. The donor card program effectively promoted family discussions and decisions about donation, even by those who were not cardholders. No other organ was considered for inclusion on the "kidney" card; such were the assumptions of the times. In Britain, these cards were publicized and widely available in many outlets, but controversy arose. Initial publicity suggested, reasonably enough, that the signing and carrying of the card gave legal permission for organ removal at the time of death. The authorities were pressed to agree that this was the case, but soon the formal legal opinion was the reverse—that the obscure "person lawfully in charge of the body" alone still had this power of permitting organ removal, after "reasonable consultation." Since this person had never been legally defined, the best, and impractical, advice was that this task fell to the hospital administrator. Donations in Britain did rise in the 1970s, and the donor card scheme was judged a success. The number of cards held by individuals reached a plateau by the 1990s, and surveys showed that 20 percent of the UK population carried such a card. With the growth of "extrarenal" transplants in the late 1970s, Britain introduced a multi-organ card (heart, liver, pancreas, and eyes) in 1981, and lungs were added to the list in 1985.

The Transplanters Diversify

The early 1970s were slack years for innovation in mainstream transplantation. No major clinical novelties emerged, and there was disappointment that many laboratory insights had failed to assist transplant efforts and be incorporated into routine transplant management. Progress seemed to be occurring mainly in the worthy work of steadily improving the management of patients, notably through better control of infection and better radiology, and the organization of transplant efforts. Some of those who had been most active earlier now seemed restless. Joseph Murray in Boston moved out of transplantation and resumed his former plastic surgery work. Starzl in Denver took on the chairmanship of the VA Hospital's Department of Surgery and observed that the "transplant crusade had become a business with intellectual growth arrest," one now merely engaged in a "shuffling of detail and adjustment of earlier attitudes."[48] He returned to his research on liver metabolism and for two or three years took a major interest in the hepatotrophic substance found in portal vein blood which sustained the liver.[49] In 1975, he took a sabbatical, which he spent at St. Mary's Hospital in London. Some transplant surgeons began turning their attention to the study of the diminished immune response after trauma and surgery. Among tissue typers, those in a fin de siècle mood concentrated on linkages with disease rather than transplantation.

But the most significant development at the time, occasionally embarrassing in retrospect, were the increasing claims in the surgical world for successful cancer control by immunotherapy—the immunological manipulation of the immune response. This goal beguiled and attracted some members of the transplantation community, and it seemed that these two disciplines might be considered two sides of the same coin. Suppressing immunity for grafting had been established; boosting it for cancer therapy had attractive symmetry. There were always cancer patients in need of treatment in the surgical units, and laboratory studies used familiar methodology and terminology, so this new vista took some transplanters away from their traditional work, for a while. By the early 1970s, both Peter Medawar, the key innovator in applied immunology, and Michael Woodruff, the exemplar of the transplant surgeon/scientist, had moved into studies of the immunology of cancer, as had Macfarlane Burnet. They were joined by others, notably Georges Mathé, the Paris hematologist involved in early human kidney and marrow transplantation. As a result, the Transplantation Society accepted this new double aspect of immunology and for a while hosted extra meetings on cancer immunology. The transplant journals also began publishing papers on cancer immunology and its uses.

The Immune Hypothesis in Cancer Research

The bold hypothesis was that emerging human and experimental tumors act as subtle grafts and that in the early stages these early tumor cells are normally removed by the surveillance of the immune system. If aberrant cancer cells do escape a host immunological response, the established cancer could then be treated by generally "boosting the immune response."[50] Little remains in clinical use now from this early, simple approach.[51]

The starting point for this work was remarkably similar to the suggestive clues and hints that had earlier linked transplant loss to an immune response. In experimental and human cancers, there is often a notable lymphocyte infiltrate and a local lymph node reaction, as in tissue transplantation. The early immunologists had ignored these graft lymphocytes, and their latter-day counterparts now perhaps made amends by not mentally airbrushing these cells out of the microscopic appearances in cancer. Moreover, Leo Loeb, who, in the 1930s, tried to draw attention to the role of the lymphocyte in transplantation, had proposed that the cellular immune system had a surveillance role of some kind. The new studies were suggesting that Loeb might have been right. Cancer patients in general and those with lymphoid cancers and Hodgkin's disease in particular have a weak immunological responsiveness. This immunological "defect," if it were a primary event, rather than secondary as the result of cancer, could be invoked as permitting the development and spread of cancer.

Many anecdotes existed about spontaneous regression of human cancer, and these patients could be seen to be offering further "experiments of Nature" of the type that had been so helpful in dissecting the normal immune response. These tales of disappearing tumors were adduced as possible immunological rejection of the malignancies, and "Coley's toxin," which New York surgeon William Coley claimed in the early twentieth century could cause sarcomas to shrink, was recalled with new interest.[52] There was also the understandable excitement when the first of many cancers appeared in immunosuppressed transplant patients. These cancers regressed when immunosuppression was withdrawn, and the finding seemed initially to support a more general link between the immune response and cancer control. It all seemed to fit.

The hopes for establishing the presence of an immunological dimension to human cancer, and hence the prospect of useful immunotherapy, were given a useful start by earlier findings. Richmond Prehn and Joan Main, who had made major contributions to experimental transplantation, reported in 1957 that there were unusual "foreign" antigens on chemically induced rat tumors.[53] Other descriptions of such tumor-specific antigens followed in the 1960s, and a major finding was that some human embryonic antigens, notably the alpha fetoprotein and carcinoembryonic antigens, which normally disappear in early childhood, persisted on some human tumors. Tumor-associated antigens surely meant that a host immune response was likely; and, if the immune response had failed on its own to control the tumor, perhaps it could be assisted to do so more effectively.

Blocking Factors

These findings were followed by confident claims that, when host lymphoid cells were tested against the cancer cells, there were weak human and experimental immune responses to tumors. Researchers suggested that this natural response was continuously present and was normally successful. Cancer development was thus seen as a failure of this host response, and soon there was a detailed immunological explanation of the failure in that "blocking antibodies" nullified this surveillance response. A few labs quickly reported these blocking agents to be present in many other situations featuring immunological unresponsiveness, including tolerance, pregnancy, bone marrow chimeras, and successful kidney transplants.[54] Leslie Brent later ruefully concluded that "blocking factors of one kind or another seemed to sweep everything before them in the early 1970s and appeared to offer a plausible explanation for the phenomenon of enhancement and many other forms of specific unresponsiveness."[55]

Other investigators could not replicate these exciting findings, said to need skill and experience to detect.

Immunotherapy

At this time, the assumption persisted that nonspecific stimulation of the alleged anticancer immune responses to tumor antigens, postulated or identified, could check tumor growth, and successful methods of nonspecific immune stimulation had been available for some time.[56] Obtaining increased antibody responses was a familiar strategy in the lab and in immunization, and a number of well-established "adjuvants" to stimulate the immune system were already available, most notably, from France, the famous BCG (Bacille de Calmette-Guérin) strain of *Mycobacterium tuberculosis*. In 1958, A. R. Prévot, working in Paris, found that the otherwise bland organism *Corynebacterium parvum* was also a remarkable immunostimulant, and, by 1959, B. N. Halpern's laboratory, also in Paris, had shown that such stimulation would cause regression of experimental animal tumors.

Further support for this strategy came in 1961. Woodruff, in Edinburgh, had obtained a large Medical Research Council grant in the early 1960s that he used not only for his well-known transplantation immunology studies, notably making antilymphocyte serum, but also for some tumor immunology work.[57] J. G. Howard, who had worked with Halpern in Paris, was part of the Edinburgh group, and, by 1965, just when Woodruff's exciting transplant work with antilymphocyte serum was gaining international attention, Howard demonstrated in studies with the rat that *Corynebacterium parvum* caused prompt regression of some transplantable cancers.[58] It was a remarkable double achievement for the Edinburgh group and seemed to emphasize that the two uses of immune manipulation were closely linked.

It was thought that immunotherapy might be most effective in dealing with micro-metastatic cancer cell deposits. It was conceded that the new strategy might not be powerful enough to deal with large, bulky tumors, but initial treatment with surgery or chemotherapy could be followed by immunotherapy to reach and deal with the residual deposits of malignant cells. Seductive new military metaphors emerged for the role of immunotherapy, such as hopes for "sniping with lethal accuracy," "mopping up unreachable strongholds," or "guided missiles rather than mortar bombs," and traditional cancer therapy could, conversely, be depicted and patronized as "a blind man hitting out with a bat."[59]

It was a time of slow progress in conventional anticancer therapy, with some hostility to the rigors of chemotherapy and radiation. There was also rising popular interest in "natural" treatment of disease in general. This mood welcomed the emergence of immunotherapy, which was soon officially called the "Fourth Modality" of cancer treatment.[60] For some, immunotherapy echoed older views of disease and therapy, especially the idea that the *terrain*, the host constitution beloved by the holistic physicians, was important after all. Remarkable enthusiasm for immunological stimulation in human cancer followed, in spite of warnings that, because of the plausibility of the idea, one perhaps too good to be false, a particularly skeptical approach and a cautious evaluation would be required.

Cancer Immunotherapy Outcomes

Moving from animal studies to humans, positive early results were indeed reported in human cancer treatment with the two biological agents BCG and *C. parvum*. In the United States, the National Cancer Act of 1971 made grants available for immunotherapy, and these funds were channeled through the new Biological Response Modifiers Program of the National Cancer Institute. By 1973, the National Institutes of Health (NIH) could report that fifty trials of human cancer immunotherapy were in progress.[61] A new society and a new journal appeared to service the subject, namely the Society for Biological Therapy and its *Journal of Biological Response Modifiers*. The journal *Transplantation* accepted papers on immunopotentiation for a while, and the CIBA Foundation, whose symposia had served transplantation so well, hosted a meeting on immunopotentiation in 1973, at Medawar's suggestion, as did the Royal Society of Medicine in London soon after.[62] Another journal, *Cancer Immunology and Immunotherapy*, started in 1976 to deal with, as the editor claimed, "the newest modality of therapy in the armamentarium of the clinical oncologist, and one of the most exciting."

By 1976, at the height of the immunotherapy enthusiasm, 347 studies in human cancer were continuing, with two-thirds using BCG and the rest involving *C. parvum* or derivatives of it. Some new agents also appeared, including levamisole, a chemical "immunomodulator." The respectability of immunotherapy continued, and, by 1979, the International Registry of Tumor Immunotherapy had made its seventh report on the various studies in progress that year.

Growing Disenchantment

But, soon after, careful investigators began to report no benefit from these strategies in human cancer. Vital support for the new movement had come from Mathé's early claim in 1969 that, in an apparently convincing controlled trial, BCG could add benefit to conventional therapy in acute lymphatic leukemia. Now the British Medical Research Council's "Concorde" trial in leukemia showed no effect when adding BCG in this way. The end was at hand for the hopes for simplistic human cancer immunotherapy. The early positive results were now overtaken by increasing numbers of negative reports. New trials ceased and older ones were terminated, as was the International Registry of Tumor Immunotherapy. The Biological Response Modifiers Program in the United States was closed, and the Society for Biological Therapy and its *Journal of Biological Response Modifiers* changed course. In 1985, the publication became the *Journal of Immunotherapy,* and its contents reverted to the always interesting animal tumor models. Use of the word *immunotherapy* was reserved for describing attempts at vaccination against specific cancers and the use of the numerous new monoclonal antibodies in the treatment of specific cancers.

This sequence of events raised not only the familiar question of the relevance of animal studies to human disease and treatment but also the difficulty in dealing with plausible new hypotheses.[63] David Weiss had a harsh verdict on the early human immunotherapy trials: "There would seem to be little excuse for the wild optimism at the outset and even less for its stubborn propagation. . . . Investigators and physicians have joined institutional administrators and media specimens in symphonies whose preludes are brainless hopefulness, their coda, when the results are in, silence or a dirge of disenchantment."[64]

One of the surgeons active in this area, Steven Rosenberg, in 1992 summed up the impasse with a statement suggesting that the immunotherapy edifice had always had a shaky foundation: "It is every immunologist's dream to use the immune system to cure cancer. It is every immunologist's nightmare that there is no such thing as an immune response to cancer in humans."[65]

Therapy on the Fringes

Others—those on the fringes of conventional medical practice—did not abandon the cause for immunotherapy and also found that claims about "stimulating the body's defenses" resonated nicely with their clients' preconceptions of what was useful, even natural, therapy. One prominent European practitioner was Josef Issels, who skillfully publicized his German private clinic and treated advanced cancer patients, including some celebrities, with a complex, holistic regimen he termed *Ganzheitstherapie,* which included fever therapy and an "autovaccine" made from the patient's own tonsils. These public claims led some British patients to demand similar treatment and forced respectable organizations to visit his clinic and study his data, but they gave universally negative reports upon their return.[66]

Misconduct and Experimental Treatments

At this time, attitudes to human experimentation were changing, and for innovation in transplantation, human subjects had been turned to in the past. There had been earlier concern when Chester Southam's group in New York went beyond even the permissive attitudes of the 1950s and injected live tumor cells from cancer patients into inmates of a mental hospital, in the hope of developing an antitumor vaccine. In another unpleasant event, a patient's melanoma was grafted experimentally to her mother, with a fatal outcome.[67] Groups exploring the ethics of medicine began to issue calls, from both the public and the profession, for ethical controls on medical research.

Added to this, this unsettled time in the world of transplantation in the 1970s saw some of the first episodes in biomedical research of scientific misconduct, a term used when claims were made known to be false. Two incidents arose from laboratory transplantation studies, and one was a defining moment in the new awareness that scientific deception was not a rare aberration, as previously supposed. The first, and lesser known of two cases, emerged when a Stanford medical student attending The Hague meeting of the Transplantation Society in 1970 noticed that, in a paper based on his student project but written and presented by his supervisor, favorable extra data had been added, and the student raised the matter after returning home. After a similar episode in the same laboratory later that year, an investigation ensued, but the local institutional verdict was that there had been "incompetence in note keeping, rather than fabrication." Further complaints regarding the same investigator reached the authorities in subsequent years, and a full National Institutes of Health inquiry, the first of its kind, charitably concluded that in his research, the surgeon tended to "anticipate results in place of waiting for the final data." There the matter rested. It was assumed that such incidents were rare and could be glossed over after temporary embarrassment.[68]

The outcome of the celebrated "painted mice" case was more conclusive. In 1973, William T. Summerlin, a favored protégé of Robert Good, by then working at the Sloan-Kettering Institute in New York, appeared to have achieved an ancient goal when he claimed permanent survival of skin grafts from black C57Bl mice on white Balb/c mice. His new method was in fact an old one, used without success before, namely tissue culture of the grafts for some days before transplantation, in the hope that surface antigens would be lost. Others were unable to replicate Summerlin's findings, and his paper and its fuzzy images of the grafts received a cool reception at the meeting of the Transplantation Society in San Francisco that year. The data, even though published in the society's *Proceedings,* might have been decently and charitably ignored as one of the unrepeatable claims which appear from time to time, but the findings had been given wide publicity as part of the necessary fund-raising by the Sloan-Kettering Institute. Complaints reached Robert Good. The mice in question were brought in for his inspection, and the supposedly surviving black skin grafts had been improved for that presentation with a black felt-tipped pen. Investigation of Summerlin and public disgrace followed.[69]

Brain Death Issues

By the mid-1970s, critical care management throughout the world routinely employed "brain-death" criteria—Harvard's or close derivatives thereof. Few intensive care units were in proximity to surgical units with transplant interests, and after the controversies during the "Year of the Heart," inquiries about obtaining organs were not always welcome. The criteria for brain death became clearer and simpler, concentrating on the preconditions of inability to breathe, deep coma, and absent reflexes. Some of the tests in the pioneer Boston brain death document were proving less useful than supposed, notably the requirements for a "flat" electroencephalogram tracing (EEG), namely an absence of brain electrical activity and an absence of spinal cord reflexes.[70]

Brain-death Criteria

Kansas, California, and the American Bar Association by 1975 had given support to the new situation, namely that one legal time of death was when the brain-death criteria were met.[71] The widely used criteria faced a legal test in the United States in 1977 in the *Golston* case, when a Massachusetts court accepted the brain-death criteria as a legal definition of death; there were similar court actions in other states.[72] In 1981, a presidential commission agreed with a report, *Defining Death,* which accepted as dead those with "irreversible cessation of all functions of the entire brain, including the brain stem." The Uniform Determination of Death Act quickly followed in 1981 using the same wording and had prominence as the fastest-known enactment in American uniform legislation—that is, laws which would apply to all states, instead of piecemeal development.

Some countries continued to be cautious in drawing up legal definitions of death.[73] By 1976, in Britain it was thought the time had come to regularize brain-death criteria, and this standardization was done not by legislation but via a consensus statement issued by a joint committee of the Colleges of Physicians and Surgeons, with input from the government's Department of Health.[74] This group had consulted widely and had made no haste to reach a final position. The guidelines, later known as the "UK Code," were accepted by the medical profession, and it studiously made no mention of transplantation.[75] The UK Code changed the terminology in use, emphasizing "brain stem" death as a more precise anatomical and functional description than "brain death." The criteria were made available for public comment, and, to the relief of the authorities, there was no public opposition and professional criticism was minimal.[76]

It was not until three years after this Colleges of Physicians and Surgeons report that the UK minister of health felt the time had come to acknowledge and advise on organ donation from brain-dead donors. The minister issued a code that gave official support to heart-beating donations, that is, the removal of organs from patients diagnosed as brain dead while ventilation and heart function continued.[77] The new approach had not been widely used; until that time, Britain had only one unit offering more than kidney transplantation.[78] Heart-beating donation was thereafter steadily agreed by intensivists, and it improved the quality of donated organs, particularly the liver and heart.

Clinical Progress Resumes

The hesitation in transplant activity that had characterized much of the 1970s finally ceased late in the decade. When Leslie Brent gave his presidential address at the 1976 meeting of the Transplantation Society, he felt it necessary to ask if progress was being made. He sensed, correctly, that something was going to happen. With professional loyalty, he suggested that the impetus would come from a basic biological insight: "The immunological jigsaw is at last about to take shape. . . . Perhaps 1976 will be seen, in retrospect, to have provided the gateway for that progress in clinical immunology that we have all been hoping and waiting for."[79]

Shortly thereafter, progress was indeed made, but the leap forward came not from solving the immunologic puzzles, nor from finding, at last, the immunologist's Holy Grail of tolerance induction. It came instead from the grinding work of mass routine testing of rather ordinary botanical material in a Swiss pharmaceutical laboratory. A new immunosuppressive drug emerged, and the fungal product cyclosporine, after a slow start, was to transform the world of organ transplantation.

18 The Arrival of Cyclosporine

AFTER THE UNCERTAIN AND AT TIMES discouraging events of the middle 1970s, the mood in the transplant world changed. In 1976, a possibly useful immunosuppressive agent made its first appearance in a pharmaceutical company laboratory and then slowly made its way into transplant management. Cyclosporine (CsA) was a difficult drug to use, but it was to bring fundamental change to transplantation, making most forms of organ grafting routine and noncontroversial.[1] The grafting of each organ increasingly had its own management routine, immunosuppression protocols, training, and interdisciplinary linkages.[2] With this expansion came new challenges and, above all, growing shortages of donor organs. Transplantation units increased in numbers and activity, and when they emerged for the first time beyond Europe and North America, the differing attitudes to cadaveric organ donation in some developing countries were clear. The pharmaceutical industry now regarded transplantation as a profitable area for investment, leading to the emergence of many new products. These were marketed aggressively, and the industry became closely and at times controversially linked to day-to-day life in the transplant units.

Cyclosporine was the first major improvement in immunosuppression since 1963, when steroids had been added to azathioprine. Also known as cyclosporin, ciclosporin(e), cyclosporin-A or by brand names Sandimmun(e) and later Neoral, cyclosporine had emerged from routine study of fungi brought from all parts of the world to the Microbiological Department of the Sandoz company in Basel, Switzerland, where researchers analyzed them for possible biological activity.[3] Sandoz had been screening soil samples since 1970, initially looking only for cytostatic activity among fungi, that is, anticancer and antibacterial properties. To this battery of studies, they then added some simple immunological tests, and shortly afterward one of their fungal products—Ovalicin—was shown to

380

be a promising immunosuppressive agent both in vitro and in experimental transplantation. Preliminary human testing, however, showed unacceptable platelet damage, a side effect not seen in experimental animal studies, and development work on the drug ceased. In 1971, after stepping up their "General Screening Programme," in which they looked at twenty new agents each week, preparation #24-556 entered the system. It came from the mycelia of a Norwegian strain of *Tolypocladium inflatum,* a fungus collected by a Sandoz researcher on a holiday visit to Scandinavia in 1970. Finding it to show some antimicrobial activity, the screeners then sent it to the immunological program in Hartmann Stähelin's lab, without any particular expectations. It showed a promising and marked reduction of antibody formation in mice in studies carried out by Jean-François Borel (born 1933). The usual "forced culture" and purification of the resulting products followed, and the active agent was shown to be a novel endecapeptide that had a very specific suppressive action against lymphocytes. A modest quantity of the active substance was made, and, designated product #27-400, it was sent for further testing in other Sandoz laboratories. Although the company managers were unenthusiastic about its commercial prospects, by the end of 1973 the immunosuppressive properties of the peptide were confirmed in other animal systems, notably experimental allergic inflammation of the brain and spinal cord. Borel hoped to save the development of his product by advocating its use in treating autoimmune diseases, and his last gram of #27-400 fortunately depressed autoimmune arthritis in rats, thus showing promise for use in that group of inflammatory diseases regarded as a priority at Sandoz.

The company's management provided funds with a view to developing the substance to treat rheumatoid disease, and since #27-400 was a cyclical peptide made from spores, it was neatly christened cyclosporine. The drug also seemed promising because of its low toxicity in animal tests, and although it was immunosuppressive, it did not depress bone marrow function. Surprisingly, these and later tests showed no kidney damage in the lab animals studied. This result later seemed to be merely luck, as nephrotoxicity was to be a major side effect of the drug in humans.

First Announcement

Six years after the study commenced at Basel, the first scientific paper on cyclosporine (CsA) was given by the Sandoz group to the meeting of the Swiss Societies for Experimental Biology in April 1976. Borel spoke a few weeks later at a meeting of the British Society for Immunology, and his results were published in that year.[4] At the BSI, the paper aroused the interest of some transplantation teams and led to a number of requests to the company for a supply of the new agent. Sandoz favored Roy Calne's Cambridge unit with a supply, and CsA was immediately studied there by David White. Experimental organ transplantation studies, notably in the rat heart model, confirmed the potential of CsA as a powerful immuno-suppressive drug.[5] The Basel and Cambridge groups also found that oral administration was possible, since the drug could be absorbed if dissolved in olive oil or corn oil, as used later.[6]

However, Sandoz managers were not convinced of the commercial po-tential of CsA, since the estimated costs of extraction, purification, and bringing this new drug to market were huge. They knew, as other drug companies had concluded in the past, that the organ transplantation mar-ket in the mid-1970s was still a small one, largely restricted to kidney trans-plantation and without serious volume sales. When the company proposed to discontinue the project, Calne and White traveled to Basel and made the case to the directors for continued production. The company relented and decided to proceed, although partly as a prestige project. The CsA-led ex-pansion of the market for immunosuppressive drugs later greatly rewarded Sandoz's early investment.

The first patients treated with CsA were reported in 1978 and were kidney graft recipients at Cambridge.[7] A second group consisted of bone marrow transplant cases at the Royal Marsden Hospital, London.[8] Calne's historic report highlighted the possibilities for the new agent, but it soon emerged that CsA unexpectedly damaged the kidneys. Since this damage mimicked rejection, transplanters logically but inappropriately increased immunosuppression, often adding other agents, and some deaths and early malignant lymphomas resulted. Blood level monitoring, helped by re-nal biopsy or fine needle aspirates, could detect and prevent toxicity. Side effects of CsA were soon mitigated by the use of lower doses, and no more tumors appeared. Calne confidently persevered with use of CsA as a single agent.[9] This "monotherapy" was not to be routine, however, after the new agent was cautiously released in 1980 for human use. Thomas Starzl in Denver, for the second time in his career, added steroids, thus developing a new combined regimen—CsA plus prednisone (later prednisolone).[10]

Clinical Experience with CsA

But the initial results with the combined regimen were inconclusive. Al-though Starzl at Denver reported success, in Boston the results were judged to be poor and side effects too numerous for routine use, and some others soon shared this negative verdict. In 1983, a European trial reported a major benefit in using CsA, but a similar Canadian multicenter trial re-ported only marginally better results, and one of the biggest centers within this trial, at Toronto, reported no benefit at all.[11] The explanation of this hesitant start for the celebrated drug was that use of CsA was an acquired skill rather than a science. After its release by the U.S. Food and Drug Administration for routine use in 1983, all units steadily converted to using it.

As clinicians gained further experience with CsA, they began to see a reliable and major improvement in organ transplantation results, with not only increasing graft survival but also a lower patient mortality. Rejection episodes seemed less abrupt, and day-to-day surveillance of the patients could thus be relaxed. A set of novel complications soon became apparent and familiar to clinicians: inappropriate hair growth, diabetes, hypertension, hyperplasia of the gums, and mild central nervous disturbances.[12] There was an increase in Epstein-Barr virus B-cell lymphomas, as well as a slight increase in thrombosis rate in the donor kidney vessels.

Significantly, however, CsA seemed to override major mismatches in tissue typing, and this finding cleared the way toward the first use of completely mismatched family members as kidney donors. It also removed the barrier to taking a kidney graft from a willing unrelated donor, notably a husband or wife. This use of "emotionally related" donors had previously been discouraged not only on ethical grounds but simply because the results were so poor.[13] This success with unrelated living kidney donation also opened the door to less admirable arrangements. The use of paid donors had always been roundly condemned on moral and clinical grounds: now only the ethical distaste remained and this scruple about organ purchase and use was not universally encountered.

Other CsA Effects

Routine, safe, and effective kidney transplantation changed many things. In particular, dialysis for chronic renal failure was increasingly seen as a temporary measure for use while awaiting kidney transplantation and for survival between transplants. Governments encouraged this cost-saving shift, and economists pointed to hidden savings resulting from successful transplantation; for example, more patients were leaving disability and social support behind and returning to work.[14]

CsA not only improved results with kidney transplants but also changed the prospects for transplanting other organs, and with this new confidence came renewed attempts at heart, liver, and other forms of transplantation.[15] Heart transplantation, once seen as posing an eternal ethical problem, now became unremarkable and routine by 1981, and the service quietly expanded, un-harassed. The number of pancreas transplants also rose after 1980. CsA improved the results of re-transplantation, and it annulled the blood transfusion effect, allowing the deliberate blood transfusions strategy to be put aside, with relief. Patient survival also increased during this time, particularly in those over the age of fifty-five, and the upper and lower age limits for patients who could receive transplants became more generous. It was wryly noted at the time that the ever-rising age limit for acceptance of senior patients for organ grafting was also the age of the increasingly senior pioneer transplant surgeons.

CsA even established kidney transplantation as a successful therapy for domestic pets, notably cats, who are prone to fatal kidney failure in late middle life. At the Boston Angell Memorial Animal Hospital, which had assisted with the general management of the historic dog kidney transplant experiments in the early 1950s, a form of emotionally bonded, living-unrelated kidney donation in cats was organized. This added to the feline recipient's already generous nine lives, and certainly added variety to the bioethicist's agenda.[16]

The human side of the successes in liver, heart, and lung transplants encouraged publication of many personal accounts by recipients, and these sold well. Some of these organ recipients had prominent positions in public life.[17] Favorable publicity came from the Transplant Games, organized for recipients of transplanted organs and begun in Portsmouth, England, in 1978. This demonstration of the vitality and fitness of patients after successful organ transplantation spoke for itself and helped encourage organ donation. Other countries followed this lead, and a biennial international World Transplant Games emerged in 1980 and flourished, later featuring a winter event in the intervening year.[18]

New Transplant Centers

With the increasing success of transplants supported by CsA, the number of new centers set up for organ transplantation increased. The structure of these specialty units was changing, however, and in kidney transplantation the early links with urology and vascular surgery were often lost. Day-to-day transplant patient management drew less on immunological research, innovation, and support. The pioneering academic units had been staffed by research-oriented, salaried surgeons, whereas the new units had technically skilled staff offering high-cost itemized surgery, notably liver transplants. In this enlarged service, the considerable costs, paid either by governments or insurers, became an issue and led to studies of pricing versus outcome.[19]

Improvements in Clinical Management

In addition to the positive impacts of CsA, organ transplantation outcomes steadily improved for a variety of other reasons. Anesthesia and critical care methods for transplant patients matured, and the management, prevention, and early diagnosis of infection also continued to improve. A new risk, however, was the emergence in the 1980s of human immunodeficiency virus (HIV), which could be transferred from donor organs to the recipient patient.[20] Although HIV could be transmitted, it proved much less of a danger to transplantation patients than other agents had been, and the HIV challenge was contained by the screening of donors.

Another measure increasingly in use in the CsA era was kidney biopsy to detect drug toxicity. Also, the microscopy for detecting changes that might signal rejection became more sophisticated and became standardized in what was known as the Banff Classification.[21] Imaging, plus interventional radiology, also continued to rise in importance in management.[22] Ultrasound scanning was increasingly dominant, and, having gained a major role in detecting collections of lymph or blood around the kidney graft, as well as obstructions of the ureter, duplex Doppler ultrasound appeared in the 1980s. With the availability of color imaging in the 1990s, scanning allowed demonstration of blood flow in the transplant artery and vein. In cases of a blocked ureter, guided ultrasound puncture of the kidney and imaging of the ureter emerged first as a diagnostic procedure and then enabled interventional treatment.

This rapid rise of interventional radiology reduced the amount of "open" transplant-related surgery and was part of a general shift in the professional boundaries of care at the time. In general surgery, increasing experience with minimally invasive techniques at this time allowed laparoscopic living-donor kidney removal to emerge, sometimes using a hand-assisted variant, and this technique lowered wound-related morbidity in the donors, in both the short and long term.[23] There was a steady improvement in graft survival, estimated by Terasaki to be about 2 percent per year, coming from this battery of advances. Boston's Francis Moore liked to point out that, after the advent of any new surgical endeavor, "things just get better"—a phenomenon difficult to analyze but suggestive of "experience in a mass of detail." Experienced surgeons transmit their unwritten surgical technique and management skills to those being trained, and these neophytes then add further nuances of their own. Although Moore had predicted in 1988 that few surgeons would master liver transplantation and he believed that "there will always be a limited number of surgeons with the skills to complete these operations successfully," a new generation of trainee surgeons seemed to pick up the once daunting procedure quite quickly.[24]

Liver Transplantation Established

Calne and Starzl had persevered with human liver transplantation throughout the difficult 1970s, and their persistence was rewarded when their results improved markedly with the use of CsA. By 1982, the results at Calne's Cambridge/King's College liver transplant unit had passed the psychologically important 50 percent one-year survival mark.[25] With these achievements, the NHS in Britain funded three more liver units, and new liver units also began to open in Europe.[26]

In some health systems, however, funding the considerable costs of liver transplantation had to wait for a decision on changing the classification of liver transplantation from "experimental" to "accepted therapy." Meanwhile, the needs of individual cases attained prominence. In November 1982, publicity about the plight of Jamie Fisk, a doomed one-year-old Massachusetts child with biliary atresia, revealed that liver transplant surgery was unavailable in Boston and that the family insurance might not cover the costs of the procedure elsewhere. After news stories across the country and an appeal for a donor, the operation was carried out at the University of Minnesota.

With liver transplantation, or the lack of a liver transplant, continuing to be newsworthy, President Ronald Reagan mentioned in one of his weekly radio broadcasts the need for a donor liver for another individual. Pleased with the success of the appeal, both clinical and political, he appointed a transplant liaison staffer at the White House, who, together with his wife Nancy Reagan (daughter of the surgeon Loyal Davis), began to deal with pleas from many individual patients needing transplantation.[27] The task of Michael Batten as transplant patient advocate at the White House was an easy one, and, in all, he dealt with about fifteen hundred requests for the president or his wife to intervene. The White House encouraged organ donation, rebuked unsympathetic insurance companies, and could obtain military air transport for organ transport. President Reagan's populist support for individual recipients contrasted, however, with his cuts in the Medicare budget at the time, plus his opposition to a blood marrow registry and to Congressman Al Gore's bill, which became the National Organ Transplant Act of 1984. Medical planners noted wryly that "when an individual human life is placed in visible, media-covered jeopardy, a tug on the public heart strings loosens public purse strings causing expenditures to save that 'identified life' which far exceeds what government is willing to spend to save an otherwise comparable 'statistical life.'"[28]

The increasing success of liver transplantation was well known, as was the cost, but because the surgery was still classified as experimental, reimbursement agencies could decline to pay. Representative Gore directed the attention of a House Science and Technology Subcommittee to the issues involved in liver transplantation, and this effort, plus intense media pressure, led to action by Surgeon General C. Everett Koop, who, as a former pediatric surgeon, was well aware of the problem of biliary atresia. In 1983, Koop mobilized the little-used mechanism of a Consensus Development Review, in which a panel largely comprising laypersons could hear the case for and against any new therapy. Surgeon-advocates were assembled from afar. Starzl, with his one-year liver transplant survival rate also now exceeding 50 percent, could make a compelling case for acceptance, as did Calne from Britain and Rudolf Pichlmayr of Germany. A 50 percent one-year survival was often taken as the tipping point for shifting treatments from the experimental to the routine category, but the pioneers could also claim that an earlier defining moment was important, too, namely stunning individual successes emerging on a regular basis.

The Consensus Development Review panel narrowly supported acceptance of the procedure as a routine therapy, and this acceptance had important consequences in the United States.[29] Now that insurance could pay the costs, liver transplantation activity increased rapidly, and liver grafting became the most expensive single medical procedure, at a cost of three hundred thousand dollars per operation in the mid-1990s. For any hospital, a liver transplant unit could bring income, profit, and prestige—it was "a gold rush, with a shortage of gold miners."[30] When nearly one hundred liver transplant units emerged in the United States, this "gold rush" was partly curbed by cautious insurers and by government, which was particularly watchful regarding Medicaid-funded liver transplantation for the indigent. Standard payments were drawn up for these higher-cost surgical procedures, and results in units with low activity were monitored. Initially, some insurance policies capped reimbursement of the liver transplant costs, and the patient might have to pledge fifty thousand dollars in personal funds up front—termed a "wallet biopsy" at the time by critics.

This funding of liver transplantation happened in a largely entrepreneurial way in the United States but in a more planned way in other health care systems. Britain found success in limiting the number of transplant units, thus giving each a desirable high volume of work and ensuring a broad-based geographic availability.

Oregon Experience with Liver Transplantation

The American debate on transplant funding continued state by state, and in Oregon in 1992, the fundamental issues of budgetary constraints, allocation of resources, and high-technology medicine collided in the public sphere. Oregon had a high proportion of citizens who met the federal criteria for poverty and hence were eligible for Medicaid health care coverage. The mood of the state's voters was resolutely against tax increases, and state officials reviewed the costs and benefits associated with the disbursement of Medicaid funds. An eleven-person committee was set up to determine priorities and invite public input, a phone survey was conducted, and citizens' town hall meetings were held. The 688 medical procedures that state Medicaid funds would cover were thus thoroughly reviewed. The lowest priority procedure was judged to be plastic surgery, second from the bottom of the list was liver transplantation, and counseling for the obese came in third from last.[31] By removing these and other low-scoring procedures from the approval list, the state committee agreed that it was more desirable to spend state Medicaid funds on common, less-costly areas of health care—a high-minded utilitarian approach of providing the greatest good to the greatest number. The committee urged Oregon employers to provide health care insurance coverage instead for treatments at the bottom of the priority list.

Protests followed, and, as always, when "individual lives" hung in the balance, these decisions on "statistical lives" seemed harsh. Compromises were made, but Oregon had opened up the debate again on budgetary constraints and choices.[32] In Massachusetts, caution was again seen in a report requested from Harvey V. Fineberg of the Harvard School of Public Health, reporting in 1984 as a state "Task Force on Organ Transplantation." The Fineberg Report solemnly posed the question of "whether society can and should support liver transplantation."[33]

Transplants across Boundaries

The early U.S. liver transplant centers were not limited by the boundaries of local kidney sharing schemes, and the biggest units sought liver donation through wide-ranging multi-organ cadaveric procurement over large areas, uncomfortably overlapping with areas covered by local kidney procurement efforts.[34] Also crossing boundaries were the patients, traditionally more informed and mobile in the United States than elsewhere, and they sought out liver transplant centers with shorter waiting times and/or better results, since information on outcomes was increasingly in the public domain via the Internet. In addition, patients with funds often arrived in the United States from abroad seeking a liver transplant at the famous centers, and they were not always turned away.

Conditions Leading to Liver Transplantations

Biliary atresia was the most common pediatric indication for liver grafting, and in the adult, various forms of acute and chronic hepatic failure gave their own pattern of need and results. Liver transplantation also found a remarkable niche use in dealing with metabolic diseases, since grafting could not only replace the general functions of the failing liver but could also annul the causative genetic defect, such as alpha-1-antitrypsin deficiency, glycogen storage disease, Wilson's Disease, tyrosinemia, and many other rare metabolic conditions. Immediate transplantation for acute liver failure also became common.

Innovations in Liver Transplantation

Liver surgery and transplantation provoked new interest in the anatomy of the liver, especially the arterial vessels and venous drainage. Not for the first time in the history of surgery, even the largest anatomy texts proved deficient when it came to anatomical variation and the various internal vascular territories. In another clinic-to-academia episode of "reverse enlightenment," surgeons had to rewrite the books on hepatic structure and organization.[35] With the newer knowledge of the liver's various lobes, adult cadaver livers, too large for young recipients, could now be confidently shaved down and used as "reduced" grafts, which then showed considerable powers of regeneration. The first reduced cadaver donor operations were described in 1977, and, by 1996, eight hundred patients had received these altered grafts.[36] Split-liver techniques followed after reports by Pichlmayr in 1988 and then by Bismuth, showing that two useful organs could be obtained from a single liver.[37]

The new anatomical findings about the liver and the split-liver techniques led to consideration of the at-first unthinkable proposal of live liver donation. The first reports of such surgery came from Brazil and Australia in 1991, attended by controversy and concern.[38] Other surgeons followed cautiously, and soon enough such cases appeared to prompt the establishment of the Hamburg International Living Donor Liver Transplant Registry. There were successful outcomes with these live donor transplants, but the danger to the donor was a central issue.[39] By the mid-1990s, the registry had learned of two donor deaths in the seven hundred cases reported, with complications in about 15 percent of donors. Donor deaths and complications in some countries, particularly where no central reporting was required, were thought to be higher. For patients in countries such as Japan, where no cadaveric donation was possible and thus no whole livers were available for transplantation, living donation was the only hope.

Lung Transplantation

Single-lung transplant cases became more frequent after the first long-term success was reported in 1986 from Toronto. By the 1990s, the indications for lung transplant had been clarified and the pattern of likely complications established. The bronchial suturing was problematic; there was leakage in the short term and narrowing later on, so appropriate strategies for dealing with these problems were devised. The donor shortage also affected this developing service, and the proportion of patients accepted for lung transplantation but dying while waiting for a donor was probably higher than for any other organ. Since young adults were often the primary recipients, particularly because of cystic fibrosis, family donors were often available, and Vaughn Starnes at the University of Southern California pioneered living-related lung transplantation.[40] Donors could give only one lobe, and, since one lobe is not sufficient lung capacity for the recipient, two lobes, one from each parent, were necessary.

Small Bowel Transplants

The small bowel transplants carried out earlier in the 1960s were forlorn attempts to treat doomed patients with sudden, extensive intestinal loss. The need was largely reduced when total "parenteral" nutrition, given intravenously, emerged in the late 1960s to deal with such massive loss of intestinal function. But experimental transplant studies continued and defined some unique features of such grafting. Most notable of these discoveries was that, contrary to physiological assumptions, loss of nerve supply and lymphatic drainage was not a serious problem.

No further human attempts at small bowel transplants were made until the CsA era. By this time, the need was increasing, since some patients who had survived for years on intravenously delivered nutrition were having technical failure after years of success. Intestinal transplantation was taken up again in 1985 in Toronto using a segment of bowel from a living-related donor.[41] The biggest series was reported later from France, at the Hôpital Necker, but only modest survival rates were obtained.[42] However, the surgical experience gained in these efforts allowed for innovation with occasional intestinal transplants between twins.

About 1988, a new strategy for transplanting bowel evolved. The procedure involved transplanting the bowel *en bloc* or in a cluster, that is, transplanting lengths of intestine along with the liver and, later, the pancreas and stomach as well. The first report of success with this approach came from David Grant in London, Ontario, and others followed.[43] This strategy was attractive from a technical point of view, and it gained further support from empirical observations in experimental liver grafting that the liver, when grafted, had a generally protective immunological effect on simultaneous grafts. Moreover, the failing parenteral nutrition syndrome, leading to consideration of intestinal grafting, often included serious liver damage.

In 1988, Starzl started a trial of these "composite" intestinal transplants, aided by encouraging results with a new agent, FK 506 (tacrolimus), and various anatomical strategies. With multivisceral transplants, his team obtained the best results using FK, reporting a 75 percent one-year survival.[44] An International Intestinal Transplant Registry emerged, signaling the establishment of the procedure, and it had reported on 180 cases by 1996.[45]

Pancreas Transplant Efforts

In the 1970s, a few pioneer centers had kept alive the hopes for pancreatic transplantation to treat diabetes, notably in the surgery departments at Minneapolis and in Munich, Lyon, and Stockholm. Treatment of diabetes with insulin was safer than transplantation, but in a minority of patients, the disease is "brittle," with uncontrolled episodes of hypoglycemia; such patients had merited consideration for transplantation since the 1960s. There were also hopes that the diffuse complications of diabetes, which progressed in spite of insulin therapy, might be contained or even reversed by a pancreatic graft.

In the first approaches, the choice was between transplanting the whole gland plus a segment of adjacent duodenum or only the pancreas; both techniques risked leakage of damaging pancreatic secretions.[46] Seeking to avoid this, in 1973, Marvin Gliedman (died 2001) first tried joining the pancreas and duct to the urinary bladder, but this bladder drainage scheme fell out of favor, only to return with the advent of CsA. From the start, surgeons attempted various strategies to destroy the parts of the pancreas making the external secretion, leaving the islets unharmed, but as with the drainage, there was no fully satisfactory solution. By 1991, though technical problems remained, some centers were achieving 80 percent one-year survival of the graft and with normal glucose tolerance. For the many diabetic patients with coexisting chronic renal failure, simultaneous pancreas and kidney transplantation gave good results.

In 1979, increasing confidence in pancreas transplant surgery allowed the first living-related segmental graft to be carried out at the pioneering unit at the University of Minnesota.[47] Surgery of this type increased, with one hundred such transplants reported in the next twenty years; it was also possible to include a simultaneous kidney graft from the same donor.[48] In 1980, the familiar signal of confidence in the future came when an international registry was established. But not until 2000 was pancreas transplantation acknowledged in the United States as "acceptable therapy," one that insurance might cover.[49]

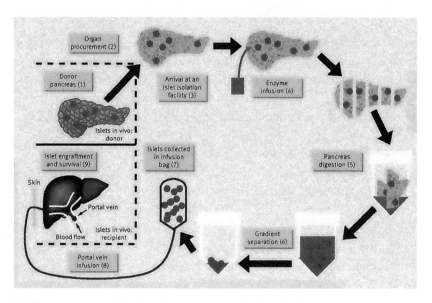

This illustrates the procedure for isolating pancreatic islets from the human pancreas. Image courtesy of E. J. P. Koning.

Pancreatic Islets

Grafts of the insulin-producing islets of Langerhans for diabetics had always been a highly attractive strategy as an alternative to the technically difficult pancreatic organ transplant. Not until the 1980s could a high yield of islets be obtained regularly from the human pancreas; this collection process involved applying the enzyme collagenase (Liberase) to the gland, then using Camillo Ricordi's dispersal device, and finally separating the islets using the St. Louis density gradient. The islets were then infused into the portal vein, where they lodged and worked well within the liver.[50] But a major constraint remained, namely that a large number of islets were required and one human donor could provide enough for only one recipient.

Another issue was that islets proved particularly subject to rejection, for which there was no clear test—something essential for day-to-day transplant work. To add to this, conventional immunosuppressive regimens damage the islet tissue, since CsA reduces blood flow to the grafts, steroids cause resistance to insulin, and azathioprine inhibits insulin secretion. For these reasons, other strategies and agents were explored, and each new immunosuppressive agent was studied with interest, with hopes rising in 1999 after good results were achieved in transplants using large numbers of donor islets or two separate donations and managed with the new immunosuppressant drugs rapamycin and mycophenolate mofetil.

In the 1950s, G. H. Algire had shown that experimental allografts would survive if surrounded by membranes impermeable to lymphoid cells. This strategy promised much, particularly in attempting islet transplantation, and the plausible hopes attracted considerable venture capital. However, design and use of suitable biohybrid "immuno-isolation" chambers, which contained enough islet tissue to give adequate insulin output, proved to be difficult, and, perhaps surprisingly, only modest progress was reported even in experimental models.[51]

Bone Marrow Needs

Bone marrow transplantation continued to build on the progress made in the 1970s. In 1977, Donnall Thomas, working at the Fred Hutchinson Cancer Center in Seattle, reported on his first one thousand bone marrow transplants from HLA-identical family donors, and he had some long-term survivors. But the bone marrow results were perhaps the only type of transplantation not showing marked improvement with the emergence of CsA. Added to this, rapid improvements in chemotherapy for blood malignancies at the time meant that, for a while, fewer patients were candidates for the riskier marrow grafting. As a result, marrow transplantation was increasingly restricted to patients with aplastic anemias, congenital disease, and failed chemotherapy efforts.[52]

But steady improvement in transplant management, especially the use of early, intensive support with platelet and white cell transfusion and the availability of newer antiviral drugs, meant that the results of marrow transplantation in acute leukemia had improved by the mid-1980s to rival those of chemotherapy. Close matching could give success, and suitable matches were sought widely, as in the early days of kidney sharing schemes. For bone marrow donation, this intensive matching effort meant building up large pools of willing, unrelated donors, typed for all the known antigens.

Britain had the first marrow donor registry. Appearing in 1974, the Anthony Nolan Registry was a charity set up by the mother of a three-year-old boy with the Wiskott-Aldrich genetic blood and immune system disorder. The charity slowly recruited volunteers and tissue-typed them, but it was some years before the first close match emerged, and, while waiting, Anthony had died without receiving a transplant.

In the United States, the primary activist for establishing marrow registries was a Colorado veterinarian, Robert Graves, whose daughter had obtained a successful unrelated marrow graft from a member of the local hospital staff in 1979, the first success in a blood malignancy using an unrelated matched donor.[53] Graves lobbied Congress for a national registry scheme, and some blood banks started informal typing of their regular blood donors. Success appeared at hand when the House passed legislation for the National Organ Transplant Act in 1984, because the bill contained an amendment to support a marrow registry. Representative Barbara Mikulski, as well as transplant-friendly House members Al Gore and Henry Waxman, had added the amendment during House debate, but the Reagan administration warned that it would veto the bill, calling the costly registry "premature." To save the bill, the registry amendment was dropped. There was another attempt to establish a registry when, in 1985, the National Institutes of Health used the "trigger" mechanism of a Technology Assessment Meeting; two years earlier, the NIH had approved routine liver transplantation with this mechanism, but, on this occasion, the strategy failed. Many supporters of the marrow register were dismayed. Graves was advised to persevere but not to "fight his way through the front door" of the House; instead, backers of the registry suggested seeking an appropriation "through the back door." An opportunity emerged in 1986, when Senator Paul Laxalt managed to slip $1.2 million into the Navy budget to pay for the registry, which provided its first match for donor marrow in 1987. In 1989, full funding from Congress allowed the freestanding National Marrow Donor Program to emerge. By the year 2000, the program had made grafts possible for twelve thousand patients.

All the international registries, in thirty countries, eventually linked their data, and by the year 2000 there were about five million willing donors typed throughout the world, with the typing data available on the Internet. Commercial organizations that banked umbilical cord blood emerged later, storing cells in case of need in later life.[54]

Heart Transplantation Resumes

Prior to the emergence of CsA, steady improvement and innovation had occurred in heart transplantation at the very few centers still trying, and only Norman Shumway was active in the United States. CsA offered the opportunity for a general resumption of adult heart transplantation, but with caution, since all clinicians involved had long memories, as did administrators and governments. Although Shumway had shown beyond doubt that good results could be obtained even in the pre-CsA era, heart transplantation was still a sensitive issue.

In the United States, many cardiac units hesitated to take up heart transplantation, and some units actively resisted. In Boston in 1980, Massachusetts General Hospital formally decided that they should not proceed with heart transplantation.[55] The hospital trustees made this decision, even though they normally concerned themselves only with legal and fiscal matters, but on this occasion they declined to support the chiefs of the hospital medical services who wished to start the operations. The trustees rationalized their decision on the grounds that the procedure was not cost effective or likely to produce novel research findings. However, more general acceptance of heart transplantation in the United States emerged in a few years, notably with publication of the supportive Battelle Report in 1984, and other units quickly built on Shumway's continuing success.[56] Combined heart-lung transplantation also emerged, being attractive because of the limited number of surgical connections needed and used primarily for patients with coexisting heart disease, cystic or pulmonary fibrosis, emphysema, and some congenital anomalies.[57] These conditions resulted in another niche opportunity for transplant innovation: on the rare occasions when heart-lung transplantation was carried out to deal only with lung disease, the recipient's normal heart was removed and could be grafted to another patient. Donor hearts from such patients were first used in Baltimore in 1989, in the so-called "domino" operation.[58]

Pediatric Heart Issues

By 1989, heart transplantation in children had become increasingly common. Quite small babies could be treated in this way, and Leonard L. Bailey (born 1946) reported particular success at the Loma Linda Center, a Seventh-day Adventist hospital in California.[59] But Bailey encountered resurgent public hostility in the case of "Baby Fae," in which he used a baboon heart graft in 1985 in a child with hypoplastic left-heart syndrome.[60] The baby lived for only twenty-one days after surgery. Bailey's administrative preparation could not be faulted, since he had persuaded twelve separate local advisory groups and committees to let him go ahead with the surgery. But the public reacted badly, and the ultimate verdict was that the operation was irresponsible.[61] These events obscured Bailey's successful series of fifty other infant heart transplants to treat serious congenital anomalies. In his work, many of the donor organs came from the bodies of newborns with anencephaly, identified by ultrasound examination well before delivery. But Bailey and others stopped the use of such donors after the complexity of the situation, both medical and ethical, emerged.[62]

Britain Resumes Heart Transplants

In Britain, there was no Shumway equivalent: heart transplantation attempts had ceased for ten years, to the relief of administrators and government. In the "Year of the Heart," the nation's chief medical officer had set up a ponderous forty-five-person committee of senior medical personnel to advise him on organ transplantation. No unwelcome advice was offered,

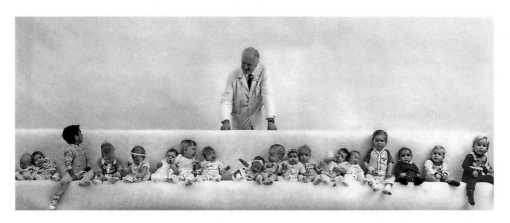

Leonard Bailey, seen here with his patients at Loma Linda Hospital, California, pioneered heart transplantation in infants. Image courtesy of Leonard Bailey.

and this inactive Transplant Regulatory Authority met but once each year and ensured that heart transplantation stayed in limbo. One rationalization was that, as had happened earlier, a resumption might threaten organ donation generally.[63] By 1977, however, attitudes had softened, and the group set out the desiderata for any cardiac unit proposing to resume transplant work. This was the only encouragement offered. Pointedly, no National Health Service funds were offered, which normally meant that nothing would happen, since no other entity funded health care in Britain. Nothing did happen for two years.

Then Terence English, a Cambridge surgeon, in 1979 obtained permission from the local health authority to go ahead with two heart transplants. Meanwhile, Magdi Yacoub (born 1935), at Harefield Hospital in London, had boldly started without official sanction.[64] The government remained actively detached, declining to contribute any new health service money and barring use of existing local budget funds for transplants, which meant that non-NHS money had to be raised for the first time for any such operations. But there was another hurdle, since in the commendably simple financing of the NHS and its salaried system, no costs for single procedures were available. A figure was somehow arrived at, and new money was obtained from personal philanthropy, notably from the founder of the Hewlett-Packard Company and various charities.[65]

The new British heart transplants, as expected, attracted considerable media attention. Good results headed off any resurgent criticism, however, and the British heart transplant units survived.[66] The timid government's "approved but not funded" stance changed, and, with proper central funding, a planned network of heart transplant units emerged in Britain. English and Yacoub, the two surgeons initially marginalized by government, now headed the first two British units and later received knighthoods; the happy ending was viewed as a parable to illustrate the travails of innovation.[67]

A more piecemeal approach emerged in Europe.[68] In the Netherlands, there was even greater resistance to resuming heart transplantation, but, in June 1984, surgeons in Rotterdam performed such surgery. With government approval, another unit soon opened, in Utrecht. France had seen some heart transplants since the early 1970s. In 1990, Denmark became the last nation in Europe to begin the surgery.

But transplantation had not fully escaped from controversy. In late 1980, the British Broadcasting Corporation program *Panorama*, at the time fond of deliberately provocative presentations, screened a belated attack on the brain-death criteria that had been generally approved four or so years earlier. Entitled "Transplants: Are the Donors Dead?" the program sought to challenge the UK brain stem death tests, and the few earlier opponents of the criteria vigorously renewed their criticism.[69] But damage was done, and, predictably, kidney and other organ donations again fell significantly. But the power of the media was again apparent after the BBC's *That's Life* screened a supportive program on liver transplantation, and donations subsequently rose.[70]

Other Donation Concerns

Also in 1984, a variety of concerns arose over organs and patients moving across national boundaries. There was surprise in some quarters when it emerged that the Southeastern Organ Procurement Foundation in the United States had sent 254 kidneys abroad in 1983 alone and that some of these organs had mysteriously found their way to private clinics in London. In the United States there was also a rise in grafts given to visiting patients from abroad. The fortunate recipients included those visitors without funds who might engage the sympathy of individual surgeons, as well as ill patients with ample funds.[71] The U.S. government itself occasionally arranged organ transplantation for important foreign nationals, particularly politicians in sympathetic countries, such as President Ferdinand Marcos of the Philippines.[72] Such use of kidneys was generally agreed to be beyond the limits of American free enterprise, and, after investigation, the American Society of Transplant Surgeons adopted an "Americans first" policy and reduced the quota of foreign nationals treated at any one center to 5 percent, a limit often circumvented.[73]

In 1985, two London surgeons and a physician at a private London clinic were found to be involved in transplanting kidneys from unrelated, paid Indian donors to well-off Indian patients, all of whom traveled to London for the surgery. A stern prohibition against any involvement in such transplants was then issued to British doctors by not only the British Transplantation Society but also the General Medical Council, such was the distaste for this type of activity, and the doctors were disciplined and barred from practice for while.[74] Britain judged the matter of paid donation to be so serious that the law was changed to require formal approval of unrelated donation. The Human Organ Transplant Act of 1989 set up a new supervisory government agency (ULTRA), which permitted transplants between emotionally bonded persons, such as husband and wife, yet sought to prevent any purely commercial arrangements.

The United States considered an alternative view for a while. A number of respectable free-market-leaning scholars were making the theoretical case for a market in human organs.[75] The debate had started when David L. Bach of Harvard University wrote to the *Lancet* in November 1984 generally supporting paid kidney donation. This opinion drew a letter of rebuke from the tissue typer Jean Dausset, who told the *Lancet* readers of a joint private letter sent one year previously from three Nobel Prize winners—himself, Peter Medawar, and George Snell—to President Reagan vigorously opposing all forms of paid donation.[76] The text of Reagan's reply was not revealed.

With the matter of payment under debate, some less admirable citizens announced detailed plans for commercial transplantation. H. Barry Jacobs of Reston, Virginia, head of his own International Kidney Exchange Ltd., proposed to bring paid donors from abroad to America to give a kidney, and he circulated his proposal to U.S. hospitals and appeared on television talk shows to promote his scheme. Jacobs had noted shrewdly that any living-related donor's American hospital care was normally chargeable to Medicare, and thus these federal funds would subsidize his plan nicely. Jacobs gave a vigorous testimony to a House committee addressing the shortage of donor organs, and in sharp exchanges with Representatives Gore and Waxman, his crisp analysis and solution suggested that "neither altruism nor a fancier computer is the answer."[77] But Jacobs's scheme was easily headed off when it was revealed that he had served jail time for Medicare fraud. A more respectable organ procurement enterprise by the talented start-up specialist William F. von Meister did survive for a short time.[78] Support also came from the magazine *Fortune,* whose editors opined that many citizens were "kidney-rich but cash poor," but the magazine's stance was criticized by many, including free-enterprise guru Milton Friedman.

UNOS Emerges

These debates on the American transplant service and other matters led to recognition that many aspects of transplantation remained unsettled. A number of these issues were finally settled with passage of the National Organ Transplant Act (1984), which resulted from the continuing efforts of Representative Al Gore. The act, among other things, provided funding to organ procurement organizations and proposed a single, nationwide donor scheme, later called the United Network for Organ Sharing (UNOS).[79] The new scheme rejected commercialism in transplantation and made the sale of organs a criminal offense.[80]

The National Organ Transplant Act's work was continued by a task force set up to look at national donor policy. Reporting in 1986, the task force invited bids for administering this new massive organ sharing organization. The success of the Southeastern Organ Procurement Foundation in Richmond meant that it had expanded steadily to cover a larger area, and other national agencies had used their robust computer systems. The contract for UNOS went to Richmond, an acknowledgment of the foundation's pioneering work in tissue typing, transplantation, and procurement, dating from the 1960s. The old sharing scheme system was transferred to the new UNOS for a nominal and agreeable fee of one dollar.

This new national organization was obliged to collect national data on outcomes, and it soon had access to the older data banks, including not only kidney transplant data, as collected by Terasaki, but also information from the Pittsburgh Liver Transplant Registry, the International Heart and Lung Transplant Society Registry, and the International Pancreas Transplant Registry. Oversight of these new registries was initially given to those who had pioneered these earlier, more personal data banks. UNOS was up and running by 1987, despite the fact that it was so unusual for a nonprofit agency in the United States to have such considerable and monopolistic powers of audit, intrusion, and control. President Reagan had opposed UNOS, and the business magazine *Fortune* had railed against the National Organ Transplant Act, asking, "Will this emerging high-tech industry [i.e., transplantation] be run efficiently by dynamic entrepreneurs of the capitalist persuasion, or will it be semi-socialized and smothered by regulators?"

UNOS charged a registration fee for each patient on the transplant waiting list. This fee was its main source of funds, save for a federal grant providing about 15 percent of the UNOS budget, a device that allowed government to have oversight and public involvement in transplantation, which Medicare and Medicaid government funds already paid for in large part.

UNOS drew up rules on organ allocation, ran day-to-day organ placement, audited the transplant results, took on research and education, added quality control, and encouraged efforts at obtaining donors. It investigated units with the poorest results, offered advice, and sometimes encouraged voluntary withdrawal of the service. UNOS made unit-specific data on transplant outcomes available on the Internet beginning in 1992, and, in line with American traditions, it allowed patients to register on more than one transplant center's waiting list.[81] Although initially unwilling to enter the sensitive area of patient selection, notably in liver grafting, UNOS introduced guidelines for allocation of livers in 1997, using the Mayo Clinic's mortality-risk scoring system, drawn up in 2000. All patients could appeal to regional committees for a review of their status. UNOS was subdivided into nine regions, seeking the best match in the local organ procurement organization (OPO) first, then in the UNOS region, then nationally. A national, seamless, nonregional scheme was advocated from time to time, but as the importance of obtaining close matching diminished, advocates of the shorter cold times possible with local matches began to win the argument.

Sharing and Shortages

In spite of increasing efforts to obtain donor organs, by the mid-1980s, most countries experienced a growing shortage of donor organs.[82] Increasingly, patients were accepted over a wider age range as well as those with other health problems. Many obtained second or further grafts after the first failed, thus reducing the number of first grafts carried out. In most countries in the 1990s, the total number of those waiting for kidney transplantation grew at a rate of 10 percent per year, while the number of transplants carried out remained static or the number of donor organs decreased.[83] The number of liver transplants had risen steadily for a while but then leveled off in most countries in the late 1990s. Heart and lung transplant numbers also failed to increase to meet the needs at about this time, and the actual need for heart, liver, and lung grafts was concealed by the deaths of patients awaiting transplants.

The factors causing the shortfall in donor numbers were complex. Road traffic accidents were commendably declining at 6 percent per year in most developed countries, aided by seatbelt legislation, compulsory helmet-wearing for motorcyclists, and campaigns and penalties against drunk driving. Homicide cases were declining in some nations, and indications for critical care were narrowing for greater efficiency. Attitudes toward donation may have been changing as well, and although surveys showed that the public were generally willing to donate, the refusal rate by relatives of suitable donors was edging up and, in the United States, could reach 50 percent. No single factor seemed dominant in explaining this reluctance.

With this trend of decreasing donations, attention turned to Spain's high donation rate of thirty-three donors per million, almost three times the level found elsewhere, notably in the United Kingdom. The "Spanish Model" of donation was of interest, since no presumed consent was in force and success may have been the result of appointing for each intensive care unit "nominated doctors" who were responsible for the local donation arrangements. The continuing high rate of fatal traffic accidents in Spain was also a factor.

Responding to the Organ Shortage

In 1983, the president of the International Society for Organ Sharing addressed their First International Symposium, and, in spite of the importance of the occasion, he had no good news: "Our problems are recurrent and we seem to have stalled in finding new solutions."[84] Nevertheless, numerous initiatives at local and national levels got under way. Governments were generally helpful and supported efforts to increase donation rates. The distribution of the traditional donor cards continued. In the United States, the Hastings Institute had begun taking an interest in transplant matters during the "Year of the Heart." In 1984, it proposed that all suitable patients be considered via a "required request" of the relatives, and, if the hospital failed to make regular inquiries regarding donation, the administration could be rebuked. Politicians changed this phraseology to requiring "routine inquiry," and, in 1985, the state of Oregon proposed the first such legislation, called "Denita's Bill," named after a young patient for whom there was difficulty obtaining a liver transplant. The approach spread, and later the Uniform Anatomical Gift Act was amended to require notification of all possible donors to local sharing schemes; when organ donation was possible, OPO staff would contact donor families. In 1995, the U.S. Congress set up a Joint Task Force on Organ and Tissue Donation, sending out seventy million cards along with the annual mailing of income tax refunds. Most states also arranged for permission for donation to be authorized at the time of drivers' license renewal. Some states set up donor registries, and some ruled that such "first-person" consent, when given in advance, was legally binding. Some states also assisted with any donor's burial expenses.

In Britain, to assist future donation, a major new "Carry the Card" campaign was launched in 1984 to revive the previous scheme, adding other encouragement via a donor declaration at drivers' license or pass-

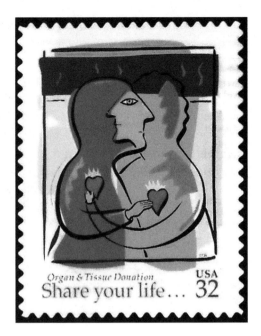

Many public initiatives, like this postage stamp campaign, were taken to increase awareness of the need for organ donors.

port application time. Extra government support via an NHS Organ Donor Registry of those willing to donate after death appeared in October 1994, and the donor card scheme was then discontinued.

From then on, this dimension of transplantation became increasingly important, and throughout the world, attention turned to analysis of the reasons for shortages of donor organs and attempts to increase the number of donations.

Other Donor Initiatives

Most countries retained traditional "opting-in" systems of organ donation in which, for deceased donation, a medical team discussed the situation with relatives, who then made a decision on whether or not to donate their loved one's organs. But some European countries had always had "opting-out" systems, and with the demand for donor organs surpassing supply by wide margins, "opt-out" systems attracted more interest. In an "opt-out" system, donor organs could be removed when, after reasonable inquiry, it was determined that the patient had never objected to donation. In 1975, the Council of Europe Resolution 78[29] encouraged such "presumed consent" schemes. This approach was for the first time made official in France, as the Caillavet Law of 1976, and some other countries in Europe introduced similar legislation. Belgium proceeded with such a plan, and

2 percent of the population registered as nondonors, suggesting, perhaps wrongly, that those who did not respond to the opportunity to opt out supported routine removal of their organs after death without further inquiry. The highest opting-out rate was among those aged twenty-five to thirty-nine and among the immigrant population. Although proponents of this opt-out mechanism claimed short-term improvement in organ donation in Belgium, organ donation rates did not seem to be affected greatly.[85] In routine donation, whatever the legal position, it was still prudent to consult the grieving relatives, and to proceed against their wishes was unwise and risked understandable protest and public dismay.[86] In Brazil, legislation for opting out was introduced but withdrawn after the public suspected that organ removal scandals were likely. In France, the Cavaillet Law was little used in practice, and the Ethics Law of 1994 replaced it, effectively removing the opt-out dimension since it made the views of a potential donor's family the dominant factor. In the Soviet Union, collectivist medical ethics had been an influence and thus autonomy was not a prominent feature, particularly in organ donation, which was traditionally viewed in the same light as a postmortem. Even after the formal end of communism and the Soviet Union, the new government of Russia enacted legislation that formalized the features of presumed consent donation.

But, in spite of international concern and activity, no one found any simple, sustainable solution to the growing need for donor organs.

Extended Donor Criteria

One response to the shortages was to make better use of all available donor organs. For example, the number of "split liver" transplants increased.[87] One move, made reluctantly, was to return to the use of "marginal" organs, that is, transplanting organs with nonstandard anatomy, known damage, or likely defects, which ill patients accepted on the grounds that a marginal organ was better than receiving no graft at all.[88] Donor hearts with obvious coronary disease might be transplanted, with or without bench surgery performed on the organ as a preliminary procedure.

Another major move toward expanding the organ supply was a return to the use of "non-heart-beating" donors, now termed "cardiac death" donors. Donations could come from patients who died outside of critical care units or were declared dead on arrival at a hospital or shortly thereafter. Death was declared after the heart had stopped, but cold perfusion of the organs was quickly carried out via catheters inserted into the femoral artery.[89] The eventual function of such kidney and lung grafts could be good, but results were poorer for livers and hearts. Perfusion machines were claimed to improve the condition of these metabolically challenged organs, and the old tests of kidney viability, popular in the 1960s, made a return in revamped forms.[90] But this type of donation was fraught with ethical concerns, difficulties over consent, and practical constraints, since trained staff had to be on standby.

Grafts of all kinds from living donors steadily rose in numbers, however, and this increase offset the lack of deceased donors.[91] There were also more instances of emotionally related donation, often for kidney transplants but for other organs as well.[92] Kidneys offered from "stranger," "altruistic," or "Samaritan" donors who simply wished to help any recipient were no longer always turned down. Pressure increased for acceptance of "cross-over" or "pooled" donor exchange of kidneys between families with willing living donors but in which a blood type or other incompatibility within the family precluded the transplant.[93] The offered kidneys could be swapped. After a cautious response from most national medical licensing authorities, in view of the ethical and human difficulties that might arise, legal permission to perform these unrelated cross-over living donor transplants emerged in the late 1990s.

Fair Sharing

The lack of donor organs increasingly highlighted the methods used to allocate organs, and, in the 1990s, some began to question whether the organs were being equitably distributed.[94] Since CsA had overridden much of the need for precise tissue matching, the traditional allocation on tissue match alone, which had precluded debates on other criteria, was less supportable. "Equity" is prominent in medical ethics, and via distributive justice, health care providers seek to give equal opportunities for treatment. In transplantation, this goal of providing equal opportunity for treatment began to clash with the usual goal of "utility," that is, optimizing donor graft outcome by maximizing the survival chances of each transplanted organ. For donated livers in particular, seeking "fair" allocation and yet attempting to maximize utility was problematic. The balance between treating urgent or nonurgent cases, and between distant or local use, was debated within the sharing organizations, and the public also took an interest, often with contrarian viewpoints. The debate was particularly polarized over whether scarce livers should go freely to those with liver failure from self-poisoning or as a consequence of past drug abuse, and whether alcoholics, even when demonstrably reformed, ought to have the chance for transplantation.[95]

Within Scandiatransplant in particular, the debate on allocation by tissue typing versus local use of kidneys was unusually intense and public, and some surgeons started to ignore the allocation protocols by typing and retaining their local kidneys. One factor was that the traditional distribution had resulted in imbalances, and, within the organization, Denmark in particular had built up a large "kidney debt," having steadily obtained more kidneys from adjacent countries by the tissue-typing allocation rules than Denmark had "exported" to the other nations in the consortium.[96] This situation was not uncommon. Within single-nation distribution systems, there were similar organ debts between transplant units, and these imported sources of organs could conceal lack of local efforts to obtain donors.

Another "debt" issue was that within single-nation organ distribution systems, some groups might be hostile to donation yet accept transplants. In the United States, the Afro-Asian population, with a higher incidence of heart and kidney disease, contributed markedly fewer donor organs than other sectors of the population. In Britain, a similar inequality of donation versus transplantation became obvious in some areas, notably the Midlands of England. There, the large immigrant-origin sector of the population had a high incidence of the normally rare blood group B and also of renal failure. They wished transplants, but their opposition to kidney donation, traditional in their faiths, meant that, through seeking a transplant, demand for group B kidneys greatly exceeded supply. All blood group B patients waiting nationally for a transplant were disadvantaged by the large subgroups' failure to donate.[97]

These statistics and attitudes naturally attracted attention from organizations representing minorities, and they took steps to encourage donation. In Britain in 1996, the Muslim Council of British Muslim Schools of Law in London issued a *fatwa* supporting transplantation.[98] For the Hindu community, transplantation was easily related to the law of "karma"—namely that good actions are rewarded in the next life. Although Christian churches no longer had much authority in secular matters, the well-attended places of worship and discourse for other faiths in Britain—the mosques of Muslims, the Hindu temples, and Sikh *gurdwaras*—were powerful sites for debating the issue of transplantation.

Orthodox Jews in the United States and elsewhere looked to their own religious scholars for advice. The rabbis faced a dilemma in dealing with the new ethical issues in transplantation. While the saving of life is a priority, there is also the traditional *"kavod hamet"*—honor to the dead—generally held to prohibit desecration of the body by dissection. Rabbinic discussions in Europe and North America showed a desire not to isolate the Jewish community over these transplant matters, and there were attempts to reconcile these two teachings by prioritizing the first. This approach came from modernizing Western Jewish ethicists like Rabbi Moshe

Tendler in the United States and Immanuel Lord Jakobovits, Britain's Chief Rabbi. After permitting and encouraging donation as a duty, these scholars went further, and, in 1986, the Rabbinical Council of America and its committee on *halakha* (Jewish law) accepted brain death as death of the body. But in Israel, older attitudes prevailed and resistance to any form of donation persists. In Antwerp, all Belgian Orthodox Jews opted out when the new national legislation on donation went into effect.

Global Transplant Activity

In the 1970s and 1980s, kidney replacement therapy spread steadily to the rest of the world from its origins in high-technology academic medicine in Europe and North America. When this complex treatment, with its associated technology, spread from the developed, and increasingly secular, nations, it met new challenges in developing countries, which often had a higher incidence of kidney disease yet lacked financial resources and technical skills needed for renal replacement therapies. In many of these countries the discourse was also different. The patients' understanding of the body was often quite different, and, in explanations of disease, disordered Galenic humoral mechanisms persisted. Faith in the remedies used by traditional healers, rather than costly Western medication, could lead to noncompliance with any treatment. Regular dialysis treatment was rarely available and, even if accessible, was often of poor quality and available only in a few centers in the cities.[99] These countries' precious health budgets, low in both absolute terms and as a percentage of the national product, were most effectively spent on efforts such as public health measures against common infectious disease.[100] The majority of patients who entered end-stage renal failure in these countries simply died, without expectation or awareness of the available treatment. Even if well-off citizens of such nations started dialysis at a private clinic abroad, on return home they found deficiencies in the medical expertise required to provide the treatment. Pure water and maintenance skills for the machines were seldom at hand, nor was the simpler peritoneal dialysis an answer, since the solutions used are remarkably expensive and challenging complications are common.

Local attitudes to organ donation were also markedly different from those common in developed nations. In many developing countries, cadaveric organ removal was out of the question for cultural reasons. Accordingly, in most of these countries the only hope for a patient in end-stage renal failure was to obtain a kidney from a living donor, an option assisted in these countries by large families, extended kinship lines, and a tradition of fulfilling one's duty to care for those within the group. Bread-winning males and mothers with children were usually exempt from the presumed duty to donate, and the choice often narrowed down, unfairly, to unmarried daughters.

Some Western medical ethical attitudes, thought to be universal or even self-evident, were instead not found across the globe; the notion of "autonomy" or the idea that each person should be free to offer or decline to offer an organ graft, was not in force in many cultures. Moreover, visitors to these developing countries sometimes found that local languages had no vocabulary to match the Western ethical concepts involved, and any discussion of these basic tenets was stilted.[101]

Despite these cultural differences, however, transplantation was increasingly taking place around the world. Wealthy patients from developing nations had initially traveled to European or North American units for transplantation. Some richer nations, often in the Middle East, could afford to send even ordinary citizens and their families abroad for transplantation. Increasingly, however, local units for transplant surgery emerged, first using Western medical personnel and then phasing in local medical staff to take over. Kidney transplantation started at the K.E.M. Hospital, Bombay, in 1968, and a unit in Vellore in southern India followed in 1971. These two units were soon doing twenty-five living-donor kidney transplants per year, since cadaveric donation met cultural objections.[102]

In the Middle East, the first dialysis unit opened in 1979 in Saudi Arabia at the Riyadh Armed Forces Hospital, and kidney transplantation commenced there in that year. In 1985, a local National Kidney Foundation was established there to coordinate renal services, and it was renamed the Saudi Center for Organ Transplantation (SCOT) in 1993.[103] The Saudi-based Middle East Society for Organ Transplantation emerged in 1983. Cadaveric donation was established there slowly, beginning in 1987, with heart transplants beginning in 1988 and liver transplantation emerging in 1994 when deceased donation emerged.[104]

Syria had similar facilities from 1983, again based in military hospitals. This interesting appearance in these nations of high-technology medical care in the military sphere came from the general obligation of most military forces to treat all serious illness in the young staff and their families, a group in which chronic renal failure features, though such care was not available to the general population. In this unstable part of the world, large armed forces are a feature.

Cadaveric Donation in the Developing World

In many developing countries, there was fundamental opposition to organ donation after death, and, in some faiths, prolonged rituals after death in any case precluded prompt donation. Although Islam is not specifically hostile to cadaveric donation, traditional cultures in Islamic countries considered it desirable to enter the afterlife intact; according to such beliefs, those who were mutilated would continue to suffer in the afterlife and continue to be disadvantaged after resurrection. It is for these reasons that the traditional punishment of cutting off a hand, ear, or nose was both a temporal and an eternal punishment, as it had been in the West until medieval times.[105]

Although it was made clear in the 1980s by some supportive secular Middle Eastern governments, notably in Iraq, that there existed no official prohibition to cadaveric organ donation, public opinion proved resistant, and a family would usually defer to religious leaders or to the conservative views of the oldest member of the family. Islamic religious leaders discussed the matter from 1982 onward, and, as was often in the case in novel situations, they looked for enlightenment not only in the wording of the Holy Qur'ān but also at the spirit of its teachings, with assistance from the nuances of the sayings of the Prophet. Much of the Islamic discussion on transplant questions and support for donation centered on the Al-Azher University in Cairo, the oldest Islamic university in the world, founded in the tenth century and headed during the late twentieth century by Sheikh Mohammed Sayyid Tantawi, known for his pro-Western stances and liberal *fatwas*, though the university lost ground with the rise of rival fundamentalist Salafi establishments.[106]

Critical care units were slow to appear in developing countries, and therefore the issue of brain death did not arise until much later, after such debates in the West. The Councils of the Islamic Jurisprudence in the Middle East did begin discussing brain death in 1989 and accepted it, but on a majority rather than unanimous decision. *Fatwas* registering approval for both living and cadaveric donation and recognizing brain death were issued, but these had only moderate impact, except in Saudi Arabia, where brain-death criteria had already come into use in 1986. In the rest of the Arab world, the Saudi "modernizers" were regarded with some suspicion, and many Muslim scholars adhered to the traditional view that the soul departs from the body only when the heart stops, and not earlier, giving a vital objection to earlier organ removal.

Other religions, notably Hinduism, Sikhism, and Confucianism, were also thought to prohibit organ removal after death, but, after discussion, the spiritual leaders did not raise formal objections. The Sikh view was particularly flexible, having no preordained position but merely a system of developing knowledge that assimilated new thought and scientific innovation.

But in Japan, major cultural objections to cadaveric donation persisted, a result of the view that dying was a seven-day process, concluding with the final exit of the soul and conversion of the deceased into an ancestor.[107] The controversial failed heart transplant in Japan in 1968, which used heart-beating donation, left a legacy of concern. Such was the cultural sensitivity that the Japanese parliament did not discuss or legalize brain death until 1997.[108]

Buying and Selling of Organs

By the 1980s, CsA made it clinically acceptable to transplant a kidney from a living nonrelated person, and this type of transplant, now giving good results, proceeded, with careful checks, in developed countries in suitable cases. But evidence continued to emerge in some countries of the use of kidney donors not only unrelated to, but also unknown to the patient, and that these donors were paid. The sum given to the kidney donor could be equivalent to the lifetime earnings of a poor person, and thus donors were easily found, particularly among those in debt, with brokers acting as shady intermediaries. Patients in kidney failure and a paid donor might have the operation locally or travel to clinics in countries with little oversight of their health care system or their medical profession or with a flexible policy on such transplants. The surgery, matching, immunosuppression, and care given in these private clinics were not always of poor quality.

The possibility of paid donation had been realized quite early, but when raised unexpectedly at The Hague meeting of the Transplantation Society in 1970 most delegates showed surprise and disbelief. Such payment for a donor organ was promptly and reflexively denounced by the society as intolerable, and any surgeons involved were warned that their activities would lead to action by the society. Many developed countries later drafted legislation forbidding any such sale of organs.[109]

Many other professional bodies, including the World Medical Association, also drew up prohibitions, but these had no force or sanctions in the poorer countries where transplant practices were largely unregulated.[110] The pope, always attentive to transplant matters, ruled in 1991 that donated organs contained part of the soul and hence were not objects to be given away to a recipient, in the absence of any emotional bond.

However, paid, living-unrelated donation was to flourish when far removed from Western ethical constraints. In the late 1970s, India was the first country to confirm the use of paid, unrelated donors, and the matter was not concealed from Western visitors.[111] The hospitals involved were mostly in Bombay and Madras, and they soon had their local apologists.[112]

In 1994, in response to international professional pressure, the embarrassed Indian government attempted to outlaw such practices, but paid donation continued unabated, since a large loophole in the legislation meant that an emotional attachment could be claimed or that a local committee could approve the donation. By the 1990s, about one-third of all donor organs in India were thought to be the result of commercial transactions, and such donation seemed unstoppable. Nor was India alone. In Israel, a country with a well-informed public and with excellent dialysis facilities, the religious opposition to cadaveric donation meant that huge waiting lists for kidney transplantation appeared. The country's underground organization for use of paid donors became increasingly well known, and the donor and recipient usually traveled to Turkey for surgery.[113] Donor kidneys also emerged in Turkey from other, more mysterious sources and were earmarked for Israeli recipients. Paid donation was soon noted in other countries, including the Philippines, Iran, Bolivia, and Peru. Exceptionally, the Iranian system was fairly open, and the officially sanctioned service of government-paid unrelated donation started in 1988. Three hospitals published their unrelated kidney donor transplant results—at Kermānshāh, Shiraz, and Tehrān.[114] In the first ten years of the service, 9,535 kidney transplants were said to have been carried out with good results, although any surgical follow-up is difficult in that region. The organizers also claimed to have met the need of all of those patients fortunate enough to obtain dialysis. Middlemen seemed absent, since the government dealt directly with the donors and made the payments.[115]

There was now a hint of sympathy from those in the Western transplant societies.[116] A shift in attitudes came at the "Ethics, Justice, and Commerce in Transplantation" meeting in Ottawa in 1989. It was agreed that "voluntary living organ and tissue donation should be encouraged when medically and ethically appropriate." This statement hinted that, in the wider world of organ transplantation, the donation had to be seen in the local cultural setting, and there was perhaps some acknowledgment that the previous Western attitudes had been paternalistic at least—or based on cultural imperialism at worst.[117] The matter, once self-evidently despicable, was now in what John Dosseter called the "gray basket."[118]

Added to the contents of this basket was the ethical issue raised by an increasingly familiar event when patients who, having waited or not caring to wait, for a transplant in Western nations, instead became "transplant tourists." Having had a prompt kidney grafting abroad, where the organ had been certainly obtained from a paid donor, they then presented themselves back to their local transplant units. They returned with brief written clinical details of their case, which might have been quite well managed. Further care could not be withheld in their home clinics. Indian and Pakistani clinics were prominent in their involvement. In 2008, the Philippines acted to ban transplants for foreign patients, noting that about five hundred such operations had been conducted in Manila in the previous year using kidneys bought from poor people, notably those from the slums of Issla Walang Bato—then known as "No-kidney island."

Other Ethical Concerns

In some countries, surgeons transplanted organs from executed criminals.[119] Although ninety nations in the world retain the death penalty, professional medical associations have usually advised against using organs in these circumstances, a view shared by most doctors.[120] But in Singapore, and more notably in China, organs were regularly obtained in this way, and 90 percent of China's reported transplants used this source. In China, prisoners' organs were not only transplanted locally but also exported. This furtive international trade ceased after media exposure, but transplantation of "transplant tourists" within China was routine and well authenticated.[121] Taiwan for a while in the 1980s obtained and used such kidneys within the country, even erecting a plaque in the prison to record the donor's actions, but this procedure later ceased.

Less believable stories of criminal organ removal for transplantation first appeared in the 1980s, and were rapidly taken up and widely believed. These included alleged use of Eastern European orphanages or abducted third world street children for organ theft. Niche "eye thieves" preying on children were also believed to exist, as was removal of kidneys from drugged victims. After careful and widespread investigation by many government authorities, notably in European countries with antitrafficking laws, no definite evidence of this illicit removal of body parts emerged. In addition, no traces of these rumored clandestine transplant operations were found, and they could scarcely have operated in complete secrecy. Increasingly, these accounts contained the typical features of "urban myths." Anthropologists began to study the tales, and they pointed out the resemblances to ancient folk tale motifs, perhaps with added modern conspiracy amplification and dissemination.[122]

Similar allegations emerged in stories that the Kosovo Liberation Army had murdered Serb captives for organ removal and trafficking, but investigations were inconclusive. These claims reemerged in 2010 in Pristina, capital of Kosovo, when a clinic and its surgeon were taken to court on organ trafficking charges. A similar clinic in Durban, South Africa, was heavily punished in 2010.

Future Needs and Solutions

By the 1990s, most organ transplants had excellent outcomes, but an impasse had been reached on increasing the organ supply. Cadaveric donation had declined and was well short of the growing need. In many parts of the world, the opposition to brain-death criteria and rarity of critical care units meant that heart and liver transplantation was simply not available, in spite of huge needs. For a solution, attention turned once more, and with determination, to the possibility of using nonhuman organs. Paul Russell, the Boston surgeon, summed up the pressures of the situation in the year 2000:

Regrettably, organs from human beings are available in numbers too small to benefit all potential recipients. Furthermore, because the transaction of transferring an organ from one individual to another is an intensely human one at every step in the process—calling on all the wisdom we have for the optimal handling and distribution of donated organs and selection of their recipients, the attentions of a wider range of savants extending from economics and the law to humanities, philosophy and even religion have been attracted. To my way of thinking, the clear shortcomings of our own species as a source of structures for the renewal of its own members can be expected to constitute a strong and continuing stimulus for further advances which will release us from this imperfect source.[123]

The conditions that limited human donation seemed resistant to all attempts at alteration. Traditionally the transplanters searching for alternatives had retained the assumption that monkey organs plus powerful immunosuppression would be the way forward. But new hopes in the twenty-first century did not rest on pharmacological input. Instead, rapid developments in genetic manipulation and cellular engineering offered radically new approaches.

19 Waiting for the Xenografts

THE 1990s were a time of continued, steady improvement in the results of organ transplantation. In the United States in mid-decade, 250 hospitals carried out kidney transplants, 160 reported heart grafting, and there were 70 liver transplant units. Cyclosporine was still important, but a number of new agents began to rival its dominant and lucrative position. Alternatives to azathioprine also appeared, and, as a result, there was an active and aggressive new commercial interest in immunosuppression.[1] The variety of immunosuppressive agents available gave doctors considerable flexibility, allowing them to individualize treatment, and different strategies evolved for different organs or tissues or for different age groups or for special groups of patients. No longer was there a single preferred regimen, and combination therapies using two or more of the available agents were actively explored in a welter of new trials. Since most organ transplants now had good outcomes, clinical and research attention switched from the traditional preoccupation with rejection to a focus on the side effects of immunosuppression. The well-known slow failure of some grafts after the first year was now also of interest, and this "chronic rejection" was now accorded attention as a new challenge.

Further Immunological Efforts

Tissue-typing methodology improved, notably from the use of flow cytometry cross-matching.[2] DNA typing offered more accurate and faster results.[3] Microchimerism in long-standing human allograft recipients was detected, and this presence of migrant donor cells persisting in the host was a major and unexpected empirical finding. Thomas Starzl strongly argued that successful graft survival depended on a subtle form of tolerance produced by these donor cells.[4] This view led to attempts at reinforcing or inducing this effect in organ grafting by a "mixed chimerism" strategy, giving donor-specific marrow cells concomitantly with the graft.[5]

413

The Holy Grail of achieving routine human tolerance induction in organ transplantation seemed reachable, yet again, and the multidisciplinary Immune Tolerance Network received a $160 million grant in 1999 for a major final push.

Chronic Rejection

There were interesting features to this steady loss of graft function after the first year.[6] All organ grafts losing function in this fashion showed a common pattern: an active fibrotic narrowing of blood vessels and duct systems, which caused individual pathological changes in the different organs.[7] In heart grafts, circumferential narrowing was found throughout the coronary vessels, "obliterative bronchiolitis" affected lung transplants, and a "vanishing bile duct syndrome" emerged after liver grafting. In the kidney, there were similar changes, as well as surface expression of senescence-associated markers on the cells.

It had been assumed that these delayed changes were immunological in nature, but closer study suggested that nonimmunological mechanisms might be important, such as the period of cold storage before transplantation, perfusion/reperfusion effects at the time of transplantation, major mismatches in size and age between the kidney graft and the recipient, and ongoing damage by immunosuppressants.[8] New attention to these factors gave hope for reducing the losses from chronic rejection.

New Immunosuppression

The expanded transplantation market was now an important one for the pharmaceutical companies, and a wealthy industrial/transplant complex was emerging. The companies looked for ways to improve on the well-established azathioprine and widened the search for products to rival CsA. Only the time-honored steroid component of the immunosuppression regimen proved indispensable for a while, despite the well-known side effects of its long-term use. There were market niches that the pharmaceutical companies wanted to fill, but stern licensing bodies continued to require expensive preliminary clinical drug trials, and there were new regulatory hurdles to surmount, including governments' increasing concern for the cost of these drugs.

Since the one-year results of transplantation were now excellent, launching a new agent meant looking for improvement in other dimensions of management, such as side effects, rejection episodes, chronic rejection, or advocating the new agent as part of a regimen for special cases, notably the niche needs of heart, lung, liver, pancreatic islet, and bone marrow transplant patients. Children's tolerance of the drugs was different, which invited the use of new protocols. With triple or even quadruple drug therapy finding favor, the possible permutations increased remarkably, sustaining the involvement of each company, and opening up the possibility of finding useful synergies, unsuspected from theory. "Big Pharma" companies and their trials were now almost embedded in the everyday life of the transplant units, and this intrusion and control had its critics.[9]

A successful alternative to azathioprine was licensed in 1995. Mycophenolate mofetil (MMF), another fungal product, was expensive and more toxic but also more powerful as an immunosuppressant than azathioprine.[10] Those patients intolerant of azathioprine immediately went on MMF therapy, and, in spite of its gastrointestinal side effects, it slowly found a place as a first-line agent in routine cases.[11]

Following the Sandoz company's commercial success with cyclosporine, the Fujisawa Pharmaceutical Company (later Astellas) also started testing microorganisms and fungi for useful activity. In 1984, the soil of the Japanese town of Tsukuba yielded a fungal strain later called *Streptomyces tsukubaensis*. From this fungus, the company produced FK 506 (tacrolimus), which proved highly successful in prolonging experimental grafts.[12] This success was followed by "fast track assessment" of the drug for use in the United States, and at the University of Pittsburgh, Starzl, who alone was licensed to study tacrolimus, soon considered it a major advance in human organ transplantation. It was tacrolimus that encouraged him to attempt human small bowel transplantation and then to use it for patients with other types of transplants.[13] It emerged as a favorite for use in liver transplantation and was notably free of some of the side effects of CsA, including the facial changes and elevation of blood lipids.[14] It did not supplant CsA immediately but initially found a place in managing those patients intolerant of CsA or when CsA was judged to have failed.[15]

These commercial successes at Sandoz and Fujisawa led a third company—Ayerst (later Wyeth-Ayerst)—to develop yet another fungal product, and this time there was no need to launch a fungus-hunting expedition. The company already had seventy-two stored soil samples obtained from the Canadian Medical Expedition's botanical survey of Rapa Nui (Easter Island), and, in 1976, Suren Sehgal began studying one of the Rapa Nui extracts: the promising substance sirolimus (branded Rapamycin or Rapamune). Although the promise of sirolimus emerged experimentally about the time of the launch of CsA, it took almost two decades before it was licensed for human use. It was then shown to be a potent immunosuppressive agent with a different chemical action and without the side effects of the other agents.[16]

The New Monoclonals

Antilymphocyte serum, the first biological agent to be used in clinical therapy, was a necessarily "polyclonal" sera derived from horses in the 1960s. It was largely replaced in the 1970s by monoclonal antibodies, which were less toxic. Genetic engineering produced "humanized" versions of these agents, and increasingly sophisticated antibodies against lymphocyte subsets were marketed with a characteristic group suffix. The first monoclonal products in regular use were muromonab (OKT3) and OKT4, which were first used clinically in 1981.[17] When steroids failed to prevent rejection, these monoclonals found their first use.

After the development of these early agents, the next human antilymphocyte monoclonals were basiliximab, daclizumab, and rituximab. An anti–CD 52 antibody, alemtuzumab (Campath), made and advocated by Roy Calne, showed promise. These antibodies steadily found use in the "induction" phase—the early period after transplantation. Experience showed that the monoclonals might be too specific and fail to affect some lymphocytes, and some continued to use the traditional, 1960s-style horse-derived "whole" sera, still available from a number of manufacturers.[18]

Homemade Immunotherapy

The early transplant surgeons had derived their own immunosuppressive methods and were proud to have introduced antilymphocyte serum at a time when none of the pharmaceutical companies were interested in organ transplantation. MALG, the Minnesota antilymphocyte globulin from John Najarian's surgical department, had sold steadily from the pioneering days of the 1960s, and, being highly regarded, it was used in 160 transplant units. The University of Minnesota had earned $79 million from MALG by 1990, but then there was a sad end to the "homemade" approach.

The regulatory environment had changed, particularly regarding reporting of side effects, and this innovative in-house production attracted the displeasure of the pharmaceutical industry and the Food and Drug Administration (FDA). MALG production was shut down abruptly in 1992, and the paperwork describing the earlier preparation and sale of the globulin was examined. After four years of unpleasant legal action, Najarian's university abandoned him to his legal fate and he went on trial in 1996 for a list of misdemeanors involving the production of MALG. Four weeks into the trial, the judge terminated the main action and dismissed it. "I don't know why we are here at all," he concluded.[19]

New Challenges

Surgical techniques for inserting first organ grafts were mature, but there were new challenges in those patients who had lost earlier grafts, notably when a third or fourth transplant was required, or when organ-splitting was possible. Minimally invasive techniques in kidney donation and transplantation emerged.[20] Hand, arm, and leg transplants, first reported in 1998, with face transplants following in 2005, were a technical and immunological tour de force as "composite tissue" grafts, in which the skin offered the toughest challenge.[21] Surgeons rejoined the large peripheral nerves involved, and the well-known reluctance of the body to regenerate peripheral nerves seemed to weaken under immunosuppression. Any failure of the nerve regrowth meant that the transplanted limb would be disabled.

But the shortage of grafts was still a major issue, and with growing numbers eligible for treatment with transplantation, the organ deficit was still growing. With little hope of supply rising to meeting the demand, attention once again turned to the ancient goal of xenografting, and the efforts to make animal organs feasible for human transplants began to show promise. But the solution to xenograft survival was not only an immunological one. The rapid developments in genetic and cellular engineering at this time offered strategies of interest to the transplant community.

Xenografting Revisited

Decades earlier, in the pioneering and optimistic 1960s, the first monkey-to-human kidney transplants were carried out, and occasional attempts with grafts of monkey livers or hearts followed. Short-term function was not unusual, but severe rejection episodes recurred and could not be controlled. In 1984, in the immediate post-CsA enthusiasm, some other similar attempts were made, but without success. The verdict was still that there was no therapeutic regimen that would ensure xenograft success.

The next xenograft attempts, in the 1990s, were quite different.[22] Until then it was widely assumed that future xenografting would involve overcoming the aggressive immune response to organs from monkeys, the animals closest to humans—"concordant transplantation," in the useful neologism Roy Calne used as early as 1970.[23] But public attitudes toward animal experimentation were changing once more. Britain's Animals Act of 1986 severely restricted all uses of primates. In any case, chimpanzees, a favored donor animal, were now an endangered species and were difficult to breed in captivity. Even if a successful xenograft strategy using primate organs could evolve, it was unlikely that the international demand could be met.

The radical alternative was to seek to modify animal donor tissue and use species not so closely related to humans—Calne's "discordant transplantation." Donor organ modification was possible because of new methods emerging in the world of cellular biology. Xenograft research and development moved rapidly up the academic transplant agenda, and biomedical companies watched the developments with interest. Controllers of start-up investment funds learned that there was a potentially large, lucrative market in engineered organs not only in developed countries but also in the huge, unmet need for the organs in developing countries, where there were so few human liver and heart donations.[24] Another potential benefit from xenografting was that the raft of ethical and clinical issues surrounding human-to-human transplantation would simply disappear.

The Challenge

Unlike a graft between the same species, a xenograft comes with a major "natural" antibody-mediated component that promptly causes hyperacute rejection; the result is damage to the arteries of the donor organ within hours. The goal of early xenografting strategies was to neutralize this antibody phase; the idea was that, if time could be bought, the cellular rejection that followed the antibody phase might be dealt with vigorously along the usual lines. Heroic regimens to remove these preformed antibodies from the blood showed some experimental promise, and such treatments involved plasmapheresis to remove antibody from the blood, immuno-absorption of antibody, the use of exotic drug agents such as cobra venom factor, or attempts to saturate donor antibody binding sites. But none of these methods found a firm place in experimental xenografting, and it was to the new genetic engineering methods that the transplanters turned.

DNA Transfers

Early experiments involving the insertion of foreign genes and DNA into bacteria or cells showed that DNA will happily transfer from species to species, settle in a new locus, and take up its normal tasks as "recombinant" DNA within organisms or cells.[25] The first practical uses of genetic engineering came in transferring human genes to the bacterium *Escherichia coli*, and, without public concern, this technology enabled the production of human insulin and a vaccine for hepatitis B.

The first approach to attempted modification of intact animals was to inject useful DNA segments into fertilized ova, hoping for integration.[26] One major success in this effort was the line of "transgenic" sheep created by microinjection of fertilized eggs with human alpha-1-antitrypsin genes (AAT). When the sheep produced by this method gave milk, it contained the AAT. The animals were then "pharmed"—that is, bred for production of this substance with potential use in treating some forms of lung disease.

Engineered Organs

The transgenic sheep work suggested the possibility of raising "discordant" animals with genetically altered organs, and the xenotransplanters turned to the pig. Pigs are hardy animals, easily handled, sexually mature at six months, and of a size similar to humans. They breed easily, and they have been tissue typed. Pigs are largely free of known pathogens affecting humans, other than one problematic retrovirus.[27] Being a common food source for humans, their experimental use seemed more acceptable to the public than use of monkeys. Moreover, pig transplant surgery was well established, notably at Calne's Cambridge University Department of Surgery.

The first genetic approach to transplant work using pigs sought to eliminate the hyperacute vascular antibody rejection phase. One attractive way was to "knock out" the attachment point of complement on the vascular cells, which proved possible in mice.[28] In pigs, another strategy also succeeded: insertion of a complement decay accelerating factor (DAF) into the pig via embryo injection. This method produced transgenic pigs suitable for organ graft studies.[29] Grafting of these modified pig hearts to monkeys did lead to less hyperacute rejection, and reasonable survival was obtained if conventional immunosuppression was added.

Xenografting Regulations

The prospect of using pig organs in human patients caused immediate concern, and the proposals attracted prompt regulatory attention. The U.S. Department of Health and Human Services issued its "Guideline on Infectious Disease Issues in Xenotransplantation."[30] In Britain, the Advisory Group on Ethics of Xenotransplantation emerged and issued a report—the Kennedy Report—in 1996.[31] The British Xenotransplantation Interim Regulatory Authority (UKXIRA) first met in May 1997 to watch developments in this field. One concern was that pig endogenous retroviruses might not only be pathogenic in humans but also enter into the human host DNA and then be inherited by the host's descendants thereafter. Some reassurance came from the absence of retroviruses in humans after use of pig tissue, notably the much-used pig heart valves, or after the brief use of pig pancreatic islet grafts in a small number of cases, or in patients

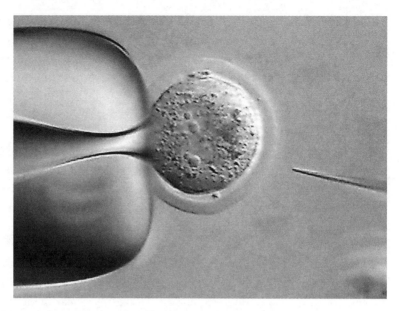

Cell fixation and injection methods allowed genetic engineering to develop. Image courtesy of Transgenic Animal Service, University of Queensland.

after pig liver perfusion was used experimentally for acute liver failure.[32] In October 1999, the UK regulatory authority cautiously encouraged the use of pig tissue but advised lifelong surveillance of any recipients.

Public opinion was generally favorable regarding these transplant developments and viewed the likely use of pigs as comic rather than threatening, but in Britain new animal rights activist groups made common cause with those already engaged in high-profile opposition to genetically modified crops. Both groups favored direct action, and there were attacks on the animal research establishments involved in genetic engineering.

Although a grand achievement had seemed likely after the development of transgenic pigs, the early promise was not quickly fulfilled.[33] Researchers soon realized that the routine use of pig organs in humans was going to be difficult and delayed, and the matter was no longer prominent on the bioethicists' agenda.

Nuclear Transfer

Gene transfer or "knock-out" for xenografting was the only major news from the genetic engineering front for a while. Attention turned to the quite different area of the possibilities for transplantation by transferring the entire central genetic apparatus of one animal cell to another via

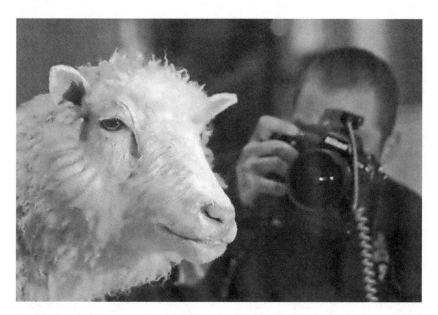

Dolly, the famous sheep cloned from cultured cells at the Roslin Institute, is now preserved at the nearby National Museum of Scotland in Edinburgh. Image courtesy of Maurice McDonald / Press Association.

whole nucleus removal and insertion. To add to this, yet another area of possibility opened up with the discoveries of the potential for stem cell use.

Nuclear transplantation of the adult cell nucleus into other cells began when Hans Spemann, Nobel Prize winner in 1935, achieved a simple form of nuclear transfer. In the 1950s, Robert Briggs, at the Institute of Cancer in Philadelphia, managed to transfer the nuclei of frog ova to the remains of a denucleated cell. Successful transfer of adult nuclei in larger animals, or "reproductive cloning," took time to emerge, and there were false dawns, both scientific and fictional.[34] Improvements in nuclear transfer techniques came in 1986, when Steen Willadsen achieved some success with nuclear transfer in large domestic species. The next innovation was crucial: adult nucleus-to-embryo transfers, successfully performed at the Roslin Institute near Edinburgh.[35] The celebrated sheep Dolly was the first animal created from nuclei of *adult* cells.[36]

These findings overturned two of the greatest certainties in classical biology, dating from August Weissman's time (1834–1914), namely that cellular differentiation was not reversible and that the nucleus steadily lost genetic material and capability with maturity. The nuclear transfer findings showed that inactive genes were retained in the adult nucleus and could be switched back on again. In theory, the cloned animal could be used for tissue to be grafted back into the nuclear donor animal, but the process was tedious and uncertain. Meanwhile, other avenues opened up.

Stem Cell Use

An embryo in its early stages comprises cells capable of development into all adult cell types. Less versatile equivalents are found in adult tissue, where they serve to repair and regenerate tissue. Fetal cord blood was also found to have cells capable of making all types of blood cells; use of these cells was soon routine in bone marrow transplantation. Other similar cells were found, even in the adult body, and developments in understanding these cells and their remarkable latent capabilities were watched with interest in transplant circles.

Embryonic cell manipulation moved rapidly, and, in 1998, the inner mass cells of the embryo (which Gail Martin called "stem cells" in 1981), were shown to be capable of developing into many specialized adult cells.[37] James Thomson at the University of Wisconsin obtained long-lasting stem cell lines from human embryos, and these cells could be stored for future use.[38] With nuclear transfer methods, it became theoretically possible to grow a new primitive kidney, which offered the distant prospect of growing organs acceptable to the nuclear donor. The use of human embryo cells caused alarm, however, and most countries soon had new legislation that allowed studies only up to about two weeks of cell culture. The United States took a harder line for a while: all such studies were prevented by legislation between 1995 and 2009.[39]

In 2007, however, further possibilities emerged that avoided the ethical concerns surrounding embryonic stem cell research. Adult stem cells, in both animals and humans, were found capable of returning to an embryonic state.[40] Useful grafts, such as bone marrow or pancreatic islets, might be created from a patient's own adult cells. Another distant prospect opened up, namely solving the ancient challenge of tissue replacement by using sources within a patient's own body.

Envoi

This account tells the story of organ and tissue transplantation up to the early part of the twenty-first century, and future historians will chronicle the events thereafter. Invention follows necessity, and for the many patients facing organ failure, the need is huge. In time, identifiable and desirable goals in medicine are usually reached. Human endeavor and ingenuity, plus some luck and attention to the unexpected, have served us well thus far and will take us further.

Conclusion
Lessons from the History of Transplantation

THE MANY LANDMARK EVENTS in the development of tissue transplantation offer data useful not only for their own sake but also for analyzing the more general mechanisms of clinical and scientific innovation. Looking at what happened and how it happened, rather than how it ought to have happened according to theory, is illuminating. The history of surgery is usually presented simply as steady technical progress in skilled hands, but the story of transplantation is a more complex one. The story has a rich mother lode of themes, topics, incidents, and case histories which offer rich pickings for historians of medicine. This is also the story of how distinguished scientists joined with erstwhile "artisans"—the surgeons—in seeking to understand and control rejection of foreign tissue.

Because progress in transplantation was not continuous, a "Whig" history, as some historians term the "onward and upward" traditional narrative, does not account for some remarkable gaps in the advance of tissue replacement. Progress not only halted at times but almost went into reverse, with insights already gained being lost. The first major hesitation in the advance of tissue replacement came with the neglect of Tagliacozzi's entirely sensible plastic surgical methods, which he published in 1599. His methods, well known at the time, then disappeared from the texts and discourse of the surgical world for two hundred years. Another remarkable discontinuity, after what is here called the "lost era," occurred after 1914, when the excellent recent gains in transplantation surgery and immunology in Europe were lost in the turmoil of World War I. In particular, Alexis Carrel's perceptive proposals in 1914 for chemical or radiation immunosuppression for organ grafting suffered neglect until revived in the 1950s, as were other insights of this lost era.

Less prolonged delays in the evolution of transplantation were the various moratoria on human organ grafting from the 1950s. A series of kidney transplants were attempted in Paris and Boston without immunosuppression, and the lessons learned were put aside until the early 1960s, when a restart was possible when immunosuppressive methods emerged. Other tentative episodes involved liver transplantation in 1966 and particularly heart transplantation after 1968, when poor results and adverse public opinion made it nearly impossible to perform heart transplants for nearly a decade.

In addition to these hesitations in the broader advance of transplantation, there were periods when "bad science," consisting mostly of uncritical observation, stymied progress. In the late 1800s, observational errors meant that skin graft assessment was faulty, leading to widespread claims for success with human-to-human grafting. The next error built on these flawed observations, namely that if homograft skin survived after grafting, then the way was open for grafting glands, even animal glands. The pitfalls here were numerous. Gland grafts could not be visually observed or otherwise assessed; microscopy had never been used in this situation. After gland grafts for treatment of diseases with a fluctuating course, such as thyroid deficiency and diabetes, spontaneous postoperative improvements were mistaken for graft function. The experimental standard of having untreated patients serve as the control group was absent, whereas observer enthusiasm was present and all powerful. Although these errors were dealt with prior to World War I, the return of postwar bad science allowed gland-grafting enthusiasm to return in the 1920s. Testis transplants for the ills of aging, though eventually ridiculed, were widely supported for a decade in respectable surgical circles.

Not even later generations were safe from beguiling projects viewed without adequate critical distance. In the low-morale period in the transplantation world in the 1970s, many became convinced that generally stimulating the immune response, a perennially seductive idea, would successfully treat human cancer, and many clinicians, including some transplanters, after anecdotal claims for success, started trials of crude methods for boosting the immune response in human cancer of all kinds. But later, more careful studies failed to show benefit, and the simplistic methods were abandoned after ten years.

At the edge of the bad science spectrum is fraud. Leaving aside the public of total eye graft claims in 1920s Vienna and the subsequent goat-gland quackery in Kansas, the world of transplantation in later, better-regulated times still had at least two serious cases of deliberate deception, including the notorious case in which black skin grafts on white mice had been enhanced with black ink.

The evolution of transplantation offers plenty of evidence that it would be a mistake to ascribe surgical progress to a single source, notably an overarching "scientific method." This method has no role in the genesis of novelty but is evoked and mobilized to prevent erroneous claims for novelty. It does so by ensuring objective analysis of sufficient observations. The roots of important scientific innovation are different and derive from creative proposals and hypotheses then subjected to repeated testing. The process is similar to artistic creativity and remains mysterious in origin; it certainly cannot be successfully sought or taught.

As this history of transplantation shows, surgical progress comes from use not of any single scientific method but from a pack of methods. Surgeons use a rich variety of strategies—heeding unusual clinical observations, taking lessons from animal experiments, picking up news from the laboratories, importing new technology, or experimenting with new pharmaceutical agents. Focused study of large human transplant data sets has a place. Significant clinical observations in organ transplantation brought to light phenomena not seen in experimental animal work, notably rejection crises and graft adaptation. Much earlier observations from the late 1700s showed for the first time that disease could be transmitted by apparently normal graft tissue. These human studies changed assumptions on fundamental pathological and immunological mechanism. A clinical paradox came in the 1970s, when transplant surgeons found that prior blood transfusion mysteriously improved organ graft survival rather than hindering it. Thus, after the reasonable no-transfusion policy was in place, clinical observation that something had "gone wrong" taught a lesson, and the no-transfusion policy was reversed since giving blood seemed to induce tolerance. In the lab, noticing experiments that "go wrong" or findings that "do not fit" has always been rewarding, since unexpected outcomes mean instead that the accepted theory was wrong and that a novel mechanism had declared itself. Medawar's freemartin twin cattle exchanged grafts when they should not have done so. Glick's class experiment with bursectomized hens "went wrong," since they failed to make antibody when they should have.

Other scientific mini-methods include good luck and serendipity, that is, finding something of significance by accident. In transplantation immunology, these documented incidents include the chance discovery of a technique for cold preservation of cells, when glycerol was inadvertently added to the reagents that had not yielded success. Even the lymphocyte mitogens—agents that activate these white cells—were first demonstrated when a cell culture was left over a weekend, rather than viewed, as usual, at twenty-four hours. Henry Claman's demonstration of the crucial lymphocyte cell cooperation between T- and B-cells was cheerfully acknowledged to have come from an unintended mixing of these cells, not previously thought to interact. Such lucky accidents may have been underreported for fear they would diminish the mystique of scientific discovery and reverence for "the method." Serious investigators often deny the existence of "Eureka" moments, so beloved in popular science writing. However, Angelo DiGeorge did have such a moment when the soon-to-be-named DiGeorge syndrome (congenital absence of the thymus) suddenly occurred to him upon hearing another speaker's data at a conference, prompting him to announce the new disease to the audience on the spot.

One lesson biomedicine has learned is to be watchful for "accidents of nature" that may provide new understandings, and transplantation is particularly in debt to such insights. Important accidents of nature include congenital deficiencies of the immune system, the study of which assisted in unraveling the workings of the system. Children born with serious susceptibility to various infectious diseases were studied in the 1960s, and such children seemed to fall into two types. These types soon neatly correlated with deficiency of cell-mediated immunity (thymus defect) or failure to make antibody (bursa-equivalent defect).

Twins as an accident of nature have certainly had an interesting role in the history of transplantation. Best known is the kidney transplant between human twins in Boston in 1954, which showed that the operation could be a technical success and sustain life; twins thus led the way to human transplantation. St. Louis plastic surgeons' use of human twins in the 1930s emphasized that all non-twin interhuman grafts failed, thus putting an end to the muddles of the 1920s. Further back, John Hunter's careful look at the puzzling anatomy of the freemartin cattle twins was important, and study of the same twin cattle led Peter Medawar to unlock the secret of their natural tolerance, which led to his celebrated description of tolerance induction mechanisms.

An overview of the history of transplantation shows that, during times of progress, paradigms later shown to be faulty had important conditioning at the time. The humoral graft rejection paradigm, that is, the antibody explanation of graft loss, was unquestioned in the mid-twentieth century. The world of immunology, vibrant at that time, favored sophisticated explanations based on antibody mechanisms. The problem was that no antibodies could be found in graft rejection. But the humoral paradigm persisted in the face of explanatory failure until its collapse; the entirely different cell-mediated rejection mechanism, based on lymphocytes, took its place in the early 1950s. Also in that decade, another humoral mechanism was reflexively favored when bone marrow cells were found to protect against radiation, when it was wrongly claimed that the cells were releasing a chemical factor. Eventually, the notion of cell seeding was accepted instead. This humoral-cellular paradigm switching was part of a wider, even ancient, debate in biology and in medicine on such mechanisms in health and disease.

The cellular role was well concealed. In physiology and anatomy up to 1950, the standard teaching was that the lymphocyte was an indolent, short-lived, immobile cell in the tissues and blood. When the lymphoid cell's origin, rapid recirculation, and long life were uncovered and its immunological role shown, the earlier teaching was abandoned with embarrassment.

Other crucial paradigm shifts are more recent. For example, it was generally held until recent times that human organ grafts do not react against the host. But the demonstration that microchimerism was playing a part in the new "two-way paradigm" led to strategies for inducing mixed chimerism and hence tolerance. A second revolutionary paradigm shift was the demise of a basic tenet of traditional biology: that cell differentiation, from embryonic forms to specialized cells, was irreversible and that the inactive genetic material was discarded as differentiation proceeded. When it was revealed that the old genetic material was retained, a new possibility of coaxing mature cells to revert to multi-potent stem cells opened up, as did the prospect for using this process to create tissue for repair. Further examples of paradigm adherence, shift, and collapse can be found in earlier periods. In Tagliacozzi's time, the reasonable mindset regarding transplantation drew on horticultural reasoning, namely that the well-established ancient methods of grafting in the plant world would also apply to animals. Since plants could be regularly and easily joined by hybridization, it was reasonably assumed that animal grafting could be achieved between disparate donors and recipients. It also followed that animal grafts would unite as in the garden, with direct end-to-end union of the vessels involved. These assumptions are embedded in John Hunter's discourse. But the animals-are-plants paradigm collapsed eventually, not only with the acceptance of homograft rejection but also with the knowledge that it was ingrowth of capillaries that restored function in free grafts.

Even the lesser paradigms were obstacles to progress. A striking example was that the pioneer kidney transplanters of the early 1960s "knew" not to cool or perfuse kidneys prior to transplantation. No one knew where the prohibition came from, but it received great respect, and only when the cardiac surgeons announced that "cool is good" for the donor heart did the kidney grafters nervously bring in flushing and cooling of their donor organs, and it was soon unthinkable not to do so.

Two other such idées fixes may not yet be entirely removed from the human mind and were excluded intermittently from the scientific literature with difficulty. One is that fetal tissues are immunologically "bland" and thus not rejected. Although this notion was already known to be false in 1912, the idea and its hopeful consequences were regularly resurrected in respectable circles up to the 1980s and were part of the plausible promotions at rejuvenation clinics. All the careful evidence is to the contrary. Another recurring hope not entirely banished is that tissue culture will remove surface constituents from cells and make them acceptable for transplantation without immunosuppression.

Historians do not often look closely at the mechanism of introduction and acceptance of new surgical procedures, but these advances are important and exhibit a recurring pattern. There are times and places for innovation. Innovative persons and their insights are not random occurrences. The few who are able to produce novelty are enabled by their milieu. The cultural confidence and creativity that nations display from time to time usually come about at times of economic strength, and vitality is seen in many of the nation's activities, not in medical science alone. In innovative centers, experimenting with new operative techniques is risky, and surgeons who do so not only encounter the usual resistance to novelty but also meet the practical objection that they could cause harm to the patients involved. Pioneering surgery is therefore carried out under a double burden and is preceded by discussion and hesitation during which conventional practitioners urge the maverick not to proceed. Furthermore, before employing a new surgical technique on human patients, it is usual to gain experience in large animal work first, a strategy not always supported by all of the public. Less supportable in retrospect was the practicing of human pioneer surgery on an available cadaver in the postmortem rooms.

Even with this preparation, the first steps into the surgical unknown often hit unknown difficulties. The originator starts and reports early cases, successful or otherwise. If there is failure, the critics feel entitled to some schadenfreude, and then there is a period of reflection, plus a moratorium, sometimes self-imposed, sometimes imposed. Later, some helpful new factor spurs a successful resumption of the surgical activity, and others cautiously follow the lead. With increasing success, earlier doubts dwindle, and, as time passes, the pioneers gain skill and confidence, and, even if the operation is difficult, surgeons in training master it with increasing ease, increasingly unaware of the earlier technical and professional challenges. Surprising numbers of cases suitable for the operation appear, and the demand for it proves greater than was previously thought. The first patients involved may have been seriously ill and ready to resort to the surgery as a last resort, but as time passes and fitter patients receive the treatment, outcomes improve. Added to these progressive steps is the mysterious "things just get better" dimension. Late, unexpected side effects and events might spark new concerns when they appear in the front-running patient survivors in the pioneer units. The new complication's successful analysis and treatment add to the reputation and authority of these units. If the new operation is complex, costs may then become an issue, especially if budgets are constrained. The point when the operation is no longer classed as experimental but routine and established is an important event in those nations where medical costs are on a fee-for-service basis, such as the United States. Later, a dispute may emerge as to who first pioneered and published the now well-established procedure or variants of it, with claims and counterclaims. This template of surgical innovation is frequently detected, as this book has shown.

A recurring theme in medical history is resistance to novelty, and new ideas and initiatives in clinical work are often only established with difficulty. Their spread and acceptance are often impeded and ring-fenced by reflex opposition at various levels. Local opposition is common, and the first documented episode was the denigration by his rivals in the 1600s of Tagliacozzi's entirely rational plastic surgery. In more recent times such opposition was prominent and is well documented. After Lawler's pioneer kidney transplant in 1950 in Chicago, he was avoided in polite company and was rebuked by his urologists' organization. The Boston kidney grafting attempts that followed quickly at that time were controversial and not described at surgical meetings nor published until much later. Even the first intertwin kidney graft in 1954, now celebrated, was carried out in spite of some local hospital hostility, and others elsewhere were discouraged from following this lead. In liver transplantation, Starzl had steady opposition from the outset. Such concerns can be called peer-group or personal resistance, but with the growth of regulatory bodies, a new level of institutional resistance emerged. At the time of the controversial heart transplants of 1968, these local and national regulatory agencies were in place, and lasting moratoriums of various kinds were imposed at high levels.

History, in analyzing the past, can be of help in considering what will happen next, and a historical awareness can lead to suggestions and predictions. The present goal in transplantation is to create a steady and adequate supply of humanized animal organs or to use versatile cells to replace defective tissues. To reach these goals, the familiar raft of methods will be in use. When, in times to come, a simple version of the various solutions is written, it may suggest that the route was obvious and progress on it was steady. Instead, at the start of the early twenty-first century, the way ahead is not clear. As always, there is a choice to make among various paths of opportunity, many doomed to be forsaken. As successful routes open up, there will be hesitations and diversions. This is the central lesson from the history of tissue and organ transplantation.

Human ingenuity usually solves human challenges, given time. In this effort, as always, the many will be guided by the few, who alone have the perception to see, and do, what others cannot.

Notes

1. Early Transplantation

1. For a full analysis, see Caroline Walker Bynum, *The Resurrection of the Body in Western Christianity, 200–1336* (New York: Columbia University Press, 1995).

2. For example, in Iraq, after the U.S. military took over the empty Abu Ghraib prison facility, former inmates appeared and sought permission to recover the remains of their hands, amputated by the Saddam Hussein regime. In 1997, a Florida court awarded $1.25 million in damages against a funeral home that had lost the legs amputated seven years earlier from a diabetic Orthodox Jew. The funeral home had agreed to store the limbs to allow their burial with the patient after death.

3. Stith Thompson, *Motif-Index of Folk-Literature*, rev. ed. (Copenhagen: Rosenkilde & Bagger, 1955–1958). See also G. Schramm, "Sun Szu-mo's Organ Transplantation: A Chinese Fairy Tale," *Deutsche Medizinische Wochenschrift* 94, no. 23 (1969): 1254; A. H. Hawkins, "A Change of Heart: The Paradigm of Regeneration in Medical and Religious Narrative," *Perspectives in Biology and Medicine* 33, no. 4 (1990): 547–59; various tales of heart loss and restoration in Milad Doueihi, *A Perverse History of the Human Heart* (Cambridge, MA: Harvard University Press, 1997), 3, 11, 16, 24, 48, 87; and Douglas B. Price, "Miraculous Restoration of Lost Body Parts: Relationship to the Phantom Limb Phenomenon and to Limb-Burial Superstitions and Practices," *American Folk Medicine: A Symposium*, ed. Wayland D. Hand (Berkeley: University of California Press, 1976), 49–71.

4. This Celtic tale is from Mary Beith, *Healing Threads: Traditional Medicines of the Highlands and Islands* (Edinburgh: Polygon, 1995), 30, 255. See also John Francis Campbell, *Popular Tales of the West Highlands* (Paisley, 1890; Edinburgh: Birlinn, 1994).

5. Barry D. Kahan, "Preface: Pien Ch'iao, the Legendary Exchange of Hearts, Traditional Chinese Medi-

cine, and the Modern Era of Cyclosporine," *Transplantation Proceedings* 20, no. 2 (1988): 3–12; Mahendra Bhandari and Ashutosh Tewari, "Is Transplantation Only 100 Years Old?" *British Journal of Urology* 79, no. 4 (1997): 495–98. For heart burial legends, see Brian R. Boylan, *The New Heart* (Philadelphia: Chilton, 1969).

6. Clarence Burton Day, *Chinese Peasant Cults: Being a Study of Chinese Paper Gods* (Shanghai: Kelly & Walsh, 1940), 39.

7. Charles Gould, *Mythical Monsters* (London, 1884); Beryl Rowland, *Animals with Human Faces: A Guide to Animal Symbolism* (London: Allen & Unwin, 1974); Pierre Brunel, ed., *Companion to Literary Myths, Heroes and Archetypes* (London: Routledge, 1992). These composites were also favored in heraldry.

8. The last public exhibition of an alleged mermaid's body was by P. T. Barnum on Broadway in 1843. Specimens of mermaids and mermen surviving in museums have been uniformly shown, usually by x-rays, to be frauds. See D. Heppell, "The Anatomy of the Mermaid," *Reports of the Proceedings of the Scottish Society of the History of Medicine* 93–94 (1992–1993): 21–26.

9. Vassilis G. Vitsaxis, *Hindu Epics, Myths and Legends in Popular Illustrations* (Delhi: Oxford University Press, 1977); Barry D. Kahan, "Ganesha: The Primeval Hindu Xenograft," *Transplantation Proceedings* 21, no. 3 (1989): 1–8. This story suggests there were no ancient cultural objections to xenografts, namely the transplanting of tissue from animals to humans.

10. Howard Clark Kee, *Miracle in the Early Christian World: A Study in Sociohistorical Method* (New Haven, CT: Yale University Press, 1983), and *Miracle and Magic in New Testament Times* (Cambridge: Cambridge University Press, 1986).

11. This "servant's ear" episode is described with variations in each of the four gospels; only in the Gospel

of Luke (reputed to be a physician) does Jesus replace the servant's ear (Luke 22:50–51). See also B. Tosatti, "Transplantation and Reimplantation in the Arts," *Surgery* 75, no. 3 (March 1974): 389–97.

12. Price, "Miraculous Restoration of Lost Body Parts," 55.

13. Barbara Fay Abou-El-Haj, *The Medieval Cult of the Saints* (Cambridge: Cambridge University Press, 1997); Benedicta Ward, *Miracles and the Medieval Mind* (London: Scolar, 1982).

14. This miracle has been extensively analyzed; see Ludwig Deubner, *Kosmas und Damian* (Leipzig: Teubner, 1907); "Cosmas and Damian," in *The Catholic Encyclopaedia* (New York: Robert Appleton, 1912, 2002); and Charles Singer and Dorothea Singer, "On a Miniature Ascribed to Mantegna, of an Operation by Cosmas and Damian," in *Contributions to Medical and Biological Research Dedicated to Sir William Osler* (New York: Paul B. Hoeber, 1919), 166–76, which has a scholarly bibliography. See also Barry D. Kahan, "Cosmas and Damian Revisited," *Transplantation Proceedings* 15, no. 4 (1983): 2211–16; Thomas Schlich, "How Gods and Saints Became Transplant Surgeons: The Scientific Article as a Model for the Writing of History," *History of Science* 33 (1995): 311–31; and D. C. Schechter, "Role of the Confraternity of St. Cosmas in the Evolution of French Surgery," *Surgery* 64, no. 5 (Nov. 1968): 1002–12. The cult of these saints in England is described in Leslie G. Matthews, "Cosmas and Damian—Patron Saints of Medicine and Pharmacy: Their Cult in England," *Medical History* 12, no. 3 (July 1968): 281–88.

15. Forty paintings of the event are reproduced in Kees W. Zimmermann, *One Leg in the Grave: The Miracle of the Transplantation of the Black Leg by the Saints Cosmas and Damian* (Maarssen, Netherlands: Elsevier, 1998).

16. For similar miracles, see Mary Hamilton, *Incubation, or the Cure of Disease in Pagan Temples and Christian Churches* (London: W. C. Henderson & Son at the University Press, St. Andrews, 1906).

17. Jacobus de Voragine's *The Golden Legend* has been reprinted many times since its first appearance as *Legenda Aurea Fiorentina* (1275). This extract comes from the Kelmscott Press edition (1900), 861–64.

18. Centuries later, in New England in 1675, the twisted-neck myth appeared again when British colonial soldiers faced the native Indians. When the bald Captain Samuel Moseley plucked off his periwig, "the better to fight with," word spread among the Indians

that he had removed one head and grown another, and they fled. See *The Present State of New England with Respect to the Indian War* (London, 1676).

19. James Craigie Robertson, *Materials for the History of Thomas Becket: Rolls Series; Chronicles and Memorials of Great Britain* (London, 1875–1885), 428. For healing at English places of pilgrimage, see Ronald C. Finucane, *Miracles and Pilgrims: Popular Beliefs in Medieval England* (New York: St. Martin's Press, 1995).

20. Modern attitudes about these early miracles range from the view that they are entirely true or entirely fanciful. A secular explanation of some limb replacement stories might be the well-known "phantom limb" sensation after amputation; see Douglas B. Price and Neil J. Twombly, *The Phantom Limb Phenomenon: A Medical, Folkloric, and Historical Study* (Washington, DC: Georgetown University Press, 1978).

21. See Charles E. Dinsmore, *A History of Regeneration Research: Milestones in the Evolution of a Science* (Cambridge: Cambridge University Press, 1991), which describes a miraculous human limb regeneration in Zaragoza, Spain, in 1640.

22. François Rabelais, *Pantagruel*, bk. II, chap. 30. The durable head-transplant-wry-neck theme emerged again in some of the Frankenstein films of the twentieth century, notably in the satirical *Torticola contre Frankensberg* (Paul Paviot, 1952).

23. Keith Thomas, *Religion and the Decline in Magic: Studies in Popular Beliefs in Sixteenth- and Seventeenth-Century England* (London: Weidenfeld & Nicolson, 1971).

24. U. B. S. Prakash, "Shushruta of Ancient India," *Surgery, Gynecology & Obstetrics* 146, no. 2 (1978): 263–72; K. B. Kansupada and J. W. Sassani, "Sushruta: The Father of Indian Surgery and Ophthalmology," *Documenta Ophthalmologica* 93 (1997): 159–67.

25. The Zeis Index is an incomparable source on early plastic surgery; see Thomas J. S. Patterson, trans., *The Zeis Index and History of Plastic Surgery 900 BC–AD 1863* (Baltimore: Williams and Wilkins, 1977). An interesting introduction is also found in John B. de C. M. Saunders, "A Conceptual History of Transplantation," in *Transplantation*, ed. John S. Najarian and Richard L. Simmons (Philadelphia: Lea & Febiger, 1972), 3–25.

26. See Erwin Heinz Ackerknecht, "Primitive Surgery," *American Anthropologist* 49, no. 1 (1947): 25–

45; and John G. Lascaratos and P. Dalla-Vorgia, "The Penalty of Mutilation for Crimes in the Byzantine Era (324–1453 A.D.)," *International Journal of Risk and Safety in Medicine* 10, no. 1 (1997): 51–56. For a late use of such punishment and surgical restoration, in colonial America in the 1760s, see M. S. Arons, M. F. Freshwater, and R. Hegel, "Abel's Auricle—A Colonial Tale of Plastic Surgery," *Connecticut Medicine* 40, no. 12 (1976): 851–55.

27. Ackerknecht, "Primitive Surgery," suggests that the puzzling absence of early excisional surgery is explained by the prevailing religious belief that there would be dire consequences if a person was not whole when entering the afterlife.

28. The Taliban mutilated and expelled a nineteen-year-old girl, cutting off her nose and ears. The Grossman Burn Foundation rescued and treated her in Los Angeles. For her story and portrait, see *Time* magazine, August 9, 2010.

29. Redcliffe N. Salaman, "Deformities and Mutilations of the Face as Depicted in the Chimu Pottery of Peru," *Journal of the Royal Anthropological Institute* 69, no. 1 (1939): 109–22; P. A. Padula and L. W. Friedmann, "Acquired Amputation and Prostheses before the Sixteenth Century," *Angiology* 38, no. 2 (Feb. 1987): 133–41.

30. Enlarged ear lobes have been noted as an aid to beauty in many early civilizations; see J. Park Harrison, "On the Artificial Enlargement of the Earlobe," *Journal of the Royal Anthropological Institute* 2 (1873): 190–99.

31. Ibn Absillsaibal translated *Suśruta* into Arabic (*Kitab-i-Susrud*) between AD 700 and 800. This surgical description of rhinoplasty in *Suśruta* is from *An English Translation of Sushruta Samhita: Based on Original Sanskrit Text*, edited and published by Kaviraj Kunja Lal Bhishagratna (Calcutta, 1907), chap. 16, paras. 19–24. A complete and satisfactory English translation of *Suśruta* does not yet exist. The Arab use of the *Suśruta* is detailed in Fuat Sezgin, *Geschichte des Arabischen Schrifttums*, vol. 3 (Leiden: Brill, 1970), 197.

32. *English Translation of Sushruta Samhita*, chap. 16.

33. This analysis is taken from Priayadaranjan Ray and Acharya Prafulla Chandra Ray, *History of Chemistry in Ancient and Medieval India* (Calcutta: Indian Chemical Society, 1956), 240–42.

34. Although early historians claimed to find evidence for the practice of skin grafting in ancient Egyptian medical works, the definitive translations do not confirm this claim; see James H. Breasted, *The Edwin Smith Surgical Papyrus*, vol. 1 (Chicago: University of Chicago Press, 1930). No early Chinese attempts at skin grafting or transplantation are found in the main works on Chinese surgical history; see Wu Lien-teh, *Manchurian Plague Prevention Service Reports* (1929–1930), 7, 93–100.

35. Celsus, *De medicina*, bk. 7, chaps. 9, 25; Galen, *Methodus medendi*, bk. 14, chap. 16.

36. See Emilie Savage-Smith, "The Practice of Surgery in Islamic Lands: Myth and Reality," *Social History of Medicine* 13 (2000): 307–21.

37. Martin S. Spink and Geoffrey L. Lewis, *Albucasis: On Surgery and Instruments; A Definitive Edition of the Arabic Text* (London: Wellcome Institute, 1973).

38. However, dog-to-human skin grafting is mentioned in fifteenth-century Persia; see Cyril Elgood, "Baha'-ul-Doulah and the Quintessence of Experience," in *Science, Medicine and History: Essays on the Evolution of Scientific Thought and Medical Practice*, ed. E. Ashworth Underwood (London: Oxford University Press, 1953), 229; and also in *Analecta Medico-Historica* 2 (1966): 62, as noticed before by Savage-Smith, "Practice of Surgery in Islamic Lands."

39. See Katherine Park and Michael R. McVaugh, *Medicine from the Black Death to the French Disease*, ed. Roger French, Jon Arrizabalaga, Andrew Cunningham, and Louis Garcia-Ballester (Aldershot, England: Ashgate, 1998), 111–55.

40. Current medical historiography avoids use of the word *empiric*, since the hints of charlatanism are not usually justified. The itinerant group, many of whom were highly regarded, could have had considerable surgical skills; see Michael McVaugh, "Cataracts and Hernias: Aspects of Surgical Practice in the Fourteenth Century," *Medical History* 45, no. 3 (July 2001): 319–40; and Sandra Cavallo, *Artisans of the Body in Modern Italy: Identities, Families and Masculinities* (Manchester: Manchester University Press, 2007).

41. Much of this account comes from the classic study by Martha T. Gnudi and Jerome P. Webster, *The Life and Times of Gaspare Tagliacozzi* (New York: Herbert Reichner, 1950). See also J. P. Webster, "Some Portrayals of Gaspare Tagliacozzi," *Plastic and Reconstructive Surgery* 41, no. 5 (May 1968): 411–26.

42. Secrecy was common in medical practice at the time, and later there came a wave of popular "books of secrets" claiming to open up the practice of medi-

cine. Most notable was *Secreti medicinali* (1561), written by the itinerant opportunist Leonardo Fioravanti. He had witnessed Italian artisans performing rhinoplasty and claimed to have successfully replaced a nose cut off in a duel. See William Eamon, *Science and the Secrets of Nature: Secrets in Medieval and Early Modern Culture* (Princeton: Princeton University Press, 1996). For an admiring biographical portrait, see Paolo Santoni-Rugiu and Riccardo Mazzola, "Leonardo Fioravanti (1517–1588): A Barber-Surgeon Who Influenced the Development of Reconstructive Surgery," *Plastic and Reconstructive Surgery* 99, no. 2 (Feb. 1997): 570–75.

43. Bartolommeo Fazio, *De viris illustribus liber nunc primum* (1456), 38. Fazio died in 1457, and his text reappeared at Florence in 1745.

44. Silvano Furlan and Riccardo F. Mazzola, "Alessandro Benedetti, a Fifteenth Century Anatomist and Surgeon: His Role in the History of Nasal Reconstruction," *Plastic and Reconstructive Surgery* 96, no. 3 (1995): 739–43.

45. McVaugh, "Cataracts and Hernias," admirably explains the surgical timidity of the day and gives details of the professional difficulties awaiting surgical failure.

46. Gaspare Tagliacozzi, *De curtorum chirurgia per insitionem* (Venice, 1597). Though the text has been much studied, particularly by Gnudi and Webster in *Life and Times of Gaspare Tagliacozzi*, a full translation is still not available. Gnudi and Webster provide a reprint of Alexander Read's 1687 translation of Tagliacozzi's work, but book 2 only.

47. A Venetian adventurer in India at this time did describe the local rhinoplasty methods, but there is no evidence that he influenced the Italian practice. See Philip J. Sykes, Paolo Santoni-Rugiu, and Riccardo F. Mazzola, "Nicolò Manuzzi (1639–1717) and the First Report of the Indian Rhinoplasty," *Journal of Plastic, Reconstructive and Aesthetic Surgery* 63, no. 2 (2010): 247–50.

48. Tagliacozzi, *Curtorum chirurgia*, bk. 2, pt. 4, p. 656, from Gnudi and Webster, *Life and Times of Gaspare Tagliacozzi*, 460.

49. In 1526, in Scotland, the abbot of Kinloss used the services of a "one-legged gardener with skills in grafting of trees and healing of wounds." Tagliacozzi quotes the grafting sections of the early Latin botanical texts by Columella (*De arboribus*) and Palladius (*De re rustica*), classical works also rediscovered during this era.

50. Tagliacozzi, *Curtorem chirurgia*, bk. 2, pt. 4, p. 646, from Gnudi and Webster, *Life and Times of Gaspare Tagliacozzi*, 457.

51. See Gnudi and Webster, *Life and Times of Gaspare Tagliacozzi*, for their translation of Tagliacozzi, *Curtorum chirurgia*, bk. 1, pt. 18, p. 61. The entirety of part 18 relates to such tissue donation from another body.

52. Robert C. van de Graaf, "Did Nicolò Manuzzi (1639–1717) Carry Out Reconstructive Nose Surgery Himself?" *Journal of Plastic, Reconstructive and Aesthetic Surgery* 63, no. 2 (2010): 254.

53. In 1587, similar accusations in Italy involved Giovanni (or Giambattista) della Porta and his Academia Secretorum Naturae. For analysis of "acceptable and unacceptable" unnatural powers at this time, see David Pingree, "Learned Magic in the Time of Frederick II," *Micrologus* 2 (1994): 39–56.

54. Alan Clive Roberts, *Facial Prostheses: The Restoration of Facial Defects by Prosthetic Means* (London: Kimpton, 1971).

55. D. C. Lee, "Tycho Brahe and His Sixteenth Century Nasal Prosthesis," *Plastic and Reconstructive Surgery* 50, no. 4 (1972): 332–37. Paré's text on prosthetic replacement is *Traitant des moyens et artifices d'ajouter ce qui defaut naturellement ou par accident* (Paris, 1575); for a commentary, see T. Gibson, "The Prostheses of Ambroise Paré," *British Journal of Plastic Surgery* 8, no. 1 (Apr. 1955): 3–8.

56. Patricia Fara, *Sympathetic Attractions: Magnetic Practices, Beliefs, and Symbolism in Eighteenth-Century England* (Princeton: Princeton University Press, 1996); Keith Thomas, *Religion and the Decline of Magic: Studies in Popular Beliefs in Sixteenth- and Seventeenth-Century England* (London: Weidenfeld & Nicolson, 1971).

57. See John M. Headley, *Tommaso Campanella and the Transformation of the World* (Princeton: Princeton University Press, 1997).

58. Athanasius Kircher, *Magnes sive de arte magnetica opus tripartitum* (Cologne, 1643), 333. Kircher gathered together all known natural knowledge in his forty-four volume work and was labeled as a "gossipy encyclopedist" by some and the "father of modern natural science" by others. See Paula Findlen, *Athanasius Kircher: The Last Man Who Knew Everything* (New York: Routledge, 2004); and John E. Fletcher, "Medical Men and Medicine in the Correspondence of Athanasius Kircher (1602–80)," *Janus* 56 (1969): 259–77.

59. Jean Baptiste van Helmont, *A Ternary of Paradoxes: The Magnetick Cure of Wounds, Nativity of Tartar in Wine, Image of God in Man*, trans. Walter Charleton (London, 1650), 13–14. See also Walter Pagel, *Joan Baptista van Helmont: Reformer of Science and Medicine* (Cambridge: Cambridge University Press, 1982). Van Helmont's report of the slave donor is the first account, albeit literary, of a paid, living, unrelated tissue donor. It is possible that a donor had died shortly after the operation, thus also giving the surgeon an excuse for the graft loss.

60. Thomas H. Browne, *Pseudodoxia epidemica* (London, 1646), bk. 2, chap. 3, line 18.

61. Robert T. Petersson, *Sir Kenelm Digby: The Ornament of England, 1603–1665* (Cambridge, MA: Harvard University Press, 1956); B. J. Dobbs, "Studies in the Natural Philosophy of Sir Kenelm Digby," *Ambix* 18, no. 1 (Mar. 1971): 1–25. See also William F. Bynum, "The Weapon Salve in Seventeenth Century English Drama," *Journal of the History of Medicine* 21, no. 1 (Jan. 1966): 8–23. The last literary use of the power of "sympathy" and transplantation was in Edmond About's novel *Le Nez d'un notaire* (Paris, 1862), translated as *The Lawyer's Nose* (London, 1879).

62. Sir Kenelm Digby, *A Late Discourse Made in a Solemn Assembly of Nobles and Learned Men at Montpellier in France* (London, 1658). See also David Hamilton and James T. Goodrich, "An Illustration of Skin Graft Rejection and Sympathetic Medicine from 1661," *Bulletin of the History of Medicine* 60, no. 2 (summer 1986): 217–21. Digby's presentation at Montpellier might be imaginatively termed the first paper on tissue transplantation given at a scholarly meeting.

63. A list of the protagonists in this matter is found in Lynn Thorndike, *A History of Magic and Experimental Science during the First Thirteen Centuries of Our Era* (New York: Columbia University Press, 1958), 7:413, 608, 8:18, 330, 633. See also Gnudi and Webster, *Life and Times of Gaspare Tagliacozzi*, 281–302.

64. The best-known edition of Butler's *Hudibras* was annotated later by Zachary Grey (London, 1764). The footnotes to lines 280–86 on page 29 give an account of Tagliacozzi and his work but repeat some of the myths surrounding his surgery. However, Grey does add that "the Serjeant Surgeon to Queen Anne told him that the operation was possible and was unjustifiably neglected."

65. M. F. Freshwater, "Pre-Baronian Tissue Transfer, or, Should the Plastic Surgery Research Council Change Its Seal?" *Connecticut Medicine* 40, no. 9 (Sept. 1976): 613–17.

66. See the collected lectures of Aberdonian Alexander Read (or Rhead or Reid), *Treatise of the First Part of Chirurgerie* (London, 1638), and his *Chirurgorum comes* (1687), pt. 4, bk. 8, p. 648. He bequeathed his library to Marischal College, Aberdeen.

67. James Cooke's *Mellificium chirurgiae, or the Marrow of Many Good Authors,* was published in 1648, and later editions were more hostile to the Tagliacozzian operation; see the third edition (London, 1662), 374. See also B. Cosman, "Another Seventeenth-Century Denigration of Gaspare Tagliacozzi," *Annals of Plastic Surgery* 1, no. 3 (May 1978): 312–14.

68. For the life of this "scientist" at a European court, see Paula Findlen, "Controlling the Experiment: Rhetoric, Court Patronage and the Experimental Method of Francesco Redi," *History of Science* 31, no. 91 (Mar. 1993): 35–64.

69. For general histories of the society, see Thomas Sprat, *History of the Royal Society* (London, 1667); Michael Hunter, *Establishing the New Science: The Experience of the Early Royal Society* (Woodbridge, England: Boydell, 1989); and *The Royal Society and Its Fellows, 1660–1700: The Morphology of an Early Scientific Institution* (Chalfont St. Giles, England: British Society for the History of Science, 1982).

70. Jobi Janszoon van Meek'ren, *Heel-en Genees-Konstige Aanmerkkingen* (Amsterdam, 1668), also published in Latin as *Observationes medico-chirurgicae* (Amsterdam, 1682). On Meek'ren, a pupil of Nicholas Tulp, see Barend Haeseker, "Mr. Job van Meekeren (1611–1666) and Surgery of the Hand," *Plastic and Reconstructive Surgery* 82 (1988): 539–46, and the related letters in *Plastic and Reconstructive Surgery* 88 (1994): 173–74 and 96 (1995): 1481.

71. For a partial account, see T. J. S. Patterson, "Experimental Skin Grafts in England, 1663–64," *British Journal of Plastic Surgery* 22 (1969): 384–85. Full details of the transplant project are found only in Thomas Birch, *History of the Royal Society* (London, 1756), 1: 303–442, from which these extracts are taken.

72. Birch, *History of the Royal Society*, 315–16.

73. Academic description of the chicken spur-to-comb implantation predates even the Royal Society's investigation, being mentioned in Aldrovandi's *Ornithologica* (1599), and by Petrus Gassendus (1641), Ole Worm (1655), and Giovanni Borelli (1656). Their source was the rural grafting in ancient times, and

the grafted animals exhibited as freaks in traveling fairs.

74. William S. Middleton, "The Medical Aspect of Robert Hooke," *Annals of Medical History* 9 (1927): 227–43; E. N. da C. Andrade, "Robert Hooke, F.R.S. (1635–1703)," *Notes and Records of the Royal Society* 15 (1960): 137–45; Stephen Inwood, *The Man Who Knew Too Much: The Strange and Inventive Life of Robert Hooke, 1635–1703* (London: Pan Books, 2002), also published as *The Forgotten Genius: The Biography of Robert Hooke 1635–1703* (San Francisco: MacAdam/Cage, 2004), but Hooke's transplant work is not noted.

75. Birch, *History of the Royal Society*, 315.

76. Ibid., 335.

77. Ibid., 428, 442.

78. Edmund King, "An Account of the Experiment of Transfusion, Practised Upon a Man in London," *Philosophical Transactions* 30 (1667): 557–59. See also Charles Webster, "The Origins of Blood Transfusion: A Reassessment," *Medical History* 15, no. 4 (Oct.

1971): 387–92. Contemporary satirists viewed blood transfusion in a more kindly light than tissue transplantation; see Thomas Shadwell, *The Virtuoso* (London, 1676).

79. Anita Guerrini, "The Ethics of Animal Experimentation in Seventeenth-Century England," *Journal of the History of Ideas* 50, no. 3 (July–Sept. 1989): 391–407. Hooke did make a brief but unsatisfactory trial of intravenous opium to assist such dog surgery, as did Robert Boyle; see Robert T. Gunther, *Early Science in Oxford*, vols. 6–7; *The Life and Work of Robert Hooke* (parts 1–2) (Oxford: Robert T. Gunther, 1930), 217.

80. Hooke to Boyle, Nov. 10, 1664, in Thomas Birch, ed., *The Works of the Honourable Robert Boyle* (London, 1772), 6:401, 498.

81. King, "Account of the Experiment of Transfusion," 559.

82. William Congreve, *Love for Love* (1695), act 4, line 555.

2. The Eighteenth Century

1. See Thomas Gibson, "The First Homografts: Trembley and the Polyps," *British Journal of Plastic Surgery* 19, no. 4 (1966): 301–7; John R. Baker, *Abraham Trembley of Geneva, Scientist and Philosopher, 1710–1784* (London: Arnold, 1952); Maurice Trembley, ed., *Correspondance inédite entre Reaumur et Abraham Trembley* (Geneva: Georg, 1943); Sylvia G. Lenhoff and Howard M. Lenhoff, *Hydra and the Birth of Experimental Biology, 1744: Abraham Trembley's Mémoires Concerning the Polyps* (Pacific Grove, CA: Boxwood, 1986). Linnaeus named the polyps *hydra* in 1746.

2. Much later, further experimentation showed a form of rejection between different species of such polyps; see R. D. Campbell and C. Bibb, "Transplantation in Coelenterates," *Transplantation Proceedings* 2, no. 2 (June 1970): 202–11.

3. Abraham Trembley, *Mémoires pour servir à l'histoire d'un genre de polypes d'eau douce à bras en forme de cornes* (Leiden, 1744).

4. Henry Baker, *An Attempt towards a Natural History of the Polype* (London, 1743). Baker's misconduct is described in Marc Ratcliff, *The Quest for the Invisible: Microscopy in the Enlightenment* (Aldershot, England: Ashgate, 2009).

5. E. L. Patrin (1788), quoted in Charles W. Bodemer, "Regeneration and the Decline of Preformationism in

Eighteenth Century Embryology," *Bulletin of the History of Medicine* 38 (1964): 20–31, 29. See also A. Vartanian, "A. Trembley's Polyp, La Mettrie and Eighteenth-Century French Materialism," *Journal of the History of Ideas* 11 (1950): 259–86.

6. The incomparable source here is Eduard Zeis, *Die Literatur und Geschichte der plastichen Chirurgie* (Leipzig, 1863), translated and edited by Thomas J. S. Patterson as *The Zeis Index and History of Plastic Surgery, 900 BC–AD 1863* (Baltimore: Williams and Wilkins, 1977). Chapter 2 deals with "the older literature on the reuniting of completely separated parts." See also the charitable article by Thomas Gibson, "Early Free Grafting: The Restitution of Parts Completely Separated from the Body," *British Journal of Plastic Surgery* 18 (1965): 1–11; and M. S. Arons, M. F. Freshwater, and R. Hegel, "Abel's Auricle—A Colonial Tale of Plastic Surgery," *Connecticut Medicine* 40, no. 12 (Dec. 1976): 851–55. For fanciful transplants in popular culture, see Rudolph Raspe, *Baron Munchausen: Narrative of his Marvellous Travels* (1785).

7. For instant successful skin grafts by the Italian quack Gambacurta of Florence, using her transplant balsam, see Dionisio A. Sancassani, *Dilucidazioni fisico-mediche* (Rome, 1731).

8. John Bell, *The Principles of Surgery*, 4 vols. (Edinburgh, 1801), 1:39.

9. On Bonnet, see Gerhard Rudolph, "Les Débuts de la transplantation expérimentale: Considérations de Charles Bonnet (1720–1793) sur la greffe animale," *Gesnerus* 34 (1977): 50–68; and Virginia P. Dawson, *Nature's Enigma: The Problem of the Polyp in the Letters of Bonnet, Trembley and Réaumur* (Philadelphia: American Philosophical Society, 1987).

10. On Spallanzani, see Marguerite Carozzi, "Bonnet, Spallanzani and Voltaire on Regeneration of Heads in Snails: A Continuation of the Spontaneous Generation Debate," *Gesnerus* 42 (1985): 265–88.

11. Henry Thomas Buckle, *On Scotland and the Scotch Intellect* (London, 1865), 359. See also John Abernethy, *An Enquiry into the Probability and Rationality of Mr Hunter's "Theory of Life"* (London, 1814).

12. C. E. Martin, "John Hunter and Tissue Transplantation," *Surgery, Gynecology & Obstetrics* 131, no. 2 (Aug. 1970): 306–10. See also T. R. Forbes, "Testis Transplantation Performed by John Hunter," *Endocrinology* 41, no. 4 (1947): 329–31; and Carl Barker-Jørgensen, *John Hunter, A. A. Berthold and Origins of Endocrinology*, Acta Historica Scientiarum Naturalium Medicinalium series, vol. 24 (Odense, Denmark: Odense University Press, 1971), 1–54.

13. John Hunter never directly quotes Tagliacozzi's surgical text in his writings, except to accept the myth that the Italian may have used homograft donors. There is a copy of Tagliacozzi's book in the (William) Hunterian Collection in the Glasgow University Library's Special Collections. The Hunterian Collection does, however, have the compendium by Jean Jacques Manget, *Bibliotheca chirurgica* (Geneva, 1721), which contains the Tagliacozzi Latin text from *De curtorum chirurgia per insitionem*, vol. 1, including the "homograft" chapter (chap. 18), though it is misprinted as chapter 8. In some editions of Manget, Tagliacozzi's skin flap illustrations are copied, though reduced in size.

14. The freemartin is described in James F. Palmer, ed., *The Complete Works of John Hunter FRS* (London, 1835), 4:38.

15. John Hunter, "An Account of a Case of an Uncommon Disease in the Omentum, and of a Double Kidney on One Side of the Body, with None on the Other," *Medical Transactions of the College of Physicians of London* 3 (1785): 250–54.

16. For the substantial literature on animals and humans with various abnormalities, see Jan Bondeson, *The Two-Headed Boy and Other Medical Marvels* (Ithaca, NY: Cornell University Press, 2000).

17. H-L. du Hamel, "Recherches sur la réunion des plaies des arbes et des Animaux; et sur les greffes ou incisions, tant végétales qu'animales," *Compte rendu de l'Académie Royale des Sciences*, Nov. 12, 1746, 345–47, reprinted in the academy's *Histoire*, 1751, 70–79. Du Hamel quotes his earlier communications to the academy on this subject in 1728, 1730, and 1731, but these have proved to be elusive.

18. Arthur Keith, "The Hunters and the Hamiltons: Some Unpublished Letters," *The Lancet* 1 (1928): 354–59.

19. See Martin, "John Hunter and Tissue Transplantation," 309, regarding Hunter's lost bone graft specimen.

20. Arthur Keith, "A Discourse on the Portraits and Personality of John Hunter," *British Medical Journal* 1 (1928): 205–9.

21. Palmer, *Complete Works of John Hunter*, 1:127.

22. Anonymous [letter], *The Lancet* 214 (1928): 359.

23. Hunter's report seems reliable and indicates that he was puzzled at this contradiction. It is tempting to conclude that he had discovered the effect of minor Y chromosome genetic differences within a supply of closely inbred animals; litter mates may have been used in his experiments. The comb may also have assisted as a partly "privileged site," namely one to which the immune response does not reach.

24. Palmer, *Complete Works of John Hunter*, 2:99.

25. For Hunter's views on tissue vitality, see Palmer, *Complete Works of John Hunter*, 2:58, 158.

26. Palmer, *Complete Works of John Hunter*, 1:99.

27. The *Oxford English Dictionary* credits John Hunter as first to use the word *transplantation* in biology, but Charles Allen certainly did so earlier. See Charles Allen, *The Operator for the Teeth*, ed. Ronald A. Coleman (1685; London: Dawsons, 1969).

28. Palmer, *Complete Works of John Hunter*, 1:99.

29. John Hunter, "Proposals for the Recovery of People Apparently Drowned," *Philosophical Transactions of the Royal Society* 66 (1776): 412–25.

30. R. King, "John Hunter and the 'The Natural History of the Human Teeth': Dentistry, Digestion, and the Living Principle," *Journal of the History of Medicine and Allied Sciences* 49, no. 4 (Oct. 1994): 504–20. Hunter's experiments and observations on teeth are described in Palmer, *Complete Works of John Hunter*, 2:56, 97–104. Palmer and others since

incorrectly credit Hunter with pioneering the operation.

31. For a historical review of tooth transplantation, see D. R. Morse, "Plantation Procedures: History, Immunology and Clinical Considerations," *Journal of Oral Implantology* 7, no. 2 (1977): 176–92; and D. C. Schechter, "The Transplantation of Teeth," *Surgery, Gynecology & Obstetrics* 132, no. 2 (1971): 305–19. Some recent reports claimed 70 percent five-year survival of "allograft" tooth transplants serving as inert bone grafts.

32. Allen, *Operator for the Teeth*, 12. The Royal Society had no standard word for their transplant experiments; members simply used ordinary descriptive language. Earlier authors, including Sir Thomas Browne, used the word *inarching*. But the word *transplant* had already made its appearance in horticulture; see the 1440 English translation of *Palladius on Husbandry*, bk. 3, 504: "transplaunte hem so & sone up wol they spring."

33. On Hunter's dentist friends, see Lloyd G. Stevenson, "The Elder Spence, William Combe and John Hunter: Sidelights on Eighteenth-Century Dentistry and Hunter's Natural History of the Human Teeth," *Journal of the History of Medicine and the Allied Sciences* 10, no. 2 (Apr. 1955): 182–96.

34. Étienne Bourdet, cited in Henry W. Noble, "Tooth Transplantation: A Controversial Story," *Newsletter of the History of Dental Research Group*, no. 11 (Oct. 2002). The earlier eighteenth-century authority on tooth transplantation was Pierre Fauchard, the "father of dentistry"; see his *Le Chirurgien dentiste* (Paris, 1728). It was republished and translated by Lilian Lindsay as *The Surgeon Dentist, or, Treatise on the Teeth* (London: Butterworth, 1946). The paid tooth donors in Paris are mentioned in Robert Bunon, *Expériences et démonstrations faites à l'hôpital de la Salpétrière* (Paris, 1746).

35. Engravings of this tooth-to-spur specimen are well known, and the original had been held in the Museum of the Royal College of Surgeons of England but was lost.

36. The choice of a living tooth donor is described in Palmer, *Complete Works of John Hunter*, 2:100.

37. Augustus J. C. Hare, *The Story of My Life* (London, 1896), 6:501.

38. W. C. Butterfield, "The Medical Caricatures of Thomas Rowlandson," *Journal of the American Medical Association* 224, no. 1 (1973): 113–17; "A Caricatur-

ist of the Eighteenth Century Anatomists and Surgeons," *Surgery, Gynecology & Obstetrics* 144, no. 4 (1977): 587–92. Criticism of living tooth donation to unrelated recipients also appears in Helenus Scott's novel, *Adventures of a Rupee* (London, 1782).

39. The removal of teeth from the dead in the Peninsular War is mentioned in Bransby B. Cooper, *The Life of Sir Astley Cooper, Bart* (London 1843), 1:399–402. The grave robbers' steady domestic trade in teeth is found in James Blake Bailey, *Diary of a London Resurrectionist 1811–1812* (London, 1896).

40. *Edinburgh Advertiser*, January 12–16, 1784.

41. This account of early tooth transplantation in America is taken from Schechter, "Transplantation of Teeth."

42. Schechter, "Transplantation of Teeth," 312, quoting the New York *Daily Advertiser*, January 28, 1789.

43. Schechter, "Transplantation of Teeth," 314.

44. See the student notes of Rae's lectures in 1782, published later as W. Rae, "Lectures on the Teeth," *British Journal of Dental Science* 1 (1857): 517–21, 520. See also Christine Hillam, "A New Set of Notes on the Lectures of William Rae (d. 1786)," *Dental Historian* 33 (1998): 50–72.

45. For the case, see the London College of Physicians, *Medical Transactions* (1785), 3:325–44, which is a report noted by Ruth Richardson, "Transplanting Teeth," *The Lancet* 354 (1999): 1740.

46. *Minute Book of the Society of Collegiate Physicians 1767–1798*, Folio 43, entry for Aug. 2, 1786, Royal College of Physicians, London.

47. Allen, *Operator for the Teeth*, 11.

48. Rae, "Lectures on the Teeth," 520.

49. The ethical concerns are found in Joseph Fox, *The History and Treatment of the Diseases of the Teeth* (London, 1806), 132. On Fox, see J. J. Herschfeld, "Joseph Fox—Pioneer Dental Investigator and Author of 'The Natural History of the Human Teeth,'" *Bulletin of History of Dentistry* 31, no. 2 (1983): 101–7.

50. A. Mitscherlich, "The Replantation and Transplantation of Teeth," *Archives of Dentistry* 1 (Apr. 1865): 169–84, 169; this article is a translation of the original article published in *Langenbeck's Archiv für Chirurgie* 4 (1865). When German tooth replacement methods did emerge later, they instead used a sterilized store of teeth from "young and healthy subjects who have died by violence."

51. This point is made twice in Palmer's intrusive footnotes to *Complete Works of John Hunter,* 2:104n, and also in Jesse Foot, *The Life of John Hunter* (London, 1794), 83.

52. The use of dead teeth as implants is still supported by some and has a respectable recent history;
see Morse, "Plantation Procedures"; and J. R. Maestri Jr., "Tooth Transplantation: An Idea Whose Time Has Past," *Bulletin of the History of Dentistry* 37, no. 2 (1989): 115–22.

3. The Reawakening

1. For a review, see C. M. Balch and F. A. Marzoni, "Skin Transplantation during the Pre-Reverdin Era, 1804–1869," *Surgery, Gynecology & Obstetrics* 144, no. 5 (1977): 766–73. For general accounts of this period, see Henk J. Klasen, *History of Free Skin Grafting: Knowledge or Empiricism?* (Berlin: Springer-Verlag, 1981); and Eduard Zeis's important *Die Literatur und Geschichte der plastischen Chirurgie* (Leipzig, 1863–1864), translated and with additions and revisions by Thomas J. S. Patterson (Baltimore: Williams and Wilkins, 1977).

2. Thomas J. S. Patterson, "The Transmission of Indian Surgical Techniques to Europe at the End of the Eighteenth Century," *Proceedings of the 23rd International Conference on the History of Medicine* (1974): 694–96.

3. M. F. Freshwater, "More about 'B. L.,' 'Mr. Lucas,' and Mr. Carpue," *Plastic and Reconstructive Surgery* 49, no. 1 (Jan. 1972): 78–79.

4. The alternative explanation, that the rediscovery of Tagliacozzi in Europe prompted a search for rhinoplasty in India, does not fit the sequence of events. Nevertheless, Zeis was not alone in thinking it odd that the ancient surgical methods in India had not been noticed until the late 1700s, a time well into the period of the British presence in India.

5. John Ferriar, *Illustrations of Sterne: With Other Essays and Verses* (London, 1798). On Ferriar, see Edward Mansfield Brockbank, *John Ferriar: Public Health Work, "Tristram Shandy," Other Essays and Verses* (London: Heinemann, 1950).

6. John Bell, *The Principles of Surgery* (Edinburgh, 1801), 1:30, 39.

7. Bell may not have had access to Tagliacozzi's original text, since none of the libraries in Edinburgh held *De curtorem chirurgia per insitionem* at this time, though there were copies in Aberdeen and St. Andrews. But the College of Physicians' library in Edinburgh did have texts that contained partial reprints of Tagliacozzi's work, without the crucial illustrations: Alexander Read, *Chirurgorum comes* (1687); Jean Jacques Manget, *Bibliotheca chirurgia* (Geneva, 1721).

8. *Bibliothèque Britannique* 13 [fifth year of publication] (1803): 282–89.

9. John Thomson, *Lectures on Inflammation: A View of the General Doctrines of Medical Surgery* (Edinburgh, 1813), 224–28, 224.

10. See Giuseppe Baronio, *Degli innesti animali* (Milan, 1804). No English version of this work appeared until the late twentieth century: see Giuseppe Baronio, *On Grafting in Animals,* trans. Joan Bond Sax, historical introduction by Robert M. Goldwyn (Boston: Boston Medical Library, 1985).

11. Baronio, *Degli innesti animali,* 38.

12. For details of Baronio's life and work see Goldwyn's introduction to Baronio, *On Grafting in Animals.* Earlier sources are Andrea Verga, "Della vita e degli scritti di Giuseppe Baronio," *Memorie del reale istituto Lombardo di scienze e lettere; Classe di scienze matematiche e naturali,* ser. 3, vol. 8 (1896): 111–31; and L. Belloni, "Dalle Riproduzioni animale di L. Spallanzani agli Innesti animale di G. Baronio," *Rivista di storia della Scienza (Physis)* 3 (1961): 37–48.

13. Giuseppe Baronio, *Opuscula di fisica animale, e chirurgia* (Milan, 1785).

14. Baronio, *On Grafting in Animals,* 36.

15. Ibid., 20. Baronio's source on Tagliacozzi's methods was Giovanni A. Brambilla, *Storia delle scoperte fisico-medico-anatomico-chirurgiche e fatte dagli uomini illustri Italiani* (Milan, 1781). This book may have started the Italian rehabilitation of Tagliacozzi a little ahead of the rest of Europe.

16. Baronio, *Degli innesti animali,* 67.

17. Free skin or tissue slice grafts show necrosis of all but the cells closest to the host, prior to capillary ingrowth, and the graft regenerates from these cells— possibly stem cells. For a review of this initial neovascularization, see M. C. Donato, D. C. Novicki, and P. A. Blume, "Skin Grafting: Historic and Practical Approaches," *Clinics in Podiatric Medicine and Surgery* 17, no. 4 (2000): 561–98.

18. M. F. Freshwater, C. T. Su, and J. E. Hoopes, "Joseph Constantine Carpue—First Military Plastic

Surgeon," *Military Medicine* 142, no. 8 (1977): 603–6. Carpue appears in *Plarr's Lives of the Fellows of the Royal College of Surgeons of England* 1 (1930): 196–99, and the Carpue family is described in *Catholic Ancestor* 4 (1992): 1.

19. The author of "Mary's Ghost" was anonymous but may have been Joshua Naples. See "The Diary of a London Resurrectionist 1811–1812," a manuscript held by the Royal College of Surgeons of England, London.

20. Joseph C. Carpue, *An Introduction to Electricity and Galvanism, with Cases Showing Their Effect in the Cure of Disease* (London, 1803). For more on Carpue's human corpse experiments with Aldini, see Charlotte Sleigh, "Life, Death and Galvanism," *Studies in History and Philosophy of Biological and Biomedical Sciences* 29, no. 2 (1998): 219–48. The trial and execution of George Foster and details of Carpue's electrical experiments afterward, are found in *The Complete Newgate Calendar* (London, 1926), 3:56–65. See also Andy Dougan, *Raising the Dead: The Men Who Created Frankenstein* (Edinburgh: Birlinn, 2008).

21. Joseph C. Carpue, *An Account of Two Successful Operations for Restoring a Lost Nose from the Integuments of the Forehead* (London, 1816). A German translation appeared in 1817, with an introduction by Carl Ferdinand von Graefe. Carpue's original text has been reprinted, with an introduction by Frank McDowell, in the Classics of Medicine Library series (Birmingham, AL, 1981). Another case of skin-flap rhinoplasty performed in London in 1825 is documented in John Symons, "'A most hideous object': John Davies (1796–1872) and Plastic Surgery," *Medical History* 45 (2001): 395–402. See also J. P. Bennett, "Sir William Fergusson and the Indian Rhinoplasty," *Annals of the Royal College of Surgeons of England* 66, no. 6 (Nov. 1984): 444–48.

22. For a thorough account of early methods of skin suturing, see B. O. Rogers, "Harelip Repair in Colonial America, a Review of 18th Century and Earlier Surgical Techniques," *Plastic and Reconstructive Surgery* 34 (Aug. 1964): 142–62.

23. Neil Chambers, ed., *Scientific Correspondence of Sir Joseph Banks* (London: Pickering and Chatto, 2007), 6:167.

24. The vigorous and tense politics of London anatomical and surgical circles in the early nineteenth century are described in Adrian J. Desmond, *The Politics of Evolution: Morphology, Medicine, and Reform in Radical London* (Chicago: University of Chicago Press, 1989).

25. There is an abundance of scholarship on the legacy of the novel *Frankenstein,* but its link with the pioneer plastic surgeons has not been suggested until now. Analysis relevant to medicine is found in Christopher Goulding, "The Real Doctor Frankenstein?" *Journal of the Royal Society of Medicine* 95, no. 5 (May 2002): 257–59; Cecil Helman, "Dr Frankenstein and the Industrial Body: Reflections on 'Spare Part' Surgery," *Anthropology Today* 4, no. 3 (June 1988): 14–16; Tim Marshall, *Murdering to Dissect* (Manchester: Manchester University Press, 1995); and Donald F. Glut's comprehensive survey, *The Frankenstein Legend: A Tribute to Mary Shelley and Boris Karloff* (Metuchen, NJ: Scarecrow Press, 1973), which notes the surgical dimension introduced into twentieth-century versions of the tale.

26. Mary Wollstonecraft Shelley, *Frankenstein, or, The Modern Prometheus* (Oxford: Oxford University Press, 1980), 55.

27. Von Graefe's *Rhinoplastik* of 1818 appeared in both German and Latin, one of the last medical works published in this bilingual tradition. Von Graefe also claimed to have supported Tagliacozzi earlier; see B. O. Rogers, "The 'Founder' of Modern Plastic Surgery: Carl Ferdinand von Graefe (1787–1840)," *The Academic Bookman* 23 (1970): 3–14.

28. Dieffenbach's *Nonnula de regeneratione et transplantatione* (Würzburg, 1822) was followed by Johann F. Dieffenbach, *Chirurgische Erfahrungen besonders über die Wiederherstellung Zerstörter Theil des menschlichen Körpers nach neuen Methoden* (Berlin, 1829–1834), translated as *Surgical Observations on the Restoration of the Nose* (London, 1832). On Dieffenbach, see Robert M. Goldwyn, "Johann Friedrich Dieffenbach (1794–1847)," *Plastic and Reconstructive Surgery* 42, no. 1 (1968): 19–28; and H. Wolff, "Das chirurgische Erbe: Zum 200. Geburtstag von Johann Friedrich Dieffenbach," *Zentralblatt für Chirurgie* 117, no. 4 (1992): 238–43.

29. Pierre-Auguste Léon Labat, *De la rhinoplastie: Art de restaurer ou de refaire complètement le nez* (Paris: Imprimerie de Ducessois, 1834); and Philippe-F. Blandin, *Autoplastie ou restauration des parties du corps qui ont été détruites à la faveur d'un emprunt fait à d'autres parties plus ou moins éloignées* (Paris, 1836).

30. Thomas Gibson, "Eduard Zeis (1807–1868): Plastic Surgical Bibliographer Extraordinary," *British Journal of Plastic Surgery* 29, no. 4 (1976): 277–82.

See also Eduard Zeis, *Handbuch der plastichen Chirurgie* (Berlin, 1838), translated as *Zeis' Manual of Plastic Surgery*, ed. and trans. Thomas J. S. Patterson (Oxford: Oxford University Press, 1988).

31. Excerpted from Carpue's evidence to the House of Commons Report from the Select Committee on Medical Education, Parliamentary Papers, vol. 13, Minutes of May 8, 1834.

32. Russell M. Jones, ed., *The Parisian Education of an American Surgeon: Letters of Jonathan Mason Warren (1832–1835)* (Philadelphia: American Philosophical Society, 1978), 185, 207.

33. Jonathan Mason Warren, "Rhinoplastic Operations," *Boston Medical and Surgical Journal* 16 (1837): 69–79; 22, no. 1 (May 1840): 264–69, operations later also described in his text *Surgical Observations, with Cases and Operations* (Boston, 1867). Warren's influence is assessed in Robert M. Goldwyn, "Jonathan Mason Warren and His Contributions to Plastic Surgery," *Plastic and Reconstructive Surgery* 41, no. 1 (Jan. 1968): 1–7. In 1846 in Boston, the Warrens, father and son, assisted dentist William Morton when he famously made the first use of ether.

34. See the interesting introduction by the Dumfries surgeon John Stevenson Bushnan to *Surgical Observations on the Restoration of the Nose* (London, 1933), his partial translation of Dieffenbach's book *Chirurgische Erfahrungen besonders über die Wiederherstellung Zerstörter Theil des menschlichen Körpers nach neuen Methoden*. Bushnan notes in his introduction that he "removed the irksome minuteness and tautology of the German author" and lists five new British cases—from London in 1818 (handled by Hutchison) and 1823 (by Travers), and the three Scottish cases—one each by Liston and Lizars in Edinburgh (1831) and one by Bushnan himself in Dumfries.

35. See, for instance, William Balfour, "Two Cases, with Observations, Demonstrative of the Powers of Nature to Reunite Parts Which Have Been, by Accident, Totally Separated from the Animal System," *Edinburgh Medical and Surgical Journal* 10 (Oct. 1814): 421–30; and *London Medical and Physical Journal* 37 (1817): 472–74. Two other accounts of similar success with replacing lost digits followed in the same issue of the London journal, one from Henry Bailey of Bedford and the other from L'Espagnal, in France. It is known that human fingers, particularly the tip in children, show a modest ability to reform and remodel after trauma; see C. M. Illingworth, "Trapped Fingers and Amputated Finger Tips in Children," *Journal of Pediatric Surgery* 9, no. 6 (Dec. 1974): 853–58.

36. Henri Dutrochet (1817), quoted in Klasen, *History of Free Skin Grafting*, 1.

37. Bünger had seen an article in a Paris journal in which Dutrochet described the use of flayed skin in India; see *Gazette de Santé* 9 (Mar. 21, 1817), reprinted as "Examples of Reunion of Parts of the Body Totally Separated from the Rest of the Body," *Plastic and Reconstructive Surgery* 44 (1969): 288–89.

38. Bünger's paper was translated and his work described in F. McDowell, trans. Hans May, "Successful Attempt of Reconstruction of a Nose from a Completely Separated Piece of Skin from the Leg, by Prof. Dr. Bünger, Marburg, Germany," *Plastic and Reconstructive Surgery* 44, no. 5 (Nov. 1969): 486–90, 487.

39. Dieffenbach, *Surgical Observations on the Restoration of the Nose*, 149.

40. François Rabelais, *Gargantua and Pantagruel* (London: Penguin Books, 2006), 429.

41. Thomas Latta, "Saline Venous Injection in Cases of Malignant Cholera, Performed While in the Vapour-Bath," *The Lancet* 19, no. 479 (Nov. 1832): 173–76, 208–9. For an account of the denigration of Latta and the neglect of his innovation, see Robert J. Morris, *Cholera, 1832: The Social Response to an Epidemic* (New York: Holmes & Meier, 1976), 166–70.

42. Morris, *Cholera, 1832*, 167.

43. Edith Frame, "Thomas Graham: A Centenary Account," *Philosophical Journal* 7, no. 2 (1970): 116–27. The first formulation of Graham's celebrated "Law of Diffusion of Gases" came in his probationary essay for fellowship of the Glasgow Faculty of Physicians and Surgeons in 1830.

4. Clinical and Academic Transplantation in Paris

1. The word *scientist* entered the language in Britain in 1833 as a description of the vocation of those attending the third meeting of the British Association for the Advancement of Science. *Sçavan* and then *savant* were the terms used in France until supplanted in the late 1800s; *biology* and *biologist* crept into usage beginning in the 1820s.

2. Claude Bernard, *An Introduction to the Study of Experimental Medicine*, ed. and trans. Henry C. Greene (1865; New York: Macmillan, 1927), 59.

3. See ibid., 184, where Claude Bernard's critics are described.

4. Acland's concern about the emergence of biomedical scientists is quoted in Roger French, *Antivivisection and Medical Science in Victorian Society* (Princeton, NJ: Princeton University Press, 1975), 43.

5. See Frances P. Cobbe, *Illustrations of Vivisection, or, Experiments on Living Animals: From the Works of Physiologists* (London, 1887), 72, 77. For a detailed account of antivivisection sentiment at the time, see Martin Willis, "Unmasking Immorality: Popular Opposition to Laboratory Science in Late Victorian Britain," in *Repositioning Victorian Sciences: Shifting Centres in Nineteenth-Century Thinking*, ed. David Clifford, Elisabeth Wadge, Alex Warwick, and Martin Willis (London: Anthem Press, 2006), 207–18.

6. *Star,* Nov. 9, 1894.

7. Bernard's biographers omit his interest in transplantation, and the transplant work on grafting at the Collège de France awaits a closer study. Of Bernard's group, only the works of Paul Bert have been translated, in précis form; see C. M. Balch and F. A. Marzoni, "Skin Transplantation during the Pre-Reverdin Era, 1804–1869," *Surgery, Gynecology & Obstetrics* 144, no. 5 (May 1977): 766–73.

8. This forgotten surgical text is Claude Bernard and Charles Huette's *Précis iconographique de médecine opératoire et d'anatomie chirurgicale* (1854), which was translated into all the European languages, as well as Japanese. The first American edition appeared in 1855. See also Robert M. Goldwyn, "Bernard and Huette: Operative Medicine," *Plastic and Reconstructive Surgery* 78, no. 1 (July 1986): 115–16. Except for these works, Bernard's clinical links have been largely overlooked.

9. Professor Gabriel Richet (personal communication) has traced these experiments to Magendie's collected lectures, *Leçons sur les phénomènes physiques de la vie*, vol. 4 (Paris, 1842), and to papers in *Comptes rendus hebdomadaires des séances de l'Académie des Sciences* 41 (1855): 628–31; 45 (1857): 562–66, 925–28. See also Charles-Édouard Brown-Séquard's article in *Journal de Physiologie* 1 (1858): 173–75.

10. The first description of a natural hemolysin is found in Leonard Landois, *Die Transfusion des Blutes* (Leipzig, 1875).

11. The only account of this limb perfusion work is the summary in Charles-Édouard Brown-Séquard, *Ex-* *perimental Researches Applied to Physiology and Pathology* (New York, 1853).

12. Edme F. A. Vulpian, "Sur la durée de la persistance des propriétés des muscles, des Neris et de la moelle épinière après l'interruption du tours du sang dans ces organes," *La Gazette Hebdomadaire de Médecine et de Chirurgie* (1861): 365–69. On Vulpian, see S. Jarcho, "Right-Sided Ulcerative Endocarditis Recognized Ante Mortem (Charcot and Vulpian 1862)," *American Journal of Cardiology* 7 (1961): 253–61. Xavier Bichat had been the first to study the responses of the human heart, removed after execution by the guillotine; see Bichat's *Les Recherches physiologiques sur la vie et la mort*, 2nd ed. (Paris, 1802).

13. J. M. D. Olmsted, *Charles-Édouard Brown-Séquard: A Nineteenth Century Neurologist and Endocrinologist* (Baltimore: Johns Hopkins University Press, 1946), 71.

14. Bert's MD thesis was "De la greffe animale" (Paris, 1863), published as "Expériences et considérations sur la greffe animale," *Journal de l'Anatomie et de la Physiologie* 1 (1864): 69. His subsequent PhD thesis was "Recherches expérimentales pour servir à l'histoire de la vitalité propre des tissus animaux" (Paris, 1866). See also Paul Bert, "Note sur quelques faits nouveaux de greffe animale," *Compte Rendu de l'Académie des Sciences* 61 (1865): 908; P. Dejours, "Une lettre de Paul Bert sur la greffe animale," *Bulletin de la Société des Sciences Historiques et Naturelles de l'Yonne* 118 (1986): 113–15; and Balch and Marzoni, "Skin Transplantation during the Pre-Reverdin Era." For a biography of Bert, see Charles Coulston Gillispie, ed., *Dictionary of Scientific Biography* (New York, 1970); and M. J. Seghers and J. J. Longacre, "Paul Bert and His Animal Grafts," *Plastic and Reconstructive Surgery* 33, no. 2 (Feb. 1964): 178–86. See also Bert's introduction to Bernard, *Introduction to the Study of Experimental Medicine*, xvi.

15. Georges Martin, *De la durée de la vitalité des tissus et des conditions d'adhérence des restitutions et transplantations cutanées (greffes animales)* (Paris, 1873); Henry Armaignac, *De la greffe animale et de ses applications à la chirurgie* (Paris, 1873). Both of these works are rare and difficult to find.

16. Investigation of the role of electrolytes, particularly potassium, was resurrected in the 1880s as a physiological investigation; see Sydney Ringer, "A Further Contribution Regarding the Influence of the Different Constituents of the Blood on the Contraction of the Heart," *Journal of Physiology* 4, no. 1 (Jan. 1883): 29–42.

17. Pierre Paul Broca's book was admired at the time and translated as *On the Phenomenon of Hybridity in the Genus Homo* (London, 1866).

18. Pierre Paul Broca, *Des anévrysmes et de leur traitement* (Paris, 1856).

19. Jacques-Louis Reverdin, "Greffe épidermique," *Bulletin de la Société Impériale Chirurgicale de Paris* 10 (1869): 511–15, reprinted as "Greffe Epidermique—Experience Faite dans le Service de M. Docteur Guyon, à l'Hôpital Necker," trans. Robert H. Ivy, in *Plastic and Reconstructive Surgery* 41, no. 1 (Jan. 1968): 79–81; see also *Gazette Médicale de Paris* 26 (1870): 544. On Reverdin, see Henri Reverdin, *Jacques-Louis Reverdin 1842–1929: Un chirurgien à l'aube d'une ère nouvelle* (Aarau, Switzerland: Sauerländer, 1971); and E. Martin, "Jacques-Louis Reverdin (1842–1929)," *Revue Médicale de la Suisse Romande* 91, no. 12 (Dec. 1971): 923–28. An interesting, detailed, and not uncritical account of the early days of skin grafting is found in Henk J. Klasen, *History of Free Skin Grafting: Knowledge or Empiricism?* (Berlin: Springer-Verlag, 1981), which has an introduction by Thomas Gibson. Easily the best early source on early skin grafting is the chapter on plastic surgery by John Ashhurst Jr. in *The International Encyclopaedia of Surgery*, vol. 1, ed. Christopher Johnston (New York, 1883), 531–49.

20. Reverdin's full paper was published in three parts: see Jacques-Louis Reverdin, "De la greffe épidermique," *Archives Générales de Médecine* 19 (1872): 276–302, 555–86, 703–11. The quotation is from page 515.

21. Dr. M. B. Mirsky of Moscow and Dr. W. A. Reid, Edinburgh pathologist, provided information on Yatsenko. Dr. Reid also translated *K voprosu o perenesenii ili privivkie otdielennich kusochkov*.

22. Pollock's role in establishing routine skin grafting was revealed by the diligent research of M. Felix Freshwater, the Florida plastic surgeon; see M. Felix Freshwater, with Thomas J. Krizek, "George David Pollock and the Development of Skin Grafting," *Annals of Plastic Surgery* 1, no. 1 (Jan. 1978): 96–102.

23. The story of the medical student, Wallace Bowles, was originally presented in James Foster Palmer, "Origin of Skin Grafting: A Reminiscence," *Medical Magazine* (London) 15 (1906): 477–81.

24. The sixteen cases were reported in George Pollock, "Cases of Skin-Grafting and Skin-Transplantation," *Transactions of the Clinical Society of London* 4 (1871): 37–47; followed quickly by George Lawson,

"On the Transplantation of Portions of Skin for the Closure of Large Granulating Surfaces," *Transactions of the Clinical Society of London* 4 (1871): 49–53. Other London publications that year include John Woodman, *Notes on Transplantation or Engrafting of Skin* (London, 1871).

25. John Woodman stated that, "like many others, I heard of this subject from announcements in the newspapers." Woodman, *Notes on Transplantation or Engrafting of Skin*, 13. This, the first transplantation press story, is elusive, and is not found in the index to the *Times* (London).

26. Charles Steele, "Clinical Lecture on the Transplantation of Skin," *British Medical Journal* 2, no. 519 (Dec. 1870): 621–23. For grafting leg ulcers, Steele used the thin skin from the medial side of the upper arm "entire thickness or in part."

27. Woodman, *Notes on Transplantation or Engrafting of Skin*, 10.

28. "Skin-Grafting," *Medical Times and Gazette* 1 (Feb. 24, 1872): 230.

29. Frank H. Hamilton, "Healing of Ulcers by Transplantation," *New York Medical Journal* n.s. 14 (1871): 225–32. He had suggested this procedure earlier, in 1847, making this claim in his text *Elkoplasty: or, Anaplasty Applied to the Treatment of Old Ulcers* (New York, 1854).

30. L. Muñoz, "Sobre el ingerto epidérmico," *Gaceta Médica de Mexico* 5 (1870): 344–48.

31. William H. Hingston, "Medico-Chirurgical Society of Montreal," *Canada Medical Journal* 7 (1871): 495.

32. S. Zebrowski, "Essais sur la greffe épidermique," *Gazette Médicale d'Orient* 16 (1872): 136–37.

33. David Page, "Observations on the True Nature of the So-Called 'Skin Grafting,'" *British Medical Journal* 2, no. 520 (Dec. 17, 1870): 655.

34. This large body of French and German work on skin grafting, neglected by the English-speaking twentieth-century surgical community, is listed in Klasen's excellent monograph, *History of Free Skin Grafting*. The early volumes of the *Index-Catalogue of the Library of the Surgeon-General's Office* (Washington, DC: U.S. Army, 1892), have a massive survey of the world medical literature, including skin grafting, to that date.

35. See, for instance, the scissors illustrated in Hermann Beigel, "Über die gynäkologische Verwend-

ung der Transplantation kleiner Hautstückchen zum Zweck der Heilung torpider Geschwüre," *Wiener Medizinische Wochenschrift* 23 (1872): 573–77.

36. Frank McDowell, "Carl Thiersch, Microscopy and Skin Grafting," *Plastic and Reconstructive Surgery* 41, no. 4 (1968): 369–70; C. F. Schwokowski, "Erinnerungen an Carl Thiersch," *Zentralblatt für Chirurgie* 121 (1996): 426–29.

37. His eponymous fame comes from his paper, C. Thiersch, "Über Hautverpflanzung," *Verhandlungen Deutsche Gesellschaft für Chirurgie* 5 (1886): 17–19.

38. J. R. Wolfe, "A New Method of Performing Plastic Operations," *British Medical Journal* 2, no. 768 (Sept. 18, 1875): 360–61. For a detailed account of Wolfe's life, see Elma P. Douglas, *The Ophthalmic: The History of the Ophthalmic Institution* (Glasgow, 1998), 83–94.

39. For George Lawson's claim to be the pioneer of thin skin grafting, see Klasen, *History of Free Skin Grafting*, 47–52.

40. This xenograft enthusiasm is from an anonymous review of the papers appearing in *Lyon Medical* in 1872 and published in the *Glasgow Medical Journal* 5 (May 1873): 361–68. For an analysis, see T. Gibson, "Zoografting: A Curious Chapter in the History of Plastic Surgery," *British Journal of Plastic Surgery* 8, no. 3 (Oct. 1955): 234–42.

41. J. H. William Meyer, "Experiments in Colored Skin Grafting," *Chicago Medical Journal and Examiner* 34 (1877): 320–22. For other instances of black-to-white human skin grafting and the reverse, including the earliest illustration of a human skin graft, which was from a black donor to a white recipient, see Thomas Bryant, "On Skin Grafting," *Guy's Hospital Reports* 17 (1872): 237–42; as well as Ashhurst, "Plastic Surgery," in *The International Encyclopaedia of Surgery*, ed. Christopher Johnston, 1:531–49. However, in the report by Dr. G. Troup Maxwell, "Grafting the Skin of a White Man upon a Negro," *Philadelphia Medical Times* 4, no. 3 (Oct. 18, 1873): 37, the author reports that the white skin (his own) was gradually lost.

42. This pioneering use of foreskin grafts was at the London Evellina Hospital; see R. Clement Lucas, "On Prepuce Grafting," *The Lancet* 124, no. 3188 (1884): 586.

43. The diary of Margaret Mathewson, an Edinburgh Royal Infirmary tuberculosis patient, was reprinted and analyzed in Martin Goldman, *Lister Ward* (Bristol: Hilger, 1987), 118–19. According to the diary, Mr.

Peddie also provided Lister with blood for transfusion.

44. Klasen, *History of Free Skin Grafting*, 36.

45. *Glasgow Herald*, Sept. 5, 1878; also reported in "Curious Charge against a Doctor," *Medical Press and Circular* n.s. 26 (1878): 211. This was an early airing of the problem of consent to surgery. Additional information provided by Dr. Derek Dow.

46. Winston Churchill, *My Early Life* (London: Macmillan, 1944), 211. His son Randolph later confirmed the presence of the scar from the skin graft attempt.

47. Alexander Miles, "Case of Extensive Burn of Leg Treated by Grafting with Skin of Dog," *The Lancet* 135, no. 3472 (1890): 594–95.

48. Thomas F. Raven, "Surgical Memoranda: Skin Grafting from the Pig," *British Medical Journal* 2, no. 879 (Nov. 3, 1877): 623.

49. W. Watson Cheyne, "Skin Grafting after Removal of the Mamma," *The Lancet* 138, no. 3540 (1891): 5–6. See also Cheyne's British Medical Association lecture in *The Practitioner* 44 (1890): 401–11.

50. Antonin Poncet, "Des greffes dermo-épidermiques et en particulier des larges lambeaux dermo-épidermiques," *Lyon Médecine* 8 (1871): 494, 520, 564.

51. Klasen, *History of Free Skin Grafting*, 97. Klasen's comment suggests that his loyalty to the surgical community was being tested by the poor quality of the early skin grafting literature, but he had some moments of insight, as this comment indicates.

52. Nonclinical medical historians are in particular difficulties when dealing with this period, because they may assume that the bulk of the literature on skin and gland grafting was based on good science and sound observation. Instead, the publications of the time have serious deficiencies and a disorderly grafting typology; only when these limitations are acknowledged can some sense be made of the anarchic transplantation literature of the period.

53. After graft loss, under the host ingrown skin, there remains a prominent pad of non-rejected, inert donor fibrous tissue—the collagen "ghost" from the graft, still exactly the same size as the original graft. This remnant, covered in very thin healthy host ingrown skin, when noticed later, has been wrongly described as a successful graft by optimistic surgeons.

54. For a bibliography of the development of bone grafting, see the early volumes of *Transplantation Bulletin*, from 1954 onward.

55. See Sir William Macewen, "Observations Concerning the Transplantation of Bone," *Proceedings of the Royal Society* 32 (1881): 232–47; his contribution was highly praised at the time. Macewen's papers are held at the Royal College of Physicians and Surgeons of Glasgow (RCPSG 10/9/5) and include a photograph of a skin graft operation. See also Julius Wolff, "Die Osteoplastik in ihren Beziehungen zur Chirurgie und Physiologie," *Archiv für Klinische Chirurgie* 4 (1863): 183–96.

56. This phenomenon was first described by Arthur Barth, "Ueber histologische Befunde nach Knochenimplantationen," *Verhandlungen der Deutschen Gesellschaft für Chirurgie* 2 (1893): 234–42.

57. For a review of the development of corneal grafting, see Benjamin W. Rycroft, ed., *Corneal Grafts* (London: Butterworth, 1955). For useful bibliographies on the history of corneal grafting compiled by A. Edward Maumenee, see *Transplantation Bulletin* 1 (1954): 107–22; 2 (1955): 73–75; and subsequent updates.

58. See Louis K. Diamond, "A History of Blood Transfusion," in *Blood, Pure and Eloquent: A Story of Discovery, of People, and of Ideas,* ed. Maxwell M. Wintrobe (New York: McGraw-Hill, 1980), 690–717. For mid-nineteenth-century transfusion methods, see James Blundell, "Observations on Transfusion of Blood," *The Lancet* no. 302 (1829): 321–24. These puzzling claims for success with unmatched blood transfusions were either because of chance matching or because, without anticoagulants, the volumes used were small. Reactions were also probably underreported.

59. For a review of early, non-skin homograft tissue transplantation, together with a list of the dubious "first" publications, mainly German, for each type of organ, see Jane M. Oppenheimer, "Taking Things Apart and Putting Them Together Again," *Bulletin of the History of Medicine* 52, no. 2 (summer 1978): 149–61; Merriley Borell, "Organotherapy and the Emergence of Reproductive Endocrinology," *Journal of the History of Biology* 18, no. 1 (spring 1985): 1–30.

60. This new surgical confidence resulted in the first case of the removal of a solitary human kidney, a tragedy that was to play a part in transplantation events much later. See W. M. Polk, "Case of Extirpation of a Displaced Kidney," *New York Medical Journal* 37 (1883): 171–78. Some pioneer kidney transplants in the 1950s were attempts to reverse this surgical disaster.

61. In experimental work at the time, an animal's own glandular tissue would be removed, but while gland grafting took place, similar glandular tissue, undetected at the time of the surgery, might enlarge and act to restore hormone production. The functioning of this undetected tissue would then lead the investigator to believe that the subsequent gland graft had been responsible for the hormonal production.

62. This famous priority dispute is analyzed in M. Michler and J. Benedum, "Die Briefe von Jacques-Louis Reverdin und Theodor Kocher an Anton v. Eiselsberg," *Gesnerus* 27 (1970): 169–84. See Kocher's defense in *Nobel Lectures: Physiology or Medicine 1901–1921* (Amsterdam: Elsevier, 1967).

63. The importance of thyroid homografting at this time is carefully described in Thomas Schlich, "Changing Disease Identities: Cretinism, Politics and Surgery (1844–1892)," *Medical History* 38, no. 4 (1994): 421–43; and also in Schlich's book, *Die Erfindung der Organtransplantation* (Frankfurt: Campus, 1998), translated as *The Origins of Organ Transplantation* (Rochester, NY: University of Rochester Press, 2010).

64. Heinrich Bircher, "Das Myxödem und die cretinische Degeneration," *Sammlung Klinischer Vorträge*, March 5, 1890, 3393–424. Bircher's patient relapsed after three months, and a second thyroid homograft was said to cure the patient.

65. John B. Lyons, *The Citizen Surgeon: A Biography of Sir Victor Horsley, F.R.S., F.R.C.S., 1857–1916* (London: Dawnay, 1966). The original paper is Victor Horsley, "Notes on a Possible Means of Arresting the Progress of Myxœdema, Cachexia, Strumipriva, and Allied Diseases," *British Medical Journal* 1, no. 1519 (Feb. 8, 1890): 287–88, and 2 (July 26, 189): 201–202; and H. Christiani, "Thyroid Grafting in Human Beings," *The Medical Press and Circular* 78 (1904): 167–70, adds a confident histological confirmation of success. Kocher stated in his Nobel Prize lecture (*Nobel Lectures: Physiology or Medicine 1901–1921*) that his results had been variable and transitory and gave priority instead to A. von Eiselsberg, "Über erfolgreiche Einheilung der Katzenschilddrüse in die Bauchdecke un Auftreten von Tetanie nach deren Extirpation," *Wiener Klinische Wochenschrift* 5 (1892): 81–85.

66. The relevant human thyroid graft papers are found in Schlich's works.

67. See the important review by C. Sengoopta, "The Modern Ovary: Constructions, Meanings, Uses," *History of Science* 38, no. 4 (Dec. 2000): 425–88; as well as B. P. Setchell, "The Testis and Tissue Transplanta-

tion: Historical Aspects," *Journal of Reproductive Immunology* 18, no. 1 (1990): 1–8. The human work was encouraged by plausible claims for testis transplant success in rabbits and guinea pigs, notably by Emil Knauer (1867–1935), work flawed by the uncertainties of the genetics of laboratory animal stocks and the persistence of ectopic glandular tissue.

68. Robert Tuttle Morris, "The Ovarian Graft," *New York Medical Journal* 62 (1895): 436–37. See also H. H. Simmer, "Robert Tuttle Morris (1857–1945): A Pioneer in Ovarian Transplants," *Obstetrics and Gynecology* 35, no. 2 (Feb. 1970): 314–28. Morris describes the ovarian grafts in his autobiography, *Fifty Years a Surgeon* (New York: Dutton, 1935).

69. Susan E. Lederer, *Flesh and Blood: Organ Transplantation and Blood Transfusion in Twentieth-Century America* (Oxford: Oxford University Press, 2008), 24–25.

70. B. F. Church, "Medical and Surgical Progress," *Southern Californian Practitioner* 17 (1902): 175.

71. For the ethical dimension of early ovarian transplantation, see Edward Reichman, "The Halakhic Chapter of Ovarian Transplantation," *Tradition* 33, no. 1 (1998): 31–70.

72. J. Halliday Croom, "A Case of Heteroplastic Ovarian Grafting, Followed by Pregnancy and a Living Child. Query—Who Was the Mother?" *Transactions of the Edinburgh Obstetrical Society* 31 (1906): 194–200. An interesting discussion followed.

73. Rabbi Y. Gordon, 15 Heshvan 5668 (October 1907), vol. 10, 9a–9b.

74. Klasen, *History of Free Skin Grafting*, 38, quotes the first reference to smallpox transfer as being the hard-to-find paper by H. D. Schaper, "Übertragung der Pocken durch Implantation während des Prodromalstadiums," *Deutsche militairärztliche Zeitschrift* 1 (1872): 53–57. For other diseases transmitted in this fashion, see Leonard Freeman, *Skin Grafting* (St. Louis: Mosby, 1912).

75. About's novel was translated as *A Solicitor's Nose* (London, 1862) and remained popular, with reprints until 1960.

76. H. G. Wells, *The Island of Dr. Moreau* (New York: Garden City Publishing, 1896), 128, 129, 130.

77. Sir Peter Chalmers Mitchell, review of *The Island of Dr. Moreau*, by H. G. Wells, *Saturday Review*, vol. 81, April 11, 1896, 368–69. The reviewer's interest was piqued in 1896 when he served as translator of Oscar Hertwig's *The Biological Problems of Today*, which included claims for the success of homografting. He also translated Ilya Metchnikoff's works on immunity at this time. See also H. G. Wells, "The Limits of Individual Plasticity," *Saturday Review*, vol. 79, January 19, 1895, 89–90.

78. See Colin Beavan, *Fingerprints: Murder and the Race to Uncover the Science of Identity* (London: Fourth Estate, 2002). Others have claimed an opposite trend, namely, loss of identity in the increasingly centralized control in the industrialized nations; see John W. Burrow, *The Crisis of Reason: European Thought, 1848–1914* (New Haven, CT: Yale University Press, 2000).

5. The Beginning of Organ Transplantation

1. Erna Lesky, *The Vienna Medical School of the 19th Century* (Baltimore: Johns Hopkins University Press, 1976), 393–415, 393.

2. A thorough history of vascular surgery is awaited. For a general account, see Steven G. Friedman, *A History of Vascular Surgery* (Mount Kisco, NY: Futura, 1989).

3. N. V. Eck in *Voenno-Meditsinskii Zhurnal* 130 (1877): 1–2. For a translation of Eck's paper, see C. G. Child, "Eck's Fistula," *Surgery, Gynecology & Obstetrics* 96 (1953): 375–76. Eck failed to notice changes in the liver that resulted, leaving it to Pavlov to report six years later.

4. For these early events in the history of vascular surgery, see Charles C. Guthrie, *Blood-Vessel Surgery and*

Its Applications (New York: Longmans, Green, 1912); Stephen H. Watts, "The Suture of Blood Vessels: Implantation and Transplantation of Vessels and Organs; An Historical and Experimental Study," *Bulletin of the Johns Hopkins Hospital* 18 (May 1907): 153–78; the series of articles by D. de Moulin, "Historical Notes on Vascular Surgery: Vascular Suture and Lateral Ligation in the Pre-Antiseptic Era," *Archivum chirurgicum Neerlandicum* 7, no. 3 (1955): 218–26; "Historical Notes on Vascular Surgery II: Development of Vascular Suture in the 19th Century, After the Introduction of Antisepsis," 7, no. 4 (1955): 321–30; and "Historical Notes on Vascular Surgery III: Development and Application during the First Fifteen Years of the Twentieth Century," 8 (1956): 31–41; see also H. B. Shumacker Jr., "Authority, Research and Publication: Reflections Based upon Some Historical Aspects of Vascular Surgery," *Annals of Surgery* 168, no. 2 (Aug. 1968): 169–82; W. A. Dale, "The Beginnings of Vascular Surgery," *Surgery* 76, no. 6 (Dec. 1974): 849–66; H. B. Shumacker and H. Y. Muhm, "Arterial Suture Techniques: Past, Present and Future," *Surgery* 66, no. 2 (Aug. 1969): 419–33; and Norman M. Rich, "Vascular Trauma," *Surgical Clinics of North America* 53, no. 6 (Dec. 1973): 1367–92. Easily the best illustrations of the history of vascular surgery are by Knute Berger, M.D., for a series of articles in the *Western Journal of Surgery, Obstetrics and Gynecology* 65 (1957), which ceased publication in 1964. Berger was a surgeon, illustrator, and later a research pathologist in Seattle.

5. Murphy's classic contribution to the field has a scholarly history of the subject; see J. B. Murphy, "Resection of Arteries and Veins Injured in Continuity: End-to-End Suture; Experimental and Clinical Research," *Medical Record* 51 (1897): 73–88. His career is described in Robert L. Schmitz and Timothy T. Oh, eds., *The Remarkable Surgical Practice of John Benjamin Murphy* (Urbana: University of Illinois Press, 1993).

6. Early surgery studies in Lyon are chronicled in Auguste-Dominique Valette, *Clinique chirurgicale de l'Hôtel-Dieu de Lyon* (Paris, 1875).

7. On Payr, see H. Schröder and G. Trebing, "Die Begegnung der Chirurgenschulen Ernst von Bergmanns und Erwin Payrs an der Universitätsklinik in Jena," *Zentralblatt für Chirurgie* 122, no. 3 (1997): 201–5; and his autobiographical notes in *Medizin der Gegenwart* 3 (1924): 121–64. Payr's links with America are found in I. R. Rutkow, "The Letters of William Halsted and Erwin Payr," *Surgery, Gynecology & Obstetrics* 161, no. 1 (July 1985): 75–87.

8. Erwin Payr, "Weitere Mittheilungen über Verwendung des Magnesiums bei der Naht der Blutgefässe," *Archiv für Klinische Chirurgie* 64 (1901): 726–40; Erwin Payr, "Zur Frage der circulären Vereinigung von Blutgefässen mit resorbirbaren Prothesen," *Archiv für Klinische Chirurgie* 72 (1904): 32–54. Payr later published a long contribution on thyroid slice transplantation: see Erwin Payr, "Transplantation von Schilddrüsengewebe in die Milz; experimentelle und klinische Beiträge," *Verhandlungen der Deutschen Gesellschaft für Chirurgie* 35 (1906): 503–99; and at length in *Archiv für Klinische Chirurgie* 80 (1906): 730–826.

9. M. Jaboulay and E. Briau, "Recherches expérimentales sur la suture et la greffe artérielles," *Lyon Médicale* 81 (1896): 97–99.

10. The best notes on Carrel's scientific work are J. M. Converse, "Alexis Carrel: The Man, the Unknown," *Plastic and Reconstructive Surgery* 68, no. 4 (Oct. 1981): 629–39; and David Hamilton, "Alexis Carrel and the Early Days of Tissue Transplantation," *Transplantation Reviews* 2 (1988): 1–15. Carrel has attracted many admiring and often uncritical biographers: Jacques Descotes, ed., *Alexis Carrel (1873–1944): Pionnier de la chirurgie vasculaire et des transplantations d'organes* (Lyon: Simep Éditions, 1966); Robert Soupault, *Alexis Carrel 1873–1944* (Paris: Plon, 1952); Joseph T. Durkin, *Hope for Our Time: Alexis Carrel on Man and Society* (New York: Harper & Row, 1965); Theodore I. Malinin, *Surgery and Life: The Extraordinary Career of Alexis Carrel* (New York: Harcourt Brace Jovanovich, 1979); and W. Sterling Edwards and Peter D. Edwards, *Alexis Carrel: Visionary Surgeon* (Springfield, IL: Thomas, 1974). The contributions to the Carrel Centennial Symposium are disappointing: see Robert W. Chambers and Joseph T. Durkin, eds., *Papers of the Alexis Carrel Centennial Conference* (Washington, DC: Georgetown University Press, 1973). The recurring concerns over the reliability of some of Carrel's scientific data are aired in J. A. Witkowski, "Alexis Carrel and the Mysticism of Tissue Culture," *Medical History* 23, no. 3 (July 1979): 279–96. Carrel's early days are often described in vivid terms. When an Italian anarchist attacked French president Sadi Carnot in his hometown of Lyon in 1894, the statesman's stab wound in the abdomen was fatal because it had damaged the portal vein. Carrel was said to have been puzzled at the time by surgeons' inability to deal with the injury. Another story is that Carrel, in his quest for a perfect suture technique, took lessons on stitching from local women in the silk industry. Carrel later encouraged these vivid accounts of his work.

11. Alexis Carrel, "La technique opératoire des anastomoses vasculaires et la transplantation des viscères," *Lyon Médicale* 98 (1902): 859–84. There is a translation of this classic paper in Toni Hau, *Renal Transplantation* (Austin, TX: Silvergirl, 1987), which nobly collected the classic early works in transplantation and has translations of the German and French contributions.

12. In Lyon, Carrel still supported the existence of miraculous healing. See Jason Szabo, "Seeing Is Believing? The Form and Substance of French Medical Debates over Lourdes," *Bulletin of the History of Medicine* 76, no. 2 (summer 2002): 199–230.

13. Emerich Ullmann, "Experimentelle Nierentransplantation," *Wiener Klinische Wochenschrift* 15 (1902): 281–82; Emerich Ullman, "Tissue and Organ Transplantation," *Annals of Surgery* 60, no. 2 (1914): 195–219 (the persistent misspelling "Ullman" seems to have arisen from this translated article). On Ullmann, see B. Török, "A Forgotten Hungarian Scientist, Dr. Imre Ullman M.D. 1861–1937," *Orvosi Hetilap* 115, no. 35 (Sept. 1, 1974): 2069–71; and E. Lesky, "Die erste Nierentransplantation: Emerich Ullmann (1861–1937)," *Münchener Medizinische Wochenschrift* 116, no. 21 (May 24, 1974): 1081–84. See also F. Largiadèr, "72 Years of Organ Transplantation: Emerich Ullmann Memorial Lecture," *European Surgical Research* 6, no. 4 (1974): 197–208; J. Nagy, "A Note on the Early History of Renal Transplantation: Emerich (Imre) Ullmann," *American Journal of Nephrology* 19, no. 2 (1999): 346–49; and W. Druml, "The Beginning of Organ Transplantation: Emerich Ullmann (1861–1937)," *Wiener Klinische Wochenschrift* 114, no. 4 (2002): 128–37.

14. A. von Decastello, "Über experimentelle Nierentransplantationen," *Wiener Klinische Wochenschrift* 15 (1902): 317–18. In the previous year, he had conducted an important study that showed a marked fall in blood lymphocyte count after tying off the thoracic duct in dogs.

15. N. Floresco, "Recherches sur la transplantation du rein," *Journal de Physiologie et de Pathologie Générale* 7 (1905): 47–59.

16. Rudolf Stich, "Zur Transplantation von Organen mittelst Gefässnaht," *Archiv für Klinische Chirurgie* 83 (1907): 494–504.

17. Quoted in de Moulin, "Historical Notes on Vascular Surgery," *Archivum chirurgicum Neerlandicum* 8 (1956): 35.

18. Mathieu Jaboulay, "La greffe de corps thyroïde et de capsules surrénales dans les maladies de ces glandes," *Lyon Médicale* 84, no. 12 (Mar. 21, 1897): 399–400.

19. Jaboulay's career is chronicled in Georges Gayet, "Jaboulay, Mathieu (1860–1913)," *Biographies Médicales de Paris* (Paris: J.-B. Baillière et Fils, 1936), 10:257–72; R. Leriche, "Jaboulay et la recherche expérimentale: Sutures et greffes vasculaires le shunt," *Lyon Chirurgical* 51, no. 1 (Jan. 1956): 21–23; F. Collet, "Testu et Jaboulay," *Cahiers de Lyon Histoire Médicale* and in an obituary in *The Lancet* 182, no. 4707 (Nov. 15, 1913): 1428–29. For his own description of his pioneering human attempt, see Mathieu Jaboulay, "Greffe de reins au pli du coude par sutures artérielles et veineuses," *Bulletin du Lyon Médical* 107 (1906): 575–77; there is a translation of this work in Hau, *Renal Transplantation*.

20. Jaboulay was the first to publish his use of a vascularized pig organ for transplantation.

21. Ernst Unger, "Über Nierentransplantationen," *Berliner Klinische Wochenschrift* 47 (1907): 1057–60, which is translated in Hau, *Renal Transplantation*. For a biography of Unger, see Enno A. Winkler, "Ernst Unger: A Pioneer in Modern Surgery," *Journal of the History of Medicine and Allied Sciences* 37, no. 3 (July 1982): 269–86; and Enno A. Winkler, *Ernst Unger 1875–1938: Eine Biobibliographie* (Berlin: Internationale Verlags-Anstalt, 1975). Unger may have been first to place a long intravenous line, passing it from his own leg into the inferior vena cava; see André J. Bruwer, ed., *Classic Descriptions in Diagnostic Roentgenology* (Springfield, IL: Thomas, 1964), 1:502–4.

22. Ernst Unger, "Über Nierentransplantationen," *Verhandlungen Berliner Medizinsche Gesellschaft* 40 (1909): 198–208.

23. Ernst Unger, "Nierentransplantationen," *Verhandlungen Berliner Medizinsche Gesellschaft* 41 (1910): 72–86. The en masse technique, as performed by Alexis Carrel, is shown in "Transplantation in Mass of the Kidneys," *Journal of Experimental Medicine* 10, no. 1 (January 1908): 98–140, 103.

24. The first microscopy carried out on homograft, rather than xenograft or autograft, kidneys, was reported by Ragnvald Ingebrigtsen (1882–1975) in Norway, when he returned to Stavanger after a period of study with Carrel in New York from 1911 to 1913. He was the first to report an accumulation of lymphocytes in such failed kidneys; see Ragnvald Ingebrigtsen, "Homoplastisk nyretransplantation," *Norsk Magazin for Lægevidenskaben* 75 (1914): 1143–46. Ingebrigtsen also looked for antibodies after the graft loss.

25. Emil Abderhalden, ed., *Handbuch der biologischen Arbeitsmethoden* (Berlin: Urban & Schwarzenberg, 1930), book 5, 267–378.

26. Zaaijer carried out the single autograft kidney, then successfully removed the remaining native kidney eighty-three days later, thus allowing the animal to survive any temporary damage to the autotransplant. His important paper, abstracted in *Deutsche Medizinische Wochenschrift* 34 (1908): 1777, appeared in the *Netherlands Tijdschrift voor Geneeskunde* 44, no. 1 (1908): 942–47. The long-term autograft is de-

scribed later, in Johannes Henricus Zaaijer, "Dauer-resultat einer autoplastischen Nierentransplantation bei einem Hunde," *Beiträge zur Klinischen Chirurgie* 93 (1914): 223–27, which contains the first illustration of the bladder attachment.

27. E. Villard and E. Perrin, "Transplantations ré-nales," *Lyon Chirurgical* 10 (1913): 109–34; and E. Villard and L. Tavernier, "La transplantation du rein," *Presse Médicale* 18, no. 52 (1910): 489. After Jaboulay's death in a rail accident in 1913, the strong Lyon tradition in vascular surgery continued under René Leriche; see Angelo M. May and Alice G. May, *The Two Lions of Lyons: The Tale of Two Surgeons, Alexis Carrel and René Leriche* (Rockville, MD: Kabel, 1992); and the collected papers given on the occasion of the centenary of the Lyon Surgical Society, published in *Annales de Chirurgie* 52, no. 3 (1998).

28. M. von Borst and E. Enderlen, "Über Transplantation von Gefässen und ganzen Organen," *Deutsche Zeitschrift für Chirurgie* 99 (1909): 54–163. On Borst's career, see C. Steffen, "The Man behind the Eponym: Max Borst (1869–1946)," *American Journal of Dermatopathology* 7, no. 1 (Feb. 1985): 25–27.

29. Borst and Enderlen, "Über Transplantation von Gefässen," 127.

30. Levi J. Hammond and Howard A. Sutton, "An Abstract Report of a Case of Transplantation of Testicle," *International Clinics* 22 (1912): 150–54; see also Thomas N. Haviland and Lawrence C. Parish, "An Early 20th-Century Testicular Transplant," *Transactions and Studies of the College of Physicians of Philadelphia* 38, no. 4 (Apr. 1971): 231–34. Adding to the mystery surrounding their work was that the *New York Times* reported on November 14, 1911, that the men had also carried out a human kidney transplant at the time, work never reported elsewhere.

31. Y. Yonekawa and J. Fandino, "Theodor Kocher, Hayazo Ito and Harvey Cushing in Berne, Switzerland," *Neurologia Medica-Chirurgica* 38, no. 5 (May 1998): 301–3.

32. W. S. Halsted, "Auto- and Isotransplantation, in Dogs, of the Parathyroid Glands," *Journal of Experimental Medicine* 11, no. 1 (Jan. 1909): 175–99. Like some others, Halsted used the "iso-" prefix instead of "homo-." The clinical need for thyroid transplantation arose from radical new thyroid surgery, which in some cases included accidental removal of the attached parathyroid glands, with serious tetany following.

33. For the acceptance, distortion, and persistence of "Halsted's Law" until the 1950s, see Michael Woodruff, *The Transplantation of Tissues and Organs* (Springfield, IL: Thomas, 1960), 25.

34. W. Baader and L. M. Nyhus, "The Life of Carl Beck and an Important Interval with Alexis Carrel," *Surgery, Gynecology & Obstetrics* 163, no. 1 (July 1986): 85–88; W. C. Beck, "Alexis Carrel and Carl Beck—A Historical Footnote," *Perspectives in Biology and Medicine* 30, no. 1 (autumn 1986): 148–51.

35. Blair O. Rogers, "Charles Claude Guthrie, M.D., Ph.D.: A Remarkable Pioneer in Tissue and Organ Transplantation," *Plastic and Reconstructive Surgery* 24, no. 1 (Oct. 1959): 380–83.

36. Quoted in L. G. Walker Jr., "The Letters and Friendship of Carrel and Cushing," *Surgery, Gynecology & Obstetrics* 167, no. 3 (1988): 253–58.

37. Isidore Cohn with Hermann B. Deutsch, *Rudolf Matas: A Biography of One of the Great Pioneers in Surgery* (Garden City, NY: Doubleday, 1960).

38. S. P. Harbison, "The Origins of Vascular Surgery: The Carrel-Guthrie Letters," *Surgery* 52 (1962): 406–18.

39. Hugh E. Stephenson and Robert S. Kimpton, *America's First Nobel Prize in Medicine or Physiology: The Story of Guthrie and Carrel* (Boston: Midwestern Vascular Surgery Society, 2000).

40. Akerman's remarks on Carrel's work are in the Nobel Foundation's *Nobel Lectures: Including Presentation Speeches and Laureates' Biographies; Physiology or Medicine 1901–1921* (Amsterdam: Elsevier, 1967). See also the interesting section on Carrel in Jon Turney, *Frankenstein's Footsteps* (New Haven, CT: Yale University Press, 1998).

41. Charles C. Guthrie, "On Misleading Statements," *Science* 29, no. 731 (Jan. 1, 1909): 29–31. Guthrie later told the Nobel Committee that the prize should have been awarded to him along with Carrel; the committee replied that joint awards were not made. That policy was soon changed, however.

42. Charles C. Guthrie, *Blood-Vessel Surgery and Its Applications* (Pittsburgh: University of Pittsburgh Press, 1912; repr., with commentaries by Samuel P. Harbison and Bernard Fisher, 1959).

43. Alexis Carrel and R. Ingebrigtsen, "The Production of Antibodies by Tissues Living Outside of the Organism," *Journal of Experimental Medicine* 15, no. 3 (Mar. 1, 1912): 287–91, with data given in two other

journals. Ingebrigtsen retained an interest in experimental kidney transplantation after his return to Norway.

44. For Carrel's views on tissue cooling, see Alexis Carrel, "The Preservation of Tissues and Its Applications in Surgery," *Journal of the American Medical Association* 59, no. 7 (1912): 523–27, 523. Carrel gives full credit to Paul Bert's much earlier Paris studies on cooling and tissue viability.

45. However, in Paris that year, M. P. Magitot showed that human corneal grafts could be preserved for some time by cold in a state of *"vie ralentie"* (slowed life) for later use: M. P. Magitot, "Possibilité de conserver à l'état de vie ralentie, pendant un temps indéterminé, la cornée transparente de l'oeil humain," *Compte Rendu de l'Académie des Sciences* 154 (1912): 75–76. This strategy was not used for decades, however.

46. Ragnvald Ingebrigtsen, "The Influence of Isoagglutinins on the Final Results of Homoplastic Transplantations of Arteries," *Journal of Experimental Medicine* 16, no. 2 (Aug. 1912): 169–77. This article from Carrel's laboratory quotes Carrel's papers extensively, but, curiously, Carrel is not a coauthor.

6. The "Lost Era" of Transplantation Immunology

1. See Arthur M. Silverstein, *A History of Immunology*, 2nd ed. (London: Academic Press, 2009); Arthur M. Silverstein and A. A. Bialasiewicz, "A History of Theories of Acquired Immunity," *Cellular Immunology* 51, no. 1 (Apr. 1980): 151–67; and W. L. Ford, "The Lymphocyte—Its Transformation from a Frustrating Enigma to a Model of Cellular Function," in *Blood, Pure and Eloquent: A Story of Discovery, of People, and of Ideas*, ed. Maxwell M. Wintrobe (New York: McGraw-Hill, 1980), 457–508. See also Pauline M. H. Mazumdar, "The Purpose of Immunity: Landsteiner's Interpretation of the Human Isoantibodies," *Journal of the History of Biology* 8, no. 1 (spring 1975): 115–33. Transplantation immunology is dealt with in Leslie Brent, *A History of Transplantation Immunology* (San Diego: Academic Press, 1997).

2. For the early terminology of immunology, see J. Lindenmann, "Origin of the Terms 'Antibody' and 'Antigen,'" *Scandinavian Journal of Immunology* 19, no. 4 (Apr. 1984): 281–85.

3. Eileen Crist and Alfred I. Tauber, "Debating Humoral Immunity and Epistemology: The Rivalry of the Immunochemists Jules Bordet and Paul Ehrlich," *Journal of the History of Biology* 30, no. 3 (autumn 1997): 321–56; Arthur M. Silverstein, *Paul Ehrlich's Receptor Immunology: The Magnificent Obsession* (San Diego: Academic Press, 2002). Ehrlich showed that antibodies could be formed in mice after immunization with the exotic and dangerous proteins ricin and abrin, unknown in the mouse world, and the concept of immunity was thereafter changed to be understood as the response to most proteins.

4. *Edinburgh Medical and Surgical Journal* 2 (1806): 382–89.

5. Quoted in B. S. Schoenberg and D. G. Schoenberg, "Of Mice and Men, of Triumph and Tragedy, of Murine Models of Malignant Disease," *Surgery, Gynecology & Obstetrics* 141, no. 6 (Dec. 1975): 933–37.

6. Edwards Crisp, "Malignant Tumor on the Pectoral Muscle of a Mouse," *Transactions of the Pathological Society of London* 5 (1854): 348. Crisp studied animal disease and pathology at the London Zoo; for an obituary, see *The Lancet* 120, no. 3093 (Dec. 9, 1882): 1010–11.

7. Michael B. Shimkin, *Contrary to Nature* (Washington, DC: U.S. Department of Health, Education, and Welfare, 1977). For Novinsky, see Michael B. Shimkin, "M. A. Novinsky: A Note on the History of Transplantation of Tumors," *Cancer* 8, no. 4 (July–Aug. 1955): 653–55. Novinsky's classic paper is M. Novinsky, "Oprivivanii rakovikh novoobrazovanii," *Medicinski Vjesnik* 16 (1876): 289–90, soon republished in Germany in *Zentralblatt fuer die medizinischen Wissenschaften* 14 (1876): 790–91.

8. H. Moreau, "Recherches expérimentales sur la transmissibilité de certains néoplasmes," *Archives de Médecine Expérimentale et d'Anatomie Pathologique* 6 (1893): 677–705.

9. From A. Borrel, "Le problème étiologique du cancer," *Zeitschrift für Krebsforschung* 7 (1909): 265–78.

10. Peter B. Medawar, "The Immunology of Transplantation," in *The Harvey Lectures*, series 52: 1956–1957 (New York: Academic Press, 1958), 144–76, 146.

11. C. O. Jensen, "Experimentelle Untersuchungen über Krebs bei Mäusen," *Zentralblatt für Bakteriologie und Parasitenkinde* 34 (1903): 28–122. See also Ilana Löwy, "Experimental Systems and Clinical Practices: Tumor Immunology and Cancer Immunotherapy 1895–1980," *Journal of the History of Biology* 27, no. 3 (autumn 1994): 403–35.

12. Quoted in Fred Himmelweit, comp. and ed., *The Collected Papers of Paul Ehrlich* (London, 1956), 3:107.

Ehrlich had quoted E. von Dungern's *Die Antikörper* (Jena, 1903) as suggesting that antibody activity was the cause of tumor loss. Ehrlich's views are stated with clarity in his three Harben Lectures in London in 1908, reprinted in Himmelweit, *Collected Papers of Paul Ehrlich*, 3:106–34. An interesting analysis is found in C. P. Rhoads, "Paul Ehrlich and the Cancer Problem," *Annals of the New York Academy of Sciences* 59, no. 2 (Sept. 1954): 190–97. Rhoads was the pioneer of nitrogen mustard chemotherapy in the post–World War II period.

13. Georg Schöne, *Die heteroplastische und homöoplastische Transplantation* (Berlin: Springer, 1912). Schöne is also remembered as the pioneer of fixation of human long bone fractures with internal rods; see *Clinical Orthopaedics* 234 (1998): 2–4. Basic information about Schöne's time with Ehrlich is lacking. Intrafamily graft studies (similar to those of Schöne) but carried out by Georg Perthes are found in *Zentralblatt für Chirurgie* 44 (1917): 641–44.

14. Erich Lexer, "Über freie Transplantationen," *Archiv für Klinische Chirurgie* 95 (1911): 827–51, a paper Medawar later described as "one of the masterpieces of the literature of transplantation." For a translation of Lexer's article, see Erich Lexer, "Free Transplantation," *Annals of Surgery* 60, no. 2 (Aug. 1914): 166–94. He brought these studies together in his two-volume monograph, *Die Freien Transplantationen* (Stuttgart: Enke, 1919, 1924). On Lexer, see H. Nathan, "Erich Lexer 1867–1937," *Die Medizinische Welt* 24, no. 52 (Dec. 28, 1973): 2088–90; and Von U. Paul, "Erich Lexer," *Zentralblatt für Chirurgie* 102, no. 1 (1976): 571–73. For a bibliography of Erich Lexer's considerable output, see H. May, *Plastic and Reconstructive Surgery* 30 (1962): 670–75. In 1907, Lexer was first to use the saphenous vein for human arterial surgical repair, and the German Society for Surgery now presents its Lexer Prize for contributions on organ replacement.

15. Lexer, "Free Transplantation," 172.

16. H. L. Underwood, "Anaphylaxis Following Skin-Grafting for Burns," *Journal of the American Medical Association* 63, no. 9 (Aug. 29, 1914): 775–76. Little is known of Underwood, in spite of inquiries. In the literature of the time, the term *anaphylaxis* was used in a much broader sense, to include most local immune responses, rather than the narrower connotation of later use.

17. Britain's Cancer Research Fund, later called the Imperial Cancer Research Fund, had been set up as a charity in 1902. After these successes, Bashford, director of its laboratory, retired on health grounds in 1914, at a time when the fund's research program had turned away from immunological studies. For his group's work, and its forgotten importance, see Joan Austoker, *A History of the Imperial Cancer Research Fund, 1902–1986* (Oxford: Oxford University Press, 1988), 43–47.

18. Ernest F. Bashford, and B. R. G. Russell, "Further Evidence on the Homogeneity of the Resistance to the Implantation of Malignant New Growths," *The Lancet* 175, no. 4516 (Mar. 19, 1910): 782–87.

19. Ernest F. Bashford, J. A. Murray, and M. Haaland, "Resistance and Susceptibility to Inoculated Cancer," *Third Scientific Report of the Cancer Research Fund* (1908): 359–97. Each report had a summary of the unit's considerable, important, and soon forgotten output. Bashford later died of alcoholism.

20. See the incisive, long, and not uncritical review of early experimental cancer studies in William H. Woglom, "Immunity to Transplantable Tumours," *Cancer Review* 4 (1929): 129–214.

21. On James Bumgardner Murphy, see Clarence C. Little, "James Bumgardner Murphy," *Biographical Memoirs of the National Academy of Sciences*, vol. 34 (Washington, DC: National Academy of Sciences: 1960), 183–203, which includes a bibliography. The neglect of Murphy's work means he is hardly mentioned in George Corner's *History of the Rockefeller Institute, 1901–1953: Origins and Growth* (New York: Rockefeller Institute Press, 1964), nor is immunology stressed in the entry for Murphy in the *Dictionary of Scientific Biography*. Less forgivable is Murphy's humble place in the first edition of Silverstein's *History of Immunology* (1989), but he made amends in his article on Murphy: Arthur M. Silverstein, "The Lymphocyte in Immunology: From James B. Murphy to James L. Gowans," *Nature Immunology* 2, no. 7 (July 2001): 569–71, with an unhelpful response from J. F. A. P. Miller following. Elsewhere Murphy has had increased attention, starting with W. L. Ford's chapter on the lymphocyte in Wintrobe's *Blood, Pure and Eloquent*. See also Brent, *History of Transplantation Immunology*, 183; and Ilana Löwy, "Biomedical Research and the Constraints of Medical Practice: James Bumgardner Murphy and the Early Discovery of the Role of the Lymphocytes in Immune Reactions," *Bulletin of the History of Medicine* 63, no. 3 (fall 1989): 356–91. Much of Murphy's transplantation work is in his neglected volume of the *Monographs of the Rockefeller Institute for Medical Research* 21 (1926): 1–168.

22. Ernest Sturm and James B. Murphy, "Homoplastic and Heteroplastic Tumor Grafts in the Brain," *Journal of the American Medical Association* 79, no. 26 (1922): 2159–60. This concept that grafts would grow in "privileged sites" in the host was proposed earlier by Julius Cohnheim (1839–1884), who had shown in 1880 that human tuberculosis bacilli would grow in the anterior chamber of the rabbit eye; see Julius Cohnheim, *Die Tuberkulose vom Standpunkt der Infektionslehre* (Leipzig, 1880), translated by Daniel H. Cullimore as *Consumption as a Contagious Disease, with Its Treatment According to the New View* (London, 1880). The Japanese work that preceded Murphy's was Y. Shirai, "On the Transplantation of the Rat Sarcoma in Adult Heterogeneous Animals," *Japan Medical World* 1, no. 2 (1921): 14–15.

23. In 1984, Morten Simonsen, pioneer in the 1960s of the study of the graft-versus-host response, graciously acknowledged the failure of modern transplantation immunologists to give credit to Murphy's forgotten observations: see M. Simonsen, "Graft-versus-Host Reactions: The History That Never Was and the Way Things Happened to Happen," *Immunological Reviews* 88 (Dec. 1985): 5–23.

24. Vera Danchakoff, a former Rockefeller Institute scientist who moved to the Wistar Institute and is now known as the "mother of stem cells," claimed to have publication precedence over Murphy in the matter. Her complaint is detailed in Vera Danchakoff, "Equivalence of Different Hematopoietic Anlages (by Method of Stimulation of Their Stem Cells)," *American Journal of Anatomy* 20, no. 3 (Nov. 1916): 255–327. Morten Simonsen later amusingly highlighted these erroneous nonimmunological explanations of the graft-versus-host response, notably that by James Ebert at the Brookhaven laboratory.

25. Murphy, *Monographs*, 163.

26. James B. Murphy and Arthur W. M. Ellis, "Experiments on the Role of Lymphoid Tissue in the Resistance to Experimental Tuberculosis in Mice," *Journal of Experimental Medicine* 20, no. 4 (Oct. 1914): 397–403. This study also pioneered the use of immunosuppression for the experimental growth of exotic organisms, a useful strategy not employed until many years later.

27. This proposed "lost era" of transplantation immunology corresponds with the "golden era" in medicine, when the germ theory achieved acceptance. Historians also identify a concurrent "Progressive Era" (1890–1920) in social care and reform.

28. For a brief note on Beard, see *Edinburgh University Journal*, vol. 15, 178. Beard is remembered for the Rohon-Beard cell, involved in an early example of "apoptosis," and his work on the thymus was supported by the local Earl of Moray Research Fund.

29. John Beard, "The True Function of the Thymus," *The Lancet* 153, no. 3934 (Jan. 21, 1899): 144–46; see also *Anatomischer Anzeiger Zentralblatt fur die Gesamte Wissenschaftliche Anatomie* 18 (1900): 550–73. Beard's work was at last recognized, but cited incorrectly, in Craig R. Stillwell, "Thymectomy as an Experimental System in Immunology," *Journal of the History of Biology* 27, no. 3 (1994): 379–401. Beard later advocated a cure for cancer using pancreatic enzymes, and this move marginalized him. See Ralph W. Moss, "Cancer, Enzymes and Trophoblast: The Legacy of John Beard, DSc," July 2009, www.cancerdecisions.com.

30. See J. Jolly, "La bourse de Fabricius et les organs lymphoepithéliauz," *Archives d'Anatomie Microscopique* 16 (1914): 363–547.

31. For these early experiments and concerned discussion about their having been forgotten, see Ford, "Lymphocyte—Its Transformation," 457–508.

32. For the flow of lymphocytes from the thoracic duct, see Arthur Biedl and Alfred von Decastello, "Über Aenderungen des Blutbildes nach Unterbrechung des Lymphzuflusses," *Archiv für die gesamte Physiologie (Pflügers)* 86 (1901): 259–90; and Benjamin F. Davis and A. J. Carlson, "Contribution to the Physiology of Lymph. IX: Notes on the Leucocytes in the Neck Lymph, Thoracic Lymph and Blood of Normal Dogs," *American Journal of Physiology* 25, no. 4 (Dec. 1909): 173–89.

33. F. K. Trapeznikoff, "Du sort des spores de microbes dans l'organisme animal," *Annales de l'Institut Pasteur* 5 (1891): 362–94. He published his monograph *Osudbie spor mikrobov* in 1891 upon his return to St. Petersburg.

34. See Günther Gillissen, "Concepts of Delayed Type Hypersensitivity," in *The Immunologic Revolution: Facts and Witnesses*, ed. Herman Friedman and Andor Szentivanyi (Boca Raton, FL: CRC Press, 1994), citations 9–15. Gillissen's chapter shows awareness of the earlier German literature.

35. B. Fellner, "Über Impfungsversuche mit Pirquetschen Papelsubstanzen am Menschen," *Wiener Klinische Wochenschrift* 32 (1919): 936–41. Merrill Chase apologetically pointed out this work fifty years after his own classic cell transfer paper with

Landsteiner in 1942; see M. W. Chase, "Early Days in Cellular Immunology," *Allergy Proceedings* 9, no. 6 (1988): 683–87.

36. See M. J. Bernstein, "A Dermatitis Caused by 'Di-Nitrochlor Benzole,'" *The Lancet* 179, no. 4632 (June 8, 1912): 1534. He noted the delay in response after the first exposure and described later the more rapid and unpleasant second reaction. He correctly blamed "a form of immunity"; the chemical was later used as a test of cell-mediated immunity levels.

37. Metchnikoff had prepared the first antiserum for use against normal cells—an antispermatozoon serum that immobilized bull sperm. The only history of such early attempts is found with difficulty, namely in C. Nava and H. O'Kane, "Antilymphocytic Serum: Historical Review (1895–1963)," *Revista de Investigación Clínica* 26, no. 1 (1974): 77–92; and more easily in Brent, *History of Transplantation Immunology*, 247–52.

38. Simon Flexner, "The Pathology of Lymphotoxic and Myelotoxic Intoxication," *University of Pennsylvania Medical Bulletin* 115 (1902): 287–95.

39. His three articles are Alwin M. Pappenheimer, "Experimental Studies on Lymphocytes: I. The Reactions of Lymphocytes under Various Experimental Conditions," *Journal of Experimental Medicine* 25, no. 5 (May 1917): 633–50; "Experimental Studies on Lymphocytes: II. The Action of Immune Sera upon Lymphocytes and Small Thymus Cells," *Journal of Experimental Medicine* 26, no. 2 (Aug. 1917): 163–79; and "Experimental Studies on Lymphocytes: Cytotoxins for Thymus and Tonsil Lymphocytes," *Proceedings of the New York Pathological Society* 17 (1917): 23–28. Bernard Amos apologetically noticed this work fifty years later.

40. Gustaf A. Lindström, *An Experimental Study of Myelotoxic Sera: Therapeutic Attempts in Myeloid Leukaemia*, Acta Medica Scandinavica series, Supplement 22 (Stockholm: Norstedt, 1927).

41. James B. Murphy, "The Effect of Adult Chicken Organ Grafts on the Chick Embryo," *Journal of Experimental Medicine* 24, no. 1 (July 1916): 1–5.

42. Stephen S. Hall conferred this title in his *A Commotion in the Blood: Life, Death, and the Immune System* (New York: Henry Holt, 1997), 129. For Carrel and Ebeling's paper, see Alexis Carrel and Albert Ebeling, "Leucocytic Secretions," *Journal of Experimental Medicine* 36, no. 6 (Dec. 1922): 645–59. Hints of the cellular chemical messenger are also found in A. E. Rich and M. R. Lewis, "Mechanism of Allergy in

Tuberculosis," *Proceedings of the Society for Experimental Biology and Medicine* 25 (1928): 596–99.

43. G. A. Currie, "Eighty Years of Immunotherapy: A Review of Immunological Methods Used for the Treatment of Human Cancer," *British Journal of Cancer* 26, no. 3 (June 1972): 141–53.

44. A detailed look at this early enthusiasm is found in Martin Gore and Pamela Riches, "The History of Immunotherapy," in *Immunotherapy in Cancer*, ed. Martin Gore and Pamela Riches (Chichester, England: Wiley, 1996), 1–10. Coley's provocative data are in William B. Coley, "The Treatment of Inoperable Sarcoma with the Mixed Toxins of Erysipelas and *Bacillus prodigious:* Immediate and Final Results in One Hundred and Forty Cases," *Journal of the American Medical Association* 31, no. 8 (Aug. 20, 1898): 389–95; and no. 9 (Aug. 27, 1898): 456–65.

45. For early immuno-stimulation attempts in human cancer, see, for instance, J. Walter Vaughan, "Cancer Vaccine and Anticancer Globulins as an Aid in the Surgical Treatment of Malignancy," *Journal of the American Medical Association* 63, no. 15 (Oct. 10, 1914): 1258–65, which quotes his earlier work. Coca's paper was published in a prestigious German journal; see Arthur F. Coca, G. M. Dorrance, and M. G. Lebredo, "'Vaccination' in Cancer: A Report of the Results of the Vaccination Therapy as Applied in Seventy-nine Cases of Human Cancer," *Zeitschrift für Immunitätsforschung* 13 (1912): 543–85.

46. Simon Flexner and J. W. Jobling, "On the Promoting Influence of Heated Tumor Emulsions on Tumor Growth," *Proceedings of the Society for Experimental Biology and Medicine* 4 (1907): 156–57.

47. See also the long, thorough analysis in John Eason, "The Pathology of Paroxysmal Haemoglobinuria," *Journal of Pathology and Bacteriology* 11, no. 2 (1906): 167–202. His obituaries in the *Lancet* and *British Medical Journal* in November 1964 do not mention the revival of this disease concept at the time and briefly describe him as "a popular clinician." After the concept of autoimmunity was rediscovered in the 1950s, credit was eventually given to J. Donath and K. Landsteiner, "Über paroxysmale Hämoglobinurie," *Münchener Medizinische Wochenschrift* 51 (1904): 1590–93.

48. Carlo Moreschi, "Neue Tatsachen über Blutkörperchenagglutination," *Zentralblatt für Bakteriologie, Parasitologie und Infektionskrankheiten* 46 (1908): 49–51. Moreschi died of smallpox at age forty-five. Coombs nobly sought out Moreschi's relatives and made them aware of the Italian scientist's priority;

see Robin R. A. Coombs, "Historical Note: The Past, Present and Future of the Antiglobulin Test," *Vox Sanguinis* 74, no. 2 (1998): 67–73.

49. Ferdinand Sauerbruch, and M. Heyde, "Über Parabiose künstlich vereinigter Warmblüter," *Münchner Medizinische Wochenschrift* 55 (1908): 153–56; B. Morpurgo, "Über Parabiose bei weissen Ratten," *Verhandlungen der Deutschen Pathologischen Gesellschaft* 13 (1909): 150–58.

50. H. Heinecke, "Experimentelle Untersuchungen über die Einwirkung der Röntgenstrahlen," *Mitteilungen aus den Grenzgebieten der Medizin und Chirurgie* 14 (1904–5): 21–94.

51. E. Benjamin and E. Sluka, "Antikörperbildung nach experimenteller Schädigung des hämatopoetischen Systems durch Röntgenstrahlen," *Wiener Klinische Wochenschrift* 21 (1908): 311–13.

52. Ludvig Hektoen and H. J. Corper, "Effect of Injection of Active Deposits of Radium Emanation on Rabbits," *Journal of Infectious Diseases* 31 (1922): 305–12. Hektoen may also have been first to demonstrate the clinical relevance of Landsteiner's blood types, that is, the dangers of blood transfusion between incompatible types.

53. James B. Murphy, "Heteroplastic Tissue Grafting Effected through Roentgen-Ray Lymphoid Destruction," *Journal of the American Medical Association* 62, no. 19 (May 9, 1914): 1459. The first American "radium bomb," used to give controlled radiation, was held at Roswell Park. Murphy, like other Rockefeller Institute scientific staff, preferred to give short summaries of work in progress in this widely read general medical periodical.

54. John J. Morton, "A Rapid Method for the Diagnosis of Renal Tuberculosis by the Use of the X-rayed Guinea Pig," *Journal of Experimental Medicine* 24, no. 4 (Oct. 1, 1916): 419–27.

55. For the visionary marrow shielding experiment, see J. Fabricious-Moeller, *Experimental Studies of Hemorrhagic Diathesis from X-ray Sickness* (Copenhagen: Levin & Munksgaards, 1922).

56. "Report on Cancer, April 1914," *Report of the Director of Laboratories to the Scientific Directors*, p. 322, RU RG439, Rockefeller University Archives, Rockefeller Archive Center, Sleepy Hollow, NY.

57. M. M. Le Noire and H. Claude, "Sur un cas de purpura attribué à l'intoxication par la benzène," *Bulletins et Mémoires de la Société Médicale des Hôpitaux de Paris* 14 (1897): 1251–60, a hard-to-find paper.

58. Laurence Selling, "A Preliminary Report of Some Cases of Purpura Hemorrhagica Due to Benzol Poisoning," *Bulletin of the Johns Hopkins Hospital* 21 (1910): 33–37; and 22 (1911): 94–101; Laurence Selling, "Benzol als Leukotoxin," *Ziegler's Beiträge für pathologische Anatomie und zur allgemeinen Pathologie* 56 (1911): 576–631. Selling thought it important to publish in Germany. He acknowledged the financial support of the Rockefeller Institute and corresponded with Flexner, its director; his work may therefore have been known to Carrel and Murphy.

59. See the careful study by H. G. Weiskotten, S. C. Schwartz, and H. S. Steensland, "The Action of Benzol: I. On the Significance of Myeloid Metaplasia," *Journal of Medical Research* 33, no. 1 (1915): 127–40.

60. W. C. White and A. M. Gammon, "The Influence of Benzol Inhalations on Experimental Pulmonary Tuberculosis in Rabbits," *Transactions of the Association of American Physicians* 29 (1914): 332–37. This paper reported on a serendipitous discovery, since the project started as an attempted cure for tuberculosis via dissolving the bacterial organism's protective capsule using the solvent benzol.

61. Frederick P. Gay and Glanville Yeisley Rusk, "Studies on the Locus of Antibody Formation: The Effect of Benzol Intoxication," *University of California Publications in Pathology* 16, no. 2 (1914): 139–45, a hard-to-find paper.

62. Frederick Stenn, "The Historical Importance of the John McCormick Institute for Infectious Diseases," *Quarterly Bulletin of the Northwest University Medical School* 35 (1961): 165–73; Thomas Neville Bonner, *Medicine in Chicago 1850–1950: A Chapter in the Social and Scientific Development of a City* (Urbana: University of Illinois Press, 1991); Ludvig Hektoen, "The Effect of Benzene on the Production of Antibodies," *Journal of Infectious Diseases* 19, no. 1 (July 1916): 69–84. The McCormick Institute was later renamed the Hektoen Institute. Another attempt using benzol comes from H. Fischer, "Tierexperimentielle Studien zum Problem der Homiotransplantation," *Archive für Klinische Chirurgie* 156 (1929): 224–50. Hektoen is described in the *Dictionary of Scientific Biography* (Detroit: Charles Scribner's Sons, 2008), 6:232–33, Gale Virtual Reference Library, and *Archives of Pathology* 52 (1951): 390, but without mention of his studies of immunosuppression. Another benzol study was F. Schiff, "Einfluss des Benzols auf die aktive Anaphylaxie des Meerschweinchens," *Zeitschrift für Immunitätsforschung und Experimentelle Therapie* 23 (1914): 61–65.

63. Ludvig Hektoen, "The Effect of Toluene on the Production of Antibodies," *Journal of Infectious Diseases* 19, no. 6 (Dec. 1916): 737–45.

64. These forgotten pioneers of chemotherapy were the Hungarian scientists G. Királyfi and A. von Korányi—see *Orvosi Hetilap* 61 (1912): 539–40, 568; see also their papers "Beeinflussung der Leukämie durch Benzol," *Berlin Klinische Wochenschrift* 49 (1912): 1357 and *Wiener Klinische Wochenschrift* 26, 1062–67. This early, creditable, science-based, but forgotten episode in cancer chemotherapy awaits a historian. Korányi was also a pioneer of assessing renal function by urine osmolarity.

65. Frank Billings, "Benzol in the Treatment of Leukemia," *Journal of the American Medical Association* 60, no. 7 (Feb. 15, 1913): 495–98. Benzene is toxic to CD34 lymphocytes.

66. P. Delore and C. Borgomano, "Leucémie aiguë au cours de l'intoxication benzénique: Sur l'origine toxique de certaines leucémies aiguës et leurs relations avec les anémies graves," *Journal de Médecine de Lyon* 9 (1928): 227–33.

67. The war experience with mustard gas is described in Milton C. Winternitz, *Collected Studies on the Pathology of War Gas Poisoning* (New Haven, CT: Yale University Press, 1920). The use of nitrogen mustard by the Germans is described in Ludwig F. Haber, *The Poisonous Cloud: Chemical Warfare in the First World War* (Oxford: Oxford University Press, 1986). The British use of poison gas is described in Albert Palazzo, *Seeking Victory on the Western Front: The British Army and Chemical Warfare in World War I* (Lincoln: University of Nebraska Press, 2000), 184–87.

68. Edward Bell Krumbhaar and H. D. Krumbhaar, "The Blood and Bone Marrow in Yellow Cross Gas (Mustard Gas) Poisoning," *Journal of Medical Research* 40, no. 3 (Sept. 1919): 497–507. Krumbhaar's biographers have missed his contributions to the development of immunosuppression; see Esmond R. Long, "Edward Bell Krumbhaar 1882–1966," *Bulletin of the History of Medicine* 31 (1957): 493–504; and S. X. Radbill, "Edward Bell Krumbhaar: Medical Historian, Bibliophile and Humanist," *Transactions and Studies of the College of Physicians of Philadelphia* 25, no. 1 (June 1957): 35–40. Krumbhaar is also known for translating Arturo Castiglioni's works, notably *A History of*

Medicine (New York: Knopf, 1941).

69. The experimental investigation of nitrogen mustard gas as an immunosuppressant is found in Ludvig Hektoen and H. J. Corper, "The Effect of Mustard Gas (Dichlorethylsulphide) on Antibody Formation," *Journal of Infectious Diseases* 28 (1921): 279–85. For a historical account, see J. Einhorn, "Nitrogen Mustard: The Origin of Chemotherapy for Cancer," *International Journal of Radiation Oncology, Biology and Physics* 11, no. 7 (July 1985): 1375–78.

70. J. Golanitzky, "Über Transplantationsversuche an farbstoffgespeicherten Tieren," *Zentralblatt für Allgemeine Pathologie und Pathologische Anatomie* 24 (1913): 809–11. This approach continued unnoticed in the 1920s; see Walter Lehmann and Heinrich Tammann, "Transplantation und Vitalspeicherung," *Beiträge zur Klinische Chirurgie* 135 (1925): 259–302; and Heinrich Tammann and M. Patrikalakis, "Weitere Versuche über homoioplastiche Hauttransplantationen bei Vitalspeicherung," *Beiträge zur Klinischen Chirurgie* 139 (1927): 550–68, which has the first illustration of skin grafting in mice.

71. Charles Todd, "On the Recognition of the Individual by Haemolytic Methods," *Journal of Genetics* 3, no. 2 (1913): 123–30. The experimental work was carried out in Egypt and had been communicated to the Royal Society in 1910.

72. In the previous year, a smaller similar meeting in London heard of progress in vascular surgery, and the *Times* (London) of August 11, 1913, reported on the "experimental kidney transplants of Dr. Ernst Jeger of Berlin." Stewart Cameron found this record of the event.

73. E. Ullmann, "Tissue and Organ Transplantation," *Annals of Surgery* 60, no. 2 (1914): 195–218.

74. Lexer, "Free Transplantation," 166.

75. *New York Times*, April 14, 1914.

76. Serving in the French military as a doctor during the war, Carrel quickly and characteristically announced a revolutionary method of wound treatment and was roundly criticized by the French surgical establishment. His new method, the Carrel-Dakin system, involved a complex new antiseptic regimen, and, though slavishly followed in many military medical facilities during the war, it was later abandoned.

7. Anarchy in the 1920s

1. Interest in this discontinuity in transplantation studies was initiated in David Hamilton, *Kidney*

Transplantation: Principles and Practice, ed. Peter J. Morris (London: Academic Press, 1979), 4; and David Hamilton, "Alexis Carrel and the Early Days of Tissue Transplantation," *Transplantation Reviews* 2 (1988): 1–15. Some immunologists, including Merrill Chase, Robin Coombs, and Morten Simonsen, had earlier expressed contrition at their own unawareness of earlier work relevant to them, and historians of immunology like Bill Ford, Leslie Brent, and Arthur Silverstein have now mentioned this gap.

2. Daniel J. Kevles, "Into Hostile Political Camps: The Reorganization of International Science in World War I," *Isis* 62, no. 1 (spring 1971): 47–60.

3. Theodore Koppányi, "Transplantation of Organs," *Scientific Monthly* 27, no. 6 (Dec. 1928): 502–5. The Theodore Koppányi Papers (Collection 6306) are in the Manuscripts and Archives Division, New York Public Library.

4. I. M. Rutkow, "The Letters of William Halsted and Erwin Payr," *Surgery, Gynecology & Obstetrics* 161 (1985): 75–87, 83.

5. See Jacques Loeb, *The Mechanistic Conception of Life* (Chicago: University of Chicago Press, 1912). On Loeb, see Charles E. Rosenberg, *No Other Gods: On Science and American Thought* (Baltimore: Johns Hopkins University Press, 1976); René J. Dubos, *The Professor, the Institute and DNA* (New York: Rockefeller University Press, 1976); and Philip J. Pauly, *Controlling Life: Jacques Loeb and the Engineering Ideal in Biology* (New York: Oxford University Press, 1987).

6. Loeb's comment is recorded in Paul de Kruif, *The Sweeping Wind: A Memoir* (New York: Harcourt, Brace & World 1962), 16. See also Paul de Kruif, *Our Medicine Men* (New York: Century, 1922).

7. These are the views of the fictitious scientist Gottlieb (based on Jacques Loeb) in Sinclair Lewis's *Martin Arrowsmith*; see I. Löwy, "Biomedical Research and the Constraints of Medical Practice," *Bulletin of the History of Medicine* 63 (1989): 356–91.

8. Osler's caution in support for clinical medical research is studied in David Hamilton, "The Leaven of Science: Osler and Medical Research," in *"Our Lords, the Sick": McGovern Lectures in the History of Medicine and Medical Humanism,* ed. Laurence D. Longo (Malabar, FL: Krieger, 2004), 103–12.

9. W. F. Goebel, "The Golden Era of Immunology at the Rockefeller Institute," *Perspectives in Biology and Medicine* 18, no. 3 (spring 1975): 419–26.

10. *Medical Research Council Annual Report* (London, 1922–1923), 10–11. These were the sentiments of the MRC's secretary, Walter Morley Fletcher, and they annoyed the British clinical community.

11. Leonard Colebrook, *Almroth Wright, Provocative Doctor and Thinker* (London: Heinemann, 1954).

12. For the growth of interwar holistic medicine and science, see Christopher Lawrence and George Weisz, *Greater Than the Parts* (New York: Oxford University Press, 1998). The views of British conservative physicians are found in Thomas Horder, *Health and a Day* (London: Dent, 1937) and, embarrassingly, in Walter Langdon-Brown, *Thus We Are Men* (London: Kegan Paul, 1938). For detailed analysis, see Christopher Lawrence, "A Tale of Two Sciences: Bedside and Bench in Twentieth-Century Britain," *Medical History* 43 (1999): 421–49; and Christopher Lawrence, "Incommunicable Knowledge: Science, Technology and the Clinical Art in Britain 1850–1914," *Journal of Contemporary History* 20, no. 4 (Oct. 1985): 503–20.

13. Quoted in W. Hengeave Ogilvie, *Recent Advances in Surgery,* 2nd ed. (London: J. & A. Churchill, 1929), 495. Lord Moynihan's millennialist views can be found in this source.

14. See Samuel Pollock Harbison, "The Origins of Vascular Surgery: The Carrel-Guthrie Letters," *Surgery* 52 (1962): 406–18.

15. S. R. Douglas, L. Colebrook, and A. Fleming, "On Skin Grafting: A Plea for Its More Extensive Application," *The Lancet* 190, no. 4897 (July 7, 1917): 5–12.

16. Davis was based at Baltimore's Union Protestant Hospital, and the quote is from his book *Plastic Surgery* (Philadelphia, 1919). His earlier paper was John Staige Davis, "Skin Transplantation: With a Review of 550 Cases at the Johns Hopkins Hospital," *Johns Hopkins Hospital Reports* 15 (1910): 307–96.

17. Fred H. Albee, *Bone-Graft Surgery* (Philadelphia: W. B. Saunders, 1915). As the standard work on this subject, it appeared in revised editions as late as 1940. Albee's biography is *A Surgeon's Fight to Rebuild Men* (New York: Dutton, 1943).

18. Harold K. Shawan, "The Principles of Blood Grouping Applied to Skin Grafts," *American Journal of Medical Science* 157, no. 4 (1919): 503–8.

19. J. C. Masson, "Skin Grafting," *Journal of the American Medical Association* 70, no. 22 (June 1, 1918): 1581–84.

20. See the excellent account in Susan E. Lederer, *Flesh and Blood: Organ Transplantation and Blood Transfusion in Twentieth-Century America* (New York: Oxford University Press, 2008).

21. Frank Ashley, "Foreskins as Skin Grafts," *Annals of Surgery* 106, no. 2 (1937): 252–56.

22. Hugh A. Baldwin, "Skin Grafting," *Medical Record* 98 (Oct. 1920): 687.

23. *New York Medical Journal* 78 (1903): 948–49.

24. Waro Kakahara, "Tissue Transplantation: Real and Bogus," *American Mercury* 17 (1925): 457.

25. E. Holman, "Protein Sensitization in Iso-Skin Grafting: Is the Latter of Practical Value?" *Surgery, Gynecology & Obstetrics* 38 (1924): 100. Holman creditably gives an extensive summary of the prewar German literature.

26. C. E. Brown-Séquard and Jacques Arsène d'Arsonval, "De l'injection des extraits liquides provenant des glandes et des tissus de l'organisme comme méthode thérapeutique," *Compte Rendu des Séances et Mémoires de la Société de Biologie* 3, no. 13 (1891): 248, 265.

27. M. Borrel, "Brown-Séquard's Organotherapy," *Bulletin of the History of Medicine* 50 (1976): 309–20.

28. See the review by B. P. Setchell, "The Testis and Tissue Transplantation: Historical Aspects," *Journal of Reproductive Immunology* 18 (1990): 1–8.

29. G. Frank Lydston, "Sex Gland Implantation," *Journal of the American Medical Association* 66, no. 20 (May 13, 1916): 1540–43. On Lydston, see W. K. Beatty, "G. Frank Lydston: Urologist, Author, and Pioneer Transplanter," *Proceedings of the Institute of Medicine, Chicago* 43 (1990): 35–69.

30. See K. M. Walker, "Hunterian Lecture on Testicular Grafts," *The Lancet* 203, no. 5242 (Feb. 16, 1924): 319–26. He added some scientific spin by measuring patients' glucose tolerance and oxygen consumption both pre- and postoperatively. He organized the British Army's early blood transfusions in World War I and wrote an account of his efforts in the official history of the war; his personal "search for truth" is found in his book *Meaning and Purpose* (London, 1944).

31. Hamilton Bailey, "Testicular Grafting," *The Lancet* 209, no. 5397 (Feb. 5, 1927): 284.

32. On Voronoff, see David Hamilton, *The Monkey Gland Affair* (London: Chatto & Windus, 1986). Publications by Voronoff include *Rejuvenation by Grafting* (London: Allen & Unwin, 1925) and *Greffes Testiculaires* (Paris: Doin, 1923). Voronoff is still patriotically defended in the French transplantation literature as a pioneer, of sorts; see René Küss, *An Illustrated History of Organ Transplantation: The Great Adventure of the Century* (Rueil-Malmaison, France: Sandoz, 1992); Alain Lellouch and Alain Segal, "Contribution à l'histoire de la gérontologie et de l'endocrinologie du début du XXème siècle," *Histoire des Sciences Médicales* 35, no. 4 (2001): 425–34; and Jean Réal, *Voronoff* (Paris: Stock Éditions, 2001).

33. An unlikely story of success in a "blind" trial of human testis grafting in Madrid is proudly mentioned in Eugen Steinach, "Biological Methods against the Process of Old Age," *Medical Journal and Record* 125 (1927): 77–81.

34. L. Dartigues, "Le rajeunissement humain par les greffes animales," *Aesculape (Paris)* 14 (1924): 129–34.

35. Max Thorek, *A Surgeon's World: An Autobiography* (New York: Somerset Books, 1943).

36. Hunt's first publication, "Experience in Testicle Transplantation," was in a respectable journal—*Endocrinology* 6 (1922): 652–54—but, by 1930, his considerable experience was less welcomed by that journal's editor, and his papers then began to appear elsewhere; see H. Lyons Hunt, "Conclusions from Observation in 600 Cases of Gland Transplantation," *Medical Record and Annals* 25 (1931): 715–17. In 1933, Hunt claimed to have done a total of 702 such transplants.

37. Leo L. Stanley, "Testicular Substance Implantation: Comments on Some Six Thousand Implantations," *California and Western Medicine* 35, no. 6 (Dec. 1931): 411–15.

38. R. G. Hoskins, "Studies on Vigor: Effects of Testicle Grafts on Spontaneous Activity," *Endocrinology* 9, no. 4 (1925): 277–96. This was a negative report, but he humbly stated that his surgical technique was at fault.

39. Quoted in "Ovarian Grafts," *British Medical Journal* 2, no. 3533 (Sept. 22, 1928): 531–32.

40. F. C. Pybus, "Notes on Suprarenal and Pancreatic Grafting," *The Lancet* 204, no. 5272 (Sept. 13, 1924): 550–51. Pybus can at least be admired for an early awareness of the need for speed in removing and implanting human donor tissue from a cadaver.

41. Frank d'Abreu, "Transplantation of Suprarenal Glands in Addison's Disease," *The Lancet* 222, no. 5757 (Dec. 30, 1933): 1478–79.

42. On the use of fetal pancreas transplants in Australia at this time, see J. C. Morris, "Pioneer Attempts to Cure Diabetes by Pancreatic Transplantation," *Medical Journal of Australia* 149 (1988): 634–36.

43. See Gerald Carson, *The Roguish World of Doctor Brinkley* (New York: Rinehart, 1960); Hamilton, *Monkey Gland Affair*; R. Alton Lee, *The Bizarre Careers of John R. Brinkley* (Lexington: University Press of Kentucky, 2002); Eric S. Juhnke, *Quacks and Crusaders: The Fabulous Careers of John Brinkley, Norman Baker, and Harry Hoxsey* (Lawrence: University Press of Kansas, 2002); and Pope Brock, *Charlatan: America's Most Dangerous Huckster, the Man Who Pursued Him, and the Age of Flimflam* (New York: Crown, 2008).

44. These hand transplants appear in short stories by Roy Wallace, "The Avenging Hand," *Weird Tales,* February 1926; and Bassett Morgan, "Demon Doom of N'Yeng Sen," *Weird Tales,* August 1929. See also the novel by Maurice Renard, *Les Mains d'Orlac* (Paris 1920), translated as *The Hands of Orlac,* twice adapted for the screen.

45. See anonymous tales like "Brian," *Chambers Journal,* November 1922; "The Seventh Devil," *Weird Tales,* November 1925; and "Horror on Owl's Hill," *Argosy All-Story Weekly,* Feb. 2, 1929. Contributions with identifiable authors are Carl Keppler's "Mr Pichegru's Discovery," *Weird Tales,* July 1929; and Bassett Morgan's "Laocoon," *Weird Tales,* July 1926. See also the series "Doctor Hackenshaw's Secrets," appearing in *Science and Invention* of May 1921 (featuring Carrel's methods used for cloning), July 1922 (human hybrids), March 1924 (human xenografting), and January 1925 (organ transplantation in the year 2000). The standard reference work on these early science fiction themes is Everett Franklin Bleiler, *Science Fiction: The Early Years* (Kent, OH: Kent State University Press, 1990).

46. Bulgakov's novel was released from censorship in 1987, one year after the first liberation of Soviet literature from state control.

47. For a full analysis see Anthony Colin Wright, *Mikhail Bulgakov: Life and Interpretations* (Toronto: University of Toronto Press, 1978), and Edythe C. Haber, *Mikhail Bulgakov: The Early Years* (Cambridge, MA: Harvard University Press, 1998).

48. Duncan Wilson, "The Early History of Tissue Culture in Britain: The Interwar Years," *Social History of Medicine* 18, no. 2 (2005): 225–43.

49. Loeb's own memoirs are in *Perspectives in Biology and Medicine* 2 (1958): 1–23. There are biographies by H. T. Blumenthal in *Science* 131 (Mar. 25, 1960): 907–8; and by Ernest W. Goodpasture in *National Academy of Sciences Biographical Memoirs* 35 (1961): 205–51, which includes his remarkable bibliography, also found in part in *Archives of Pathology* 50 (1950): 657–86. For obituaries of Loeb, see W. S. Hartroft, *Archives of Pathology* 70 (Aug. 1960): 269–74; and the tribute by Peyton Rous, "Leo Loeb (1869–1959)," *Cancer* 13 (May–June 1960): 437–38. See also Jan A. Witkowski, "Experimental Pathology and the Origins of Tissue Culture: Leo Loeb's Contribution," *Medical History* 27, no. 3 (July 1983): 269–88. These authors have missed his importance in transplantation studies.

50. His early works are Leo Loeb, *Ueber Transplantation* (Leipzig, 1897); "Über Transplantation eines Sarkoms der Thyreoidea bei einer weissen Ratte," *Virchows Archive für Pathologische Anatomie und Physiologie* 167 (1901): 175–91; "On Transplantation of Tumors," *Journal of Medical Research* 6, no. 1 (July 1901): 28–38; and "Further Investigations in Transplantation of Tumors," *Journal of Medical Research* 8, no. 1 (June 1902): 44–73. His other important works are Leo Loeb, "Transplantation and Individuality," *Physiological Reviews* 10 (1930): 547–616, published when he was sixty-five, and his book *The Biological Basis of Individuality* (Springfield, IL: Thomas, 1945), which appeared when he was seventy-nine.

51. Witkowski, "Experimental Pathology and the Origins of Tissue Culture," has emphasized Loeb's important place in developing early tissue culture methods.

52. See Juan Rosai, *Guiding the Surgeon's Hand: The History of American Surgical Pathology* (Washington, DC: American Registry of Pathology, 1997), chap. 7.

53. Loeb, "Transplantation and Individuality."

54. Ibid., 572.

55. This was Loeb's final, prescient, clear conclusion in ibid., 557.

56. Leo Loeb, "The Individuality-Differential and Its Mode of Inheritance," *American Naturalist* 54, no. 630 (1920): 58–59.

57. Loeb, "Transplantation and Individuality," 556. If we substitute "aberrant-protein-plus-MHC" for Loeb's "homoiotoxin" coming from the graft, then Loeb's proposed internal surveillance mechanism is not far from the Nobel Prize–winning MHC restriction and combination mechanisms uncovered in the 1970s.

58. Cora Hesselberg and Leo Loeb, "Successive Transplantation of Thyroid Tissue into the Same Host," *Journal of Medical Research* 38, no. 1 (Mar. 1918): 33–53. See also Georg Schöne, *Die heteroplastische und homöoplastische Transplantation* (Berlin: Springer, 1912), chap. 7; and B. Morpurgo, "Untersuchungen über die individuelle Konstitution an Parabiose rat-

ten," *Frankfurter Zeitschrift für Pathologie* 34 (1926): 337–49.

59. Leo Loeb, "Ueber die Entstehung eines Sarkoms nach Transplantation eines Adenocarcinoms einer japanischen Maus," *Zeitschrift für Krebsforschung* 7 (1908): 80–110. This lengthy article is a classic.

60. Mitosi Tokuda, "An Eighteenth Century Japanese Guide-Book on Mouse-Breeding," *Journal of Heredity* 26, no. 12 (1935): 481–84.

61. The notebooks of Abbie Lathrop, who had no formal scientific education, are preserved at the Jackson Laboratory Archives, Bar Harbor, Maine. See M. B. Shimkin, "A. E. C. Lathrop (1868–1918): Mouse Woman of Granby," *Cancer Research* 35, no. 6 (June 1975): 1597–98.

62. This important paper is A. E. C. Lathrop and Leo Loeb, "The Influence of Pregnancies on the Incidence of Cancer in Mice," *Proceedings of the Society for Experimental Biology* 11 (Oct. 1913): 38–40. Although this work confirmed Beatson's clinical finding in Glasgow in 1896 of the benefit of ovary removal in human breast cancer, clinical use of hormonal therapy to treat this malignancy was greatly delayed despite the obvious logic in its use.

63. Loeb's generous tribute to Lathrop was soon published in *Journal of Medical Research* 40 (1919): 496.

64. Herbert C. Morse III, *Origins of Inbred Mice* (New York: Academic Press, 1978); Jean Holstein, *The First Fifty Years at the Jackson Laboratory* (Bar Harbor, ME: Jackson Laboratory, 1979). See also Clyde E. Keeler, *The Laboratory Mouse: Its Origin, Heredity and Culture* (Cambridge, MA: Harvard University Press, 1931); and M. Potter, "History of the BALB/c Family," *Current Topics in Microbiology and Immunology* 122 (1985): 1–5. For the use of the guinea pig, see Stacy L. Pritt, "The History of the Guinea Pig (*Cavia porcellus*) in Society and Veterinary Medicine," *Veterinary Heritage* 21, no. 1 (May 1998): 12–16.

65. For Little's biography and bibliography, see National Academy of Sciences, *Biographical Memoirs* 46 (1975): 24–63; and the excellent entry in *American National Biography* (Oxford, 1999). The Jackson Laboratory has an oral history collection with material relating to these times.

66. Karen A. Rader, *Making Mice: Standardizing Animals for American Biomedical Research, 1900–1955* (Princeton, NJ: Princeton University Press, 2004).

67. Clarence C. Little and E. E. Tyzzer, "Further Experimental Studies on the Inheritance of Susceptibility to a Transplantable Tumor, Carcinoma (J. W. A.) of the Japanese Waltzing Mouse," *Journal of Medical Research* 33, no. 3 (Jan. 1916): 393–453. This outcome was later explained simply as nonrejection of parental tissue by the hybrid made from two parental inbred strains.

68. Tyzzer and Loeb had earlier made a similar suggestion after conducting an experiment using partly inbred animals; see E. E. Tyzzer, "A Study of Inheritance in Mice with Reference to Their Susceptibility to Transplantable Tumors," *Journal of Medical Research* 21, no. 3 (Oct. 1909): 519–73; and Leo Loeb and Moyer S. Fleisher, "Untersuchungen über die Vererbung der das Tumorwachstum bestimmenden Faktoren," *Zentralblatt für Bakteriologie* 67 (1912): 135–48. See also Moyer S. Fleisher and Leo Loeb, "Transplantation of Tumors in Animals with Spontaneously Developed Tumors," *Surgery, Gynecology & Obstetrics* 17 (1913): 203–6.

69. The Cold Spring Harbor story and criticism of the conventional "Bar Harbor" version of the history of inbred mice and mouse genetics are found in Karen Ann Rader, "The Origins of Mouse Genetics: Beyond the Bussey Institute," *Mammalian Genome* 8, no. 7 (July 1997): 464–66.

70. See Bentley Glass, "Geneticists Embattled: Their Stand against Rampant Eugenics and Racism in America during the 1920s and 1930s," *Proceedings of the American Philosophical Society* 130, no. 1 (1986): 130–54. Every possible cancer in a family, confirmed or merely suspected, was included in the tally.

71. Clarence Cook Little, "The Relations of Genetics to the Problem of Cancer Research," *Harvey Lectures 1921–1922* 17 (1923): 65–88; Clarence Cook Little, "The Genetics of Tissue Transplantation in Mammals," *Journal of Cancer Research* 8 (1924): 75–95; J. J. Bittner, "A Review of Genetic Studies on the Transplantation of Tumours," *Journal of Genetics* 31 (1935): 471–87. See also L. C. Strong, "Transplantation Studies on Tumours Arising Spontaneously in Heterozygous Individuals," *Journal of Cancer Research* 13 (1929): 103–15.

72. Little "gave his support to immigration restriction and involuntary sterilization and tacitly accepted the racism of major elements of the eugenics movement." Roberta Gallant Clark, "The Social Uses of Scientific Knowledge: Eugenics in the Career of Clarence Cook Little, 1919–1954" (MA thesis, University of Maine, 1986).

73. Jean Holstein, *The First Fifty Years at the Jackson Laboratory* (Bar Harbor, ME: Jackson Laboratory, 1979).

74. The geneticist J. B. S. Haldane was first to bring such animals to Britain, traveling back to London with his newly purchased mice on the *Mauritania* in 1932. Haldane's nephew, Avrion Mitchison, traveling on the same ship in the 1950s, brought an additional supply of inbred mice back to Britain. When Mitchison delivered these to the pet deck, the ship's staff produced their notes on caring for the mice Haldane brought on board in 1932.

75. Little, "Genetics of Tissue Transplantation in Mammals" (1924).

76. Slye's running battle with Little is chronicled in J. J. McCoy, *The Cancer Lady: Maud Slye and Her Hereditary Studies* (Nashville: T. Nelson, 1977). Little had earlier made harsh comments about Karl Pearson and the London biometricians. For Little's similar attack on the Mendelian Alfred Sturtevant, the "*Drosophila* prodigy," see Rader, *Making Mice*, 329.

77. The original description of the inbreeding effort is in Helen Dean King, *Studies on Inbreeding* (Philadelphia: Wistar Institute, 1919). See also Bonnie Tocher Clause, "The Wistar Rat as a Right Choice: Establishing Mammalian Standards and the Ideal of a Standardized Mammal," *Journal of the History of Biology* 26, no. 2 (summer 1993): 329–49; and Marilyn Bailey Ogilvie, "Inbreeding, Eugenics and Helen Dean King (1869–1955)," *Journal of the History of Biology* 40, no. 3 (2007): 467–507.

78. See, for instance, the references in H. S. Jennings, "Formulae for the Results of Inbreeding," *American Naturalist* 48, no. 575 (Nov. 1914): 693–96.

79. There was a solitary attempt in 1923 to use a sheep kidney transplanted to a patient who suffered kidney failure after a failed attempt at suicide with mercuric chloride. Harold Neuhof's performed the surgery at Bellevue Hospital in New York, and it was reported in detail in the *New York Times* on January 6, 1923. Neuhof had some experience with tissue transplantation, mostly bone and cartilage, and was an enthusiast for homografting of skin. His text *The Transplantation of Tissues* was published in 1923 and gives brief detail of the kidney transplant case.

80. Some of the Mayo Clinic work is described in S. Sterioff and N. Rucker-Johnson, "Frank C. Mann and Transplantation at the Mayo Clinic," *Mayo Clinic Proceedings* 62, no. 11 (Nov. 1987): 1051–55, but they understate the clinic's involvement. Mann encouraged the research fellows to submit the work toward a PhD degree from the University of Minnesota, a move that was unusual for young surgeons at the time.

81. Holger Hansen and Mervyn Susser, "Historic Trends in Deaths from Chronic Kidney Disease in the United States and Britain," *American Journal of Epidemiology* 93, no. 6 (June 1971): 413–24.

82. John Berry Haycroft, "On the Action of the Secretion Obtained from the Medicinal Leech on the Coagulation of the Blood," *Proceedings of the Royal Society of London, 1883–1884* 36 (1884): 478–87; and C. Jacoby, "Über hirudin," *Deutsch Medicine Wochenschrift* 30 (1904): 1786–94.

83. For a thorough history of dialysis and the artificial kidney, see J. Stewart Cameron, *A History of the Treatment of Renal Failure by Dialysis* (Oxford: Oxford University Press, 2002).

84. *Times* (London), Aug. 11, 1913, article was noticed by J. Stewart Cameron. The session at which Abel presented his device was chaired by Rudolf Matas, and it included reports of experimental kidney transplants by the German surgeon Jeger.

85. See brief personal notes in Leonard G. Rowntree, *Amid Masters of Twentieth Century Medicine: A Panorama of Persons and Pictures* (Springfield, IL: Thomas, 1958).

86. For the story of the publishing priority dispute that arose over this test, see Moses Swick, "Urographic Media," *Urology* 4 (1974): 750–57. Swick was belatedly nominated for a Nobel Prize and also later accidentally discovered the usefulness of Uroselectan (used as a contrast medium during x-ray imaging) while studying its antibacterial properties in patients with syphilis. The development of renal imaging is well described in André J. Bruwer, *Classic Descriptions in Diagnostic Roentgenology* (Springfield, IL: Thomas, 1964).

87. Thomas Horder, "On the Need for Standardisation in Clinical Pathology," *The Lancet* 2 (1928): 136–39, 137.

88. John Collie, ed., *Recent Progress in Medicine and Surgery 1919–1933* (London: H. K. Lewis, 1933), 311.

89. Mann's general approach to transplantation is given in his valuable chapter "Transplantation of Organs," in *Contributions to the Medical Sciences: In Honor of Dr. Emanuel Libman* (New York: International Press, 1932). Mann's protégés are featured in *Physicians of the Mayo Clinic and Mayo Foundation* (Minneapolis: University of Minnesota Press, 1937), which gives comprehensive bio-bibliographies. For Mann's own publications, see Maurice B. Visscher, "Frank Charles Mann," *National Academy of Sciences:*

Biographical Memoirs (1963): 161–73; 38 (1965): 161–204; and Hiram E. Essex, "Dr. Frank C. Mann," *Physiologist* 6 (1963): 66–69. Mann's gastroenterological work is the subject of a special edition of *American Journal of Digestive Diseases* 5 (1960): 283–394. See also Frank C. Mann, James T. Priestley, J. Markowitz, and Wallace M. Yater, "Transplantation of the Intact Mammalian Heart," *Archives of Surgery* 26, no. 2 (1933): 219–24. This study arose out of a plan to study the pharmacological responses of the denervated heart.

90. C. Deederer, "Transplantation of the Kidney and the Ovary," *Journal of the American Medical Association* 70 (1918): 6–9, and *Surgery, Gynecology & Obstetrics* 31, 45–50. This work included early use of phenolsulfonphthalein (phenol red) as a kidney function test. Deederer moved afterward to the Jones Clinic nearby and to New York later, publishing an interesting essay on the practicalities of human kidney transplantation; see C. Dedera [sic], "Can a Life Be Saved by the Transplanting of an Organ?" *Medical Journal and Record*, Nov. 4, 1925. His memoirs are in his *Man the Known* (Miami: Deederer Publications, 1947).

91. C. S. Williamson, "Some Observations on the Length of Survival and Function of Homogeneous Kidney Transplants," *Journal of Urology* 10 (1923): 275–87; C. S. Williamson, "Further Studies on the Transplantation of the Kidney," *Journal of Urology* 16 (1926): 231–53. Williamson is best remembered for the Mann-Williamson experimental duodenal ulcer preparation in dogs. Williamson also published on the management of acute hepatic failure and on thoracic duct drainage methods.

92. "Function of the Autogenous Kidney Transplant," *American Journal of Medical Sciences* 171, no. 3 (1926): 407–19; Kenji Ibuka, "Function of the Homogenous Kidney Transplant," 420–32. Wu's PhD thesis was abridged and published as Patrick P. T. Wu and Frank C. Mann, "Histologic Studies of Autogenous and Homogenous Transplants of the Kidney," *Archives of Surgery* 28, no. 5 (May 1934): 889–908.

93. See L. Lux, G. M. Higgins, and Frank C. Mann, "Functional Homografts of the Rat Adrenal Gland Grown in Vitro," *Anatomical Record* 70 (1937): 29–43, 29.

94. The pioneer experimental liver transplanter C. Stuart Welch in 1955 acknowledged Mann's influence, and both noticed that the liver atrophied after porto-caval shunting.

95. L. G. Rowntree, "Stories of Rejuvenation by Grafting of Glands Merely Myth," *Northwestern Health Journal* 11 (1926): 6–7, 22–23. In the 1930s, he took a brief interest in solving the puzzle of the thymus gland's role.

96. Mann quoted in Sterioff and Rucker-Johnson, "Frank C. Mann and Transplantation at the Mayo Clinic," 1055.

97. Harvey B. Stone, James C. Owings, and George O. Gey, "Transplantation of Living Grafts of Thyroid and Parathyroid," *Annals of Surgery* 100, no. 4 (Oct. 1934): 613–28; the *New York Times* lauded this paper on December 11, 1933, and October 17, 1934. Gey was highly regarded at Johns Hopkins as a pioneer of tissue culture, and William P. Longmire Jr. trained in this unit, publishing with Stone into the early 1950s. Stone contributed on homografting to the Southern Medical Society until 1964; see J. D. Hardy, "Transplantation of Tissues and Organs: Review of the First 100 Years of the Southern Surgical Association," *Annals of Surgery* 207, no. 6 (June 1988): 776–87. Stone has some admirers, notably Thomas Starzl, as well as Clyde Barker, who found reduced immunological responses to parathyroid tissue in some situations; see A. Naji and Clyde F. Barker, "The Influence of Histocompatibility and Transplantation Site on Parathyroid Allograft Survival," *Journal of Surgical Research* 20 (1976): 261–67. Stone's presidential address on homografting to the American Surgical Association (see *Annals of Surgery* 115, no. 6 [June 1942]: 883–91) is worth reading since it accurately set a road map for the next decade. Finally, in some niche models, removal of passenger cells from grafts can reduce alternative pathway immunogenicity, but the strategy is not of general application.

98. This unusually careful study of endocrine grafting is Lydia Lux, George M. Higgins, and Frank C. Mann, "Functional Homeografts of the Rat Adrenal Gland Grown *in Vitro*," *Anatomical Record* 70, no. 1 (Dec. 1937): 29–43.

8. Progress in the 1930s

1. Kidney transplantation studies were continuing in Bucharest and were published in a Lyon journal; see Aurel Avramovici, "Les transplantations du rein (étude expérimentale)," *Lyon Chirurgical* 21 (1924): 734–57.

2. H. Velu, "État actuel de nos connaissances sur le greffe testiculaire," *Presse Médicale* 39 (1931): 1496; *Bulletin de l'Académie véterinaire Française* 4 (1931): 166–69. Velu is one of the neglected figures in early transplantation immunology. His impressive collected works are found in Henri Velu, *Vingt-cinq ans de recherches veterinaries au Maroc, 1913–1938: Titres et travaux scientifiques de Henri Velu* (Casablanca: Française, 1938).

3. See Professor Petit's critique in the discussion after Velu's *Bulletin* paper, cited above, p. 169.

4. Carl R. Moore, "The Physiologic Effects of Non-Living Testis Grafts," *Journal of the American Medical Association* 94, no. 24 (1930): 1912–15.

5. The events are fully described in David Hamilton, *The Monkey Gland Affair* (London: Chatto & Windus, 1986), 125–28. The American Medical Association continued throughout the 1930s to receive inquiries on the efficacy of Voronoff's and Brinkley's work, to which a standard letter critical of testis transplantation was sent in reply. For a good account of these times, see Jessica Jahiel, "Rejuvenation Research and the American Medical Association in the Early Twentieth Century: Paradigms in Conflict" (PhD diss., Boston University, 1992).

6. That Loeb's early supply of animals may not have been fully inbred, thus explaining his findings, has been briefly noted in Robert Good, "Runestones in Immunology," *Journal of Immunology* 117, no. 5 (Nov. 1, 1976): 1413–28; and in Leslie Brent, *A History of Transplantation Immunology* (San Diego: Academic Press, 1997), 63–65. However, both suggest that Loeb alone had bad luck, as if there were good and bad batches, rather than that *all* inbred rat supplies were defective at the time.

7. Incomplete genetic uniformity even with many generations of inbreeding was noted in at least one rat strain and analyzed in Donald Michie and Norman F. Anderson, "A Strong Selective Effect Associated with a Histocompatibility Gene in the Rat," *Annals of the New York Academy of Sciences* 129, no. 1 (1966): 88–93. They suggested that a natural elimination of "inbred" homozygote embryos in utero at each generation assisted species diversity.

8. Loeb's study of the unsatisfactory inbred mouse supplies came much later, well after publication of his *Physiological Reviews* paper. The data appear only in his book, *The Biological Basis of Individuality* (Springfield, IL: Thomas, 1945), 98–106.

9. Information from Muriel T. Davisson, director of genetic resources, Jackson Laboratory, Bar Harbor, ME.

10. On Evarts Graham, see Charles Barber Mueller, *Evarts A. Graham: The Life, Lives, and Times of the Surgical Spirit of St. Louis* (Hamilton, ON: BC Decker, 2002); and R. C. Brock, "Evarts A. Graham," *Annals of Thoracic Surgery* 9, no. 3 (Mar. 1970): 272–79. At Washington University, Carrel's former colleague C. C. Guthrie had been on the faculty since 1905 and would bring to the table not only his own views on organ grafting but also Carrel's.

11. Eric J. Stelnicki, V. Leroy Young, Tom Francel, and Peter Randall, "Vilray P. Blair, His Surgical Descendants, and Their Roles in Plastic Surgical Departments," *Plastic and Reconstructive Surgery* 103, no. 7 (1999): 1990–2009. For an overview of this specialty, see J. M. Converse, "Plastic Surgery: The Twentieth Century; The Period of Growth (1914–1939)," *Surgical Clinics of North America* 47, no. 2 (Apr. 1967): 261–78.

12. The celebrated St. Louis group of skin grafters is described in Bradford Cannon, Joseph E. Murray, and Elvin G. Zook, "The Influence of the St. Louis Quadrumvirate on Plastic Surgery," *Plastic and Reconstructive Surgery* 95, no. 6 (1995): 1118–22. See also Bradford Cannon, *James Barrett Brown: Biography* (St. Louis, 1967). Barrett Brown was at Washington University, graduating in 1923, and thus was one of Leo Loeb's students. Blair and Brown re-established routine "split thickness" skin grafting in 1929, and Brown succeeded Blair as chief of plastic surgery in the 1930s. Brown was in Britain during World War II; see chap. 9.

13. D. Robison, *Earl Calvin Padgett: Biography* (St. Louis, 1990).

14. Padgett's memoir, *Skin Grafting: From a Personal and Experimental Viewpoint* (Springfield, IL: Thomas, 1942), acknowledges Loeb's influence throughout. For confirmation of Padgett's high opinion of Loeb's book, see Kathryn L. Stephenson, "As I Remember: Earl C. Padgett," *Annals of Plastic Surgery* 6, no. 2 (Feb. 1981): 142–57. Stephenson, one of the first female plastic surgeons, coauthored *Plastic and Reconstructive Surgery* with Padgett in 1948. The Padgett-Hood dermatome is still manufactured in Kansas City.

15. Earl C. Padgett, "Is Iso-Skin Grafting Practicable?" *Southern Medical Journal* 25, no. 9 (Sept. 1932): 895–900; his discussion relies heavily on Loeb's teachings.

16. "Beating the bushes" is amusingly described in Stephenson, "As I Remember."

17. This important information on Snell was found by Carole Prietto, archivist at Washington University, St. Louis. Following this St. Louis academic post, Snell was unemployed for a while and moved around Texas offering flying lessons. He might well have encountered tales of Brinkley's rural Midwest gland-graft activities.

18. See the note in *American Review of Soviet Medicine* 5 (1947–1948): 127.

19. S. S. Yudin, "Transfusion of Cadaver Blood," *Journal of the American Medical Association* 106, no. 12 (Mar. 21, 1936): 997–99. Yudin made every effort to have his work known in the West, which led to political difficulties later, as detailed in H. Swan, "S. S. Yudin: A Study in Frustration," *Surgery* 58 (Sept. 1965): 572–85. For the Soviet use of cadaveric blood, see V. P. Filatov, "The History of Blood Transfusions: Soviet Contribution," *Bulletin de la Société Internationale de Chirurgie* 14 (1955): 257–65; and H. Swan and D. C. Schechter, "The Transfusion of Blood from Cadavers: A Historical Review," *Surgery* 52 (Sept. 1962): 545–60.

20. Swan and Schechter, "Transfusion of Blood from Cadavers," 548.

21. Shamov's career is described in G. G. Karavanov and N. N. Oborin, "K istorii razvitiia metoda perelivaniia krovi na Ukraine (vklad V. N. Shamova i ego shkoly)" [History of the development of the method of blood transfusion in Ukraine (contribution of V. N. Shamov and his school)], *Klinicheskaia Khirurgiia* 12 (Dec. 1973): 56–62.

22. Later, in 1955, Vladimir Demikhov set up an organ transplant laboratory at the Sklifosovskiy Emergency Research Institute. (The institute's name has been transliterated in various ways.)

23. The vitality of orthodox Soviet immunology at this time is described in T. I. Ulyankina, "Origin and Development of Immunology in Russia," *Cellular Immunology* 126, no. 1 (Mar. 1990): 227–32.

24. This thorough and visionary paper was published as Ü. Woronoy, "Die Immunität bei Organtransplantation. I: Mitteilung: Über spezifische komplementbindende Antikörper bei freier Transplantation der Testes," *Archiv für Klinische Chirurgie* 171 (1932): 361–85. It was common for Soviet scientists to publish in German journals at the time. The variant on Voronoy's name here may have ensured bibliographi-

cal burial for this crucial paper. In the text, Voronoy describes making soluble extracts of kidney to inject into dogs; the serum from these immunized animals gave a positive Bordet-Gengou reaction when tested against the kidney antigens.

25. Yu. Yu. Voronoy, "Sobre el bloqueo del aparato réticuloendotelial del hombre en algunas formas de intoxicación por el sublimado y sobre la transplantación del riñón cadavérico como método tratamiento de la anuria consecutiva aquella intoxicación" [On the blockage of the reticulo-endothelial system in some kinds of corrosive sublimate poisoning and the transplantation of the kidney from the cadaver as a method of treatment of that anuria] *El Siglo Médico* 97 (1936): 296–97. Biographical information on Emilio de la Peña, the translator, was kindly supplied by Professor J. Ortuña of Madrid. Peña was a Madrid urologist who traveled to the innovative centers in the Soviet Union and maintained the resulting professional links. An English translation by Ronald G. Landes is in Toni Hau, *Renal Transplantation* (Austin, TX: Silvergirl, 1987), 24–25. For an account of Voronoy and his work, see David Hamilton and W. A. Reid, "Yu. Yu. Voronoy and the First Human Kidney Allograft," *Surgery, Gynecology & Obstetrics* 159, no. 3 (Sept. 1984): 289–94. The hard-to-find original Russian paper of 1934 appeared in full in M. B. Mirskii, "Sovetskii khirurg Iu. Iu. Voronoi—pioner allotransplantatsii trupnoi pochki v klinike" [The Soviet surgeon Iu. Iu. Voronoi—a pioneer of allotransplantation in the clinic], *Klinicheskaia Khirurgii* 5 (May 1973): 76–81.

26. Up to this time, there were three rival nomenclatures in use for blood types: Landsteiner's ABO terminology and the terminologies of Jansky and Moss, which both used Roman numerals. The ABO terminology was accepted as the standard by the League of Nations in 1930.

27. The English translation of the Spanish-language version of the paper appearing in Hau, *Renal Transplantation*, 24–25, confusingly states first that Group C blood was used for the new transfusion and then later indicates that it was Group A blood.

28. Quoted in Reid and Hamilton, "Yu. Yu. Voronoy and the First Human Kidney Allograft," translation by W. A. Reid.

29. The early human kidney transplants in Paris and Boston in the 1950s, and even later, broke the classical "rules" of blood grouping, not necessarily with disastrous results. Both Hume and Starzl transplanted blood type B kidneys into type O or A recipients in

early cases, without immediate reaction; see Guy P. J. Alexandre, Dominique Latinne, Marianne Carlier, Maurice Moriau, Yves Pirson, Pierre Gianello, and Jean Paul Squifflet, "ABO-Incompatibility and Organ Transplantation," *Transplantation Reviews* 5 (1991): 230–41.

30. Ironically, a variant on "reverse incompatibility" did emerge much later, when Starzl showed that in blood-type mismatched human liver grafting, antihost antibodies appeared briefly, doubtless made by graft cells. See G. Ramsey, J. Nusbacher, Thomas E. Starzl, et al., "Isohemagglutinins of Graft Origin after ABO-Unmatched Liver Transplantation," *New England Journal of Medicine* 311, no. 18 (Nov. 1, 1984): 1167–70.

31. Samuel W. Lambert, "The Vagaries of a Vivisectionist Turned Clinical Surgeon and the Story of the Lady Who Lay with a Pig for Five Nights and Five Days on Professional Advice," *Proceedings of the Charaka Club* 9 (1938): 38–43. The case might have referred to a 1932 attempt using a sheep kidney at Bellevue Hospital. Samuel Lambert, dean of New York's College of Physicians and Surgeons, was a prominent contributor to the club's publications.

32. See Carrel's uninspired contribution, "The Physiological Substratum of Malignancy," in *Contributions to the Medical Sciences: In Honor of Dr. Emanuel Libman* (New York: International Press, 1932), 289–95.

33. Carrel's oversubscribed public lecture in New York was noted in *New York Herald Tribune,* December 14, 1935. His book *Man the Unknown* had fifty reprints and editions and many translations; the last known reprinting was the Spanish edition of 1953. Some sentiments in the book prompted allegations of Nazi collaboration when he later settled in occupied Paris.

34. Paul Henry de Kruif, *The Sweeping Wind: A Memoir* (New York: Harcourt, Brace & World, 1962), 22.

35. See A. Carrel and C. A. Lindbergh, *The Culture of Organs* (New York: Hoeber, 1938), as well as David M. Friedman's flawed account, *The Immortalists: Charles Lindbergh, Dr. Alexis Carrel and Their Daring Quest to Live Forever* (New York: Ecco, 2007).

9. Understanding the Mechanism

1. Thomas Gibson and Peter B. Medawar, "The Fate of Skin Homografts in Man," *Journal of Anatomy* 77 (July 1943): 299–310; see also Peter Medawar, *Memoir of a Thinking Radish* (Oxford: Oxford University Press, 1986). Medawar's version of some events has been added to, and modified, by R. E. Billingham,

Of the perfusion experiments, E. N. Willmer's text, *Cells and Tissues in Culture: Methods, Biology and Physiology* (London: Academic Press, 1965), cautiously reported that "as no one has been able to obtain any similar results, this claim must be discounted." After consulting Lindbergh, Theodore I. Malinin built a similar perfusion machine in the 1960s and claimed some success; see Malinin, *Surgery and Life: The Extraordinary Career of Alexis Carrel* (New York: Harcourt Brace Jovanovich, 1979). For the chicken heart cell debacle, see Jan A. Witkowski, "Dr. Carrel's Immortal Cells," *Medical History* 24, no. 2 (Apr. 1980): 129–42.

36. For an excellent review of early perfusion machines, see H.-G. Zimmer, "Perfusion of Isolated Organs and the First Heart-Lung Machine," *Canadian Journal of Cardiology* 17, no. 9 (Sept. 2001): 963–69. Zimmer was unimpressed with the Carrel/Lindbergh device. See also Friedman, *Immortalists*.

37. A. N. Richards and Cecil K. Drinker, "An Apparatus for the Perfusion of Isolated Organs," *Journal of Pharmacology and Experimental Therapeutics* 7 (1915): 467–83.

38. Carrel quoted in Bob Johnson, "Kidney Preservation by Continuous Perfusion," in *Organ Preservation: Basic and Applied Aspects*, ed. David E. Pegg, Ib Abildgaard Jacobsen, and N. A. Halasz (Lancaster, England: MTP Press, 1982), 215.

39. Padgett was first with a twin skin exchange in 1932, reported as E. C. Padgett, "Is Iso-Skin Grafting Practicable?" *Southern Medical Journal* 25, no. 9 (Sept. 1932): 895–900; it was followed by J. B. Brown, "Homografting of Skin: With Report of Success in Identical Twins," *Surgery* 1 (1937): 558–63.

40. Although much legal comment continues on the landmark *Bonner v. Moran* case, details of the operation are scanty. The operation itself was not condemned, the surgical issues being secondary to the considerations on informed consent; see *Bonner v. Moran*, 126 F.2d 121, 75 U.S. App. D.C. 156; and Russell Scott, *The Body as Property* (New York: Viking, 1981), 101–4.

"Reminiscences of a 'Transplanter,'" *Transplantation Proceedings* 6, no. 4 (Dec. 1974): supplement 1, 5–17, which marked an early use of this job title.

2. Florey's early interest in the lymphocyte is found in Gwyn Macfarlane, *Howard Florey: The Mak-*

ing of a Great Scientist (Oxford: Oxford University Press, 1979), 266. Much of the mystery surrounding the lymphocyte was solved later, at Oxford, by Jim Gowans and Avrion Mitchison in the 1950s.

3. It was during a session of this difficult rat surgery that Ernst Chain, for the fourth time, approached Florey with yet another request that Florey test Chain's first supply of penicillin for toxicity in mice. Irritated at the interruption, Florey rebuked Chain, who then enlisted John Barnes to do the famous, negative toxicity testing of penicillin, again to Florey's annoyance; see Trevor I. Williams, *Howard Florey: Penicillin and After* (Oxford: Oxford University Press, 1984), 106.

4. When Medawar later in life suffered a stroke, he ruefully suggested that he might have been better off persisting with this early interest in nerve regeneration.

5. Medawar, as quoted in Peter J. Morris, *Kidney Transplantation: Principles and Practice* (London: Academic Press, 1979), viii. Medawar generally disliked anecdotes, and his use of this one suggests the importance of the incident to him.

6. P. Hupkens, H. Boxma, and J. Dokter, "Tannic Acid as a Topical Agent in Burns: Historical Considerations and Implications for New Developments," *Burns: Journal of the International Society for Burn Injuries* 21, no. 1 (Feb. 1995): 57–61.

7. For the tannic acid report, see War Wounds Committee, FD1/6300, Medical Research Council Archives, UK Public Record Office, London (hereafter, MRC Archives).

8. On Colebrook, see E. J. L. Lowbury, "Leonard Colebrook (1883–1967)," *British Medical Journal* 287, no. 6409 (1983): 1981–83; *Biographical Memoirs of Fellows of the Royal Society* 71 (1971): 91–138; and William C. Noble, *Coli, Great Healer of Men: The Biography of Dr. Leonard Colebrook* (London: Heinemann Medical, 1974). Colebrook's papers, including his Glasgow notebooks, are held at the Wellcome Library, Contemporary Medical Archives Centre, CMAC No. 465, PP/COL, London.

9. During World War I, Gillies was an advisor on surgery to the Ministry of Health, but his biography gives little detail on these events; see Reginald Pound, *Gillies, Surgeon Extraordinary* (London: M. Joseph, 1964).

10. Personal communication from the late Tom Gibson.

11. McIndoe had been appointed civilian consultant in plastic surgery to the Royal Air Force in 1938; see Leonard Mosley, *Faces from the Fire: The Biography of Sir Archibald McIndoe* (London: Weidenfeld and Nicolson, 1962); and Hugh McLeave, *McIndoe: Plastic Surgeon* (London: Muller, 1961). The pilots undergoing long-term facial reconstructions indulged in black humor, including forming the "Guinea Pig Club." The East Grinstead hospital thereafter had a tradition of transplantation research, and pioneering corneal transplant work was done there; see Ernest J. Dennison, *A Cottage Hospital Grows Up: The Story of the Queen Victoria Hospital, East Grinstead* (London: Blond, 1963).

12. The linking of Medawar and Colebrook is described by his widow; see Vera Colebrook, "Leonard Colebrook: Reminiscences on the Occasion of the 25th Anniversary of the Birmingham Burns Units," *Injury* 2, no. 3 (1971): 182–84.

13. Peter B. Medawar, "Sheets of Pure Epidermal Epithelium from Human Skin," *Nature* 148, no. 783 (Dec. 27, 1941): 783. Medawar used trypsin before its important introduction into tissue culture.

14. Brown was featured in a radio play dealing with military plastic surgery; see Arthur Miller, "Lips for the Trumpet," *Medical Heritage* 1, no. 6 (1985): 414–20. See also Joseph Murray, "Reminiscences on Renal Transplantation," in *Organ Transplantation*, ed. Satya N. Chatterjee (Boston: Wright, 1982), 1–13. In Europe, Brown was a "tent mate" of Loyal Davis, later editor of *Surgery, Gynecology & Obstetrics*. Davis supported the early organ transplant efforts and was the father of Nancy Reagan, who, while in the White House, gave personal support to donor procurement schemes.

15. Autobiographical notes are found in John Marquis Converse, "Experimental Human Skin Allografts, the HLA Complex, and a Nobel Prize," *Plastic and Reconstructive Surgery* 70, no. 2 (Aug. 1982): 255–62. On Converse, see Blair O. Rogers, "John Marquis Converse, 1909–1981," *Annals of Plastic Surgery* 8, no. 4 (Apr. 1982): 342–58; and Frank McDowell, "Plastic Surgery in the Twentieth Century," *Annals of Plastic Surgery* 1, no. 2 (1978): 217–24. Converse later obtained a major grant for transplantation research from the U.S. Atomic Energy Commission in 1950. His five-volume text, *Reconstructive Plastic Surgery: Principles and Procedures in Correction, Reconstruction and Transplantation*, was first published in 1964. Material on Converse is held in the archives of the American Society of Plastic and Reconstructive Surgeons, held in Harvard University's Countway Library, Boston.

16. See W. H. Reid, "Reflecting on 35 Years at the Glasgow Burns Unit," *Burns* 25, no. 1 (Feb. 1999): 57–61. The Edinburgh Burns Unit was older; see D. C. Simpson and A. B. Wallace, "Edinburgh's First Burn Hospital," *Journal of the Royal College of Surgeons of Edinburgh* 2, no. 2 (Dec. 1956): 134–43.

17. A simple but important observation on the bacterial flora of burns is in Robert Cruikshank, "The Bacterial Infection of Burns," *Journal of Pathology and Bacteriology* 41, no. 2 (1935): 367–69.

18. For Clark's obituary, see *British Medical Journal* 1, no. 4863 (March 20, 1954): 707.

19. Curiously, Sir Charles Illingworth, though a highly successful head of department, later failed to see the potential of organ transplantation and, like many other surgeons in the 1960s, was hostile to the early attempts, both experimental and human. However, Tom Gibson was later invited to rejoin Illingworth's department, when both were quite senior.

20. From Thomas Gibson, "The 'Second Set' Phenomenon as First Shown in Skin Allografts: An Historical Case Which Shows Also the Behaviour of Cell Free Collagen," *British Journal of Plastic Surgery* 39, no. 1 (Jan. 1986): 96–102, 96.

21. Colebrook eventually devised the "Glasgow" sulfanilamide-base CTAB No. 9 cream, which was widely used thereafter by the British military and copied for the U.S. Army, at James Barrett Brown's suggestion. Colebrook also drew up the much-needed first aid advice that then appeared in the military manuals.

22. Gibson was a keen photographer and helped make this film on the treatment of burns funded by the Medical Research Council. No copies exist, perhaps because other films in the series had scenes of drug experiments on army volunteers.

23. Gibson, "'Second Set' Phenomenon as First Shown in Skin Allografts."

24. Gillies to Drury, July 14, 1942, FD1/6493, MRC Archives. Wartime secrecy has hidden the details of the episode resulting in the "Aberdeen convoy of severe cases," but forty-one seriously burned survivors of an incident reached Stracathro Hospital, south of Aberdeen, for further treatment and convalescence, having probably been "tanned" in Aberdeen first.

25. James Barrett Brown's textbook, coauthored with Frank McDowell, *Skin Grafting of Burns* (Philadelphia: Lippincott, 1943), mentions many of the Glasgow medical men he met.

26. A. N. Drury, secretary, MRC, to Colebrook, Apr. 26, 1942, FD1/6493, MRC Archives.

27. Colebrook diary, A.8 May 1942, Colebrook Papers, CMAC, Wellcome Library.

28. Some accounts suggest instead that Colebrook took the initiative and brought Medawar reluctantly to Glasgow, but the tone and wording of Medawar's letters to the MRC run counter to this claim.

29. Blacklock, the pathologist, was reluctant to help Medawar because of wartime staff shortages. Though this lack of support for Medawar's histological work seems regrettable, throughout his later career Medawar insisted on doing much of his own technical work, to avoid others' errors. Blacklock's attitude ultimately denied him some long-lasting fame, since in the alphabetical listing of authors commonly used then, the famous paper that resulted from Medawar's research in Glasgow would instead have been Blacklock, Gibson, and Medawar. Alfred Clark, the visiting senior surgeon who proved unhelpful to the research effort, also missed a prominent place in the transplantation citation pantheon, because, had he taken part, he would have been first or second author.

30. The July 2 conference agenda is found in FD1/6492, MRC Archives.

31. The female burn victim is easily identified as case No. 31 in the group of plasma-transfused patients described in the Glasgow Burns Unit's report: *Studies of Burns and Scalds: Reports of Burns Unit, Royal Infirmary, Glasgow, 1942–43*, Medical Research Council Special Report Series 249 (London: His Majesty's Stationery Office, 1944).

32. Felix Rapaport showed later that such prolonged skin graft survival was possible between fully matched siblings; under those circumstances, grafts lasted for twenty-two to twenty-five days.

33. Gibson and Medawar, "Fate of Skin Homografts in Man," 376.

34. Gibson, "'Second Set' Phenomenon as First Shown in Skin Allografts," 98. Medawar, in a letter to the MRC on September 6, 1942 (FD1/6492, MRC Archives), commented on some "immunological evidence" Gibson obtained. This letter thus dates Gibson's serology work to the time of Medawar's visit or shortly after.

35. Leonard Colebrook, *A New Approach to the Treatment of Burns and Scalds* (London: Fine Technical Publications, 1950). Publication of this book was

stimulated by the possibility of mass casualties from nuclear war.

36. Medawar reported on his visit: Medawar to the MRC, September 6, 1942, FD1/6492, MRC Archives.

37. In a 1944 paper (Peter B. Medawar, "The Behaviour and Fate of Skin Autografts and Skin Homografts in Rabbits," *Journal of Anatomy* 78 (Oct. 1944): 176–99), Medawar goes further and graciously credits a personal communication from Gibson in 1942 as the origin of the crucial acquired active immunity hypothesis in their 1943 paper, "The Fate of Skin Homografts in Man." Gibson is the first author, but this lacks significance since the style of the day was to list authors alphabetically.

38. The head of the Department of Anatomy was George Wyburn, and his department had taken an early interest in the subject of cartilage, bone, and corneal grafting; see J. Wyburn and P. Bacsich, "The Grafting of Animal Tissues," *Endeavour* 7 (1948): 165–69; and J. Hutchison, "The Fate of Experimental Autografts and Homografts," *British Journal of Surgery* 39, no. 158 (May 1952): 552–61.

39. R. J. Scothorne and Ian A. McGregor, "Cellular Changes in Lymph Nodes and Spleen Following Skin Homografting in Rabbits," *Journal of Anatomy* 89 (1955): 283–92. Interestingly, Medawar had also looked at lymph node responses to nearby homografts but later confessed (to the author of this book) that he could make no sense of the changes seen until Scothorne and McGregor solved the puzzle. Much later, when interest revived, Gibson wrote a series of important papers on the history of skin transplantation.

40. Medawar's work on regeneration appeared in 1942 in the *Journal of Anatomy* as papers coauthored with J. Z. Young, E. Guttmann, and Ludwig Guttmann, the last being the recognized authority on spinal cord injuries. In moving into the study of homograft behavior, Medawar's commitment was so great that he joined the worthy band of those who failed to write up their PhD theses and moved on to other projects.

41. Peter B. Medawar, "Notes on the Problem of Skin Homografts," *Bulletin of War Medicine* 4 (1943): 1–4. The word *anaphylaxis* was still used at that time as a broad term for the various forms of immune responses.

42. This account of the controversies was assisted by an unpublished manuscript written by the late Ian McGregor, submitted to the *Lancet* shortly before his death, and sent for peer review to Tom Starzl. Mc-

Gregor was a plastic surgeon in Glasgow and a pupil of Tom Gibson. See Ian A. McGregor and R. Watson, "History of the West of Scotland Plastic Surgery Unit: 1940–1986," *British Journal of Plastic Surgery* 51, no. 5 (July 1998): 333–42. See also Ian A. McGregor, "Thomas Gibson's Contribution to Immunology," *Plastic and Reconstructive Surgery* 71, no. 3 (1983): 440. Brown's supporters point to what might have been said at a conference presentation promptly published in June 1942 as James Barrett Brown and Frank McDowell, "Epithelial Healing and the Transplantation of Skin," *Annals of Surgery* 115, no. 6 (Jun. 1942): 1166–81. In any case, the "second set" probe was not new; it was an insight whose time had come.

43. For Medawar's antireductionism, see David Hamilton, "Peter Medawar and Clinical Transplantation," *Immunology Letters* 21, no. 1 (1989): 9–13. See also Gwyn Macfarlane, *Alexander Fleming: The Man and the Myth* (London: Chatto & Windus, 1984), 59, 270. It is possible that this was the mood in Oxford, since Fleming in London had given up work on penicillin twelve years earlier, being discouraged, among other things, by penicillin's lack of effectiveness in his test tube model. It came as a surprise when at Oxford, in 1941, Florey showed a powerful effect of penicillin to protect the *whole* animal from infection.

44. Leslie Brent, *A History of Transplantation Immunology* (San Diego: Academic Press, 1997), 156, notes that even in their classic 1956 paper on tolerance, Medawar's group stated that tolerance was effected through deletion of "antibody-forming cells."

45. Medawar, "Behaviour and Fate of Skin Autografts and Skin Homografts in Rabbits"; Peter B. Medawar, "A Second Study of the Behaviour and Fate of Skin Homografts in Rabbits," *Journal of Anatomy* 79 (1945): 157–76.

46. Peter B. Medawar, "Tests by Tissue Culture Methods on the Nature of Immunity to Transplanted Skin," *Quarterly Journal of Microscopical Science* 89 (Sept. 1948): 239–52, 252. He may have been fortunate in this analysis, since free antibody is quickly neutralized by such tissue. In Birmingham, Medawar's new interest was an old puzzle, one also of interest to Leo Loeb, namely skin pigment migration, and this interest led to a flirtation with transferable, inheritable "plasmagenes."

47. Avrion Mitchison's D.Phil. thesis announcing the cellular mechanism of homograft rejection had a cool reception from Peter Gorer, the serologist who was the external examiner.

48. Medawar report to the MRC, FD1/696D, MRC Archives.

49. The word *rejection* was used by some speakers at the Second Transplantation Conference, in 1956; see *Annals of the New York Academy of Sciences* 64 (1957): 735. Interestingly, Emile Holman used the word *rejection* occasionally in his 1924 paper (E. Holman, "Protein Sensitization in Iso-Skin Grafting: Is the Latter of Practical Value?" *Surgery, Gynecology & Obstetrics* 38 [1924]: 100–106), and the word is used throughout David Hume's classic 1953 paper on human kidney transplantation.

50. His major review is Blair O. Rogers, "Guide and Bibliography for Research into the Skin Homograft Problem," *Plastic and Reconstructive Surgery* 7, no. 3 (Mar. 1951): 169–201, which has 429 references; see also Blair O. Rogers, "The Problem of Skin Homografts," *Plastic and Reconstructive Surgery* 5, no. 4 (Apr. 1950): 269–82. Rogers was still a student when Jerome P. Webster (the plastic surgeon, bibliophile, and historian) suggested that he start on this bibliography of transplantation studies.

51. A thorough review of the medical care after this disaster is found in *Annals of Surgery* 117 (1943): 801–965, later published as *Management of the Cocoanut Grove Burns at the Massachusetts General Hospital* (Philadelphia: Lippincott, 1943).

52. The Cocoanut Grove fire and its consequences are described in Francis "Franny" Moore's autobiography, *A Miracle and a Privilege: Recounting a Half Century of Surgical Advance* (Washington, DC: Joseph Henry Press, 1995).

53. W. P. Longmire and S. W. Smith, "Homologous Transplantation of Tissues: A Review of the Literature," *Archives of Surgery* 62, no. 3 (Mar. 1951): 443–54. See also William P. Longmire Jr., *Starting from Scratch: The Early History of the UCLA Department of Surgery* (Pasadena, CA: Castle Press, 1984).

54. For the continuing low-key transplantation interest at Johns Hopkins, see W. P. Longmire, H. B. Stone, A. S. Daniel, and C. D. Goon, "Report of Clinical Experience with Homografts," *Plastic and Reconstructive Surgery* 2, no. 5 (Sept. 1947): 419–26. This paper denied that human homografts survived permanently. For Stone's unhelpful earlier views, see Harvey B. Stone, James C. Owings, and George O. Gey, "Transplantation of Living Grafts of Thyroid and Parathyroid," *Annals of Surgery* 100, no. 4 (Oct. 1934): 613–28.

55. A. McIndoe, and A. Franceschetti, "Reciprocal Skin Homografts in a Medico-Legal Case of Exchanged Identical Twins," *British Journal of Plastic Surgery* 2, no. 4 (Jan. 1950): 283–89.

56. Naomi Mitchison (died 1998) was the sister of J. B. S. Haldane and mother of Avrion Mitchison.

57. See P. J. Gaillard, "Transplantation of Cultivated Parathyroid Gland Tissue in Man," in *Preservation and Transplantation of Normal Tissues,* ed. Gordon E. W. Wolstenholme and Margaret P. Cameron (London, 1954).

58. See Alan S. Parkes, *Off-Beat Biologist: The Autobiography of Alan S. Parkes* (Cambridge: Galton Foundation, 1985), 152. Parkes probably innocently used "pen-bred," that is, partly inbred rats, with all the genetic pitfalls.

59. Some claims for successful human skin homografting continued to appear in the literature until 1949; see John Edward Kearns and Stephen E. Reid, "Successful Homotransplantation of Skin from Parents to Son," *Plastic and Reconstructive Surgery* 4, no. 6 (Nov. 1949): 502–7. Ovary graft survival within corneal "wraps" was described by Castellanos and Sturgis at Harvard, and they later used millipore chambers. For reports of successful pituitary gland grafting in 1951, see note 69.

60. The second-last claim for successful human gland homografting without immunosuppression was Herbert Conway, William F. Nickel, and James W. Smith, "Homotransplantation of Thyroid and Parathyroid Glands by Vascular Anastomoses," *Plastic and Reconstructive Surgery* 23 (May 1959): 469–79. Conway, a plastic surgeon, was an editor of this journal, and at this point was no longer part of mainstream transplantation efforts. For the final surgical verdict on this issue, see Stanley W. Jacob and J. Englebert Dunphy, "'Successful' Parathyroid Transplantation: A Review of the Literature," *American Journal of Surgery* 105, no. 2 (Feb. 1963): 196–204.

61. John R. Brooks, in his book *Endocrine Tissue Transplantation* (Springfield, IL: Thomas, 1962), firmly dismissed all claims for survival of non-immunosuppressed endocrine gland grafts. Brooks's own work was on experimental pancreatic transplantation.

62. See Arthur J. Birch, "Steroid Hormones and the Luftwaffe: A Venture into Fundamental Strategic Research and Some of Its Consequences: The Birch Reduction Becomes a Birth Reduction," *Steroids* 57, no. 8 (Aug. 1992): 363–77; Nicolas Rasmussen, "Steroids in Arms: Science, Government, Industry, and the Hor-

mones of the Adrenal Cortex in the United States, 1930–1950," *Medical History* 46, no. 3 (July 2002): 299–324; and "Die deutsche Luftwaffe und das Cortison," in *Sternstunden der Medizin: Eine Dokumentation der herausragenden Fortschritte seit 1945*, ed. Max Conradt (Reinbek: Einhorn-Presse, 1997).

63. H. F. Polley and C. H. Slocumb, "Behind the Scenes with Cortisone and ACTH," *Mayo Clinic Proceedings* 51, no. 8 (1976): 471–77. The earlier events are found in Edward C. Kendall's memoir, *Cortisone* (New York: Scribner, 1971).

64. G. Hetenyi Jr. and J. Karsh, "Cortisone Therapy: A Challenge to Academic Medicine in 1949–1952," *Perspectives in Biology and Medicine* 40, no. 3 (spring 1997): 426–39.

65. David Cantor, "Cortisone and the Politics of Drama," in *Medical Innovations in Historical Perspective,* ed. John V. Pickstone (New York: St. Martin's Press, 1992), 163–84.

66. Cortisone file, FD 1/633, MRC Archives. The arrangement by the Merck Company with British representatives was reached over dinner at the Athenaeum club in London, and it was agreed to keep the plan secret. This lack of transparency was possible in the immediate postwar period.

67. "Prolonged Treatment with Cortisone and A.C.T.H.," *British Medical Journal* 1, no. 4873 (May 29, 1954): 1249–50. The cool official attitude to cortisone is obvious in the editorial.

68. John H. Glyn, "The Discovery of Cortisone: A Personal View," *British Medical Journal* 317, no. 7161 (1998): 822.

69. M. James Whitelaw, "Physiological Reaction to Pituitary Adrenocorticotropic Hormone (ACTH) in Severe Burns," *Journal of American Medical Association* 145, no. 2 (Jan. 13, 1951): 85–88. The claims for antihistamines were made by D. G. Foster and E. M. Hanrahan, "Observations on a Skin Homograft after 60 Days of Pyribenzamine Therapy," *Bulletin of the Johns Hopkins Hospital* 82 (1948): 501–2: white skin to a black recipient was used. The success of ACTH and cortisone therapy in rheumatoid arthritis led to dreary claims for similar success using pituitary gland grafts; see Gunnar Edström and Stig Thune, "Further Investigations of Pituitary Gland Implantation in Rheumatoid Arthritis," *Annals of Rheumatic Diseases* 10, no. 2 (June 1951): 163–70.

70. Frederick G. Germuth Jr. and Barbara Ottinger, "Effect of 17-hydroxy-11-dehydrocorticosterone (Com-

pound E) and of ACTH on Arthus Reaction and Antibody Formation in the Rabbit," *Proceedings of the Society for Experimental Biology and Medicine* 74, no. 4 (Aug. 1950): 815–23.

71. J. A. Morgan, "The Influence of Cortisone on the Survival of Homografts of Skin in the Rabbit," *Surgery* 30, no. 3 (1951): 506–15. For a reduction in the effect on the tuberculin response, see S. Harris and T. N. Harris, "Effect of Cortisone on Some Reactions of Hypersensitivity in Laboratory Animals," *Proceedings of the Society for Experimental Biology and Medicine* 74, no. 1 (May 1950): 186–89.

72. Helene Wallace Toolan, "The Possible Role of Cortisone in Overcoming Resistance to the Growth of Human Tissues in Heterologous Hosts," *Annals of the New York Academy of Sciences* 59, no. 3 (1955): 394–400.

73. Longmire used newly hatched chickens because he found that the host homograft reaction was weak in the first few days, with some prolonged spontaneous graft survivals. The chicks were thus a sensitive test ground for any agent influencing graft survival. The historic paper from the "chicken lab," soon reanalyzed in terms of tolerance induction, is Jack A. Cannon and William P. Longmire, "Studies of Successful Skin Homografts in the Chicken," *Annals of Surgery* 135, no. 1 (Jan. 1952): 60–68. For regrafting from the same donor chicken, see Robert A. Weber, Jack A. Cannon, and William P. Longmire Jr., "Observations on the Regrafting of Successful Homografts in Chickens," *Annals of Surgery* 139, no. 4 (Apr. 1954): 473–77. For Cannon's varied career and Terasaki's involvement, see Longmire, *Starting from Scratch.*

74. Cannon and Longmire, "Studies of Successful Skin Homografts in the Chicken," 68.

75. R. E. Billingham, P. L. Krohn, and Peter B. Medawar, "Effect of Cortisone on Survival of Skin Homografts in Rabbits," *British Medical Journal* 1, no. 4716 (May 26, 1951): 1157–58. The dose used was a commendably high one, equivalent to three hundred milligrams of cortisone daily for human patients.

76. Peter B. Medawar and Elizabeth M. Sparrow, "The Effects of Adrenocortical Hormones, Adrenocorticotrophic Hormone and Pregnancy on Skin Transplantation Immunity in Mice," *Journal of Endocrinology* 14, no. 3 (Nov. 1956): 240–56.

77. In clinical work, combinations of two drugs, even triple regimens, have given other successes, notably in the treatment of tuberculosis, hepatitis, and AIDS

and to prevent organ rejection after transplantation. Laboratory research attitudes favor the study of single agents, to give analytical simplicity, and thus synergies are seldom sought.

10. Experimental Organ Transplantation

1. Jean Hamburger, "Note préliminaire sur les greffes rénales," *Journal d'Urologie Médicale et Chirurgicale* 53 (1947): 563–67. Charles Dubost assisted in this work and in 1951 was the first to attempt aortic aneurysm replacement by a human homograft.

2. J. Oudot, "Transplantation rénale," *Presse Médicale* 56 (1948): 319. Oudot, also a pioneer in aortic reconstruction, had published from 1947 to 1951 on surgical methods of dealing with human renal artery abnormalities, notably resulting in hypertension. He was also surgeon to the Mount Annapurna expedition in the Himalayas.

3. For an overview of this and other French contributions, see M. Meradier, "Contribution française à l'essor de nouvelles disciplines chirurgicales," *Bulletin de l'Académie Nationale de Médecine* 180, no. 1 (Jan. 1996): 13–31. This period can be seen as part of a belle époque in French science and cultural life in the immediate postwar period. Innovation in vascular and transplant surgery was prominent and hearkened back to the era of Lyon dominance via René Leriche and Alexis Carrel.

4. Morten Simonsen and F. Sørensen, "Homoplastic Kidney Transplantation in Dogs," *Acta Chirurgica Scandinavica* 99, no. 1 (Oct. 31, 1949): 61–72, quotes at 54 and 69; Morten Simonsen, "Biological Incompatibility in Kidney Transplantation in Dogs: I. Experimental and Morphological Investigations," and "Biological Incompatibility in Kidney Transplantation in Dogs: II. Serological Investigations," both in *Acta Pathologica et Microbiologica Scandinavica* 32, no. 1 (July 1953): 1–35 and 35–84, respectively. Simonsen, like Medawar and Mitchison, seemed unaware of Peter Gorer's patient work from 1936 on the antibodies arising from tumor grafts in mice, which he concluded were a response to the normal tissue antigens of the graft.

5. Simonsen's announcement of the graft-versus-host response came in 1957, but his standard popliteal lymph node assay did not evolve until 1970; see Morten Simonsen, "The Early Days of the Two-Way Paradigm for the Allograft Reaction," *Transplantation Proceedings* 27, no. 1 (1995): 18–21. Sir Roy Calne and Ken Porter later used labeled cells to show conclusively that the lymphoid cells in a rejecting kidney came from the host. Simonsen's reaction to the discovery much later of the muted GvH of microchime-

rism following human organ transplantation was that it "warmed his old heart." Ibid., 20.

6. James Calnan, *The Hammersmith: The First Fifty Years of the Royal Postgraduate Medical School at Hammersmith Hospital* (Lancaster: MTP, 1985); Christopher C. Booth, "Medical Science and Technology at the Royal Postgraduate Medical School: The First 50 Years," *British Medical Journal* 291, no. 6511 (1985): 1771–79. See also Jessie Dobson and Cecil Wakeley, *Sir George Buckston Browne* (Edinburgh: Livingstone, 1957). Francis Galton had earlier attempted to set up a similar venture at Down House to study genetics.

7. W. J. Dempster, "Kidney Homotransplantation," *British Journal of Surgery* 40 (Mar. 1953): 463.

8. W. J. Dempster, "The Effects of Cortisone on the Homotransplanted Kidney," *Archives Internationales de Pharmacodynamie et de Thérapie* 95 (1953): 253–82.

9. His main work is Dempster, "Kidney Homotransplantation," 447–65. Dempster did find that rabbit skin graft survival could be prolonged by irradiation. The effect was quite marked on first grafts but had no effect on the survival of a second set of grafts from the same donor; see W. J. Dempster, B. Lennox, and J. W. Boag, "Prolongation of Survival of Skin Homotransplants in the Rabbit by Irradiation of the Host," *British Journal of Experimental Pathology* 31, no. 5 (Oct. 1950): 670–79. But a careful study in rats inexplicably failed to show skin graft prolongation by radiation; see N. Rabinovici, "The Fate of Skin Homotransplants Performed on Previously X-Rayed Rats," *Plastic and Reconstructive Surgery* 2, no. 5 (Sept. 1947): 413–18, and interest thus faded.

10. L. Persky and S. Jacob, "Effect of ACTH and Cortisone on Homogenous Kidney Transplants," *Proceedings of the Society for Experimental Biology and Medicine* 77, no. 1 (May 1951): 66–68. Largely unnoticed at the time, or later, was Wilford Neptune's single lung experimental transplants in dogs, in which ACTH prolonged survival from six days to twenty-five days, an effect reported to the 1952 National Cancer Institute's Tissue Transplantation Conference.

11. William J. Dempster, *An Introduction to Experimental Surgical Studies* (Oxford: Blackwell, 1957), 178.

12. Dempster then became a lofty and critical observer of the evolution of human organ transplanta-

tion; see Leslie Brent, "Transplantation: Some British Pioneers," *Journal of the Royal College of Physicians of London* 31 (1997): 434–44. Dempster and Simonsen shared left-wing political views, and this stance, popular in European academia at the time, for a while resulted in the denial of both their visa applications to visit America, even when invited to give lectures.

13. Christopher C. Booth, *Doctors in Science and Society: Essays of a Clinical Scientist* (London: British Medical Journal, 1987), 274.

14. For an excellent review of the early events, see D. K. C. Cooper, "Experimental Development of Cardiac Transplantation," *British Medical Journal* 4, no. 5624 (Oct. 19, 1968): 174–81.

15. Among Demikhov's achievements were early attempts at the use of artificial hearts and at human coronary artery surgery, and his achievements were slowly recognized after the cold war thaw; see H. B. Shumacker, "A Surgeon to Remember: Notes about Vladimir Demikhov," *Annals of Thoracic Surgery* 58, no. 4 (Oct. 1994): 1196–98. For his neglected Soviet work, see Vladimir P. Demikhov, "Homoplastic Transplantation of the Heart and Lungs in Warm-Blooded Animals," in *Problems of Thoracic Surgery* (Medgiz, 1949). His heart transplants are mentioned in his book *Experimental Transplantation of Vital Organs*, trans. from Russian by Basil Haigh (New York: Consultants Bureau, 1962). Medawar encountered Demikhov in Moscow in 1966 and was unimpressed with the Russian's claim that surgical skill rather than immunosuppression brought success with homografts. Calne also gives an account of Demikhov's behavior at this 1966 lecture by Medawar; see Roy Calne, *The Ultimate Gift: The Story of Britain's Premier Transplant Surgeon* (London: Headline, 1998), 85. See also I. E. Konstantinov, "A Mystery of Vladimir P. Demikhov: The 50th Anniversary of the First Intrathoracic Transplantation," *Annals of Thoracic Surgery* 65, no. 4 (Apr. 1998): 1171–77. Demikhov's experiment was carried out on December 25, 1951.

16. E. Marcus, S. N. T. Wong, and A. A. Luisada, "Homologous Heart Grafts: Transplantation of the Heart in Dogs," *Surgical Forum* 2 (1951): 212–17.

17. W. G. Bigelow, W. K. Lindsay, and W. F. Greenwood, "Hypothermia: Its Possible Role in Cardiac Surgery," *Annals of Surgery* 132, no. 5 (Nov. 1950): 849–66. Bigelow's autobiography is *Cold Hearts: The Story of Hypothermia and the Pacemaker in Heart Surgery* (Toronto: McClelland and Stewart, 1984).

18. The bathtub Swan used for his pioneering use of hypothermia in cardiac surgery is now lodged in the Smithsonian Institution, Washington, DC.

19. Wilford B. Neptune, Brian A. Cookson, and Charles P. Bailey, "Complete Homologous Heart Transplantation," *Archives of Surgery* 66, no. 2 (Feb. 1953): 174–91. Neptune later used cortisone and ACTH in this model with some graft prolongation but did not consider the effect to be of significant interest.

20. W. R. Webb and H. S. Howard, "Restoration of Function of the Refrigerated Heart," *Surgical Forum* 8 (1957): 302–6.

21. The "hypothermia era" in cardiac surgery is described in Stephen L. Johnson, *The History of Cardiac Surgery 1896–1955* (Baltimore: Johns Hopkins University Press, 1970), 113–19; and Ulrich Tröhler, "From Rehn's Risky Cardiac Suture (1896) to Routine Cardiac Transplantation (1996): Historical and Ethical Perspectives," *Journal of Cardiovascular Surgery* 39 (1998): 7–22. See also the excellent review by Mark S. Shiroishi, "Myocardial Protection: The Rebirth of Potassium-Based Cardioplegia," *Texas Heart Journal* 26, no. 1 (1999): 71–86. The tortuous road to the introduction of hypothermia in pre-pump cardiac surgery is closely described in Clarence Dennis, "A Heart-Lung Machine for Open-Heart Operations: How It Came About," *Transactions of the American Society for Artificial Internal Organs* 35, no. 4 (1989): 767–77. See also Michael F. A. Woodruff, *The Transplantation of Tissues and Organs* (Springfield, IL: Thomas, 1960), 516. For Thomas E. Starzl's view, see his book *The Puzzle People* (Pittsburgh: University of Pittsburgh Press, 1992), 66. Another group reported cold preservation of the bowel for transplantation, with use of "cold saline"; see the much-quoted Richard C. Lillehei, Bernard Goott, and Fletcher A. Miller, "The Physiological Response of the Small Bowel of the Dog to Ischemia Including Prolonged in Vitro Preservation of the Bowel," *Annals of Surgery* 150, no. 4 (1959): 543–59. Other gastroenterologists, such as Owen Wangensteen, took an early interest in hypothermia because it extended the time available for experimental liver surgery.

22. Charles Rob and Rodney Smith, *Operative Surgery: Service Volume* (London: Butterworths, 1965), pt. 15, p. 19.

23. Woodruff, *Transplantation of Tissues and Organs*, 516.

24. See Jerome P. Webster, "Refrigerated Skin Grafts," *Annals of Surgery* 120 (1944): 431–48; and D. N. Matthews, "Storage of Skin for Autogenous

Grafts," *The Lancet* 245, no. 6356 (1945): 775–78—another wartime initiative.

25. See the interesting paper by Fred C. Reynolds and David R. Oliver, "Clinical Evaluation of the Merthiolate Bone Bank: A Preliminary Report," *Journal of Bone and Joint Surgery* 31A, no. 4 (1949): 792–99. In the discussion after the paper, some participants clearly still believed that the cells within homograft bone survived and, accordingly, that only fresh bone should be used.

26. See "Proceedings of the Tissue Bank Symposium," *Transplantation Proceedings* 8, no. 2 (1976): supplement 1, 1–257.

27. This prescient review is Allan D. Vestal, Rodman E. Taber, and W. J. Shoemaker, "Medico-Legal Aspects of Homotransplantation," *University of Detroit Law Journal* 18 (1955): 171–94, pagination later corrected to 271–94.

28. The earliest instances of litigation for unauthorized tissue use were in Scotland: see *Conway v. Dalziel*, Session Cases (1901) vol. 3, Fifth Series 3F, 918–23. Much later, in Britain, public opinion on organ donation shifted in 2001 when the extent of unauthorized postmortem tissue retention by pathologists came to light, a discovery arising out of an investigation at the Alder Hey Hospital, Liverpool.

29. *Palenzke v. Bruning*, 98 Ill. App. 644 (1900).

30. The surprising "lack of property" (legal ownership) of a dead body is unchallenged and dates from the reluctant view of the eminent judge in the British case of *Williams v. Williams* 20 Ch.D. 659 in 1881.

31. E. G. L. Bywaters, "50 Years On: The Crush Syndrome," *British Medical Journal* 301, no. 6766 (Dec. 22, 1990): 1412–15. Similar syndromes had been well described earlier, notably after earthquakes, and also in the official German medical history of World War I; see Ori S. Better, "History of the Crush Syndrome: From the Earthquakes of Messina, Sicily 1909 to Spitak, Armenia 1988," *American Journal of Nephrology* 17 (1997): 392–94.

32. See Jost Benedum, "Georg Haas 1886–1971: Pionier der Hämodialyse," *Revue Suisse de Médecine Praxis* 75, no. 14 (1986): 390–94; and for a thorough review, J. Stewart Cameron, *A History of the Treatment of Renal Failure by Dialysis* (Oxford: Oxford University Press, 2002).

33. Kolff described his first machine in his monograph, *De kunstmatige nier* (Kampen, Netherlands: J. H. Kok, 1946).

34. For Merrill's defensive, almost apologetic, account of the place of dialysis treatment at that time, see his classic article, John P. Merrill, "The Use of the Artificial Kidney in the Treatment of Uremia," *Bulletin of the New York Academy of Medicine* 28, no. 8 (Aug. 1952): 523–31.

35. Professor Gabriel Richet, Paris, personal communication.

36. Homer William Smith, *The Kidney: Structure and Function in Health and Disease* (New York: Oxford University Press, 1951). This classic was known at the time as "The Green Book."

37. The harmful effects of potassium had been known since Sidney Ringer's pioneering work on heart contractility in solutions prepared with known composition. The first clinical warning that potassium ingestion might be harmful in chronic renal failure was Wilson G. Smillie, "Potassium Poisoning in Nephritis," *Archives of Internal Medicine* 16, no. 2 (Aug. 1915): 330–39.

38. *British Medical Journal* 1 (1941): 491.

39. Paul E. Teschan, "Building an Acute Dialysis Machine in Korea," *Transactions of the American Society for Artificial Internal Organs* 39, no. 4 (1993): 957–61. Earlier, during wartime, Kolff had similar freedom from institutional resistance. See Paul E. Teschan, "Acute Renal Failure during the Korean War," *Renal Failure* 14, no. 3 (1992): 237–39; Teschan's classic paper, presented at the American Society Artificial Internal Organs meeting in 1955, is reproduced in *Transactions of the American Society for Artificial Internal Organs* 44, no. 4 (1998): 260–62.

40. D. Hamilton, "Developing the Artificial Kidney in Britain: Frank Maudsley Parsons at Leeds," *University of Leeds Review* 27 (1985): 89–96; Frank M. Parsons, "Origins of Haemodialysis in the United Kingdom," *British Medical Journal* 299, no. 6715 (Dec. 23–30, 1989): 1557–60.

41. See Rene Küss's comments quoted in Tony Stark, *Knife to the Heart: The Story of Transplant Surgery* (London: Macmillan, 1996), 31.

42. W. J. Dempster, A. M. Joekes, and N. Oeconomos, "The Function of Kidneys Autotransplanted to the Iliac Vessels," *Annals of the Royal College of Surgeons of England* 16, no. 5 (May 1955): 324–36.

43. Yu. Yu. Voronoy, "Transplantation of a Conserved Cadaveric Kidney as a Method of Biostimulation in Severe Nephritides" [in Russian], *Vrachebnoe Dyel* 9 (1950): 813–16. He gives brief details of only two of the five cases.

44. Vladimir P. Filatov, *My Path in Science and Tissue Therapy: Teaching on Biogenic Stimulators,* trans. G. H. Hanna (Moscow: Foreign Languages Publishing House, 1957; London: Central Books, 1958). Filatov had supporters in the West; see Rudolph Friedrich, *Frontiers of Medicine* (New York: Liveright, 1961); and Bruce M. Carlson, "Regeneration Research in the Soviet Union," *Anatomical Record* 160, no. 4 (1968): 665–74. A gloomy verdict on later Soviet transplantation is given in Medawar's confidential report to the British Council after his visit to the Soviet Union with Roy Calne and Jim Gowans in 1966, as part of a scientific exchange scheme.

45. D. Paton and M. Martinez, "Corneal Tissue Preservation for Penetrating Keratoplasty: Past, Present and Future," *International Surgery* 49, no. 5 (1968): 428–35. The authors mention that as late as 1968, ophthalmologists visiting Russia noted the deification of Filatov and were surprised that the Filatov Institute in Odessa, though having access to fresh corneal tissue, still opted to store the whole eye at normal temperatures for four or five days prior to use, as had Filatov decades before.

46. For early psychoneuroimmunology (PNI) studies, see Debra J. Bibel, *Milestones in Immunology: A Historical Exploration* (Madison, WI: Science Tech Publishers, 1988), 310–12. Links are regularly claimed between mental activity and immune responses, but via the endocrine system.

47. The extension of Pavlov's theories to include reflex control of the function of the internal organs, including the kidney, is described in Konstantin M. Bykov, *The Cerebral Cortex and the Internal Organs,* trans. W. Horsley Gantt (New York: Chemical Publishing, 1957). See also Elena A. Korneva, Viktor M. Klimenko, and Elenora K. Shkhinek, *Neurohumoral Maintenance of Immune Homeostasis,* trans. and ed. Samuel A. Corson and Elizabeth O'Leary Corson (Chicago: University of Chicago Press, 1978).

48. See Mikhail Gerasimovich Ananév, ed., *New Soviet Surgical Apparatus and Instruments and Their Application* (New York: Pergamon, 1961). Soviet stapling work is mentioned in Woodruff, *Transplantation of Tissues and Organs,* 420. Anastasy Lapchinsky described the apparatus in detail at the Fourth Tissue Homotransplantation Conference in New York in 1960. For a thorough review acknowledging the Soviet contributions in this area of surgical instrumentation, see Felicien M. Steichen and Mark M. Ravitch, "History of Mechanical Devices and Instruments for Suturing," *Current Problems in Surgery* 19, no.

1 (1982): 1–52, later published as *Stapling in Surgery* (Chicago: Year Book Medical Publishers, 1984). Ravitch had visited the Soviet Union in 1958 and later satirized the Soviet transplant efforts in *Perspectives in Biology and Medicine* 19 (summer 1975): 501–4.

49. Richard H. Lawler, James W. West, Patrick H. McNulty, Edward J. Clancy, and Raymond P. Murphy, "Homotransplantation of the Kidney in the Human: Supplemental Report of a Case," *Journal of the American Medical Association* 147, no. 1 (Sept. 1951): 45–46. Details of this transplant patient's case are found in Jürgen Thorwald, *The Patients* (New York: Harcourt Brace Jovanovich, 1972), 92–101, and the publicity is described in Stark, *Knife to the Heart,* 25. Lawler recalled the events later in *Medical World News,* April 14, 1972, 52–56, claiming "I just wanted to get it started."

50. Quoted in Stark, *Knife to the Heart,* 29.

51. The first French case, transplanted at the Créteil hospital, is described in detail in Thorwald, *Patients,* 102–11, including the important influence of the Lawler case on the French patient's parents.

52. The resulting papers are M. Servelle, P. Soulié, J. Rougeulle, G. Delahaye, and M. Touche, "Greffe d'un rein de supplicié d'une malade avec rein unique congénital, atteinte de néphrite chronique hypertensive azotémique," *Bulletin Société Médicale des Hôpitaux de Paris* 67 (1951): 99–106; C. Dubost, N. Oeconomos, A. Nenna, J. Vaysse, et al., "Résultats d'une tentative de greffe rénale," *Bulletin Société Médicale des Hôpitaux de Paris* 67 (1951): 1372–82; and R. Küss, J. Teinturier, and P. Milliez, "Quelques essais de greffe de rein chez l'homme," *Mémoires de l'Académie de Chirurgie* 77 (1951): 755–64. There is a useful translation of the Küss paper in Toni Hau's collection of historic papers *Renal Transplantation* (Austin, TX: Silvergirl, 1987).

53. On Küss, see Paul I. Terasaki, ed., *History of Transplantation: Thirty-Five Recollections* (Los Angeles: UCLA Tissue Typing Laboratory, 1991), 37–60.

54. For tributes to Jean Hamburger, see *Kidney International* 21 (1982): supplement 11, 1–75. See also Thomas E. Starzl, "France and the Early History of Organ Transplantation," *Perspectives on Biology and Medicine* 37, no. 1 (1993): 35–47; and G. Richet, "Hamburger's Achievements with Early Renal Transplants," *American Journal of Nephrology* 17 (1997): 315–17. Roy Calne, *The Ultimate Gift: The Story of Britain's Premier Transplant Surgeon* (London: Headline, 1998), opined that Hamburger, the lofty physi-

cian, only "brought in surgeons to mend the pipes."
Ibid., 46.

55. This declamatory letter of 1952, which the newspapers did not publish, is printed in full in Thorwald,
Patients, 112.

56. L. Michon, J. Hamburger, N. Oeconomos, P. Deli-
notte, Gabriel Richet, J. Vaysse, and B. Antoine, "Une
tentative de transplantation rénale chez l'homme,"
Presse Médicale 61, no. 70 (Nov. 4, 1953): 1419–23.
This includes the first report of the histopathology of
early kidney graft rejection. Gabriel Richet of Paris
provided additional information about this case in a
personal communication.

57. The day-to-day events surrounding the case are
available in Thorwald, *Patients*, 112–29. The media
interest and intrusion rivaled the response later to
the first heart transplant, performed in South Africa in November 1967. This was one of a number of
Christmas period pioneer transplant operations—
notably the first Boston twin kidney donation in 1954
and Barnard's second heart transplant in 1967. This
holiday is a time when surgical innovators have opportunities.

58. See Francis D. Moore, *Give and Take: The Development of Tissue Transplantation* (Philadelphia: Saunders, 1964), revised and reissued as *Transplant: The
Give and Take of Tissue Transplantation* (New York: Simon and Schuster, 1972). For an extended obituary of
Moore, see the *New Yorker*, May 5, 2003, 71–81.

59. On Hume, see Terasaki, *History of Transplantation*, 117–20. Hume died in an air accident in 1973, at
age fifty-six, and for the remarkable tributes to him,
see "The David M. Hume Memorial Symposium of
1974," *Transplantation Proceedings* 6, no. 4 (1974):
supplement 1.

60. On Merrill, see "The John P. Merrill Celebration
Symposium," *Artificial Organs* 11, no. 6 (Dec. 1987):
437–85. For an analysis of Merrill's classic 1952 paper, "The Use of the Artificial Kidney in the Treatment of Uremia," see *Journal of Urban Health* 75,
no. 4 (1998): 911–21.

61. Cited in Moore, *Transplant*, 40.

62. David M., Hume, John P. Merrill, Benjamin
F. Miller, and George W. Thorn, "Experiences with
Renal Homotransplantation in the Human: Report
of Nine Cases," *Journal of Clinical Investigation* 34,
no. 2 (1955): 327–82. Both Merrill and Joseph Murray
later stated that there were six or eight additional unpublished transplants performed from 1953 to 1955,
which presumably showed no encouraging features.

For an account of the times, see Hume's posthumous
article, "Early Experiences in Organ Homotransplantation in Man and the Unexpected Sequelae Thereof,"
American Journal of Surgery 137, no. 2 (1979): 152–61.
A useful table listing the early human kidney transplants is found in Woodruff, *Transplantation of Tissues
and Organs*, 521–25; see also A. M. Joekes, K. A. Porter, and William J. Dempster, "Immediate Post-
Operative Anuria in a Human Kidney Transplant,"
British Journal of Surgery 44, no. 188 (May 1957):
607–15. For another account of these times, see Joseph E. Murray, "Organ Transplantation (Skin, Kidney, Heart) and the Plastic Surgeon," *Plastic and Reconstructive Surgery* 47, no. 5 (May 1971): 425–31.

63. Matson had previously supplied these "expendable" human kidneys to give the tissue culture cells
for the use of Enders, Weller, and Robbins in their
Nobel Prize–winning polio virus tissue culture work.
Matson responded to the Boston transplant team's request for kidneys by flippantly saying that he was glad
to assist work toward another Nobel Prize. Matson
did not live to hear of this event—Joseph Murray's
award; see Joseph E. Murray, *Surgery of the Soul* (Canton, MA: Science History Publications for the Boston
Medical Library, 2001), 95.

64. There was no consensus on the role of human
blood types at this time, and Woodruff stated in his
1960 book, *Transplantation of Tissues and Organs*, that
ABO matching was of no value in organ transplantation. Merrill at this time still had a concern about "reverse incompatibility," that is, that recipient red cells
would be agglutinated in the donor kidney and thus
that some mismatches might paradoxically be favorable.

65. Dempster assisted with this operation, and the
thigh position was used; see Joekes, Porter, and
Dempster, "Immediate Post-Operative Anuria in a
Human Kidney Transplant," 607–15.

66. See Gordon Murray, *Medicine in the Making* (Toronto: Ryerson, 1960), later published in Britain under the title *Surgery in the Making* (London: Johnson,
1964); and Murray, *Quest in Medicine* (Toronto: Ryer
son, 1963); see also G. D. W. Murray and R. Holden,
"Transplantation of Kidneys, Experimentally and in
Human Cases," *American Journal of Surgery* 87, no. 4
(Apr. 1954): 508–15.

67. Murray and Holden, "Transplantation of Kidneys,
Experimentally and in Human Cases," 509.

68. Murray's reputation is slowly being rehabilitated;
see William Clarke, "A Canadian Giant: Dr. Gordon

Murray and the Artificial Kidney," *Canadian Medical Association Journal* 137 (1987): 246–48; and Shelley McKellar, *Surgical Limits: The Life of Gordon Murray* (Toronto: University of Toronto Press, 2003).

69. MacLean quotation from Mark M. Ravitch, *A Century of Surgery: The History of the American Surgical Association* (Philadelphia: Lippincott, 1981), 1019. For Woodruff's Hunterian Lecture, see *Annals of the Royal College of Surgeons of England* 11, no. 3 (1952): 173–94.

70. See Roger Baker, Robert Gordon, John Huffer, and George H. Miller, "Experimental Renal Transplantation: I. Effect of Nitrogen Mustard, Cortisone

and Splenectomy," *Archives of Surgery* 65, no. 5 (Nov. 1952): 702–5. The authors dismissed the marked effect of these substances as a nonspecific one, perhaps related to poor nutrition of the treated dogs. No memory remains in Washington or Chicago of this group or their work.

71. B. Benacerraf, B. N. Halpern, G. Biozzi, and S. A. Benos, "Quantitative Study of the Granulopectic Activity of the Reticulo-Endothelial System: Effect of Cortisone and Nitrogen Mustard on Regenerative Capacity of the R.E.S. after Saturation with Carbon," *British Journal of Experimental Pathology* 35, no. 2 (Apr. 1954): 97–106.

11. Transplantation Tolerance and Beyond

1. Peter B. Medawar, *Memoir of a Thinking Radish: An Autobiography* (Oxford: Oxford University Press, 1986), 110.

2. Ray D. Owen's original finding was reported as "Immunogenetic Consequences of Vascular Anastomoses between Bovine Twins," *Science* 102, no. 2651 (1945): 400–401; and later in "Quintuplet Calves and Erythrocyte Mosaicism," *Journal of Heredity* 37, no. 10 (Oct. 1946): 291–97. Owen reviewed his work much later, by invitation, at the Royal Society's 1956 meeting on tolerance: "Erythrocyte Antigens and Tolerance Phenomena," *Proceedings of the Royal Society*, series B, 146, no. 922 (Nov. 13, 1956): 8–18. Medawar replaced Owen's use of the word *mosaic* with *chimaera*. For a generous tribute to Owen from Medawar's colleagues, see Leslie Brent, "The Discovery of Immunologic Tolerance," *Human Immunology* 52, no. 2 (Feb. 1997): 75–81.

3. F. R. Lillie, "The Theory of the Free-Martin," *Science* 43, no. 1113 (Apr. 28, 1916): 611–13. Lillie had arranged for local abattoirs to send him any interesting material.

4. R. A. Good has emphasized the historical role of the immunology of such "experiments of Nature," including immunity to smallpox, Edward Jenner's observations on cowpox, industrial contact sensitivity, Heinz Küstner's own allergy to fish, Ogden Bruton's cases of agammaglobulinemia, Angelo DiGeorge's athymic patients, and the antibodies multiparous women raise against the fetus. These observations in human patients all gave key clues to fundamental mechanisms: see Robert A. Good, "The Minnesota Scene: A Crucial Portal of Entry to Modern Cellular Immunology," in *The Immunologic Revolution: Facts and Witnesses*, ed. Andor Szentivanyi and Herman Friedman (Boca Raton, FL: CRC Press, 1994).

5. Owen's PhD student was Sherman Ripley, from South Africa. He had the necessary microprobe skills for neonatal injection, but his main, unrelated project was based in the neurobiology section at CalTech. Ripley briefly mentions his successful induction of chimerism in the 1951 *Annual Report of the CalTech Biology Division*. Ray Owen, personal communication.

6. Frank Macfarlane Burnet and Frank Fenner, *The Production of Antibodies*, 2nd ed. (Melbourne: Macmillan, 1949), 136.

7. Medawar, *Memoir of a Thinking Radish*, 111. The cattle work is described in R. E. Billingham, G. H. Lampkin, P. B. Medawar, and H. L. Williams, "Tolerance to Homografts, Twin Diagnosis, and the Freemartin Condition in Cattle," *Heredity* 6 (1952): 201–12.

8. Harvey Stone and Burnet had also used the word *tolerance*, and Gorer had used it in 1936, but in the broader sense of the word, when describing any long-term survival of a graft. *Tolerance* was used in this nonspecific sense, particularly in the clinical literature, during the 1960s and 1970s.

9. Jack A. Cannon and William P. Longmire Jr., "Studies of Successful Skin Homografts in the Chicken: Description of a Method of Grafting and Its Application as a Technic of Investigation," *Annals of Surgery* 135, no. 1 (Jan. 1952): 60–68.

10. In a report to the MRC in 1954, Medawar noted that at Oxford four strains of mice were available after "20 generations of inbreeding."

11. Tolerance induction has proved to be difficult in outbred animals, including wild mice; see A. Sogioka, M. Morita, J. Fujita, A. Hasumi, and T. Shiroishi, "Graft Acceptance and Tolerance Induction in Mouse

Liver Transplantation Using Wild Mice," *Transplantation Proceedings* 33, no. 1 (2001): 137–39.

12. Mitchison at Oxford had started using inbred mice in his cell transfer work in 1953; he obtained his CBA mice from Edinburgh.

13. Medawar and Mitchison converted some of their immunological findings into mathematical language in their early papers, but this traditional Oxford approach faded. However, visitors to Medawar's laboratory, notably R. A. Fisher and clinicians like Paul Russell, reproached the team for failing at first to use statistical methods to compare the usually self-evident differences in survival between the groups of mice. Eventually, Medawar began to employ a suitable life-table formula to appease the pedants; see R. E. Billingham in Paul I. Terasaki, ed., *History of Transplantation: Thirty-Five Recollections* (Los Angeles: UCLA Tissue Typing Laboratory, 1991), 73.

14. R. E. Billingham, L. Brent, and P. B. Medawar, "'Actively Acquired Tolerance' of Foreign Cells," *Nature* 172, no. 4379 (Oct. 3, 1953): 603–6. The full version of the paper was delayed and eventually published in 1956 as "Quantitative Studies on Tissue Transplantation Immunity: III. Actively Acquired Tolerance," *Philosophical Transactions of the Royal Society*, series B, 239, no. 666 (Mar. 15, 1956): 357–414. In all of the trio's publications, Medawar took the traditional view that the authors' names should be listed in alphabetical order.

15. This tolerance work was the basis for much of Leslie Brent's PhD thesis. Much of the crucial data was lost, however, as a result of car theft in 1954; the findings had to be reconstructed.

16. Snell quoted in Terasaki, *History of Transplantation*, 26.

17. Burnet believed that his clonal selection theory was more worthy of an award than his contribution to tolerance. Medawar and Burnet's Nobel Prize addresses are found in *Science* 133 (1961): 303–11. Brent, in his "Discovery of Immunologic Tolerance," considered that he believed Owen should have shared the prize.

18. At University College London, Alex Comfort, a Russian speaker, alerted Medawar to the 1953 Czechoslovakian paper. The original is M. Hašek, "Vegetavni hybridisace zivocichu spojenim krevnich obehu v embryonalnim vyvojhi," *Československá Biologie* 2 (1953): 256; the later English-language version is M. Hašek and T. Hraba, "Immunological Effects of Experimental Embryonal Parabiosis," *Nature* 175,

no. 4461 (Apr. 30, 1955): 764–65. Czechoslovak transplantation studies were highly regarded at the time and merited a special bibliography in volumes 2 and 5 of *Transplantation Bulletin*, compiled by the energetic R. Klen of Hradec Králové.

19. The best account of Lysenkoism is Valery Soyfer, *Lysenko and the Tragedy of Soviet Science* (New Brunswick, NJ: Rutgers University Press, 1994), and the local misery in Czechoslovakia is described in "The Grim Heritage of Lysenkoism: Four Personal Accounts," *Quarterly Review of Biology* 65, no. 4 (Dec. 1990): 413–79.

20. Brent's contacts with Hašek and his admiration for Hašek's struggles in Czechoslovakia are poignantly described in Leslie Brent, *A History of Transplantation Immunology* (London: Academic Press, 1997), 191–95, 228–29; by Snell in Terasaki, *History of Transplantation*, 30; an obituary in *Immunogenetics* 21 (1985): 21; and in a memorial volume, P. Iv'nyi, ed., *The Realm of Tolerance* (New York: Springer Verlag, 1989). See also B. Cinader, "Tolerance as a Regulatory Process," *Immunologic Revolution*, ed. Szentivanyi and Friedman, 53–72; Snell in Terasaki, *History of Transplantation*, 35; and the curious note by Georges Mathé, "Transplantation, Immunity, Tolerance and Grafts: Dempster, Hasek 'et les autres,'" *Biomedicine & Pharmacotherapie* 46, no. 2–3 (1992): 49–52. Medawar's group from 1947 had included the biologist George Szabo, a Hungarian political refugee, and Igor Egorov, who left the Soviet Union in the late 1970s, working first with D. B. Amos and then with Snell at Bar Harbor.

21. Medawar, letter to Rogers, August 6, 1951, personal communication.

22. The crucial proposal of "cell-mediated immunity" is given in N. A. Mitchison, "Passive Transfer of Transplantation Immunity," *Proceedings of the Royal Society*, series B, 142 (1954): 72–87; and briefly in *Nature* 171 (1953): 267. Hints of such transfer were reported in K. Landsteiner and M. W. Chase, "Experiments on Transfer of Cutaneous Sensitivity to Simple Compounds," *Proceedings of the Society for Experimental Biology and Medicine* 49 (1942): 688–90. For an account of these times, see William L. Ford, "The Lymphocyte—Its Transformation from a Frustrating Enigma to a Model of Cellular Function," in *Blood, Pure and Eloquent: A Story of Discovery, of People, and of Ideas*, ed. Maxwell M. Wintrobe (New York: McGraw-Hill, 1980), 457–508.

23. For the wartime interest in contact sensitivity, see Philip G. H. Gell, "Sensitisation to 'Tetryl,'" *British*

Journal of Experimental Pathology 25 (1944): 174–92, 191. For Gell, see Arthur M. Silverstein, Baruj Benacerraf, "In Memoriam: Philip Gell (1914–2001)," *Cellular Immunology* 213 (Oct. 10, 2001): 1–3. In Birmingham in 1965, Sells and Gell wrote the classic article on lymphocyte transformation by anti-allotype serum: "Studies on Rabbit Lymphocytes in Vitro: I. Stimulation of Blast Transformation with an Anti-allotype Serum," *Journal of Experimental Medicine* 122 (1965): 423–40.

24. Mitchison, "Passive Transfer of Transplantation Immunity," 87. Mitchison did not quote the important earlier views of James Bumgardner Murphy and Loeb on the lymphocyte.

25. Clyde Barker contributed significantly toward expanding the list of privileged sites and giving an understanding of them; see Clyde F. Barker and R. E. Billingham, "Immunologically Privileged Sites and Tissues," in *Corneal Graft Failure*, CIBA Symposium No. 15 (Amsterdam: Elsevier, 1973).

26. G. H. Algire, J. M. Weaver, and R. T. Prehn, "Growth of Cells in Vivo in Diffusion Chambers. I: Survival of Homografts in Immunized Mice," *Journal of the National Cancer Institute* 15, no. 3 (1954): 493–507.

27. See Brent in Terasaki, *History of Transplantation*, 93. The antibody-only hypothesis had a late boost when Robert A. Good reported that children with the newly discovered defect of agammaglobulinemia, who were incapable of forming antibodies, would not reject skin grafts. Robert A. Good and Richard L. Varco, "Successful Homograft of Skin in a Child with Agammaglobulinemia," *Journal of the American Medical Association* 157, no. 9 (Feb. 1955): 713–16.

28. The authority on these "privileged sites" was H. S. N. Greene, whose numerous papers are listed in Michael Woodruff, *The Transplantation of Tissues and Organs* (Springfield, IL: Thomas, 1960), 654.

29. Medawar, *Memoir of a Thinking Radish*, 83. For Medawar's other assessment of these times, see *The Harvey Lectures 1956–1957* (New York: Academic Press, 1958), 144–76.

30. Rupert Billingham and Willys K. Silvers, eds., *Transplantation of Tissues and Cells* (Philadelphia: Wistar Institute Press, 1961).

31. Brent, *History of Transplantation Immunology*, quotes the abrasive Little's verdict. Brent also ignores Loeb's capability as a scientist as judged by his record of innovation in other areas.

32. William C. Boyd, *Fundamentals of Immunology*, 3rd ed. (New York: Interscience Publishers, 1956), 76.

33. Joseph Murray maintained this view in his post–Nobel Prize memoirs, *Surgery of the Soul* (Canton, MA: Science History Publications for the Boston Medical Library, 2001), 109.

34. For a note on Hildemann, see Brent, *History of Transplantation Immunology*, 106.

35. See the comprehensive "Symposium on Phylogeny of Transplantation Reactions," *Transplantation Proceedings* 2 (1970): 179–341.

36. The development of the various physiological saline solutions awaits a historian, but meantime see J. Alfred Lee, "Sydney Ringer (1834–1910) and Alexis Hartmann (1898–1964)," *Anaesthesia* 36 (1981): 1115–21.

37. C. Polge, A. U. Smith, and A. S. Parkes, "Revival of Spermatozoa after Vitrification and Dehydration at Low Temperatures," *Nature* 164, no. 4172 (Oct. 15, 1949): 666. See also their paper presented at the CIBA conference, the proceedings of which were published as *Preservation and Transplantation of Normal Tissues*, ed. G. E. W. Wolstenholme and M. P. Cameron (London, 1954). An account of Parkes's low temperature work is found in his *Off-Beat Biologist: The Autobiography of Alan S. Parkes* (Cambridge: Galton Foundation, 1985), 458. The group used the word *biocryology* at first, settling for the present term, *cryopreservation*, in 1958.

38. H. H. G. Eastcott, A. G. Cross, A. G. Leigh, and D. P. North, "Preservation of Corneal Grafts by Freezing," *The Lancet* 263, no. 6805 (Jan. 30, 1954): 237–39.

39. For accounts of Peter Gorer, see Medawar's detailed tribute in *Biographical Memoirs of Fellows of the Royal Society* 7 (1961): 95–109; and D. Bernard Amos, "Recollections of Dr. Peter Gorer," *Immunogenetics* 24, no. 6 (1986): 341–44. He died at the age of fifty, of lung cancer. Amos described him as "a wealthy chain-smoking aristocrat who seldom appeared before lunchtime." Ibid., 341.

40. Medawar's tribute to Gorer, in *Biographical Memoirs of Fellows of the Royal Society* 7 (1961): 98.

41. Snell's reminiscences are in Terasaki, *History of Transplantation*, 21–35.

42. On Snell, see Jan Klein, "In Memoriam: George D. Snell (1903–1996): The Last of the Just," *Immunogenetics* 44, no. 6 (1996): 409–18; and the obituaries by I. Hilgert, "In Memoriam: Flowers for George D. Snell

(1903–1996)," *Folia Biologica* 43, no. 1 (1997): 1–3; and G. Hoecker, "Memories of George Davis Snell (1904–1996)," *Immunogenetics* 46, no. 1 (1997): 3–4.

43. P. A. Gorer, S. Lyman, and George D. Snell, "Studies in the Antigenic Basis of Tumour Transplantation: Linkage between a Histocompatibility Gene and 'Fused' in Mice," *Proceedings of the Royal Society*, series B, 135, no. 881 (1948): 499–505.

44. George D. Snell, "Methods for the Study of Histocompatibility Genes," *Journal of Genetics* 49, no. 2 (Oct. 1948): 87–108. This paper contains an appendix with a thorough analysis of histocompatibility genetics, in the English mathematical biology tradition of the time, written by J. B. S. Haldane.

45. George D. Snell, A. M. Cloudman, E. Failor, et al., "Inhibition and Stimulation of Tumor Homoiotransplants by Prior Injections of Lyophilized Tumor Tissue," *Journal of the National Cancer Institute* 6 (June 1946): 303–16.

46. The jousting continued until about 1960; see the papers of the Liege Conference, a symposium sponsored by the Commission administrative du patrimoine universitaire de Liège and the Council for International Organizations of Medical Sciences, March 18–21, 1959, published as *Biological Problems of Grafting*, ed. Fritz Albert and Peter B. Medawar (Oxford: Blackwell Scientific Publishing, 1959).

47. D. Bernard Amos, P. A. Gorer, B. M. Mikulska, R. E. Billingham, and Elizabeth M. Sparrow, "An Antibody Response to Skin Homografts in Mice," *British Journal of Experimental Pathology* 35, no. 2 (Apr. 1954): 203–8.

48. D. Bernard Amos, "The Agglutination of Mouse Leucocytes by Iso-Immune Sera," *British Journal of Experimental Pathology* 34, no. 4 (Aug. 1953): 464–70. Amos creditably noticed Gustaf Lindström's 1927 paper on an early antilymphocyte sera and mentioned that there might be antileukocyte antibodies after multiple human blood transfusions. Jean Dausset in Paris meanwhile was puzzling over the multispecific antileukocyte serum from such a case.

49. P. A. Gorer and P. O'Gorman, "The Cytotoxic Action of Antibodies in Mice," *Transplantation Bulletin* 3 (1956): 142–43. For Edward Boyse's career, see Caroline Richmond, "Edward Arthur Boyse," *British Medical Journal* 335, no. 7618 (2007): 518.

50. Gorer in *Biological Problems of Grafting*, ed. Fritz Albert and Peter B. Medawar (Oxford: Blackwell Scientific Publishing, 1959), 55.

51. J. L. Gowans, "The Lymphocyte: A Disgraceful Gap in Medical Knowledge," *Immunology Today* 17, no. 6 (June 1996): 288–91, 288.

52. J. Ottesen, "On the Age of Human White Cells in Peripheral Blood," *Acta Physiologica Scandinavica* 32, no. 1 (Oct. 20, 1954): 75–93.

53. J. L. Gowans, "The Effect of the Continuous Re-Infusion of Lymph and Lymphocytes on the Output of Lymphocytes from the Thoracic Duct of Unanaesthetised Rats," *British Journal of Experimental Pathology* 38, no. 1 (Feb. 1957): 67–81. One of Gowans's important papers of 1959 was turned down by one referee, citing possible transfer of isotope between cells as the explanation.

54. For an account of these times, see J. L. Gowans, "The Recirculating Small Lymphocyte," *Transplantation Proceedings* 23, no. 1 (Feb. 1991): 7–8; and Gowans, "The Lymphocyte," 288–91.

55. Morten Simonsen, "The Impact on the Developing Embryo and Newborn Animal of Adult Homologous Cells," *Acta Pathologica et Microbiologica Scandinavica* 40, no. 6 (1957): 480–500.

56. Morten Simonsen, "Graft versus Host Reactions: Their Natural History, and Applicability as Tools of Research," *Progress in Allergy* 6 (1962): 349–467. He neatly eliminated the host-versus-graft element by injecting parental cells into F1 hybrid crosses. These parental cells would react against the F1 hybrid animal's host tissues, notably the spleen, but the F1 hosts were unable to eliminate the attacking cells, which were not recognized as foreign.

57. D. E. Uphoff, "Genetic Factors Influencing Irradiation Protection by Bone Marrow: I.: The F1 Hybrid Effect," *Journal of the National Cancer Institute* 19, no. 1 (July 1957): 123–30. Trentin had earlier noticed "poor survival" of the chimeric mice used in his skin graft experiments.

58. Peter Medawar, introduction to *Preservation and Transplantation of Normal Tissues*, ed. G. E. W. Wolstenholme and M. P. Cameron, 19. For Medawar's increasing confidence later, see the rest of his introduction to that volume of the CIBA conference proceedings from 1953. For a readable account of the immunology of these times, see David Wilson, *The Science of Self: A Report of the New Immunology* (London: Longman, 1972); and *The Listener*, Aug. 2, 1979, Aug. 9, 1979.

59. M. F. Woodruff, "Can Tolerance to Homologous Skin Be Induced in the Human Infant at Birth?" *Transplantation Bulletin* 4, no. 1 (1957): 26–28.

60. "Proceedings: Tissue Transplantation Conference New York 1952," *Journal of the National Cancer Institute* 14 (1953): 667–704. Eichwald had hoped that the surgeons and immunologists would find common ground professionally and socially, but at that time they did not.

61. Eichwald was editor of *Transplantation Bulletin* from 1953 to 1962, when it was superseded by *Transplantation*. He then served as editor for many more years. He also assisted on the editorial boards of a number of other journals, including *Transplantation Proceedings*. For his reminiscences, see Terasaki, *History of Transplantation*, 199–213.

62. Air travel between Europe and North America commenced in a small way about 1955. When Woodruff attended the 1962 transplant conference in New York, he was still traveling by sea, on the SS *France*.

63. The CIBA Foundation symposium of 1953 was published as *Preservation and Transplantation of Normal Tissues*, ed. G. E. W. Wolstenholme and M. P. Cameron (London, 1954). Less well known is the meeting at London in 1956 on tolerance: see McFarlane Burnet, "Concluding Remarks," *Proceedings of the Royal Society of London*, series B, no. 146 (Nov. 13, 1956): 90–92. Hašek also organized a conference on tolerance later at Liblice, a castle near Prague, in 1961.

64. A brief account of this series of meetings is given by the foundation's archivist, Nancy Spufford, in the *Novartis Foundation Bulletin*, March 1999. An interesting, detailed overview is found in F. Peter Woodford, *The CIBA Foundation: An Analytical History 1949–1974* (Amsterdam: Elsevier, 1974).

65. John Marquis Converse, "Experimental Human Skin Allografts, the HLA Complex, and a Nobel Prize," *Plastic and Reconstructive Surgery* 70, no. 2 (Aug. 1982): 255–62, 256.

66. Rapaport's memoirs are in Terasaki, *History of Transplantation*, 497–510.

67. Attending were Allgöwer, Billingham, Brent, Conway, Dammin, Gorer, Grabar, Hardin, Kaliss, Medawar, Simonsen, Stark, Toolan, Werder, and Kahn.

68. For their overview of the work of the early conferences, see John Marquis Converse and Felix T. Rapaport, "The Evolution of Tissue Homotransplantation Research," *Annals of the New York Academy of Sciences* 87 (May 31, 1960): 6–9.

69. Anastasy G. Lapchinsky, "Recent Results of Experimental Transplantation of Preserved Limbs and Kidneys and Possible Use of This Technique in Clinical Practice," *Annals of the New York Academy of Sciences* 87 (May 31, 1960): 539–71; see also *Transplantation Proceedings* 5 (1973): 773–79. Lapchinsky's tasteless two-headed dog experiments fascinated the general public but not the transplant community.

70. The New York series of meetings featuring only invited speakers was discontinued in 1962. Regular meetings restarted with the biennial meetings of the Transplantation Society in 1967, as reported from 1969 in special issues of the journal *Transplantation Proceedings*, the journal of a federation of national transplantation societies. The American Society for Artificial Internal Organs was founded in 1955. Its early proceedings have valuable papers on the use of the artificial kidney, and the annual presidential address contains valuable contemporary comment.

71. In the mid-1950s, the Medical Research Council in Britain offered grant support to Medawar to make common cause with plastic surgeons in a new, ill-defined research initiative on skin homografting. Medawar made excuses and declined; see "Working Party on Skin Grafting," FD7/1125, MRC Archives, UK Public Record Office, London.

72. Michael F. A. Woodruff, "Hunterian Lecture," *Annals of the Royal College of Surgeons of England* 11 (1952): 173.

73. The case is described in detail in C. Snyder, "Alois Glogar, Karl Bräuer, and Eduard Konrad Zirm," *Archives of Ophthalmology* 74, no. 6 (Dec. 1965): 871–74.

74. Vladimir P. Filatov, "La cornée de cadaver matériel de transplantation," *Annales d'Oculistique* 171 (1934): 721–34. See also his monograph, *Opticheskaya peresadka rogovitsy i tkanevaya terapiya* (Moscow, 1945).

75. See the remarkable account of the history of corneal grafting by David Paton in Mark J. Mannis and Avi A. Mannis, *Corneal Transplantation: A History in Profiles* (Oostende, Belgium: J. P. Wayenbourgh, 1999), 247, 249. For a detailed bibliography of early studies on corneal grafting, see A. E. Maumenee, *Transplantation Bulletin* 1 (1954): 107–22, with additions in later volumes. See also Benjamin W. Rycroft, *Corneal Grafts* (London: Butterworth, 1955). Louis Paufique, *Les Greffes de la cornée* (Paris: Masson, 1948), had international influence.

76. J. W. Tudor Thomas, "Donor Material for Corneal Grafts," *Transactions of the Ophthalmological Society of the United Kingdom* 67 (1947): 308.

77. Ibid., 303.

78. Quoted in *Proceedings of the Royal Society of Medicine* 62 (1969): 25–27.

79. C. R. Graham, "Eye Banking: A Growth Story," *Transplantation Proceedings* 17, no. 6 (Dec. 1985): 105–11; Wing Chu, "The Past Twenty-Five Years in Eye Banking," *Cornea* 19, no. 5 (Sept. 2000): 754–65. The developments to 1976 are described in *Transplantation Proceedings* 8 (1985): supplement 2.

80. The administrative events are found in "Papers Relating to Corneal Grafting Act," File BD 58/500–506, UK Public Record Office.

81. B. W. Rycroft, "The Corneal Grafting Act, 1952," *British Journal of Ophthalmology* 37, no. 6 (June 1953): 349–52.

82. See Murray's disappointing memoirs, *Surgery of the Soul.* More technical material is found in Terasaki, *History of Transplantation*, 121–44. For Murray's place in plastic surgery, see "An Interview with Joseph E. Murray, M.D., Conducted by Joel M. Noe, M.D.," *Annals of Plastic Surgery* 12, no. 1 (1984): 84–89.

83. Joseph E. Murray, John P. Merrill, and J. Hartwell Harrison, "Kidney Transplantation between Seven Pairs of Identical Twins," *Annals of Surgery* 148, no. 3 (Sept. 1958): 343–57. For an account of these times, see Joseph E. Murray, Nicholas L. Tilney, and R. E. Wilson, "Renal Transplantation: A Twenty-Five Year Experience," *Annals of Surgery* 184, no. 5 (1976): 565–73.

84. See John Marquis Converse and Gaston Duchet, "Successful Homologous Skin Grafting in War Burn Using Identical Twin as Donor," *Plastic and Reconstructive Surgery* 2, no. 4 (July 1947): 342–44.

85. After Brigham Hospital asked for help from the Boston Police Department on fingerprinting the twins, word of the proposed operation got out immediately.

86. From *Urology* 10, no. 1 (1977): supplement, 8. This "rehearsal" of a novel surgical procedure using a convenient cadaver, common at the time, is now regarded with embarrassment.

87. The John A. Hartford Foundation, now active in support of studies of aging, also funded kidney transplantation development in Boston at this time, including paying the patient's Brigham hospital bills, and even for the patient Edith Helm's prolonged stay during her normal pregnancy.

88. There is much detail on this case in Jürgen Thorwald, *The Patients* (New York: Harcourt Brace Jovanovich, 1972), 130–44. Merrill had realized that pregnancy was possible after a transplant and reasonably considered that it posed a serious danger to both patient and child. He had told Edith Helm's husband, but not the patient, that she could not have children. The husband misunderstood and assumed that Merrill meant that his wife had been surgically sterilized.

12. Hopes for Radiation Tolerance

1. This situation differed from that of classical Medawarian tolerance since the recipient regained cellular immunity when donor marrow cells, via the thymus, permitted lymphoid repopulation of peripheral T-cells. The role of the thymus was not recognized until 1960, a few years after these radiobiological insights arose in the mid-1950s. After 1960, researchers realized that if the thymus is removed and followed by lethal irradiation and marrow infusion, the animal is permanently depleted of T-cells—as in the so-called "B mouse."

2. For contemporary comment on medical effects of the use of atomic weapons against Japan, see "Atom Bomb Disease," *The Lancet* 248, no. 6410 (July 6, 1946): 14; and later analysis in Samuel Berg, "History of the First Survey on the Medical Effects of Radioactive Fall-Out (Nishiyama Valley, Nagasaki, 1945)," *Military Medicine* 124 (Nov. 1959): 782–85.

3. The Atomic Energy Research Establishment at Harwell had been established in 1946, and the biological studies group there was originally called the Radiation Protection Unit. J. F. Loutit, the first director, brought in a lasting neologism when he changed the name to Radiobiological Research Unit. By 1967, the unit still took 6 percent of the MRC budget; when the international political climate was more peaceful, the unit's grant was halved.

4. The later development at Oak Ridge of radioisotopes for clinical use is recorded in Ralph T. Overman, "Oak Ridge Remembered: 1944–1949," *Journal of Nuclear Medicine* 18, no. 8 (Aug. 1977): 759–63.

5. See the *Ciba Foundation Symposium on Experimental Tuberculosis: Bacillus and Host*, ed. G. E. W. Wolstenholme and Margaret P. Cameron (London: Churchill, 1955).

6. For the early studies reporting methods to treat radiation victims, see Leon O. Jacobson, E. L. Simmons, E. K. Marks, and J. H. Eldredge, "Recovery from Radiation Injury," *Science* 113, no. 2940 (May 4, 1951):

510–11; and Egon Lorenz, Delta Uphoff, T. R. Reid, and E. Shelton, "Modification of Irradiation Injury in Mice and Guinea Pigs," *Journal of the National Cancer Institute* 12, no. 1 (Aug. 1951): 197–201. The latter group of authors initially supported a cellular mechanism for marrow restoration but changed their analysis later. There are good summaries of these events in Michael Woodruff, *The Transplantation of Tissues and Organs* (Springfield, IL: Thomas, 1960): 452–56; Leslie Brent, *A History of Transplantation Immunology* (London: Academic Press, 1997); and in detail in Alison Kraft, "Manhattan Transfer: Lethal Radiation, Bone Marrow Transplantation and the Birth of Stem Cell Biology, ca. 1942–1961," *Historical Studies in the Natural Sciences* 39, no. 2 (spring 2009): 171–218.

7. Leon O. Jacobson, "Evidence for a Humoral Factor (or Factors) Concerned in Recovery from Radiation Injury: A Review," *Cancer Research* 12, no. 5 (May 1952): 315–25.

8. Leonard J. Cole, Maurice C. Fishler, and Victor P. Bond, "Subcellular Fractionation of Mouse Spleen Radiation Protection Activity," *Proceedings of the National Academy of Sciences* 39, no. 8 (Aug. 1953): 759–72. Although this group over many years showed that subcellular transfer of marrow activity and protection was possible, their central findings have not been confirmed. It may be that some cells escaped the homogenization or even that surviving nuclei and cytoplasmic ghosts recombined to form normal cells, as was later found to be possible with the use of nuclear transfer techniques. Hunters Point later required a major cleanup of radioactive waste.

9. For a biography of John Loutit and a list of his publications, see *Biographical Memoirs of Fellows of the Royal Society* 40 (1994): 237–52. Loutit also worked with Peter Gorer in successfully revising the terminology of tissue transplantation. The Harwell team presented this cellular hypothesis at an October 1952 meeting of the Royal Society of Medicine in London; see D. W. H. Barnes and J. F. Loutit, "Protective Effects of Implants of Splenic Tissue," *Proceedings of the Royal Society of Medicine* 46, no. 4 (Apr. 1953): 251–52; see also D. W. H. Barnes and J. F. Loutit, "Spleen Protection: The Cellular Hypothesis," in *Proceedings of the Radiobiology Symposium*, ed. Zénon Marcel Bacq and Peter Alexander (London: Butterworths, 1955), 134–40; and *Nucleonics* 12 (1954): 68–71.

10. J. M. Main and R. T. Prehn, "Successful Skin Homografts after the Administration of High Dosage X Radiation and Homologous Bone Marrow," *Journal of the National Cancer Institute* 15, no. 4 (Feb. 1955): 1023–29. By using F1 hybrid rescue marrow, they missed demonstrating a graft-versus-host response for the first time. Later, in 1976, Prehn became director of the Jackson Laboratory in Bar Harbor.

11. Main and Prehn's findings were confirmed one year later by J. J. Trentin, "Mortality and Skin Transplantability in X-Irradiated Mice Receiving Isologous, Homologous or Heterologous Bone Marrow," *Proceedings of the Society for Experimental Biology and Medicine* 92, no. 4 (Aug. 1956): 688–93. Main and Prehn were unaware of the short-term, nonspecific period of immunosuppression, and Trentin recorded "late deaths" in his chimeras, doubtless due to unrecognized GvH.

12. D. L. Lindsley, T. T. Odell Jr., and Frances G. Tausche, "Implantation of Functional Erythropoietic Elements Following Total Body Irradiation," *Proceedings of the Society for Experimental Biology and Medicine* 90, no. 2 (Nov. 1955): 512–15. This work had been greatly assisted by advice and reagents provided by Ray Owen, still involved in untangling the neonatal tolerance mechanism at the time. Owen still used the word *mosaic*, which he introduced from his famous cattle work, and others that year used the word *pseudohybrid*.

13. Peter C. Nowell, Leonard J. Cole, John G. Habermeyer, and Patricia L. Roan, "Growth and Continued Function of Rat Marrow Cells in X-Radiated Mice," *Cancer Research* 16, no. 3 (Mar. 1956): 258–61; O. Vos, J. A. G. Davids, W. W. H. Weyzen, and D. W. van Bekkum, "Evidence for the Cellular Hypothesis in Radiation Protection by Bone Marrow Cells," *Acta Physiologica Pharmacologica Neerlandica* 4, no. 4 (Mar. 1956): 482–86; N. A. Mitchison, "The Colonisation of Irradiated Tissue by Transplanted Spleen Cells," *British Journal of Experimental Pathology* 37, no. 3 (June 1956): 239–47.

14. Mitchison's priority in use of this term in adult-acquired chimerism is pointed out in *Organ Transplantation: Current Clinical and Immunological Concepts*, ed. Leslie Brent and Robert A. Sells (London: Baillière Tindall, 1989), 278.

15. C. E. Ford, J. L. Hamerton, D. W. H. Barnes, and J. F. Loutit, "Cytological Identification of Radiation-Chimaeras," *Nature* 177, no. 4506 (Mar. 10, 1956): 452–54.

16. Loutit began using irradiation and bone marrow transplantation therapy in malignancy models,

and he successfully eradicated leukemia in mice, a pioneering study for which he was awarded the prize of the Leukaemia Society; see D. W. Barnes and J. F. Loutit, "Treatment of Murine Leukaemia with X-Rays and Homologous Bone Marrow," *British Journal of Haematology* 3, no. 3 (July 1957): 241–52. This work was highlighted in Denis English and Hans-G. Klingemann, "The Foundations of Cellular Therapy: Barnes and Loutit, 1957," *Journal of Hematotherapy and Stem Cell Research* 10, no. 3 (2001): 323–34.

17. J. W. Ferrebee and J. P. Merrill, "Spare Parts: A Review with a Forward Look," *Surgery* 41, no. 3 (Mar. 1957): 503–7. Ferrebee was the activist in this "think piece" and also joined in on an article with E. D. Thomas, "Radiation Injury and Marrow Replacement: Factors Affecting Survival of the Host and the Homograft," *Annals of Internal Medicine* 49, no. 5 (Nov. 1958): 987–1003. Merrill was well aware of the power of radiation, having served as flight surgeon to the 509th Bomb Group, whose planes dropped the atom bombs on Japan.

18. J. F. Loutit, personal communication with the author. The study that arose from Merrill's European visit was on xenogeneic marrow protection; see P. Grabar, J. Courcon, P. L. Ilberg, J. F. Loutit, and John P. Merrill, "Étude immuno-électrophorétique du sérum de souris irradiées par des doses létales de rayons X et protégées par des cellules de la moelle osseuse de rats," *Comptes Rendus Hebdomadaires des Séances de l'Académie des Sciences* 245, no. 10 (Sept. 2, 1957): 950–52, published later as P. Grabar, J. Courcon, John P. Merrill, P. L. T. Ilbery, and J. F. Loutit, "Immuno-Electrophoretic Study of the Serum of Mice Irradiated by Lethal Doses of X-Ray and Protected by Rat Bone Marrow," *Transplantation Bulletin* 5, no. 2 (Apr. 1958): 58–60.

19. J. A. Mannick, H. L. Lochte, C. A. Ashley, E. D. Thomas, and J. W. Ferrebee, "A Functioning Kidney Homotransplant in the Dog," *Surgery* 46 (Oct. 1959): 821–28. The recipient did not show GvH effects; the donor marrow may have been fortuitously compatible with the recipient.

20. G. Mathé, H. Jammet, B. Pendic, L. Schwarzenberg, J. F. Duplan, B. Maupin, R. Latarjet, M. J. Larrieu, D. Kalic, and Z. Djukic, "Transfusions et greffes de moelle osseuse homologue chez des humains irradiés a haute dose accidentellement," *Revue Française d'Études: Clinique et Biologique* 4, no. 3 (Mar. 1959): 226–38; see also G. Mathé, J. L. Amiel, L. Schwarzenberg, A. Cattan, and M. Schneider, "Haematopoietic Chimera in Man after Allogenic (Homologous) Bone Marrow Transplantation," *British Medical Journal* 2, no. 5373 (Dec. 28, 1963): 1633–35.

21. Full details of the case were not published until 1960; see James B. Dealy Jr., Gustave J. Dammin, Joseph E. Murray, and John P. Merrill, "Total Body Irradiation in Man: Tissue Patterns Observed in Attempts to Increase the Receptivity of Renal Homografts," *Annals of the New York Academy of Sciences* 87 (May 1960): 572–85; and Joseph E. Murray, John P. Merrill, Gustave J. Dammin, James B. Dealy, C. W. Walter, M. S. Brooke, and R. E. Wilson, "Study on Transplantation Immunity after Total Body Irradiation: Clinical and Experimental Investigation," *Surgery* 48 (July 1960): 272–84. Merrill's thinking at this time is recalled briefly in John P. Merrill, "The Development of Human Kidney Transplantation—Personal Recollections," *Pharos* 47, no. 2 (spring 1984): 22–24. A brief account of the early cases is in J. W. Ferrebee and E. D. Thomas, "Radiation Injury and Marrow Replacement: Factors Affecting Survival of the Host and the Homograft," *Annals of Internal Medicine* 49, no. 5 (Nov. 1958): 987–1003. Ferrebee had also written an editorial on transplantation in 1957, entitled "Spare Parts," *New England Journal of Medicine* 257, no. 11 (Sept. 12, 1957): 524–25. Thomas's first paper on marrow grafting had been E. Donnall Thomas, Harry L. Lochte Jr., Wan Ching Lu, and Joseph W. Ferrebee, "Intravenous Infusion of Bone Marrow in Patients Receiving Radiation and Chemotherapy," *New England Journal of Medicine* 257 (1957): 491–96.

22. Donnall Thomas had returned from Cooperstown to assist in this case.

23. The Boston group seem to have prevented this irradiation work from merging with the unpleasant secret human radiation experiments then encouraged by the U.S. government; see Ronald Neumann, "The U.S. Advisory Committee on Human Radiation Experiments," *European Journal of Nuclear Medicine* 22, no. 6 (June 1995): 589–91.

24. See Dealy et al., "Total Body Irradiation in Man," 577. The staff protests are found in Nicholas Tilney, *Transplant: From Myth to Reality* (New Haven, CT: Yale University Press, 2003), 72. Adding to the concern at this time were the deaths of two patients at another hospital in Boston after attempted bone marrow transplantation for blood disorders.

25. From Merrill's Sydney Watson Smith Lecture in Edinburgh in 1961, which shows that his long-term planning was still linked to and directed toward achieving Medawarian tolerance; see *Symposium: Some Aspects of Renal Disease* (Edinburgh: Royal Col-

lege of Physicians, 1961), 76–91, a work noticed by the late John McConachie of Lossiemouth.

26. John P. Merrill, Joseph E. Murray, J. Hartwell Harrison, Eli A. Friedman, James B. Dealy, and Gustave J. Dammin, "Successful Homotransplantation of the Kidney between Nonidentical Twins," *New England Journal of Medicine* 262, no. 25 (June 23, 1960): 1251–60. At nine months, a biopsy of the transplanted kidney showed some signs of rejection, so small doses of irradiation and cortisone were successfully given.

27. Six months after the kidney transplant, the recipient's test skin graft from his donor was rejected, but the kidney survived, offering further proof that human kidney grafting was less of a hurdle than skin grafting and thus marginalizing the historically important input from plastic surgeons. Willard Goodwin recalled that, when thinking of starting kidney transplantation surgery in California in the early 1960s, he was told "not to waste your time on kidneys: skin is where the action is." Goodwin in Paul Terasaki, ed., *History of Transplantation: Thirty-Five Recollections* (Los Angeles: UCLA Tissue Typing Laboratory, 1991), 215.

28. For Riteris's testimony, see "The Basis for Ethical Decisions on Clinical Transplantation as Viewed by a Transplant Recipient," *Transplantation Proceedings* 5, no. 2 (June 1973): 1039–42. There is additional background in Jürgen Thorwald, *The Patients* (New York: Harcourt Brace Jovanovich, 1971), 145–69. Joseph Murray, *Surgery of the Soul* (Canton, MA: Science History Publications for Boston Medical Library, 2001), 97, surprisingly and wrongly states that Riteris was given bone marrow after the radiation.

29. This case is described in meticulous detail in Thorwald, *Patients*, 145–67.

30. Jean Hamburger, J. Vaysse, J. Crosnier, M. Tubiana, C. M. LaLanne, B. Antoine, J. Auvert, J.-P. Soulier, J. Dormont, C. Salmon, M. Maisonnet, and J.-L. Amiel, "Transplantation d'un rein entre jumeaux non-monozygotes après irradiation du receveur," *Presse Médicale* 67 (1959): 1771–75. This Paris transplant was carried out after the Boston case had been successful, and the Paris team always acknowledged the encouragement and support from Merrill. The French case history was published before the similar Boston report. Also, the Paris case offers yet another example in which the patients involved in the pioneer transplants were not passive guinea pigs, as sometimes suggested, but instead actively sought to receive any risky therapeutic measure as an alternative to certain death.

31. The doses of radiation were 260 and 200 rad, each given over six hours with the patient in the fetal position. A germ-free box was used during transport, and strict isolation was generally in force. Donor hypothermia was used while obtaining the transplant, possibly the first introduction of this strategy; see Thorwald, *Patients,* 158.

32. Morten Simonsen, "On the Acquisition of Tolerance by Adult Cells," *Annals of the New York Academy of Sciences* 87 (1960): 382–90. Simonsen, an immunologist, was greatly interested in the "crisis" at three weeks in the Paris case and suggested at the time that a subtle GvH might be occurring, but his comment fell on deaf ears.

33. J. Hamburger, J. Vaysse, J. Crosnier, J. Auvert, C. M. LaLanne, and R. T. Overman Jr., "Six tentatives d'homotransplantation renale chez l'homme après irradiation du receveur," *Revue Française d'Etudes: Clinique et Biologique* 7 (1962): 20–39. The same data appear in "Renal Homotransplantation in Man after Radiation of the Recipient: Experience with Six Patients since 1959," *American Journal of Medicine* 32 (June 1962): 854–71. Hamburger's team was last to abandon the use of the low-dose, irradiation-only regimen. See also René Küss, Marcel Legrain, Georges Mathé, R. Nedey, and M. Camey, "Homologous Human Kidney Transplantation: Experience with Six Patients," *Postgraduate Medical Journal* 38 (1962): 528–31. The same data appear in "Homologous Transplantations of the Human Kidney Experience with Four Patients," *Transactions of the American Society for Artificial Internal Organs* 7 (1961): 116–22; as was the case with Hamburger's reports, publication in English was now accepted. See also Küss in Terasaki, *History of Transplantation*, 37–60. In the total Paris experience of twenty-five radiation cases, in twelve of these transplants the mother was the donor to a child, and in nine, a brother or sister gave a kidney. The Paris physician Marcel Legrain had worked in Boston with Merrill.

34. Hume inventively tried added local graft irradiation; see David M. Hume, Joseph H. Magee, H. Myron Kauffman, Max S. Rittenbury, and George R. Prout, "Renal Homotransplantation in Man in Modified Recipients," *Annals of Surgery* 158, no. 4 (Oct. 1963): 608–44.

35. René Küss, *An Illustrated History of Organ Transplantation: The Great Adventure of the Century* (Rueil-Malmaison, France: Sandoz, 1992), 53. Küss gives an important account, from the Paris viewpoint, of their success in the radiation-only phase of human kidney

transplantation in the early 1960s. Admiration for this forgotten French effort is found in Thomas E. Starzl, "France and the Early History of Organ Transplantation," *Perspectives in Biology and Medicine* 37, no. 1 (1993): 35–47. Around this time, Hamburger and the others in Paris decided to publish in English-language journals for the first time. They did so reluctantly in 1962 since government policy was to preserve national pride via use of the French language and to let the world find its way to France's highly successful contributions to culture and science. But French scientists were aware that this view was increasingly unrealistic in an anglophone world, and Hamburger in particular decided that the policy meant that French medical contributions, notably in nephrology and transplantation, were being overlooked.

36. The resistance to proposals for kidney transplantation in Edinburgh, also encountered elsewhere, are described in Michael Woodruff, *Nothing Venture Nothing Win* (Edinburgh: Scottish Academic Press, 1997), 139.

37. About 150 cases of homograft bone marrow transplantation using radiation were reported in the literature between 1959 and 1962, and there were many more unreported, unsuccessful cases. The results were uniformly bad, and attempts virtually ceased from 1962 until 1968. The dismal results of the early bone marrow transplants are reviewed in Mortimer M. Bortin, "A Compendium of Reported Human Bone Marrow Transplants," *Transplantation* 9, no. 6 (June 1970): 571–80.

13. The Emergence of Chemical Immunosuppression

1. The first use of the word *immunosuppression* was in Joseph E. Murray, John P. Merrill, J. Hartwell Harrison, Richard E. Wilson, and Gustave J. Dammin, "Prolonged Survival of Human-Kidney Homografts by Immunosuppressive Drug Therapy," *New England Journal of Medicine* 268, no. 24 (June 13, 1963): 1315–23, and this word has connotations of continuous and nonspecific management of a latent force. Previously used phrases included Robert Good's "suppression of the immune response," Robert Schwartz and William Dameshek's "anti-immune therapy," and "immunologic suppression," as used by Victor Richards in "Transplantation and the Surgeon," *American Journal of Surgery* 105, no. 2 (Feb. 1963): 147–50.

2. Historical accounts of cancer chemotherapy are surprisingly poor, but see John R. Heller, "Cancer Chemotherapy, History and Present Status," *Bulletin of the New York Academy of Medicine* 38 (May 1962): 348–63; Jane C. Wright, "Clinical Cancer Chemotherapy," *New York State Journal of Medicine* 61 (Jan. 15, 1961): 249–80; and Jane C. Wright, "Cancer Chemotherapy: Past, Present and Future—Part I," *Journal of the National Medical Association* 76, no. 8 (Aug. 1984): 773–84.

3. Hermann Büscher's chilling book on World War I poison gases was forgotten until World War II, when it was translated for the military by Nell Conway as *Green and Yellow Cross* (Cincinnati: O. Kettering Laboratory of Applied Physiology, 1944). See also Milton C. Winternitz, ed., *Collected Studies on the Pathology of War Gas Poisoning* (New Haven, CT: Yale University Press, 1920). For British preparations for chemical warfare in World War I, see Albert Palazzo, *Seek-*

ing Victory on the Western Front: The British Army and Chemical Warfare in World War I (Lincoln: University of Nebraska Press, 2000).

4. The role of the mustard gas in the *John Harvey* disaster was successfully downplayed at the time. The effect on white blood cell count was noted, but the rushed postmortems paid scant attention to the bone marrow. Details emerged slowly after the war; see S. F. Alexander, "Medical Report on the Bari Harbor Mustard Casualties," *Military Surgeon* 101, no. 1 (July 1947): 1–17. See also Judith Perera and Andy Thomas, "Britain's Victims of Mustard-Gas Disaster," *New Scientist*, January 30, 1986, 26–27.

5. In a bizarre episode in 1943, while Macfarlane Burnett was having lunch with Linus Pauling in California, masked soldiers interrupted and advised evacuation because mustard gas was blowing in the wrong direction from a local test site.

6. On this early use of nitrogen mustard for chemotherapy, see Alfred Gilman, "The Initial Clinical Trial of Nitrogen Mustard," *American Journal of Surgery* 105 (May 1963): 574–78; and J. Einhorn, "Nitrogen Mustard: The Origin of Chemotherapy for Cancer," *International Journal of Radiation Oncology, Biology and Physics* 11, no. 7 (July 1985): 1375–78. Gilman shared a Nobel Prize in 1994 for studies on cellular transduction signals.

7. Gilman, "Initial Clinical Trial of Nitrogen Mustard," 577. Goodman and Gilman's text on pharmacology of 1943 was considered to be a risky publishing venture in a small market but became a classic also known for its historical insights. See also Cornelius P. Rhoads, "Nitrogen Mustards in the Treatment

of Neoplastic Disease: Official Statement," *Journal of the American Medical Association* 131, no. 8 (June 15, 1946): 656–58.

8. Other anticancer drugs to attract use and transplant interest were methotrexate, first used in 1956 for solid tumors, actinomycin C, first used in some malignancies in 1953, and cyclophosphamide, available beginning in 1959.

9. The one attempt at experimental immunosuppression with nitrogen mustard was described in Roger Baker, Robert Gordon, John Huffer, and George H. Miller Jr., "Experimental Renal Transplantation: Effect of Nitrogen Mustard, Cortisone and Splenectomy," *Archives of Surgery* 65, no. 5 (Nov. 1952): 702–5.

10. Robert Schwartz, J. Stack, and William Dameshek, "Effect of 6-Mercaptopurine on Antibody Production," *Proceedings of the Society for Experimental Biology and Medicine* 99, no. 1 (Oct. 1958): 164–69.

11. Robert Schwartz and William Dameshek, "Drug-Induced Immunological Tolerance," *Nature* 183, no. 4676 (June 13, 1959): 1682–83. William Dameshek (1900–1969) had earlier identified the first known autoimmune disease (acquired hemolytic anemia) and was known in Boston for a famous debate at the Boston City Hospital with William B. Castle (son of the geneticist William E. Castle) on the role of the spleen in hemolysis.

12. Publication of this important paper was delayed into the following year; see Robert Schwartz and William Dameshek with Janice Donovan, "The Effects of 6-Mercaptopurine on Homograft Reactions," *Journal of Clinical Investigation* 39, no. 6 (June 1, 1960): 952–58, 957. Meanwhile, Robert Good's group in Minnesota had achieved a similar finding and rapidly published it in December 1959; see William Meeker, Richard Condie, Daniel Weiner, Richard L. Varco, and Robert A. Good, "Prolongation of Skin Homograft Survival in Rabbits by 6-Mercaptopurine," *Proceedings of the Society for Experimental Biology* 102 (1959): 459–61. See also Gertrude Belle Elion, S. Callahan, S. Bieber, G. H. Hitchings, and R. W. Rundles, "A Summary of Investigations with 2-amino-6-[(1-methyl-4-nitro-5-imidazolyl)thio]purine (B.W. 57–322)," *Cancer Chemotherapy Reports* 8 (July 1960): 36–43. For an account of these times, see Robert S. Schwartz, in *Design and Achievements in Chemotherapy*, ed. G. H. Hitchings (n.p.: Burroughs Wellcome, 1976). See also Gertrude Belle Elion, "The Pharmacology of Azathioprine," *Annals of the New York Academy Sciences* 685 (June 23, 1993): 400–407.

Schwartz, like many other research teams at this time, had support from the U.S. Atomic Energy Commission.

13. K. A. Porter and Joseph E. Murray, "Successful Homotransplantation of Rabbit Bone Marrow after Preservation in Glycerol at -70° C.," *Cancer Research* 18, no. 1 (Jan. 1958): 117–19. This study may have been the first crucial use of cryopreservation in transplantation studies. Later, Porter's London hospital laboratory at St. Mary's was the first to store human lymphocytes for tissue-typing studies.

14. K. A. Porter and Joseph E. Murray, "Homologous Marrow Transplantation in Rabbits after Triethylenethiophosphoramide," *Archives of Surgery* 76, no. 6 (June 1958): 908–11. Porter later worked with Thomas Starzl transatlantically, examining all tissues from his human and experimental transplants.

15. Calne was one of many pioneer transplanters who recalled that Medawar's invited lectures inspired them to take up their interest in this subject. However, Calne also recalled later that, when he first heard Medawar speak and someone asked about the relevance of tolerance to clinical transplantation, Medawar replied "absolutely nothing." This may have been a Medawarian, sarcastic Oxford put-down, meaning the opposite, rather than a serious verdict. See Roy Calne, *The Ultimate Gift: The Story of Britain's Premier Transplant Surgeon* (London: Headline, 1998), 21.

16. For the technical difficulties, see Calne in Paul I. Terasaki, ed., *History of Transplantation: Thirty-Five Recollections* (Los Angeles: UCLA Tissue Typing Laboratory, 1991), 230; and Calne, *Ultimate Gift*, 37–40.

17. Roy Yorke Calne, "The Rejection of Renal Homografts," *The Lancet*, 275, no. 7121 (1960): 417–18. This historic, and characteristically terse, paper reported two kidney homograft survivals, of twenty-one and forty-seven days, obtained with use of 6-MP, but it does not say how many animals were used in the work. Calne was first to monitor white blood cell counts when using chemical immunosuppression. For another account of these times, see Roy Yorke Calne, "The Development of Immunosuppressive Therapy," *Transplantation Proceedings* 13, no. 1 (Mar. 1981): supplement 1, 44–49.

18. Calne, "Rejection of Renal Homografts," 418.

19. Dempster's letter is "Rejection of Renal Homografts," *The Lancet* 275, no. 7123 (Mar. 5, 1960): 551. Dempster was perhaps piqued that Calne had not sought his advice, in spite of the older surgeon's ex-

perience in the previous decade with similar grafting at the same experimental facilities at Buckston
Browne in Downe. Calne's view was that Dempster
was considered "difficult to approach"; see Calne in
Terasaki, *History of Transplantation*, 231. The American surgeon Sam Kountz spent a year with Dempster
at Hammersmith, and although the two had serious scientific and professional disagreements, they
wrote up a paper together: William J. Dempster and
S. L. Kountz, "Recent Concepts of the Cause of Functional Arrest of Homotransplanted Kidneys," *Review
of Surgery* 23, no. 1 (1966): 5–28.

20. C. F. Zukoski, H. M. Lee, and David M. Hume,
"The Effect of 6-Mercaptopurine on Renal Homograft Survival in the Dog," *Surgery, Gynecology & Obstetrics* 112 (June 1961): 470–72.

21. Calne, *Ultimate Gift*, 46, gives an amusing account of the rivalry he encountered between the two
Paris transplant units.

22. Calne's early cases were later presented rather
reluctantly as John Hopewell, Roy Yorke Calne, and
Isobel Beswick, "Three Clinical Cases of Renal Transplantation," *British Medical Journal* 1, no. 5380 (Feb.
15, 1964): 411–13. The arrangements for the surgery
were ahead of the times, namely in the use of cadaveric kidneys, continuous chemical immunosuppression, and even the artificial kidney for preparation in
one case. Hopewell later organized a London sharing scheme for cadaver kidneys—the London Transplant Club—and he was active in setting up the British Transplantation Society (BTS) in 1972. The BTS
supervised a pioneering audit of individual center
results at a time when such intrusion was novel and
generally resisted. For a history of the BTS, see Mary
G. McGeown, *The British Transplantation Society: A
Brief History* (London, 2001).

23. Transplantation research in Boston and elsewhere
had major support from the John A. Hartford Foundation, and their grants, fruitful and otherwise, are described in interesting detail in Judith S. Jacobson, *The
Greatest Good: A History of the John A. Hartford Foundation* (New York: The Foundation, 1984), 179–92.

24. Gertrude Belle Elion (1918–1999) was reluctantly
taken on as an assistant to George Hitchings (1905–
1998) as a favor in 1944 by the male-dominated Burroughs Wellcome organization—"Okay, there's a war
going on"; see *Sunday Times News Review*, March 6,
1994. Elion, Hitchings, and James Black shared a
Nobel Prize in 1988 for their pioneering pharmacological work. For obituaries of Elion, see *Science* 284

(May 28, 1999): 1480; and *Nature* 398, no. 6726
(Apr. 1, 1999): 380.

25. Murray's account of this episode instead indicates
that he encouraged Calne's azathioprine work. Murray says that Merrill advocated continuing with radiation studies, doubtless because of Merrill's knowledge of the success with low-dose irradiation in Paris
at the time. See Joseph E. Murray, *Surgery of the Soul:
Reflections on a Curious Career* (Canton, MA: Science History Publications for Boston Medical Library,
2001), 105–7. Like Calne, Murray had used 6-MP
clinically, but only in one patient in 1960, and without success.

26. Roy Yorke Calne and Joseph E. Murray, "Inhibition of the Rejection of Renal Homografts in Dogs
by Burroughs Wellcome 57-322," *Surgical Forum* 12
(1961): 118–20. In this study, they also tried cortisone in combination with BW 57-322 in two cases
but failed to find the synergism noted later. For other
strategies attempted then but ultimately discarded,
see Roy Yorke Calne, "Inhibition of the Rejection of
Renal Homografts by Purine Analogues," *Transplantation Bulletin* 28 (Oct. 1961): 65–81. See also Roy
Yorke Calne, G. P. Alexandre, and Joseph E. Murray,
"A Study of the Effects of Drugs in Prolonging Survival of Homologous Renal Transplants in Dogs," *Annals of the New York Academy of Sciences* 99 (Oct. 24,
1962): 743–61.

27. The Boston dog transplanters obtained skilled
veterinarian support from Boston's Angell Memorial
Animal Hospital when problems arose. That hospital, decades later, pioneered a kidney transplant program for cats.

28. Considerable background on the one patient who
survived three months as well as the debate on management are found in Murray, *Surgery of the Soul*,
115–17, but Murray's memory of the important azathioprine dose is incorrect. The donor had died during open heart surgery. The case is also described in
Jürgen Thorwald, *The Patients* (New York: Harcourt
Brace Jovanovich, 1971), 184–99.

29. David M. Hume, Joseph H. Magee, H. Myron
Kauffman, Max S. Rittenbury, and George R. Prout,
"Renal Homotransplantation in Man in Modified
Recipients," *Annals of Surgery* 158, no. 4 (Oct. 1963):
608–44.

30. Joseph E. Murray, John P. Merrill, J. Hartwell Harrison, Richard E. Wilson, and Gustave J. Dammin,
"Prolonged Survival of Human-Kidney Homografts
by Immunosuppressive Drug Therapy," *New England*

Journal of Medicine 268, no. 24 (June 13, 1963): 1315–23. For an account of these times, see Joseph E. Murray, Nicholas L. Tilney, and Richard E. Wilson, "Renal Transplantation: A Twenty-Five Year Experience," *Annals of Plastic Surgery* 184, no. 5 (Nov. 1976): 565–73; and the proceedings of the symposium to mark twenty-five years of transplantation at the Peter Bent Brigham Hospital in *Transplantation Proceedings* 13 (1981): supplement 1.

31. See Calne's chapter, written in 1963, in *The Scientific Basis of Surgery*, ed. William Tait Irvine (London: Churchill, 1965), 456–67, 464.

32. Willard E. Goodwin, Matt M. Mims, and Joseph J. Kaufman, "Human Renal Transplantation III: Technical Problems Encountered in Six Cases of Kidney Homotransplantation," *Transactions of the American Association of Genito-Urinary Surgeons* 54 (1962): 116–23.

33. Willard E. Goodwin, Joseph J. Kauffman, Matt M. Mims, Roderick D. Turner, Richard Glasscock, Ralph Goldman, and M. M. Maxwell, "Human Renal Transplantation: I. Clinical Experience with Six Cases," *Journal of Urology* 89 (Mar. 1963): 13–24. Case 3 is the historic one showing good kidney function and then a rejection episode reversed by prednisone. Goodwin maintained an interest in the advances in transplantation thereafter and was the key organizer of the National Research Council meeting in Washington in late 1963. Goodwin's career is described in William P. Longmire, *Starting from Scratch: The Early History of the UCLA Department of Surgery* (Pasadena, CA: Castle Press, 1984), 153–60; Terasaki, *History of Transplantation*, 215–26; and Thomas E. Starzl, *The Puzzle People* (Pittsburgh: University of Pittsburgh Press, 1992).

34. Thomas L. Marchioro, H. K. Axtell, M. F. LaVia, William R. Waddell, and Thomas E. Starzl, "The Role of Adrenocortical Steroids in Reversing Established Homograft Rejection," *Surgery* 55 (Mar. 1964): 412–17. This paper on the dog studies was held up for a year by referees and thus appeared after the report of the similar success in Denver with steroid use to prevent human kidney transplant patient rejection (see Starzl et al., "Reversal of Rejection" in note 36 below); this paper had also been delayed.

35. Goodwin arrived in Denver during Starzl's second attempt at liver transplantation, and the relevant entry in Goodwin's personal journal is reprinted in Starzl, *Puzzle People,* 102. For Goodwin's reports on his travels, which he titled "Urologists' Correspondence Club," see W. E. Goodwin, "Recollections: Early Experiences in Kidney Transplantation," *Transplantation Proceedings* 13, no. 1 (Mar. 1981): supplement 1, 29–31. C. C. Congdon sent out similar newsletters in the earlier period when radiation biology was developing quickly.

36. Thomas E. Starzl, Thomas L. Marchioro, and William R. Waddell, "The Reversal of Rejection in Human Renal Homografts with Subsequent Development of Homograft Tolerance," *Surgery, Gynecology & Obstetrics* 117 (1963): 385–95. This crucial paper had first been offered to the *Journal of the American Medical Association* but was held up once more by critical reviewers. A modified version then went to *Surgery, Gynecology & Obstetrics,* whose editor, Loyal Davis, chairman of the Department of Surgery at Northwestern University, Chicago, was more sympathetic then and thereafter to transplantation studies. Davis is described in Thomas E. Starzl, "Loyal Davis, Surgery of the Liver and Transplantation of the Kidney," *Surgery, Gynecology & Obstetrics* 157, no. 2 (Aug. 1983): 160–63.

37. Thomas E. Starzl, "Personal Reflections in Transplantation," *Surgical Clinics of North America* 58, no. 5 (Oct. 1978): 879–93, both quotations on 881.

38. See "Human Kidney Transplant Conference" (National Academy of Sciences–National Research Council, September 26–27, 1963), *Transplantation* 2 (1964): 147–65, 581–600. Documents relevant to the conference are held in the archives of the National Academy of Sciences but are disappointing. The proceedings, occasionally acrimonious, were recorded, but the tapes have disappeared. Personal accounts of the events are found in Starzl, *Puzzle People,* 109–11; and in René Küss, *An Illustrated History of Organ Transplantation* (Rueil-Malmaison, France: Sandoz, 1992), 58–61.

39. W. E. Goodwin and D. C. Martin had published a summary of all kidney transplant cases until 1963 in the hard-to-find *Urological Survey* 13 (1963): 229–48. For the pre-1960 transplants, they used Woodruff's detailed compilation in his book *The Transplantation of Tissues and Organs* (Springfield, IL: Thomas, 1960).

40. Hume et al., "Renal Homotransplantation in Man in Modified Recipients."

41. Starzl later commented dryly that his charts prevented "failure of recording of laboratory examinations known to have been ordered but from which the results were misplaced" and that "trends are easily observed and recurrent patterns can be easily identified and quantified which might otherwise be lost in

a maze of detail." He added that "accurate and unbiased information is frequently requested by visitors." Thomas Starzl, *Experience in Renal Transplantation* (Philadelphia: Saunders, 1964), 10. Starzl had many visitors immediately after the Washington meeting, notably Porter, Calne, Hume, Poisson, Küss, Shackman, and Terasaki. Murray, *Surgery of the Soul*, also claims credit for these soon-to-be essential wall charts.

42. This need for ABO matching came as a result of empirical observations and new awareness that ABO factors were carried on nucleated human cells; see R. R. A. Coombs, D. Bedford, and L. M. Rouillard, "A and B Blood-Group Antigens on Human Epidermal Cells: Demonstrated by Mixed Agglutination," *The Lancet* 267, no. 6921 (1956): 461–63; and Claes Högman, "The Principle of Mixed Agglutination Applied to Tissue Culture Systems," *Vox Sanguinis* 4, no. 1 (Feb. 1959): 12–20.

43. For early evidence of the value of cooling in experimental kidney transplantation, see G. M. Bogardus and R. J. Schlosser, "The Influence of Temperature upon Ischemic Renal Damage," *Surgery* 39, no. 6 (June 1956): 970–74. It was also thought that any delay in homograft function might be the result of immunological factors rather than ischemia: "It is equally possible that the immediate function of the homograft is more dependent than genetically identical tissue upon minimization of ischemia." Starzl, *Experience in Renal Transplantation*, 49.

44. The mid-1960s was also when hopes for deep freezing of the recently deceased and "life extension" organizations emerged and claimed satisfactory and expensive preservation of loved ones in liquid nitrogen, stating with sincerity that functional revival would have to await improvements in the thawing process.

45. Julio E. Figueroa, Satoru Nakamoto, Eugene F. Poutasse, and Willem J. Kolff, "Renal Homotransplantation in Man," *Annals of Internal Medicine* 61, no. 2 (Aug. 1964): 188–206.

46. Murray's contributions, clinical and organizational, were rewarded with a Nobel Prize in 1990, shared with E. Donnall Thomas; see Francis D. Moore, "A Nobel Award to Joseph E. Murray, M.D.: Some Historical Perspectives," *Archives of Surgery* 127, no. 5 (May 1992): 627–32. Controversy over these awards is usually muted but was more public on this occasion, particularly when there were so many likely candidates; see Tony Stark, *Knife to the Heart: The Story of Transplant Surgery* (London: Macmillan, 1996), 53–55; and John Hopewell, "Nobel Prizes Given for Clinical Research," *British Medical Journal* 301 (Nov. 17, 1990): 1165. The exclusion of the French pioneers led to expressions of anger in the French lay and scientific press, and elsewhere expectations had been raised by misleading leaks from the near-final Nobel Prize committee meetings.

47. Murray, a devout Catholic, said that Medawar's suggestion "was like the Pope telling the Bishops what to do." Murray, *Surgery of the Soul*, 119. Medawar was not at this clinically oriented NRC meeting.

48. This quotation comes from the interesting comments on the issues of the day invited by J. R. Elkinton, the Quaker editor of *Annals of Internal Medicine*, reported in "Moral Problems of Artificial and Transplanted Organs," *Annals of Internal Medicine* 61 (Aug. 1964): 355–63, 357.

49. For the snags in dealing with pooled results, see R. D. Guttmann, "The Graft Survival Curve: Ideology and Rhetoric," *Transplantation Proceedings* 24, no. 6 (Dec. 1992): 2407–10.

50. The activists in this matter were the physicians William Drukker of Amsterdam, Stanley Shaldon from London, and David Kerr of Newcastle; see David N. S. Kerr, "EDTA to ERA," *Nephrology, Dialysis and Transplantation* 4, no. 5 (1989): 411–15. The boundaries of "Europe" in this context were later interpreted broadly. Reporting of data on dialysis outcome was a condition of EDTA membership, and this discipline proved highly successful; see A. J. Wing and F. P. Brunner, "Twenty-Three Years of Dialysis and Transplantation in Europe: Experiences of the EDTA Registry," *American Journal of Kidney Diseases* 14, no. 5 (Nov. 1989): 341–46.

51. Nathan P. Couch, "Supply and Demand in Kidney and Liver Transplantation: A Statistical Survey," *Transplantation* 4, no. 5 (Sept. 1966): 587–95. At the Brigham Hospital, Murray, Couch, and Richard E. Wilson began taking turns sleeping in the hospital so as to be available in case a deceased patient's organs were available for donation.

52. Joseph E. Murray and J. Hartwell Harrison, "Surgical Management of Fifty Patients with Kidney Transplants Including Eighteen Pairs of Twins," *American Journal of Surgery* 105 (Feb. 1963): 205–18, 206.

53. Calne, *Ultimate Gift*, 56. See ibid., 105, on hurried and risky air journeys in pursuit of donor organs for transplantation.

54. The first recorded interhospital cooperation was when Massachusetts General transferred a donor liver to Brigham Hospital in late 1963 for possible use by Moore. For the importance of such cooperation at the time, see Nathan P. Couch, William J. Curran, and Francis D. Moore, "The Use of Cadaver Tissues in Transplantation," *New England Journal of Medicine* 271, no. 14 (Oct. 1, 1964): 691–95, 693n.

55. See Starzl, *Puzzle People*, 879–93; Goodwin and Martin in *Urological Survey* 13 (1963): 229–48; and Francis D. Moore, "Transplantation—A Perspective," *Transplantation Proceedings* 12, no. 4 (Dec. 1980): 539–50.

56. Simonsen noted that a surmountable, short-term crisis also occurred in nonlethal graft-versus-host reactions, followed by abeyance of the immunological attack.

57. The puzzle of "adaptation" was regularly highlighted by Medawar and Woodruff but was not back in favor until the 1990s—in relation to microchimerism. Their views are recalled enthusiastically in Thomas E. Starzl, "History of Clinical Transplantation," *World Journal of Surgery* 24, no. 7 (2000): 759–82.

58. The troublesome cytomegalovirus (CMV), often transferred with the donor organs, was first identified in Robert E. Kanich and John E. Craighead, "Cytomegalovirus Infection and Cytomegalic Inclusion Disease in Renal Homotransplant Recipients," *American Journal of Medicine* 40, no. 6 (June 1966): 874–82.

59. On the new "transplantation pneumonia," see David Rifkind, Thomas E. Starzl, Thomas L. Marchioro, William R. Waddell, David T. Rowlands, and Rolla B. Hill Jr., "Transplantation Pneumonia," *Journal of American Medical Association* 189 (1964): 808–12, and the review by Rolla B. Hill, David T. Rowlands, and David Rifkind, "Infectious Pulmonary Disease in Patients Receiving Immunosuppressive Therapy," *New England Journal of Medicine* 271, no. 20 (Nov. 12, 1964): 1021–27. This paper reviewed overt and latent lung infection in the thirty-two deaths out of sixty-one patients at Denver from 1961 to February 1964. This 1964 report was selected as a citation classic in *Reviews in Medical Virology* 9, no. 1 (1999): 3–14. The transplant experience was invaluable later when dealing with similar challenges arising during the AIDS epidemic.

60. Hill et al., "Infectious Pulmonary Disease in Patients Receiving Immunosuppressive Therapy," 1025.

61. The first reported and treated case of RASt is in William T. Newton, Raymond M. Keltner, and Stewart W. Shankel, "Acquired Renovascular Hypertension in a Patient with Renal Allotransplantation," *American Journal of Surgery* 113, no. 2 (Feb. 1967): 292–94.

62. The story of the rising importance of imaging in transplant management is detailed by David Hamilton in *Ultrasound of Abdominal Transplantation*, ed. Paul Sidhu and Grant Baxter (Stuttgart: Thieme, 2002), 1–12.

63. T. H. Mathew, P. Kincaid-Smith, J. Eremin, and V. C. Marshall, "Percutaneous Needle Biopsy of Renal Homografts," *Medical Journal of Australia* 1, no. 1 (Jan. 6, 1968): 6–7. Biopsies with the relatively large Vim-Silverman needle remained controversial for a while, but transplant biopsy eventually became safe and routine, and in the cyclosporine era such biopsies became the commonest of all forms of renal biopsy. Hume et al., "Renal Homotransplantation in Man in Modified Recipients," reported needle-biopsy of transplanted kidneys on two occasions, but the hemorrhage after the second attempt seems to have discouraged further such attempts by his and other teams at this time. The Boston team had earlier closely followed some of the azathioprine cases with frequent open biopsies under local anaesthetic, as did Starzl.

64. Avascular necrosis of bone was noticed at Denver and mentioned in Starzl's *Experience in Renal Transplantation*, 206. It is described in full in Jaime F. Bravo, Jerome H. Herman, and Charley J. Smyth, "Musculoskeletal Disorders after Renal Homotransplantation," *Annals of Internal Medicine* 66, no. 1 (1967): 87–104. Necrosis was noted in six cases out of twenty-seven patients surviving six months with kidney transplants at Montreal by R. L. Cruess, J. Blennerhassett, F. R. MacDonald, L. D. MacLean, and J. Dossetor, "Aseptic Necrosis Following Renal Transplantation," *Journal of Bone and Joint Surgery* 50A, no. 8 (Dec. 1968): 1577–90; and by Kevin D. Harrington, William R. Murray, Samuel L. Kountz, and Folkert O. Belzer, "Avascular Necrosis of Bone after Renal Transplantation," *Journal of Bone and Joint Surgery* 53A, no. 2 (Mar. 1, 1971): 203–15, which reviews possible explanations of the puzzle.

65. The first case of the common post-transplant hyperparathyroidism may be the Boston report by Richard E. Wilson, Daniel S. Bernstein, Joseph E. Murray, and Francis D. Moore, "Effects of Parathyroidectomy and Kidney Transplantation on Renal Osteodystrophy," *American Journal of Surgery* 110 (Sept.

1965): 384–93; and Richard E. Wilson, Constantine L. Hampers, Daniel S. Bernstein, James W. Johnson, and John P. Merrill, "Subtotal Parathyroidectomy in Chronic Renal Failure: A Seven-Year Experience in a Dialysis and Transplant Program," *Annals of Surgery* 174, no. 4 (Oct. 1971): 640–54.

66. This "chronic rejection" was noted on open biopsies of successful transplants; see Ken A. Porter, J. B. Dossetor, Thomas L. Marchioro, W. S. Peart, J. M. Rendall, Thomas E. Starzl, and Paul I. Terasaki, "Human Renal Transplants: I. Glomerular Changes." *Laboratory Investigation* 16, no. 1 (Jan. 1967): 153–81.

67. Starzl, *Experience in Renal Transplantation;* and Thomas E. Starzl, Thomas L. Marchioro, Ken A. Porter, Tanous D. Faris, and Thomas A. Carey, "The Role of Organ Transplantation in Pediatrics," *Pediatric Clinics of North America* 13 (1966): 381–422. The Richmond report is G. M. Williams, H. M. Lee, and D. M. Hume, "Renal Transplants in Children," *Transplantation Proceedings* 1, no. 1 (Mar. 1969): 262–66.

68. John S. Najarian, Richard L. Simmons, Marion B. Tallent, Carl M. Kiellstrand, Theodore J. Buselmeier, Robert L. Vernier, and Alfred F. Michael, "Renal Transplantation in Infants and Children," *Annals of Surgery* 174, no. 4 (Oct. 1971): 583–601.

69. A review of the pioneering kidney transplants in diabetics is given in John S. Najarian, D. E. Sutherland, Richard L. Simmons, R. J. Howard, C. M. Kjellstrand, S. M. Mauer, W. Kennedy, R. Ramsay, J. Barbosa, and F. C. Goetz, "Kidney Transplantation for the Uremic Diabetic Patient," *Surgery, Gynecology & Obstetrics* 144, no. 5 (May 1977): 682–90. Najarian gives an account of these times in his autobiography, *The Miracle of Transplantation: The Unique Odyssey of a Pioneer Transplant Surgeon* (Beverly Hills, CA: Medallion Publishing/Phoenix Books, 2009).

70. The first such pregnancy, in a transplanted twin, was in 1958. The first birth to a patient with a cadaver kidney was not until 1970. See Ginny L. Bumgardner and Arthur J. Matas, "Transplantation and Pregnancy," *Transplantation Reviews* 6 (1992): 139–62.

71. L. D. MacLean, J. B. Dossetor, M. H. Gault, J. A. Oliver, F. G. Inglis, and K. J. MacKinnon, "Renal Transplantation Using Cadaveric Donors," *Archives of Surgery* 91, no. 2 (Aug. 1965): 288–306; Donald C. Martin, Milton Rubini, and Victor J. Rosen, "Cadaveric Renal Homotransplantation with Inadvertent Transplantation of Carcinoma," *Journal of the American Medical Association* 192, no. 9 (May 31, 1965): 752–54; and J. J. McPhaul and D. A. McIntosh, "Tis-

sue Transplantation Still Vexes" (letter), *New England Journal of Medicine* 272, no. 2 (Jan. 14, 1965): 105.

72. Although news of single cases of de novo lymphoid malignancy circulated, published reports on these tumors were delayed until the trend had become clear. Michael Woodruff mentioned five cases known to him while attending a cancer symposium in Dundee, Scotland, in May 1968, and an annotation followed in the *Lancet* 291, no. 7555 (Jun. 15, 1968): 1298–99. The first formal paper, on two cases, is P. B. Doak, J. Z. Montgomerie, J. D. K. North, and F. Smith, "Reticulum Cell Sarcoma after Renal Transplantation and Azathioprine and Prednisone Therapy," *British Medical Journal* 4, no. 5633 (Dec. 21, 1968): 746–48. Details of the Denver patients' lymphoid tumors were published as I. Penn, W. Hammond, L. Brettschneider, and Thomas E. Starzl, "Malignant Lymphomas in Transplant Patients," *Transplantation Proceedings* 1 (1969): 106–12.

73. Thomas E. Starzl, Ken A. Porter, S. Iwatsuki, J. T. Rosenthal, B. W. Shaw, R. W. Atchison, M. A. Nalesnik, M. Ho, B. P. Griffith, T. R. Hakala, R. L. Hardesty, R. Jaffe, and H. T. Bahnson, "Reversibility of Lymphomas and Lymphoproliferative Lesions Developing under Cyclosporin-Steroid Therapy," *The Lancet* 323, no. 8377 (Mar. 17, 1984): 583–87.

74. I. Penn, C. G. Halgrimson, and Thomas E. Starzl, "De Novo Malignant Tumors in Organ Transplant Recipients," *Transplantation Proceedings* 3, no. 1 (1971): 773–78.

75. Starzl, *Puzzle People*, 96.

76. J. A. Cannon, "Brief Report," *Transplantation Bulletin* 3 (1956): 7.

77. C. S. Welch, "A Note on Transplantation of the Whole Liver in Dogs," *Transplantation Bulletin* 2 (1955): 54–55. Welch ascribed the graft atrophy to rejection, but in retrospect, loss of normal portal blood flow also contributed. Welch's work and career are described in Starzl, *Puzzle People*.

78. Francis D. Moore, Louis L. Smith, Thomas K. Burnap, Frederick D. Dallenbach, Gustave J. Dammin, Ulrich F. Gruber, William C. Shoemaker, Richard W. Steenburg, Margaret R. Ball, and John S. Belko, "One Stage Homotransplantation of the Liver Following Total Hepatectomy in Dogs," *Transplantation Bulletin* 6, no. 1 (1959): 103–7, and a fuller account in *Annals of Surgery* 152 (1960): 374–87. See also Thomas E. Starzl, Harry E. Kaupp, Donald R. Brock, Robert E. Lazarus, and Robert V. Johnson, "Reconstructive Problems in Canine Liver Homotransplantation with

Special Reference to the Postoperative Role of Hepatic Venous Flow," *Surgery, Gynecology & Obstetrics* 111 (1960): 733–43. Starzl and Moore both started their experimental liver transplant work in mid-1958, and the major effort by Moore in Boston, now forgotten, is described with admiration by Calne in Terasaki, *History of Transplantation*, 101–2, though it is said Moore had less technical skill than the others.

79. The early cases were published later in a scholarly monograph also describing his later experience: Thomas E. Starzl, *Experience in Hepatic Transplantation* (Philadelphia: Saunders, 1969).

80. Kurt von Kaulla, a member of Starzl's team later showed that the bleeding problem could be controlled with epsilon aminocaproic acid (EACA), which was later replaced by aprotinine.

81. Vladimir Petrovich Demikhov, *Experimental Transplantation of Vital Organs*, trans. Basil Haigh (New York: Consultants Bureau, 1962). There was a good historical survey at the time by David A. Blumenstock and Joseph W. Ferrebee, "Transplantation of the Lung—Retrospect and Prospect," *Vascular Surgery* 8, no. 5 (Nov.–Dec. 1974): 266–72.

82. James D. Hardy, Watts R. Webb, Martin L. Dalton Jr., and George R. Walker Jr., "Lung Homotransplantation in Man: Report of the Initial Case," *Journal of the American Medical Association* 186, no. 12 (Dec. 21, 1963): 1065–74. Hardy's retrospective assessments on his heart and lung transplants are found in James D. Hardy, "Human Organ Replacement—Then and Now," *Transactions & Studies of the College of Physicians of Philadelphia* 7 (1985): 159–76. The diseased organs from these cases are preserved in the Smithsonian Institution, Washington, DC. Much human detail on these cases is found in Thorwald, *Patients*, 217–50.

83. See C. R. Wildevuur and J. R. Benfield, "A Review of 23 Human Lung Transplantations by 20 Surgeons," *Annals of Thoracic Surgery* 9, no. 6 (June 1970): 489–515; C. M. Montefusco and F. J. Veith, "Lung Transplantation," *Surgical Clinics of North America* 66, no. 3 (June 1986): 503–15. The first long-term survivor—ten months—was a patient transplanted at Ghent in Belgium in 1969 by F. Derom, and Frank Veith had a similar result two years later. There is a scholarly account of lung transplantation in Sara J. Shumway and Norman E. Shumway, *Thoracic Transplantation* (Cambridge, MA: Blackwell, 1995).

84. W. D. Kelly, R. C. Lillehei, F. K. Merkel, et al., "Allotransplantation of the Pancreas and Duode-

num Along with the Kidney in Diabetic Nephropathy," *Surgery* 61, no. 6 (June. 1967): 827–37. For the early history of pancreatic transplantation, see David E. R. Sutherland and Carl G. Groth, "History of Pancreas Transplantation" in *Pancreas and Islet Transplantation*, ed. Nadey S. Hakim, Robert J. Stratta, and Derek Gray (Oxford: Oxford University Press, 2002), 1–15. Kelly, active at this time, went into private practice shortly afterward.

85. The results to 1970 are reviewed in Richard C. Lillehei, Richard L. Simmons, John S. Najarian, Carl M. Kjellstrand, and Frederick C. Goetz, "Current State of Pancreatic Transplantation," *Transplantation Proceedings* 3, no. 1 (Mar. 1971): 318–24; and Richard C. Lillehei, Richard L. Simmons, John S. Najarian, Richard Weil, Hisanori Uchida, Jose O. Ruiz, Carl M. Kjellstrand, and Frederick C. Goetz, "Pancreatico-Duodenal Allotransplantation: Experimental and Clinical Experience," *Annals of Surgery* 172, no. 3 (Sept. 1970): 405–36; and later by John E. Connolly, "Pancreatic Whole Organ Transplantation," *Surgical Clinics of North America* 58, no. 2 (Apr. 1978): 383–90.

86. Paul E. Lacy and M. Kostianovsky, "Method for the Isolation of Intact Islets of Langerhans from the Rat Pancreas," *Diabetes* 16, no. 1 (Jan. 1967): 35–39.

87. S. Moskalewski, "Studies on the Culture and Transplantation of Isolated Islets of Langerhans of the Guinea Pig," *Proceedings of the Koninklijke Nederlandse Akademie van Wetenschappen*, series C, *Biological and Medical Sciences* 72 (1969): 157–71; W. F. Ballinger and Paul E. Lacy, "Transplantation of Intact Pancreatic Islets in Rats," *Surgery* 72, no. 2 (Aug. 1972): 175–86.

88. Temporary enthusiasm for the procedure was reviewed at the time in Erle E. Peacock, W. P. Webster, and G. D. Penick, "Transplantation of the Spleen," *Transplantation Proceedings* 1, no. 1 (Mar. 1969): 239–45.

89. The relevant papers are Keith Reemtsma, B. H. McCracken, J. U. Schlegel, M. A. Pearl, C. W. Pearce, C. W. DeWitt, P. E. Smith, R. L. Hewitt, R. L. Flinner, and Oscar Creech Jr., "Renal Heterotransplantation in Man," *Annals of Surgery* 160 (1964): 384–408; Claude R. Hitchcock, Joseph C. Kiser, Robert L. Telander, and Edward L. Seljeskog, "Baboon Renal Grafts," *Journal of the American Medical Association* 189, no. 12 (Sept. 21, 1964): 934–37; and Thomas E. Starzl, Thomas L. Marchioro, G. N. Peters, C. H. Kirkpatrick, W. E. C. Wilson, Ken A. Porter, D. Rifkind, D. A. Ogden, C. R. Hitchcock, and W. R. Waddell, "Renal Heterotransplantation from

Baboon to Man: Experience with 6 Cases," *Transplantation* 2, no. 6 (1964): 752–76. This article's title showed a late survival of the term *heterograft*, suggesting some clinical resistance to changes in terminology. See George D. Snell, "The Terminology of Tissue Transplantation," *Transplantation* 2 (Sept. 1964): 655–57.

90. For details of the events surrounding Reemtsma's second xenograft recipient, see Thorwald, *Patients*, 200–213. Reemtsma served in Korea during the war there and is said to have been the model for the surgeon Hawkeye Pierce in the 1970s movie and television series *M*A*S*H*.

91. The British Medical Research Council's "monkey kidney file" is in FD 23/833, UK Public Record Office.

92. For a retrospective on Hardy's heart xenograft, see "The First Heart Transplant in Man," *Transplantation Proceedings* 1 (1969): 717–21. More personal detail is given in Thorwald, *Patients*, 217–50. At this time also, various artificial devices to assist or replace the human heart were designed and tested, notably by Willem Kolff in Cleveland. These pumps showed early promise, and in 1964 the National Institutes of Health set up an artificial heart program, but it made very slow progress.

93. Hitchings's view of the press was in his response to editor J. R. Elkinton's request for views on transplant ethical concerns as gathered in his *Annals of Internal Medicine* 61 (1964): 361. In Edinburgh, reporters posed as relatives or clergy to gain the transplant stories and pictures.

94. Right Honourable Lord Justice Edmund Davies, "A Legal Look at Transplants," *Proceedings of the Royal Society of Medicine* 62, no. 7 (Jul. 1969): 633–40, 633. The judge was speaking after the heart transplant controversies. According to the *British Medical Journal*, commenting on the Human Tissue Act of 1961, "It is much to be regretted that the terms of its drafting were so inadequately thought out." "News and Notes: Kidney Donation and the Law," *British Medical Journal* 3, no. 5875 (Aug. 11, 1973): 360.

95. For early Boston legal initiatives on cadaveric donation, see Nathan P. Couch, William J. Curran, and Francis D. Moore, "The Use of Cadaver Tissues in Transplantation," *New England Journal of Medicine* 271, no. 14 (Oct. 1, 1964): 691–95.

96. At the opening of the Wright Fleming Institute at St. Mary's Hospital in 1966, the immunologist James Mowbray organized a group photograph of a mix of transplant patients, doctors, and journalists. The only

ill figure to stand out was a journalist on steroids for disseminated sclerosis. Mowbray started providing good news for the media, and the *Daily Express* and British Broadcasting Corporation proved especially friendly media. The BBC's medical correspondent, David Wilson, even wrote a supportive book, *The Science of Self: A Report of the New Immunology* (London: Longman, 1972). Later, Terasaki published the stories of a group of individual high-achieving transplant patients: Paul I. Terasaki and Jane Schoenberg, *Transplant Success Stories* (Los Angeles: UCLA Tissue Typing Laboratory, 1993).

97. P. A. Gorer, "Transplantese," *Annals of the New York Academy Sciences* 87 (May 31, 1960): 604–7, 604. The term *isogeneic* grafting was encouraged for grafting between identical individuals, with *syngeneic*, commonly used in inbred animal work, as an alternative. *Autograft* and *autografting* remained in use for grafts and grafting from one part of the body to another.

98. For these further discussions on terminology, see Peter A. Gorer, J. F. Loutit, and H. S. Micklem, "Proposed Revisions of 'Transplantese,'" *Nature* 189, no. 4769 (Mar. 25, 1961): 1024–25; Snell, "Terminology of Tissue Transplantation"; and Peter A. Gorer, J. F. Loutit, and H. S. Micklem, "Proposed Revision of 'Transplantese,'" *Transplantation Bulletin* 28, no. 6 (1961): 139–40. For the German revision, see "Deutschsprachige Transplantations—Nomenclature," *Deutsche Medizin Wochenschrift* 94 (1969): 56.

99. Snell, "The Terminology of Tissue Transplantation." Snell had always preferred use of adjectives, as in "homologous" or "allogeneic" graft, rather than nouns, as in "homograft" or "allograft."

100. This change of terminology presents a problem to writers of transplantation history. In this book, I have used *allograft* only after this word permanently entered the literature. But inconsistently I have used *xenograft* from the start of the book, rather than the historically correct, but awkward, *heterograft*.

101. In the discussion recorded after Hume presented his paper "Renal Homotransplantation in Man in Modified Recipients" at the American College of Surgeons meeting in spring 1963, William Waddell did not use the term *rejection crisis* when reporting the Denver experience. It thus seems that the use of *rejection crisis* emerged in day-to-day discourse about mid-1963. A *"crise"* three weeks after human kidney transplantation was described by Hamburger's team in 1959.

102. For the continuing inability of the physicians, as late as 1998, to agree on a standard phrase for chronic kidney failure, see the letters in the *British Medical Journal* 315, no. 1021 (Oct. 18, 1997): 1021; and 316, no. 7131 (Feb. 21, 1998): 632.

103. Medawar stated that "I myself am always oppressed by large conferences, and it is many years since I have been to anything but fairly small discussion groups." Medawar to Rogers, September 16, 1963, quoted in Blair Rogers, personal communication with the author.

14. Support from Hemodialysis and Immunology in the 1960s

1. The author of this book, considered by himself to be receptive to new ideas, reacted with distaste on first hearing in 1961 of the attempts to keep end-stage renal failure patients alive by regular hemodialysis.

2. The classic paper on this work is Wayne E. Quinton, David Dillard, and Belding H. Scribner, "Cannulation of Blood Vessels for Prolonged Hemodialysis," *Transactions of the American Society for Artificial Internal Organs* 6 (April 10–11, 1960): 104–13, but the paper was never presented, since the authors instead gave a different paper at the conference: B. H. Scribner, R. Buri, J. E. Z. Caner, R. Hegstrom, and J. M. Burnell, "The Treatment of Chronic Uremia by Means of Intermittent Hemodialysis: A Preliminary Report," *Transactions of the American Society for Artificial Internal Organs* 6 (1960): 114–22. Scribner had heard of the availability of Teflon tubing from a hospital telephone engineer.

3. Teflon (polytetrafluoroethylene), a polymer of the simple carbon and fluorine molecule CF_2, is inert, resists thermal, chemical, enzymatic, or biological damage and, above all, has an extraordinarily low coefficient of friction. Industrial use, particularly for nonstick pans, began in 1957, and the material was found to be helpful in a number of clinical situations. See F. Becmeur, S. Geiss, S. Laustriat, J. Bientz, L. Marcellin, and P. Sauvage, "History of Teflon," *European Urology* 17, no. 4 (1990): 299–300.

4. Jürgen Thorwald, *The Patients* (New York: Harcourt Brace Jovanovich, 1972), 170–83, records in detail the historic treatment of Clyde Shields, the first patient to be given regular dialysis. The book also mentions how the patient and his wife pressured the medical team to use the experimental shunt in his treatment.

5. The unusual swap of presentations on the Scribner shunt has led to a bibliographical muddle. The pioneering paper actually presented at the ASAIO meeting is Scribner et al., "Treatment of Chronic Uremia by Means of Intermittent Hemodialysis," but this classic is often ignored in favor of Quinton et al., "Cannulation of Blood Vessels for Prolonged Hemodialysis," which was printed but never presented; see

Scribner's comments in the reprint of the article in *Journal of the American Society of Nephrology* 9, no. 4 (Apr. 1, 1998): 719–26. Use of these shunts for other reasons in non-dialysis patients failed because renal failure patients have a subtle clotting defect.

6. Robin Eady, later professor of experimental dermatopathology at St. Thomas's Hospital, London, was dying of renal failure in 1962 but managed to obtain one of the early places in the Seattle program in February 1963. He moved to Canada later that year to join the staff, and be treated, at the new Artificial Kidney Laboratory program in Edmonton, returning to the Royal Free Hospital in London when regular dialysis was established in Britain in 1964.

7. Cimino, as a student phlebotomist, had noticed that it was easy to get blood samples from Korean War veterans who had developed traumatic arteriovenous fistulas. For a history, see T. Kapoian and R. A. Sherman, "A Brief History of Vascular Access for Hemodialysis: An Unfinished Story," *Seminars in Nephrology* 17, no. 3 (May 1997): 239–45.

8. A useful review of the literature on this matter is in J. R. Elkinton, "Ethical and Moral Problems in the Use of Artificial and Transplanted Organs," in *To Live and to Die: When, Why, and How,* ed. Robert Hardin Williams (New York: Springer-Verlag, 1973).

9. See the accounts in David Rothman, *Strangers at the Bedside: A History of How Law and Bioethics Transformed Medical Decision Making* (New York: Basic Books, 1991); and M. L. Tina Stevens, *Bioethics in America: Origins and Cultural Politics* (Baltimore: Johns Hopkins University Press, 2000).

10. For instance, in the early 1940s, penicillin was initially in short supply. For the comparable case of "iron lung" shortages during the polio epidemics, see Philip A. Drinker and Charles F. McKhann III, "The Iron Lung: First Practical Means of Respiratory Support," *Journal of the American Medical Association* 255, no. 11 (Mar. 21, 1986): 1476–80.

11. The philosopher Henry David Thoreau (1817–1862) was an uncompromising critic of American materialism.

12. S. Toulmin, "How Medicine Saved the Life of Ethics," *Perspectives in Biology and Medicine* 25, no. 4 (summer 1982): 736–50. The pioneering Ciba Foundation symposium followed; see Gordon E. W. Wolstenholme and Maeve O'Connor, eds., *Ethics in Medical Progress: With Special Reference to Transplantation* (London: Churchill, 1966), later reprinted under the title *Law and Ethics of Transplantation* (London: Churchill, 1968).

13. Sargent Shriver claimed priority in introducing the neologism *bioethics* in 1970 when planning the Kennedy Institute of Ethics; see Robert Martensen, "The History of Bioethics: An Essay Review," *Journal of the History of Medicine and Allied Sciences* 56, no. 2 (2001): 168–75.

14. See "How Much Is Human Life Worth?" *Wall Street Journal,* August 22, 1963; and Nicholas Rescher, "The Allocation of Exotic Medical Lifesaving Therapy," *Ethics* 79, no. 3 (1969): 173–96. Careful legal discussion is found in two long, thorough, unsigned articles: "Patient Selection for Artificial and Transplanted Organs," *Harvard Law Review* 82, no. 6 (1969): 1322–42; and "Scarce Medical Resources," *Columbia Law Review* 69, no. 4 (1969): 620–92. Both reviews note that medical case law was moving from its traditional restricted base in medical litigation and edging toward influencing routine clinical decisions.

15. The law courts have examined only one case in which a choice was made between human lives. In 1884, crew members of a lifeboat were charged with killing a boy for food to preserve the lives of the remaining members. But the English jury agreed with the defense's claim that the boy was already dead when his body was used; see *Regina vs. Dudley and Stephens,* Queens Bench Division (1884) 14, 273. This famous case of the last voyage of the *Mignonette* is analyzed in A. W. Brian Simpson, *Cannibalism and the Common Law: The Story of the Tragic Last Voyage of the* Mignonette *and the Strange Legal Proceedings to Which It Gave Rise* (Chicago: University of Chicago Press, 1984).

16. The difficulties and tensions arising from the expansion of regular hemodialysis facilities in Boston are mentioned in Nicholas L. Tilney, *Transplant: From Myth to Reality* (New Haven, CT: Yale University Press, 2003), 150. See also "Selection of Patients for Haemodialysis," *British Medical Journal* 1, no. 5540 (Mar. 11, 1967): 622–24.

17. Page's critique is in *Modern Medicine,* October 14, 1963. Kolff gives further detail of Page's opposition to regular dialysis, a view shared by other distinguished Cleveland physicians, in his reminiscences in Paul I. Terasaki, ed., *History of Transplantation: Thirty-Five Recollections* (Los Angeles: UCLA Tissue Typing Laboratory, 1991), 245.

18. For some aspects of Mary Shelley's *Frankenstein* (1818), see Lester D. Friedman, "Sporting with Life: 'Frankenstein' and the Responsibility of Medical Research," *Medical Heritage* 1, no. 3 (1985): 181–85. There are further nuances in the famous gothic horror story since as a subplot, analogous to the hepatitis epidemic, the monster unintentionally brings death and misfortune to those he encounters. The humble outcast's nocturnal raids for food were also depriving the villagers of "scarce resources."

19. Page theatrically attacked what were, he claimed, proposals for an "artificial uterus"—an unfair description of Kolff's plan for an oxygenator to prevent recurrent spontaneous abortion resulting from placental insufficiency.

20. The high "suicide" rate widely quoted by critics of regular dialysis treatment did not refer to the usual forms of self-destruction but instead included deaths caused by noncompliance, failure to heed dietary restrictions, or voluntary termination of the new treatment.

21. J. Russell Elkinton, "Moral Problems in the Use of Borrowed Organs, Artificial and Transplanted," *Annals of Internal Medicine* 60, no. 2 (Feb. 1964): 309–13. Elkinton then contacted the leading physicians and transplant surgeons and invited comments. The replies, which included responses from Medawar, Murray, Merrill, Reemstma, and Starzl, were published as an interesting compilation in J. R. E., ed., "Moral Problems of Artificial and Transplanted Organs," *Annals of Internal Medicine* 61 (Aug. 1, 1964): 355–63. Elkinton was later one of the authors of a Quaker document devoted to medical ethics, and his brief autobiography is *Bird on a Rocking Chair: A Miscellany of Occasional Essays from Family and Professional Life, 1957–1987* (Lincoln, MA: Cottage Press, 1988).

22. *Medical Tribune,* April 10, 1961.

23. The formal report came from the Committee on Chronic Kidney Disease, set up to advise the Bureau of the Budget, but the name of the distinguished nephrologist who chaired it, Carl W. Gottschalk, was quickly attached to it. See George E. Schreiner, "How End-Stage Renal Disease (ESRD)-Medicare Developed," *Seminars in Nephrology* 17, no. 3 (May 1997): 152–59. See also Carl W. Gottschalk, Robert W. Ber-

liner, and Gerhard H. Giebisch, *Renal Physiology: People and Ideas* (Bethesda, MD: American Physiological Society, 1987); and Richard A. Rettig, "The Politics of Transplantation," in *Organ Transplantation Policy: Issues and Prospects*, ed. James F. Blumstein and Frank A. Sloan (Durham, NC: Duke University Press, 1989), 191–227.

24. Richard A. Rettig, *The Federal Government and Social Planning for End-Stage Renal Disease: Past, Present, and Future* (Santa Monica, CA: Rand, 1983). See also Jerome Aroesty and Richard A. Rettig, *The Cost Effects of Improved Kidney Transplantation*, document R-3099-NIH/RC (Santa Monica, CA: Rand, 1984); and Jonathan Oberlander, *The Political Life of Medicare* (Chicago: University of Chicago Press, 2003). Similar British administrative interest is found in *Report of the Joint Committee on Maintenance Dialysis and Transplantation in the Treatment of Chronic Renal Failure* (London: Royal College of Physicians of London, 1972). There is further comment in Jennifer Stanton, "The Cost of Living: Kidney Dialysis, Rationing and Health Economics in Britain 1965–1996," *Social Science and Medicine* 49, no. 9 (1999): 1169–82; Jennifer Stanton, *Innovations in Health and Medicine: Diffusion and Resistance in the Twentieth Century* (London: Routledge, 2002); and "The Office of Health Economics," in William Laing, *Renal Failure: A Priority in Health?* (London: Office of Health Economics, 1978).

25. Kidney transplantation costs were much less than those for hemodialysis and were not identified separately at this time in the United Kingdom. Such transplant units were not formally set up and did not require approval if they arose through local efforts. Transplantation running costs were met from local health authority budgets without much discussion, and the procedures and patient care were usually provided by existing, salaried staff. Moreover, the combined regimen of azathioprine and steroids was relatively inexpensive. These simple arrangements changed in the United Kingdom after controversy later arose over heart transplantation and led to central direction, control, and costing.

26. The British government files on regular dialysis are in MH 150/8, UK Public Record Office.

27. On Starzl's hepatitis, see his *The Puzzle People: Memoirs of a Transplant Surgeon* (Pittsburgh: University of Pittsburgh Press, 1992), 117. The melancholy events in the virulent Edinburgh renal unit outbreak of hepatitis were used in Colin Douglas's novel, *The Houseman's Tale* (Edinburgh: Canongate, 1974), and

are chronicled at the Edinburgh Renal Unit Web site, www.edren.org. Calne tells of his escape, not only from death, but also from a liver biopsy, in *The Ultimate Gift: The Story of Britain's Premier Transplant Surgeon* (London: Headline, 1998) 39.

28. The British Rosenheim Report of 1973 gave advice on dealing with hepatitis. See Max L. Rosenheim, *Advisory Group on Hepatitis and the Treatment of Chronic Renal Failure* (London: HMSO, 1973).

29. Eli Friedman, M.D., personal communication with the author.

30. Almost unnoticed was Nicolas Avrion Mitchison's finding of "low-zone tolerance" in the intact animal: N. A. Mitchison, "Induction of Immunological Paralysis in Two Zones of Dosage," *Proceedings of the Royal Society*, series B, 161 (Dec. 15, 1964): 275–92.

31. For an excellent review, see William L. Ford, "The Lymphocyte—Its Transformation from a Frustrating Enigma to a Model of Cellular Function" in *Blood, Pure and Eloquent*, ed. Maxwell M. Wintrobe (New York: McGraw-Hill, 1980), 457–508; and Leslie Brent, *A History of Transplantation Immunology* (London: Academic Press, 1997).

32. The first description of lymphoblast transformation came from Peter C. Nowell, "Phytohemagglutinin: An Initiator of Mitosis in Cultures of Normal Human Leukocytes," *Cancer Research* 20, no. 4 (May 1960): 462–66. His memoirs are "From Chromosomes to Oncogenes: A Personal Perspective," chap. 24 in *The Causes and Consequences of Chromosomal Aberrations*, ed. Ilan R. Kirsch (Boca Raton, FL: CRC Press, 1993).

33. John R. David, H. S. Lawrence, and L. Thomas, "Delayed Hypersensitivity *in Vitro*: III. The Specificity of Hapten-Protein Conjugates in the Inhibition of Cell Migration," *Journal of Immunology* 93, no. 2 (Aug. 1964): 264–73. Details of the race to identify MIF are given in Debra Jan Bibel, *Milestones in Immunology: A Historical Exploration* (Madison, WI: Science Tech Publishers, 1988), 212–14.

34. Fritz H. Bach and Kurt Hirschhorn, "Lymphocyte Interaction: A Potential Histocompatibility Test *in Vitro*," *Science* 143, no. 3608 (Feb. 21, 1964): 813–14. See also Barbara Bain, Magdalene R. Vas, and Louis Lowenstein, "The Development of Large Immature Mononuclear Cells in Mixed Leukocyte Cultures," *Blood* 23, no. 1 (1964): 108–16.

35. J. F. A. P. Miller, "Immunological Function of the Thymus," *The Lancet* 278, no. 7205 (Sept. 30, 1961):

748–49. The story of seventy years of mistimed thymectomies and the failure to uncover the crucial role of the thymus is told carefully in Craig R. Stillwell, "Thymectomy as an Experimental System in Immunology," *Journal of the History of Biology* 27, no. 3 (1994): 379–401. The embryologist John Beard, working in the "lost era" of immunology, had correctly understood the function of the thymus.

36. For Miller's account of his discovery, and his robust priority dispute on the matter with Robert Good, see Jacques F. A. P. Miller, "The Immunological Function of the Thymus," *Transplantation Proceedings* 23, no. 1 (Feb. 1991): 9–10; as well as his "Immunological Function of the Thymus and Thymus-Derived Cells," in *The Immunologic Revolution: Facts and Witnesses,* ed. Andor Szentivanyi and Herman Friedman (Boca Raton, FL: CRC Press, 1994), 169–80; "Uncovering Thymus Function," *Perspectives in Biology and Medicine* 39, no. 3 (spring 1996): 338–52; and "Discovering the Origins of Immunological Competence," *Annual Review of Immunology* 17, no. 1 (1999): 1–17.

Good's studies and his own claim for the discovery are reported in Szentivanyi and Friedman, *Immunologic Revolution,* 105–68, and in Good's historical introduction to David Bergsma and Robert A. Good, eds., *Immunologic Deficiency Diseases in Man* (New York: National Foundation–March of Dimes, 1968). The high-profile dispute continued in several issues of *Immunology Today,* volume 12: Jacques F. A. P. Miller, "The Discovery of the Immunological Function of the Thymus," no. 1 (Jan. 1991): 42–45; Branislav D. Janković, "The Discovery of the Immunological Function of the Thymus," no. 7 (July 1991): 247–48; and Robert A. Good, "Experiments of Nature in the Development of Modern Immunology," no. 8 (Aug. 1991): 283–86. There is also a detailed account in Brent, *History of Transplantation Immunology,* 16–20.

37. Bruce Glick, Timothy S. Chang, and R. George Jaap, "The Bursa of Fabricius and Antibody Production," *Poultry Science* 35 (1956): 224–25. Immunologists of the time ruefully admitted that this journal was not a must-read for them, nor was it abstracted in *Index Medicus.* The full story of this major discovery, buried in this obscure journal, is found in Good's article in Szentivanyi and Friedman, *Immunologic Revolution,* 126–27; and in Bibel, *Milestones in Immunology,* 129–31.

38. The useful phrase "experiments of nature" was a favorite of Irvine McQuarrie, Robert Good's mentor; see Irvine McQuarrie, *The Experiments of Nature, and Other Essays* (Lawrence: University Extension Division, University of Kansas, 1944).

39. See, for instance, H. Sherwood Lawrence, "Similarities between Homograft Rejection and Tuberculin-Type Allergy: A Review of Recent Experimental Findings," *Annals of New York Academy of Sciences* 64, no. 5 (Mar. 22, 1957): 826–35; William D. Kelly, Donald L. Lamb, Richard L. Varco, and Robert A. Good, "An Investigation of Hodgkin's Disease with Respect to the Problem of Homotransplantation," *Annals of the New York Academy of Sciences* 87 (1960): 187–202; and Robert A. Good, "Runestones in Immunology: Inscriptions to Journeys of Discovery and Analysis," *Journal of Immunology* 117, no. 5, pt. 1 (Nov. 1, 1976): 1413–28.

40. For this accidental revelation of cellular cooperation, see Claman in Szentivanyi and Friedman, *Immunologic Revolution.* The other similar events were the discovery of cryopreservation, mitogens, and the role of thymus and bursa. Other such immunological advances may have been serendipitous but were not acknowledged: Billingham criticized his mentor Medawar for not reporting any unplanned findings in their joint work—see Billingham in Terasaki, *History of Transplantation,* 77.

41. Martin C. Raff, "Theta Isoantigen as a Marker of Thymus-Derived Lymphocytes in Mice," *Nature* 224, no. 5217 (1969): 378–79. The mutant, thymusless "nude" mouse appeared first during routine lab breeding in Glasgow and was important in the developments at this time; see E. M. Pantelouris, "Observations on the Immunobiology of the 'Nude' Mouse," *Immunology* 20, no. 2 (Feb. 1971): 247–52. The first of many T-cell subsets emerged with the identification of helper cells (CD4), as reported in by H. Cantor and E. A. Boyse, "Functional Subclasses of T Lymphocytes Bearing Different Ly Antigens: I. The Generation of Functionally Distinct T-Cell Subclasses Is a Differentiative Process Independent of Antigen," *Journal of Experimental Medicine* 141, no. 6 (June 1, 1975): 1376–89. The description of suppressor cells offered explanations, but no assistance, in transplantation. See R. K. Gershon, "T Cell Control of Antibody Production," *Contemporary Topics in Immunobiology* 3 (1973): 1–40.

42. Good in *Immunologic Revolution,* ed. Szentivanyi and Friedman, 135.

43. A detached account of DiGeorge's enthusiastic intervention is given in Max D. Cooper, Raymond D. A. Peterson, and Robert A. Good, "A New Concept

of the Cellular Basis of Immunity," *Journal of Pediatrics* 67 (1965): 907–8.

44. Terasaki, *History of Transplantation*, 215.

45. See the comments by Brigham Hospital's Charles B. Carpenter on his fellow immunologists' attitudes to transplantation in the 1960s in Joseph E. Murray, John P. Merrill, and J. Hartwell Harrison, with comments by Joseph E. Murray and Charles B. Carpenter, "Milestones in Nephrology: Renal Homotransplantation in Identical Twins," *Journal of the American Society of Nephrology* 12, no. 1 (Jan. 2001): 201–4.

46. Peter B. Medawar, "Transplantation of Tissues and Organs," *British Medical Bulletin* 21, no. 2 (1965): 97–99, 98. Medawar had an interesting reservation, namely that the likely expansion in the numbers of kidney transplant units would take the service away from larger institutions and might break the professional and organizational links with basic science departments. He wrote of this "indiscriminate growth" and that "it was a pity that organ transplantation is not confined to the half dozen experienced and expert teams who have a thorough grasp of the biological, surgical and ethical problems."

47. J. R. E., ed., "Moral Problems of Artificial and Transplanted Organs," 357.

48. "Human Kidney Transplant Conference" (National Academy of Sciences–National Research Council, September 26–27, 1963), *Transplantation* 2 (1964): 148.

49. See Brent's view from the laboratory on these interactions in Brent, *History of Transplantation Immunology*, 422–27.

15. Progress in the Mid-1960s

1. For thoughtful reviews of the events in early tissue typing, see Ilana Löwy, "The Impact of Medical Practice on Biomedical Research: The Case of Human Leucocyte Antigens Studies," *Minerva* 25, no. 1–2 (spring–summer 1987): 171–200; and Nancy L. Reinsmoen and Frances E. Ward, "The History of HLA and Transplantation Immunology," in *History of Organ and Cell Transplantation*, ed. Nadey S. Hakim and Vassilios E. Papalois (London: Imperial College Press, 2003), 1–54.

2. Karl Landsteiner, "Individual Differences in Human Blood," *Science* 73, no. 1894 (Apr. 17, 1931): 403–9.

3. For an interesting contemporary analysis of these in vivo matching methods, see Paul S. Russell, Samuel D. Nelson, and Gordon J. Johnson, "Matching Tests for Histocompatibility in Man," *Annals of the New York Academy of Sciences* 129 (Dec. 1966): 368–85.

4. R. Shackman and J. E. Castro, "Prelusive Skin Grafts in Live-Donor Kidney Transplantation," *The Lancet* 306, no. 7934 (Sept. 20, 1975): 521–24.

5. Medawar's lifelong interest in seeking practical solutions to human transplantation was behind this project, and his return to the use of outbred animals, rather than inbred, is of interest.

6. These risky sensitizations and skin grafting experiments in Boston, reported in 1961, were carried out on military volunteers and supported by army research funds. They were probably the last such studies of their kind, as public opinion turned against such human experimentation on "captive" groups. During the Boston work, John Merrill became sensitized by self-injection with lymphocytes, leading to a nasty blood transfusion reaction during a hip replacement operation later. Ruggero Ceppellini in Italy had been raising his typing sera by small blood transfusions given to patients in psychiatric institutions, and he also ceased such work.

7. The first use of the phrase "tissue type" was by Paul Terasaki in 1968; the term previously in use was "leukocyte typing" or similar words. At this time, speculation on the normal biological role of individuality was avoided. In 1974, Rolf Zinkernagel and Peter Doherty demonstrated "MHC restriction" in viral responses, and one of the speculations is that this polymorphic genetic region is responsible for varieties of body odor. Diversity of odor might aid mothers identifying their offspring in crowded animal colonies, and the system could have utility in detecting and preventing harmful inbreeding; see Claus Wedekind and Sandra Füri, "Body Odour Preferences in Men and Women: Do They Aim for Specific MHC Combinations or Simple Heterozygosity?" *Proceedings of the Royal Society of London*, series B, 264 (Oct. 22, 1997): 1471–79.

8. Jean Dausset and A. Nenna, "Présence d'une leuco-agglutinine dans le sérum d'un cas d'agranulocytose chronique," *Comptes Rendus des Séances da la Société de Biologie* 146, nos. 19–20 (1952): 1539–41. For Dausset's contribution, see Peter B. Medawar, "The Nobel Awards for Medicine or Physiology," *Nature* 289, no. 5796 (1981): 345; and Lois Wingerse, "Nobel Recognition for Transplant Pioneers," *New Scientist* 88 (198): 148–49. For an account of these times, see

J. J. van Rood, "Tissue Typing and Organ Transplantation," *The Lancet* 293, no. 7606 (June 7, 1969): 1142–46; Jean Dausset, "The Challenge of the Early Days of Human Histocompatibility," *Immunogenetics* 10, no. 1 (1980): 1–5; and J. J. van Rood, "1996 Medawar Prize Lecture—Looking Back and Forward," *Transplantation Proceedings* 29, no. 1–2 (Feb.–Mar. 1997): 39–42. Dausset recalls that there was at first little contact between the scattered pioneers of these tests and that their methodology was simple—"sans computer, plastic trays and tubes and no photocopier."

9. Harrington's triumphant immunological explanation of the well-known platelet disease thrombocytopenia came in 1951.

10. Jean Dausset, A. Nenna, and H. Brecy, "Leuko-agglutinins: V. Leukoagglutinins in Chronic Idiopathic or Symptomatic Pancytopenia and in Paroxysmal Nocturnal Hemoglobinuria," *Blood* 9, no. 7 (July 1954): 7, 696–720; and "Immuno-hématologie des plaquettes et des leucocytes," *Presse Médicale* 61, no. 75 (Nov. 21, 1953): 1533–35. At this time, Miescher in Switzerland also used the term "groupes leucocytaires"—see P. A. Miescher and M. Fauconnet, "Mise en évidence de différents groupes leucocytaires chez l'homme," *Schweizerische Medizinische Wochenschrift* 84 (1954): 597–99. Dausset's MAC tissue antigens are now known as HLA-A2 and A28. Much of the later development of tissue typing can be traced in the *Histocompatibility Testing* publications supported by the National Academy of Sciences. In addition, any decisions on standard nomenclature were published from 1968 in the *Bulletin of the World Health Organization*.

11. Rose Payne, "Leukocyte Agglutinins in Human Sera," *Archives of Internal Medicine* 99, no. 4 (1957): 587–606; Rose Payne and Mary R. Rolfs, "Fetomaternal Leukocyte Incompatibility," *Journal of Clinical Investigation* 37, no. 12 (Dec. 1, 1958): 1756–63. Payne's career is described in Julia Bodmer and Walter Bodmer, "Rose Payne 1909–1999," *Tissue Antigens* 54, no. 1 (Jul. 1999): 102–5.

12. J. J. van Rood, J. G. Eernisse, and A. van Leeuwen, "Leukocyte Antibodies in Sera from Pregnant Women," *Nature* 181, no. 4625 (1958): 1735–36.

13. Jean Dausset, in *History of HLA: Ten Recollections*, ed. Paul I. Terasaki (Los Angeles: UCLA Tissue Typing Laboratory, 1990), 3–19. The entry of the term *histocompatibility* into the literature is dated to the article by George D. Snell, "The Terminology of Tissue Transplantation," *Transplantation* 2 (Sept. 1964): 655–57, but Snell had credited Gorer with this neologism.

14. Chella S. David, "The Mystery of HLA-B27 and Disease," *Immunogenetics* 46, no. 1 (1997): 73–77.

15. Van Rood first presented his pioneering findings at the autumn meeting of the British Society for Immunology in 1965. Shortly afterward, van Rood presented his data at the Paris meeting of the Transplantation Society (attended by the author of this book), and all but the experts found the matter, so familiar now, difficult to comprehend.

16. This collection of volunteer skin grafting data was not published quickly or prominently; see Jean Dausset, F. T. Rapaport, J. Colombani, and N. Feingold, "A Leucocyte Group and Its Relationship to Tissue Histocompatibility in Man," *Transplantation* 3, no. 6 (Nov. 1965): 701–5; and Jean Dausset and F. T. Rapaport, "Immunology and Genetics of Transplantation," in *Seminars in Nephrology*, ed. Ernest Lovell Becker (New York: Wiley, 1977), 97–138. See also Donald L. Ballantyne and John Marquis Converse, *Experimental Skin Grafts and Transplantation Immunity: A Recapitulation* (New York: Springer-Verlag, 1979). A picture of skin grafts on Dausset's own arm appears is his book, *Titres et travaux scientifiques* (Châtelaudren, France: Impr. de Châtelaudren, 1968).

17. This francophone friendship and collaboration is described in the article "*Transplantation Proceedings* Editors Decorated by President Jacques Chirac of France at the Elysée Palace in Paris (June 30, 2000)," *Transplantation Proceedings* 32, no. 8 (Dec. 2000): 2563–66.

18. Fritz Bach raised ethical concerns over his own skin graft/tissue-typing experiments using volunteer blood donors; see Fritz H. Bach and William A. Kisken, "Predictive Value of Results of Mixed Leukocyte Cultures for Skin Allograft Survival in Man," *Transplantation* 5, suppl. 4 (July 1967): 1046–52. Human volunteer studies were rapidly diminishing at this time, and Thomas Starzl decided to discontinue use of prisoners as kidney donors; see G. E. W. Wolstenholme and Maeve O'Connor, *Ethics in Medical Progress: With Special Reference to Transplantation* (London: Churchill, 1966), 76.

19. See the interesting account in William P. Longmire Jr., *Starting from Scratch: The Early History of the UCLA Department of Surgery* (Pasadena, CA: Castle Press, 1984).

20. Paul I. Terasaki, "Antibody Response to Homografts: II. Preliminary Studies of the Time Appearance of Lymphagglutinins after Homografting," *American Surgeon* 25 (1959): 896–99.

21. P. A. Gorer and P. O'Gorman, "The Cytotoxic Activity of Isoantibodies in Mice," *Transplantation Bulletin* 3 (1956): 142–43. Gorer admirably noticed Pappenheimer's thymocyte cytotoxicity test (developed in 1917 during the "lost era"), which used trypan blue exclusion; see chap. 8.

22. Paul I. Terasaki and John D. McClelland, "Microdroplet Assay of Human Serum Cytotoxins," *Nature* 204, no. 4962 (1964): 998–1000.

23. Paul I. Terasaki, D. L. Vredevoe, Ken A. Porter, M. R. Mickey, Thomas L. Marchioro, T. D. Faris, T. J. Herrmann, and Thomas E. Starzl, "Serotyping for Homotransplantation: V. Evaluation of a Matching System," *Transplantation* 4 (1966): 688–99. This bibliographical standardization of the papers from many units was an attempt to give cohesion to the studies coming from the dispersed tissue-typing community.

24. J. J. van Rood, A. van Leeuwen, and J. W. Bruning, "The Relevance of Leucocyte Antigens," *Journal of Clinical Pathology* 20 (1967): 504–12. The first use of HLA to type for platelet transfusion was by van Rood in 1964.

25. For these encouraging retrospective series, see Thomas E. Starzl, Thomas L. Marchioro, Paul I. Terasaki, Ken A. Porter, T. D. Faris, T. J. Herrmann, D. L. Vredevoe, M. P. Hutt, D. A. Ogden, and W. R. Waddell, "Chronic Survival after Renal Homotransplantation," *Annals of Surgery* 162, no. 4 (Oct. 1965): 749–85; and Ramon Patel, Max R. Mickey, and Paul I. Terasaki, "Serotyping for Homotransplantation—Analysis of Kidney Transplants from Unrelated Donors," *New England Journal of Medicine* 279, no. 10 (Sept. 5, 1968): 501–6. This paper established "tissue typing" as the standard term for the practice.

26. The improved, simpler methods of cell preservation included the use of Ficol-Hypaque to separate leukocytes, followed by DMSO/liquid nitrogen storage; see E. Cohen and A. W. Rowe, "A Frozen Leucocyte Bank," *Transfusion* 3, no. 5 (1963): 427.

27. This, the first prospective cadaveric donor transplantation study, is by J. J. van Rood, A. van Leeuwen, J. W. Bruning, and K. A. Porter, in *Advances in Transplantation*, ed. Jean Dausset, Jean Hamburger, and Georges Mathé (Copenhagen: Munksgaard, 1968), 213. See also R. Pearce, J. J. van Rood, A. van Leeuwen, and J. A. van der Does, "Leucocyte Typing and Kidney Transplantation in Unrelated Donor-Recipient Pairs," *Transplantation Proceedings* 1, no. 1 (Mar. 1969): 372–435. The St. Mary's Hospital cell reserve usually not only had spleen cells from the donors but also an unusual quantity of recipient cells, as recipient splenectomy was favored at this time.

28. Paul I. Terasaki, D. L. Vredevoe, M. R. Mickey, Ken A. Porter, Thomas L. Marchioro, T. D. Faris, and Thomas E. Starzl, "Serotyping for Homotransplantation: VII. Selection of Kidney Donors for Thirty-Two Recipients," *Annals of the New York Academy of Sciences* 129 (1966): 500–520.

29. For a review of the changing verdict on the value of tissue typing, see P. J. Morris, "Analyses of Histocompatibility—Cadaver Renal Transplantation," *Transplantation Proceedings* 3, no. 2 (June 1971): 1030–35.

30. Later reviewed in P. J. Morris, M. R. Mickey, D. P. Singal, and Paul I. Terasaki, "Serotyping for Homotransplantation: XXII. Specificity of Cytotoxic Antibodies after Renal Transplantation," *British Medical Journal* 1, no. 5646 (Mar. 22, 1969): 758–59. On a closed-circuit television demonstration of kidney transplantation being performed by Goodwin in 1964, a memorable, immediate immunological failure occurred.

31. F. Kissmeyer-Nielsen, Steen Olsen, V. P. Peterson, and O. Fjeldborg, "Hyperacute Rejection of Kidney Allografts, Associated with Pre-Existing Humoral Antibodies against Donor Cells," *The Lancet* 288, no. 7465 (1966): 662–65, a paper initially rejected by the referee.

32. There is a civilized priority dispute over this discovery; see Thomas E. Starzl, *The Puzzle People: Memoirs of a Transplant Surgeon* (Pittsburgh: University of Pittsburgh Press, 1992), 123, and the relevant papers, Paul I. Terasaki, Thomas L. Marchioro, and Thomas E. Starzl, "Serotyping of Human Lymphocyte Antigens," in *Histocompatibility Testing* (Washington, DC: National Academy of Sciences, 1965), 83–96; Ramon Patel and Paul I. Terasaki, "Significance of the Positive Crossmatch Test in Kidney Transplantation," *New England Journal of Medicine* 280, no. 14 (Apr. 3, 1969): 735–39; and G. Melville Williams, David M. Hume, R. Page Hudson, Peter J. Morris, Kyoichi Kano, and Felix Milgrom, "Hyperacute Renal-Homograft Rejection in Man," *New England Journal of Medicine* 279, no. 12 (Sept. 19, 1968): 611–18. For further comment on recognition of the early cases of hyperacute rejection, see Paul Terasaki, "1996 Medawar Prize Lecture," *Transplantation Proceedings* 29, no. 1 (Feb. 1997): 33–38.

33. Fritz H. Bach, "D. Bernard Amos: Humanist, Scientist and Friend," *Human Immunology* 57, no. 1

(Sept. 15, 1997): 51–53. Dausset says more dramatically that "the results were so discordant that they were destroyed [by Ceppellini]." Dausset in Terasaki, *History of HLA*, 3. A publication did result, however—*Histocompatibility Testing: A Report of a Conference and Workshop Sponsored by the Division of Medical Sciences, National Academy of Sciences, National Research Council, 7–12 June, 1964* (Washington, DC: National Academy of Sciences, 1965). For Ceppellini's role at this time, see Fritz H. Bach, "Ruggero Ceppellini (1917–1988)," *Immunology Today* 9, no. 11 (1988): 335–37. Earlier in the century, using similar workshops, there were international efforts to standardize the Wasserman Test for syphilis.

34. Batchelor's account in Terasaki, *History of Transplantation*, 181.

35. Ramon Patel, Richard Glassock, and Paul I. Terasaki, "Serotyping for Homotransplantation: XIX. Experience with an Interhospital Scheme of Cadaver-Kidney Sharing and Tissue Typing," *Journal of the American Medical Association* 207, no. 7 (1969): 1319–24.

36. See Benjamin A. Bradley, ed., *U.K. Transplant Service Review, 1982: Ten Years of Service to Transplantation* (Bristol: UK Transplant Service, 1982).

37. In 1987, when longer cold times allowed less urgent transfers and matching was less highly regarded, the use of the St. John Air Ambulance Wing ceased. By this time, the air wing had been flying surgeons to multi-organ donations, and after some incidents, insurance difficulties had arisen and commercial alternatives had to be used. For Calne's aerial brushes with death, see Roy Calne, *The Ultimate Gift* (London: Headline, 1998), 105. For Starzl's near-misses, see Starzl, *Puzzle People*, 262, which also describes the deaths of two pilots during training with the company providing donor flights.

38. See the excellent reviews by R. G. W. Johnson, "Kidney Perfusion by Continuous Perfusion," in *Organ Preservation: Basic and Applied Aspects*, ed. David E. Pegg, Ib. A. Jacobsen, and N. A. Halasz (Hingham, MA: MTP Press, 1982); and H.-G. Zimmer, "Perfusion of Isolated Organs and the First Heart-Lung Machine," *Canadian Journal of Cardiology* 17, no. 1 (Sept. 2001): 963–69.

39. Soviet surgeons had been involved in such perfusion work for many years, with the stimulus coming from Vladimir Filatov's claim that preserved organs had stimulating properties when grafted. The Soviet perfusion/refrigeration apparatus was described in

Anastasy Lapchinsky's paper at the 1960 New York Academy of Sciences meeting.

40. See the pioneering work by Arthur Sicular and Francis D. Moore, "The Postmortem Survival of Tissues," *Journal of Surgical Research* 1, no. 1 (1961): 9–22. One of many similar tests is reported in Paul I. Terasaki, Donald C. Martin, and R. B. Smith, "A Rapid Metabolism Test to Screen Cadaver Kidneys for Transplantation," *Transplantation* 5, no. 1 (Jan. 1967): 76–78.

41. J. Englebert Dunphy's Department of Surgery at San Francisco had considerable influence in American clinical transplantation. Dunphy trained and encouraged surgeons Belzer, Samuel Kountz, and John S. Najarian, and they had Rose Payne, at Stanford, as tissue typer. Najarian moved to Minneapolis in 1967, Kountz went to New York in 1972, and Belzer joined the University of Wisconsin in 1974. Oscar Salvatierra joined Dunphy in 1972.

42. Folkert O. Belzer, B. Sterry Ashby, Paul F. Gulyassy, and Malcolm Powell, "Successful Seventeen-Hour Preservation and Transplantation of Human-Cadaver Kidney," *New England Journal of Medicine* 278, no. 11 (Mar. 14, 1968): 608–10.

43. Surgical practice soon abandoned both the "natural" pulsatile version of the heart-lung machines used in cardiac surgery and the hyperbaric oxygen treatment tanks for treating various ills at this time.

44. Folkert O. Belzer, B. Sterry Ashby, and J. Englebert Dunphy, "24-Hour and 72-Hour Preservation of Canine Kidneys," *The Lancet* 290, no. 7515 (Sept. 9, 1967): 536–39. The British company Vickers made these machines, and the other companies involved were Travenol, Van Waters, and Gambro.

45. Starzl, *Puzzle People*, 151–53, describes this surprising public interest in perfusion machines. The relevant paper is Lawrence Brettschneider, Pierre M. Daloze, Claude Huguet, Kenneth A. Porter, Carl G. Groth, Noboru Kashiwagi, David E. Hutchison, and Thomas E. Starzl, "The Use of Combined Preservation Techniques for Extended Storage of Orthotopic Liver Homografts," *Surgery, Gynecology & Obstetrics* 126 (Feb. 1968): 263–74.

46. R. Keeler, J. Swinney, R. M. R. Taylor, and P. R. Uldall, "The Problem of Renal Preservation," *British Journal of Urology* 38, no. 6 (1966): 653–56. The Newcastle group experimented, without success, with subzero organ storage.

47. Potassium cardioplegia was abandoned in cardiac surgery in the late 1950s in favor of other methods,

but it made a return with an improved potassium-rich "intracellular" perfusion fluid, devised in 1975 by Hans Bretschneider of Göttingen (no relation to Larry Brettschneider); see W. A. Gay Jr., "Potassium-Induced Cardioplegia: Evolution and Present Status," *Annals of Thoracic Surgery* 48, no. 3 (Sept. 1989): 441–43.

48. B. L. Lindström, "Lars-Erik Gelin: In Memoriam," *Scandinavian Journal of Urology and Nephrology* (Supplement) 64 (1981): 1–5.

49. G. M. Collins, Maria Bravo-Shugarman, and Paul I. Terasaki, "Kidney Preservation for Transport," *The Lancet* 294, no. 7632 (Dec. 6, 1969): 1219–22. Similar findings were reported at this time in D. C. Martin, G. A. Smith, and D. O. Fareed, "Experimental Renal Preservation," *Surgical Forum* 20 (1969): 529–31.

50. Terasaki, *History of HLA*, 519.

51. K. Dreikorn, J. H. Horsch, and L. Röhl, "48- to 96-Hour Preservation of Canine Kidneys by Initial Perfusion and Hypothermic Storage Using the Euro-Collins Solution," *European Urology* 6, no. 4 (1980): 221–24. For the later UW solution, see Jan A. Wahlberg, Robert Love, Lars Landegaard, James H. Southard, and Folkert O. Belzer, "72-Hour Preservation of the Canine Pancreas," *Transplantation* 43, no. 1 (Jan. 1987): 5–7; Neville V. Jamieson, Ralf Sundberg, Susanne Lindell, Kerstin Claesson, Jon Moen, Paul K. Vreugdenhil, G. D. Derek, James H. Southard, and Folkert O. Belzer, "Preservation of the Canine Liver for 24–48 Hours Using Simple Cold Storage with UW Solution," *Transplantation* 46, no. 4 (Oct. 1988): 517–22; and Robert M. Hoffman, Robert J. Stratta, Anthony M. D'Alessandro, Hans W. Solunger, Munci Kalayoglu, John D. Pirsch, James H. Southard, and Folkert O. Belzer, "Combined Cold Storage-Perfusion Preservation with a New Synthetic Perfusate," *Transplantation* 47, no. 1 (Jan. 1989): 32–37.

52. Roy Yorke Calne, H. J. O. White, D. E. Yoffa, R. M. Binns, R. R. Maginn, R. M. Herbertson, P. R. Millard, V. P. Molina, and D. R. Davis, "Prolonged Survival of Liver Transplants in the Pig," *British Medical Journal* 4, no. 5580 (Dec. 16, 1967): 645–48.

53. Roy Yorke Calne, R. A. Sells, J. R. Pena, D. R. Davis, P. R. Millard, B. M. Herbertson, R. M. Binns, and D. A. L. Davies, "Induction of Immunological Tolerance by Porcine Liver Allografts," *Nature* 223, no. 5205 (1969): 472–76.

54. The rise of microsurgery is dealt with in Harry J. Buncke, "Microsurgery—Retrospective," *Clinics in*

Plastic Surgery 13, no. 2 (Apr. 1986): 315–18; and in Susumu Tamai, "History of Microsurgery—From the Beginning until the End of the 1970s," *Microsurgery* 14, no. 1 (1993): 6–13. The main events in its use in human cases are listed in *Microsurgery* 17 (1996): 582–87. Re-implantation of human digits was first reported in 1963 by Zhong Wei Chen; see his obituary in *British Medical Journal* 328, no. 7446 (Apr. 24, 2004): 1019. For the emergence of the operating microscope, see Carl-Olof Nylén, "The Otomicroscope and Microsurgery, 1921–1971," *Acta Otolaryngologica* 73, no. 6 (June 1972): 453–54; and Timothy C. Kriss and Vesna Martich Kriss, "History of the Operating Microscope: From Magnifying Glass to Microneurosurgery," *Neurosurgery* 42, no. 4 (1998): 899–907. The new methods in microsurgery are detailed in the group of papers by Carton, Raton, and others in *Surgical Forum* 11 (1960): 238–43. Calne had tried the stent methods in his unsuccessful rat work before starting his classic 1960 work on 6-MP in dog kidney grafting. C. A. Carton, L. A. Kessler, B. Seidenberg, and E. S. Hurwitt, "Experimental Studies in the Surgery of Small Blood Vessels: IV. Nonsuture Anastomosis of Arteries and Veins, Using Flanged Ring Prostheses and Plastic Adhesive," *Surgical Forum* 11 (1960): 238–39; R. S. Ratan, M. Leon, J. B. Lovette, B. S. Levowitz, G. J. Magovern, and E. M. Kent, "Modified Nonsuture Anastomosis of Coronary Artery and Internal Mammary Artery in Dogs," *Surgical Forum* 11 (1960): 239–41; G. P. Holt and F. J. Lewis, "A New Technique for End-to-End Anastomosis of Small Arteries," *Surgical Forum* 11 (1960): 242–43.

55. J. H. Jacobsen and E. L. Suarez, "Microsurgery in the Anastomosis of Small Vessels," *Surgical Forum* 11 (1960): 243–45.

56. Reviewed later in Sun Lee, "An Improved Technique of Renal Transplantation in the Rat," *Surgery* 61, no. 5 (1967): 771–73. Lee's pioneering paper in *Surgery* in 1961 was initially turned down as "unoriginal."

57. Charles P. Abbott, Edward S. Lindsey, Oscar Creech Jr., and Charles W. DeWitt, "A Technique for Heart Transplantation in the Rat," *Archives of Surgery* 89, no. 4 (Oct. 1964): 645–52.

58. For an account of small vessel surgery, see also Sun Lee, David H. Frank, and Sang Y. Choi, "Historical Review of Small and Microvascular Vessel Surgery," *Annals of Plastic Surgery* 11, no. 1 (July 1983): 53–62; and Sun Lee, "Historical Significance on Rat Organ Transplantation," *Microsurgery* 11, no. 2 (1990): 115–21. For information on the emergence of

fine sutures, see Wendell L. Hughes, "The Evolution of Ophthalmic Sutures," *Annals of Plastic Surgery* 6, no. 1 (Jan. 1981): 48–65. See also Sun Lee and S. J. Li, "Clinical and Experimental Microsurgery in China: An Historical Note," *Journal of Microsurgery* 3, no. 3 (1982): 180–83. There is a tribute to Sun Lee by Robert Zhong in *Microsurgery* 23, no. 5 (Oct. 2003): 412–13. Lee later worked at the Scripps Clinic in southern California.

59. AS to AS2 rat kidney grafts showed spontaneous acceptance across this strong combination, and when, in 1972, the cogenic/co-isogenic mice Snell had developed to differ by only one H2 antigen became available for routine use, these mice also showed unexpected graft behavior never encountered in the outbred situation.

60. Frank P. Stuart, Tatsuo Saitoh, and Frank W. Fitch, "Rejection of Renal Allografts: Specific Immunologic Suppression," *Science* 160 (June 28, 1968): 1463–65; M. E. French and J. R. Batchelor, "Immunological Enhancement of Rat Kidney Grafts," *The Lancet* 294, no. 7630 (Nov. 22, 1969): 1103–6.

61. For attempts at human organ graft enhancement, see Leslie Brent, "Tolerance and Enhancement in Organ Transplantation," *Transplantation Proceedings* 4, no. 3 (Sept. 1972): 363–68.

62. Nicholas L. Tilney and Joseph E. Murray, "Thoracic Duct Fistula in Human Being Renal Transplantation," *Surgical Forum* 17 (1966): 234–36; C. Franksson and R. Blomstrand, "Drainage of the Thoracic Lymph Duct during Homologous Kidney Transplantation in Man," *Scandinavian Journal of Urology and Nephrology* 1 (1967): 123–31. See also Takao Sonoda, Minato Takaha, and Takamitsu Kusunoki, "Prolonged Thoracic Duct Drainage," *Archives of Surgery* 93, no. 5 (1966): 831–33.

63. A. M. Cruickshank, "Antilymphocytic Serum," *British Journal of Experimental Pathology* 22 (1941): 126–36. Cruickshank followed the lead of W. B. Chew and John S. Lawrence "Antilymphocytic Serum," *Journal of Immunology* 33. no. 4 (1937): 271–78. They in turn credited the strategy to Metchnikoff and Simon Flexner in the "lost era" of transplantation immunology. The full story of antilymphocyte sera remains to be told, but, in the meantime, there is the hard-to-find C. Nava and H. O'Kane, "Antilymphocytic Serum: Historical Review," *Revista de Investigación Clínica* 26, no. 1 (Jan.–Mar. 1974): 77–92; and Leslie Brent, *A History of Transplantation Immunology* (London: Academic Press, 1997), 247–52.

64. Alexander A. Bogomolets, "Antireticular Cytotoxic Serum," *Annual Review of Soviet Medicine* 1 (1943): 101–12; there is a short biography of Bogomolets in *Annual Review of Soviet Medicine* 1 (1943–1944): 173–75. The preparation of the serum is described by P. D. Marchuk in scholarly detail in *Annual Review of Soviet Medicine* 1 (1943–1944): 113–29. For an account of similar multipurpose sera at the time, see Ilana Löwy, "The Terrain Is All," in *Greater Than the Parts: Holism in Biomedicine, 1920–1950*, ed. Christopher Lawrence and George Weisz (New York: Oxford University Press, 1998), 257–82.

65. Woodruff gives an account of his antilymphocyte serum research from 1959 onward in his text, *The Transplantation of Tissues and Organs* (Springfield, IL: Thomas, 1960), 100, and in his autobiography, *Nothing Venture Nothing Win* (Edinburgh: Scottish Academic Press, 1996). The formal papers are Michael F. A. Woodruff and N. F. Anderson, "The Effect of Lymphocyte Depletion by Thoracic Duct Fistula and Administration of Antilymphocytic Serum on the Survival of Skin Homografts in Rats," *Annals of the New York Academy of Sciences* 120 (1964): 119–28, earlier announced in *Nature* 200, no. 4907 (1963): 702. The whole serum was heat treated to remove complement and absorbed with red cells to remove the anti–red cell antibodies also generated.

66. Byron H. Waksman, Simone Arbouys, and Barry G. Arnason, "The Use of Specific 'Lymphocyte' Antisera to Inhibit Hypersensitivity Reactions of the 'Delayed' Type," *Journal of Experimental Medicine* 114, no. 6 (Dec. 1961): 997–1022.

67. Anthony P. Monaco, Mary L. Wood, and Paul S. Russell, "Studies on Heterologous Anti-Lymphocyte Serum in Mice: III. Immunologic Tolerance and Chimerism Produced Across the H-2 Locus with Adult Thymectomy and Anti-Lymphocyte Serum," *Annals of the New York Academy of Sciences* 129 (1966): 190–209.

68. R. H. Levey and Peter B. Medawar, "Some Experiments on the Action of Antilymphoid Antisera," *Annals of the New York Academy of Sciences* 129 (1966): 164–77; and "Nature and Mode of Action of Antilymphocytic Antiserum," *Proceedings of the National Academy of Sciences* 56, no. 4 (1966): 1130–37. See also E. M. Lance and Peter B. Medawar, "Quantitative Studies on Tissue Transplantation Immunity: IX. Induction of Tolerance with Antilymphocytic Serum," *Proceedings of the Royal Society*, series B, 173, no. 1033 (July 22, 1969): 447–73. The researchers emphasized that a simple two-pulse immunization, plus the usual

absorptions, was not only adequate but optimal and that the usual "more is better" approach that dictated use of multiple immunizations in conventional vaccine production was counterproductive. For the wide use of antilymphocyte serum in experimental work, see the proceedings of the CIBA conference, arranged with unusual urgency, in G. E. W. Wolstenholme and Maeve O'Connor, eds., *Anti-Lymphocytic Serum* (London: Churchill, 1967).

69. E. M. Lance and Peter B. Medawar, "Survival of Skin Heterografts under Treatment with Antilymphocytic Serum," *The Lancet* 291, no. 7553 (June 1, 1968): 1174–76. This was one of the few occasions on which Medawar agreed to quick publication of his work.

70. The 1967 Santa Barbara conference was the first meeting in the style of the regular transplantation conferences as organized later by the Transplantation Society.

71. Thomas E. Starzl, Thomas L. Marchioro, Ken A. Porter, Y. Iwasaki, and G. J. Cerilli, "The Use of Heterologous Antilymphoid Agents in Canine Renal and Liver Homotransplantation and in Human Renal Homotransplantation," *Surgery, Gynecology & Obstetrics* 124, no. 2 (Feb. 1967): 301–18.

72. John S. Najarian, Richard L. Simmons, Henry Gewurz, Allan Moberg, Frederick Merkel, and George E. Moore, "Anti-Serum to Cultured Human Lymphoblasts: Preparation, Purification and Immunosuppressive Properties in Man," *Annals of Surgery* 170, no. 4 (1969): 617–32. The cell line used came from George Moore at Roswell Park. He tested his sera on volunteer patients with multiple sclerosis. The Food and Drug Administration disliked his homemade medication, but Najarian survived the legal action.

73. Support for the Primate Center came from its work on bone marrow transplantation and the general assumption that, in the future, human xenografting would use monkey organs. Accordingly, there was great interest in primate blood grouping and tis-

sue typing; see the symposium on "Transplantation Genetics of Primates," *Transplantation Proceedings* 4 (1972): 1–121.

74. A full account of the work of the ponderous "Working Party on Antihuman Lymphocyte Serum" is found in file FD 7/1237 of the UK Public Record Office. The much-delayed report on the MRC trial appeared in "Medical Research Council Trial of Antilymphocyte Globulin in Renal Transplantation: A Multicenter Randomized Double-Blind Placebo Controlled Clinical Investigation," *Transplantation* 35, no. 6 (June 1983): 539–45.

75. When Calne was facing local opposition to his first liver graft attempt, he had the support of Francis Moore. Moore was unexpectedly visiting Cambridge that day, and he assisted Calne with the successful operation; see Calne, *Ultimate Gift*, 96.

76. At this time, Starzl also described successful liver transplantation for two patients with Wilson's disease. See also Roy Yorke Calne, "Observations on Experimental and Clinical Liver Transplantation," *Transplantation Proceedings* 4, no. 4 (Dec. 1972): 773–79.

77. J. D. N. Nabarro, "Selection of Patients for Haemodialysis: Who Best to Make the Choice?" *British Medical Journal* 1, no. 5540 (Mar. 11, 1967): 622; S. C. Farrow, D. J. Fisher, and D. B. Johnson, "Dialysis and Transplantation: The National Picture over the Next Five Years," *British Medical Journal* 3, no. 5828 (Sept. 16, 1972): 686–90.

78. Starzl, *Puzzle People*, 92.

79. "The Ninth Report of the Human Renal Transplant Registry," *Journal of the American Medical Association* 220, no. 2 (1972): 253–60. Nicholas Tilney dates the slow change of policy in Boston to the late 1960s; see Joseph E. Murray, Nicholas L. Tilney, and R. E. Wilson, "Renal Transplantation: A Twenty-Five Year Experience," *Annals of Plastic Surgery* 184 (1976): 565–73.

16. Brain Death and the "Year of the Heart"

1. On the growth of intensive care, see "NIH Workshop on Withholding and Withdrawing Mechanical Ventilation," *American Review of Respiratory Disease* 140, no. 2 (1989): supplement, 1–24.

2. Other prominent issues in medical ethics at this time included the debate on how to allocate scarce dialysis resources to patients and human experimentation scandals. George Miller's *Moral and Ethical Im-*

plications of Human Organ Transplants (Springfield, IL: Thomas, 1971) appears to be the first of many in this genre. For good general historical accounts of medical ethics, see David J. Rothman, *Strangers at the Bedside: A History of How Law and Bioethics Transformed Medical Decision Making* (New York: Basic Books, 1991); and M. L. Tina Stevens, *Bioethics in America: Origins and Cultural Politics* (Baltimore: Johns Hopkins University Press, 2000).

3. See Pius XII, "The Prolongation of Life: Allocution to the International Congress of Anesthesiologists (Nov. 24, 1957)," *The Pope Speaks* 4, no. 4 (1958): 393–98.

4. For the 1960s literature on legal questions relating to declaration of death, see Gary S. Belkin, "Brain Death and the Historical Understanding of Bioethics," *Journal of History of Medicine and Allied Sciences* 58, no. 3 (2003): 325–61. For occasional legal disputes involving questions of the order of death in inheritance cases, see N. P. Jeddeloh, "The Uniform Anatomical Gift Act and a Statutory Definition of Death," *Transplantation Proceedings* 8, no. 2, suppl. 1 (June 1976): 245–49.

5. Hannibal Hamlin, "Life or Death by EEG," *Journal of the American Medical Association* 190, no. 2 (Oct. 12, 1964): 121.

6. James D. Hardy, Carlos M. Chavez, Fred D. Kurrus, William A. Neely, Sadan Eraslan, M. Don Turner, Leonard W. Fabian, and Thaddeus D. Labecki, "Heart Transplantation in Man: Developmental Studies and Report of a Case," *Journal of the American Medical Association* 188, no. 13 (June 29, 1964): 1132–40, 1133.

7. In Britain in 1963, news of heart-beating donations at Newcastle and Leeds caused considerable government concern. The matter had not reached the media, but a civil servant noted, "My misgivings about this case are in no way relieved. Prudence was lacking in the surgeon's action." File MH 150/43.7, UK Public Record Office. The events were mentioned in the *Times* (London), July 26, 1963, but, astonishingly, it was only legal commentators who pursued the issue; see "When Do We Die?" *Medico-Legal Journal* 31 (1963): 195–96; and *Medicine, Science and the Law* 4 (1964): 59.

8. G. E. W. Wolstenholme and Maeve O'Connor, eds., *Ethics in Medical Progress: With Special Reference to Transplantation* (London: Churchill, 1966). The resulting book is now highly regarded as a landmark in the development of medical ethics and was reprinted as *Law and Ethics of Transplantation* (London: Churchill, 1968).

9. Guy Alexandre described this 1963 ventilator-supported donation in Wolstenholme and O'Connor, *Ethics in Medical Progress*. The case now has celebrity in the world of neurology; see Calixto Machado, "Historical Neurology—The First Organ Transplant from a Brain-Dead Donor," *Neurology* 64, no. 11 (2005): 1938–42; and "Correspondence—Reply from the Author: The First Organ Transplant from a Brain-Dead Donor," *Neurology* 66, no. 3 (2006): 460–61. The "heart-beating" donations at Newcastle and Leeds may have occurred some weeks before the Belgian brain-dead donation case.

10. Quoted in Wolstenholme and O'Connor, *Ethics in Medical Progress*, 157. See also Starzl's opposition to brain-dead, heart-beating donations in the "Colloquium on Ethical Dilemmas from Medical Advances," *Annals of Internal Medicine* 67 (1967): supplement 7, 36, an "ethics" meeting organized by the American College of Physicians.

11. Norman E. Shumway, William W. Angell, and Robert D. Wuerflein, "Progress in Transplantation of the Heart," *Transplantation* 5, suppl. 4 (July 1967): 900–903; see also *Journal of the American Medical Association* 202 (1967): 31–32. Both articles show reluctance to consider heart-beating donation. For an earlier view, see Norman E. Shumway, "Transplantation of the Heart," *Surgery, Gynecology & Obstetrics* 117 (1963): 361–62.

12. See Starzl's "A Clinician's Point of View," in Wolstenholme and O'Connor, *Ethics in Medical Progress*, 32–42.

13. This account is taken mainly from Belkin, "Brain Death and the Historical Understanding of Bioethics," and from the excellent study of Henry Beecher's personal papers, held in Boston's Countway Library, in Vincent J. Kopp, "Henry Knowles Beecher and the Redefinition of Death," *Bulletin of Anesthesia History* 15, no. 4 (Oct. 1997): 6–9. See also Gary Belkin, "Death before Dying: Mind, Body, Ethics and the Harvard Brain Death Committee" (PhD thesis, Harvard University, 2000). Other assessments of Beecher's varied career, which included initiating the debate on informed consent, are in J. S. Gravenstein, "Henry K. Beecher: The Introduction of Anaesthesia into the University," *Anesthesiology* 88, no. 1 (Jan. 1998): 245–53; the reply by Douglas Bacon, "Henry K. Beecher, M.D.: An Historical Perspective?" *Anesthesiology* 89, no. 3 (Sept. 1998): 792–93; Vincent J. Kopp, "Henry Knowles Beecher and the Development of Informed Consent in Anesthesia," *Anesthesiology* 90, no. 6 (June 1999): 1756–65; and John B. Bunker, "Henry K. Beecher," in *The Genesis of Contemporary American Anesthesiology*, ed. Perry P. Volpitto and Leroy D. Vandam (Springfield, IL: Thomas, 1982), 105–19.

14. Kopp, "Henry Knowles Beecher and the Redefinition of Death," 6.

15. Ibid.

16. Murray's stance on use of heart-beating donation at the time is not clear: his published memoirs are silent on the issue, and, in a lecture in June 1968, his close surgical senior colleague Francis D. Moore indicated that Murray was hostile to using "brain death" criteria; see Francis D. Moore, "Medical Responsibility for the Prolongation of Life," *Journal of the American Medical Association* 206, no. 2 (Oct. 7, 1968): 384–86. Murray left transplantation work soon afterward, and it may be that he and others at Brigham Hospital were not enthusiastic about heart-beating donation.

17. Kopp, "Henry Knowles Beecher and the Redefinition of Death," 8.

18. The *JAMA* Ad Hoc Committee report had only one reference—Pius XII's address to the International Congress of Anesthesiologists, "The Prolongation of Life," possibly inserted at the suggestion of Joseph Murray, a devout Catholic.

19. That the transplanters were the activists in advocating for the brain death criteria is strongly believed by some historians: see the flawed analysis in Margaret M. Lock, *Twice Dead: Organ Transplants and the Reinvention of Death* (Berkeley: University of California Press, 2002).

20. Christiaan Neethling Barnard, "The Operation: A Human Cardiac Transplant; An Interim Report of a Successful Operation Performed at Groote Schuur Hospital, Cape Town," *South African Medical Journal* 41, no. 48 (Dec. 30, 1967): 1271–74. In the 1950s, South Africa had been one of the few countries to reform its laws regarding donor tissue. See On the Postmortem Examination and Removal of Human Tissue Act (30 of 1952); for comment, see T. W. Price, "Legal Rights and Duties in Regard to Dead Bodies, Post-Mortems, and Dissections," *South African Law Journal* 68 (1951): 403–41.

21. Barnard had published four papers on transplantation prior to his heart transplant, including J. R. W. Ackermann and Christiaan Neethling Barnard, "Successful Storage of Kidneys," *British Journal of Surgery* 53, no. 6 (1966): 525–32. Following his heart transplants, he wrote little and did not attend surgical conferences.

22. Richard R. Lower and Norman E. Shumway, "Studies on Orthotopic Homotransplantation of the Canine Heart," *Surgical Forum* 11 (1960): 18–19.

23. For an account of the Palo Alto work, see Eugene Dong, Norman E. Shumway, and Richard R. Lower, "A Heart Transplant Narrative: The Earliest Years,"

in *History of Transplantation: Thirty-Five Recollections,* ed. Paul I. Terasaki (Los Angeles: UCLA Tissue Typing Laboratory, 1991). Shumway had left Minnesota in 1957 and, after a brief period of private practice, joined the academic staff at Stanford in 1959.

24. See E. M. Tansey and Lois A. Reynolds, eds., *Early Heart Transplant Surgery in the UK: Witness Seminar Transcript,* vol. 3 of *Wellcome Witnesses to Twentieth Century Medicine* (London: Wellcome Trust, 1999). Shumway pointed out that the London surgeons M. H. Cass and R. Brock developed the important atrial cuff technique.

25. The early experimental heart transplantation experience was described at the time in D. K. C. Cooper, "Transplantation of the Heart and Both Lungs: I. Historical Review," *Thorax* 24, no. 4 (July 1969): 383–98; and D. K. C. Cooper, "Experimental Development of Cardiac Transplantation," *British Medical Journal* 4, no. 5624 (Oct. 19, 1968): 174–81. Later reviews are S. L. Lansman, M. A. Ergin, and R. B. Griepp, "The History of Heart and Heart-Lung Transplantation," *Cardiovascular Clinics* 20, no. 2 (1990): 3–19; and C. McGregor, "Evolution of Heart Transplantation," *Cardiology Clinics* 8, no. 1 (1990): 3–10. For the development of combined heart-lung transplantation, see S. W. Jamieson, "Heart-Lung Transplantation," in *Progress in Transplantation,* vol. 2, ed. Peter J. Morris and Nicholas L. Tilney (Edinburgh: Churchill Livingstone, 1985), 147–66. See also Albert Brest, ed., *Heart Substitutes: Mechanical and Transplant* (Springfield, IL: Thomas, 1966). The drama and controversy resulting from the first human heart transplants in the late 1960s concealed the existence of the respectable and careful experimental work done earlier.

26. For an account of his times, see James D. Hardy, "Human Organ Replacement—Then and Now," *Transactions and Studies of the College of Physicians of Philadelphia* 7, no. 3 (1985): 159–76. Hardy's memoirs are *The World of Surgery, 1945–1985: Memoirs of One Participant* (Philadelphia: University of Pennsylvania Press, 1986).

27. The Groote Schuur Hospital's cardiac clinic was a large and innovative one, led by the talented, supportive, and Hammersmith-trained Maurice Nellen; for his role, see his obituary in the *Daily Telegraph* (London), August 31, 2000.

28. In this historic case, there had been time for Barnard to tissue-type the donor and recipient, and, by chance, there was a good match. A supply of anti-lymphocyte globulin was obtained from Denver and added to the conventional immunosuppression.

29. Earlier, in June 1966, Kantrowitz had sought to use the heart from a dying anencephalic baby, but a hospital committee decided against use of "heart-beating donation" in this case, in spite of the absence of most of the brain. They ruled that any heart donation should be delayed until conventional death, that is, after the heart stopped beating. For a detailed retrospective account of his involvement at the time, see Adrian Kantrowitz, "America's First Human Heart Transplantation: The Concept, the Planning, and the Furor," *ASAIO Journal* 44, no. 4 (1998): 244–52.

30. The excellent result achieved with Blaiberg's graft can be attributed to good luck of all kinds, including a close tissue match. Philip Blaiberg's *Looking at My Heart* (New York: Stein and Day, 1968) was the first of the genre of personal accounts by heart transplant recipients. Publishers elsewhere welcomed similar heart transplant patients' accounts, and science-fiction writers found new themes in various aspects of the transplant process.

31. The political nuances of Barnard's operation are listed in a very hostile briefing from the British ambassador in South Africa to the Foreign Office, FCO 25/721, UK Public Record Office. But the Soviet Union's *Pravda*, after a swipe at South Africa, conceded that creative forces could still exist in reactionary lands.

32. Joseph Murray's rueful explanation of the intense public interest in heart transplants was that "they don't put kidneys on Valentine's Day cards." For a general discussion of cultural attitudes about the heart, see Milad Doueihi, *A Perverse History of the Human Heart* (Cambridge, MA: Harvard University Press, 1997).

33. Mondale proposed a "Commission on Health, Science, and Society" that would have oversight in ethical, social, and political matters related to medical care. This commission was to include lay persons and was generally welcomed, except by U.S. doctors' organizations. Barnard's ebullient remarks are quoted in Rothman, *Strangers at the Bedside*, 172.

34. For popular accounts of the high-profile Texas heart surgeons and their involvement in cardiac replacement, see Harry Minetree, *Cooley: The Career of a Great Heart Surgeon* (New York: Harper's Magazine Press, 1973); Thomas Thompson, *Hearts: Of Surgeons and Transplants, Miracles and Disasters along the Cardiac Frontier* (New York: McCall, 1971) and published in Britain as *Hearts: DeBakey and Cooley, Surgeons Extraordinary* (London: Joseph, 1972); Denton A. Cooley, *Reflections and Observations* (Austin, TX: Eakin Press,

1984); and Tony Stark, *Knife to the Heart: The Story of Transplant Surgery* (London: Macmillan, 1996).

35. Cooley's star patient was Everett Thomas, and his case is closely described in Jürgen Thorwald, *The Patients* (New York: Harcourt Brace Jovanovich, 1972), 294.

36. For a vivid account of the doomed patients camped out in the neighborhood of the hospital at Houston, see Thompson, *Hearts*, 169.

37. Roy Calne recalled that "the cardiac surgeons denied the existence of it [rejection]. They imagined all they needed to do was make one phone call to people doing kidney grafting, or not even bother with that." Quoted from the transcript of *The History of Surgery*, a BBC series, held in the Wellcome Archives for Contemporary Medicine, London. However, the Wellcome Witness account of the London heart transplants (Tansey and Reynolds, *Early Heart Transplant Surgery in the UK*) suggests instead that, rather than too little advice in these two cases, there were too many individuals, including scientists, involved in a complex management group. The sophisticated immunological analysis and exotic explanations of the chest complications seem to have blinded the surgeons to the recognition of common, treatable, serious events in these cases, notably pulmonary emboli.

38. For the controversial first use of the artificial heart, see Minetree, *Cooley;* and Thompson, *Hearts*. There is insider detail in Nicholas L. Tilney, *Transplant: From Myth to Reality* (New Haven, CT: Yale University Press, 2003).

39. Moore's strange rebuke was published in an article based on his address to the American Medical Association in June 1968; see Francis D. Moore, "Medical Responsibility for the Prolongation of Life," *Journal of the American Medical Association* 206, no. 2 (Oct. 7, 1968): 384–86.

40. File MH 150/413 and GC/238/8 and 9, UK Public Record Office. Detailed reminiscences of the day-by-day events surrounding the London heart transplants are found in Tansey and Reynolds, *Early Heart Transplant Surgery in the UK*. There is also considerable detail in Ayesha Nathoo, *Hearts Exposed: Transplants and the Media in 1960s Britain* (Basingstoke: Palgrave Macmillan, 2009). For one journalist's experience of these times, see R. Bedford, "Medicine and the Media: The Need to Strengthen the Bridge," *Journal of the Royal College of Physicians of London* 13, no. 1 (Jan. 1979): 7–14. Some further details are found in Tilney, *Transplant*, 173–74.

41. For these events, see Sara J. Shumway and Norman E. Shumway, *Thoracic Transplantation* (Cambridge, MA: Blackwell Science, 1995), chap. 1. In liver transplantation donation, Starzl was, by 1969, edging toward use of heart-beating donation, after initial opposition. As in many other centers, the change was incremental, rather than sudden, and these gradual steps are described in Thomas E. Starzl and Charles W. Putnam, *Experience in Hepatic Transplantation* (Philadelphia: Saunders, 1969), 16–21.

42. The ever-present fear of premature burial is described in Jan Bondeson, *Buried Alive: The Terrifying History of Our Most Primal Fear* (New York: Norton, 2001). Easily the earliest airing of the matter is the substantial book by Jacques Winslow, *The Uncertainty of the Signs of Death, and the Danger of Precipitate Interments and Dissections, Demonstrated* (London, 1746). For a full bibliography of this human preoccupation, see Jan Bondeson, *A Cabinet of Medical Curiosities* (Ithaca, NY: Cornell University Press, 1997), 247. For a scholarly analysis, see both T. K. Marshall, "Premature Burial," *Medico-Legal Journal* 35 (1967): 14–24; and Marc Alexander, "'The Rigid Embrace of the Narrow House': Premature Burial and the Signs of Death," *Hastings Center Reports* 10, no. 3 (June 1980): 25–31. See also J. P. Payne, "On the Resuscitation of the Apparently Dead," *Annals of the Royal College of Surgeons* 45, no. 2 (1967): 98–107; and Lloyd G. Stevenson, "Suspended Animation and the History of Anesthesia," *Bulletin of the History of Medicine* 49, no. 4 (1952): 482–511. The humane societies set up in the eighteenth century offered rescue to those "apparently drowned."

43. Stark, *Knife to the Heart,* 98; Mark Dowie, *"We Have a Donor": The Bold New World of Organ Transplanting* (New York: St. Martin's Press, 1988), 159–60. The *Tucker's Administrator v. Lower* case was not heard until 1972, and, by then, the jury and judge were ready to accept the medical claim for a diagnosis of death on brain death criteria, though in this case it had been made shortly after admission and when ventilation stopped.

44. See the generally critical letters to the *British Medical Journal* 1 (1968): 177, 254, 378, 577, and continuing with 1 (1969): 631, and 2 (1969): 296.

45. See the views of N. P. Jeddeloh, "The Uniform Anatomical Gift Act and a Statutory Definition of Death," *Transplantation Proceedings* 8, no. 2, suppl. 1 (1976): 245–49.

46. The Law Lords' cautious view came about indirectly, from a murder case in which the ventilator switch-off was alleged to have been the cause of death; see *Regina v. Malcherek* and *Regina v. Steel*, All England Law Reports (1981) 2 All ER, 422–29. Their lordships' common-sense ruling was that "when a medical practitioner, adopting methods which are generally accepted . . . discontinues treatment, that does not prevent the person who inflicted the original injury from being responsible for the victim's death. Putting it in another way, the discontinuation of treatment in those circumstances does not break the chain of causation between the initial injury and the death." Ibid., 428–29.

47. At the meeting, Calne and Woodruff provided medical input and the nursing profession was also represented. In an unusual move, two medical journal editors and some religious leaders were also invited. This innovation set the pattern for lay involvement in later investigations into areas of medicine with an ethical dimension.

48. This recommendation meant that a unique arrangement was in force for a while in Britain, namely that liver *recipients* would be moved to the donor hospital for the transplant operation. Some memorable never-to-be-repeated liver donations and liver transplants were carried out in small English hospitals. Calne describes this unhappy period in his biography, *The Ultimate Gift: The Story of Britain's Premier Transplant Surgeon* (London: Headline, 1998), 100. Other people unhappy with the new guidelines were the distressed blood bank directors in different parts of England who were reacting to Calne's itinerant transplant activities, which could require massive blood transfusions. See file BN 13/110, UK Public Record Office. Some ad hominem complaints from the blood banks made Calne consider legal action.

49. Advice from the MacLennan Committee, *The Advisory Group on Transplantation Problems . . .* , Cmnd 4106 (London: HMSO, 1969).

50. A memo to the prime minister from his civil servants warning him to delay publication is in file PREM 13/2802, UK Public Record Office. In addition, a bill introduced by Gerald Nabarro to establish routine "opt-out" only organ donation rules was withdrawn; see files MH 150/396 and 397, UK Public Record Office. A delay to the totally unrelated, noncontroversial Brodrick Committee work on death certification also resulted and is described in file MH 150/400, UK Public Record Office.

51. For a similar British Medical Association advisory report, see "Report of the Special Committee on Organ Transplantation," *British Medical Journal* 1, no. 5698 (Mar. 21, 1970): 750–51.

52. Beecher, always blunt, was soon supportive of heart-beating donation, and he was saddened by the necessity of a delay that was "of no benefit to anyone. . . . The proper course seems clear, but it takes a brave man to embark on the 'right' course." Henry K. Beecher, "After the Definition of Irreversible Coma," *New England Journal of Medicine* 281, no. 19 (1969): 1070–71.

53. Tansey and Reynolds, *Early Heart Transplant Surgery in the UK*, 35.

54. The first of many novels using the heart transplantation controversies was Collier Young's innocuous work, *The Todd Dossier* (1969). But John Boyd's *The Organ Bank Farm* (1970) described cannibalization of abducted lunatics, and John Hejinian's *Extreme Remedies* (1974) showed transplanters as vultures picking on the not-quite dead. Most damaging was Robin Cook's *Coma* (1977), also adapted for film.

Curt Siodmak's *Donovan's Brain* (1969) was pure science fiction, as was Robert Heinlein's *I Will Fear No Evil* (1970) and Margaret Jones's *The Day They Put Humpty Together Again* (1968), retitled *Transplant* when the American edition was published (1969). First in the whimsical genre of transfer of personality, good and bad, with a graft, notably the heart, was Robert Silverberg's *To Live Again* (1969).

55. After his success with *Coma*, Robin Cook returned to the use of transplant themes in *Brain* (1982) and *Blindsight* (1993). The notion of a transfer of personality or other human traits via an organ graft continued to be an attractive theme for novelists; see Alexander McCall Smith, *Friends, Lovers, Chocolate* (2005).

56. Peter Medawar, "The Future of Transplantation Biology and Medicine," *Transplantation Proceedings* 1, no. 1 (Mar. 1969): 666–69, 666.

17. The Plateau of the Early 1970s

1. For a year-on-year study of kidney transplant outcomes, see Paul I. Terasaki, G. Opelz, and M. R. Mickey, "Analysis of Yearly Kidney Transplant Survival Rates," *Transplantation Proceedings* 8, no. 2 (June 1976): 139–44.

2. For a useful memoir on the events in transplantation in the mid-1970s, see Folkert O. Belzer, "Immunosuppressive Agents—A Personal Historical Perspective," *Transplantation Proceedings* 20, no. 3, suppl. 2 (June 1988): 3–7.

3. E. Donnall Thomas, "Landmarks in the Development of Hematopoietic Cell Transplantation," *World Journal of Surgery* 24, no. 7 (2000): 815–18.

4. This apocalyptic quote comes from Niels Jerne, "The Complete Solution of Immunology," *Australasian Annals of Medicine* 18, no. 4 (1969): 345–48.

5. T. E. Starzl, "My Thirty-Five Years of Organ Transplantation," in *History of Transplantation: Thirty-Five Recollections*, ed. Paul I. Terasaki (Los Angeles: UCLA Tissue Typing Laboratory, 1990), 145–82, 170.

6. Starzl has suggested that a subtle, favorable graft-versus-host response does occur in organ transplantation as donor cells intermingle with the recipient's cells, producing microchimerism.

7. Fritz H. Bach, Richard J. Albertini, Patricia Joo, James L. Anderson, and Mortimer M. Bortin, "Bone-Marrow Transplantation in a Patient with the Wiskott-Aldrich Syndrome," *The Lancet* 292, 7583 (Dec. 28, 1968): 1364–66; R. A. Gatti, H. J. Meuwis-

sen, H. D. Allen, R. Hong, and R. A. Good, "Immunological Reconstitution of Sex-Linked Lymphopenic Immunological Deficiency," *The Lancet* 292, no. 7583 (Dec. 28, 1968): 1366–96. See also R. Storb, R. B. Epstein, J. Bryant, H. Ragde, and E. Donnall Thomas, "Marrow Grafts by Combined Marrow and Leukocyte Infusions in Unrelated Dogs Selected by Histocompatibility Typing," *Transplantation* 6, no. 4 (July 1968): 587–93.

8. Karel A. Dicke, J. I. M. van Hooft, and D. W. van Bekkum, "The Selective Elimination of Immunologically Competent Cells from Bone Marrow and Lymphatic Cell Mixtures: II. Mouse Spleen Cell Fractionation on a Discontinuous Albumin Gradient," *Transplantation* 6, no. 4 (July 1968): 562–70. See also Arne Böyum, *Separation of Leucocytes from Blood and Bone Marrow*, Supplement 97, *Scandinavian Journal of Clinical and Laboratory Investigation*, vol. 21 (Oslo: Universitetsforlaget, 1968).

9. G. W. Santos, L. L. Sensenbrenner, P. J. Burke, M. Colvin, A. H. Owens Jr., W. B. Bias, and R. E. Slavin, "Marrow Transplantation in Man Following Cyclophosphamide," *Transplantation Proceedings* 3, no. 1 (Mar. 1971): 400–404.

10. R. Storb, R. B. Epstein, T. C. Graham, and E. Donnall Thomas, "Methotrexate Regimens for Control of Graft-versus-Host Disease in Dogs with Allogeneic Marrow Grafts," *Transplantation* 9, no. 3 (Mar. 1970): 240–46. Mixed lymphocyte culture (MLC) studies became essential prior to marrow donation, and the

development of tests for matching HLA/DR antigens later contributed to unrelated bone marrow donation.

11. F. Derom, F. Barbier, S. Ringoir, J. Versieck, G. Rolly, G. Berzsenyi, P. Vermeire, and L. Vrints, "Ten-Month Survival after Lung Homotransplantation in Man," *Journal of Thoracic and Cardiovascular Surgery* 61, no. 6 (June 1971): 835–46.

12. The early Stanford heart transplant results are in R. B. Griepp, E. D. Stinson, Eugene Dong, D. A. Clark, and Norman E. Shumway, "Hemodynamic Performance of the Transplanted Human Heart," *Surgery* 70, no. 1 (July 1971): 88–96, and their later success is reported in Stuart W. Jamieson, Edward B. Stinson, and Norman E. Shumway, "Cardiac Transplantation in 150 Patients at Stanford University," *British Medical Journal* 1, no. 6156 (Jan. 13, 1979): 93–95.

13. The classic paper on transvenous cardiac biopsy is P. K. Caves, E. B. Stinson, M. E. Billingham, and Norman E. Shumway, "Percutaneous Transvenous Endomyocardial Biopsy in Human Heart Recipients," *Annals of Thoracic Surgery* 16, no. 4 (1973): 325–36. The new bioptome, or biopsy device, was based on one developed in Japan.

14. The classic papers on the benefits of pretransplant blood transfusion are G. Opelz and Paul I. Terasaki, "Histocompatibility Matching Utilizing Responsiveness as a New Dimension," *Transplantation Proceedings* 4, no. 4 (1972): 433–37; and "Analysis of Yearly Kidney Transplant Survival Rates," *Transplantation Proceedings* 8, no. 2 (June 1976): 139–44.

15. David Hume had hinted at this paradoxical response to blood transfusion in 1954, but the first clear evidence was reported in P. J. Morris, A. Ting, and J. Stocker, "Leukocyte Antigens in Renal Transplantation: I. The Paradox of Blood Transfusions in Renal Transplantation," *Medical Journal of Australia* 2, no. 24 (Dec. 14, 1968): 1088–90. See also earlier hints of this unexpected response in J. B. Dossetor, K. J. MacKinnon, M. H. Gault, and L. D. MacLean, "Cadaver Kidney Transplants," *Transplantation* 5, suppl. 4 (July 1967): 844–53; and in P. Michielsen, "Hémodialyse et transplantation rénale," *E.D.T.A. Proceedings* 3 (1966): 162–63.

16. K. C. Cochrum, D. Hanes, D. Potter, F. Vincenti, W. Amend, N. Feduska, H. Perkins, and O. Salvatierra, "Donor-Specific Blood Transfusions in HLA-D-Disparate One-Haplotype-Related Allografts," *Transplantation Proceedings* 11, no. 4 (Dec. 1979): 1903–7. Salvatierra was roundly criticized in private and at transplantation meetings for attempting this strategy.

17. Terasaki's regional tissue-typing service also allowed for follow-up of the transplanted patients. Accordingly, as well as his analysis of the role of tissue typing, he could look at the effect of many other influences, including blood transfusion, perfusion methods, and year-by-year changes in survival rates. Terasaki's data constituted the only large-scale American data set, until the United Network for Organ Sharing (UNOS) took over in 1987. The European Dialysis and Transplant Association started its excellent data collection effort in 1965; see W. Drukker, "The Founding of the EDTA: Facts and Lessons," *Nephrology, Dialysis, Transplantation* 4, no. 5 (1989): 401–7.

18. For the murky politics of the withdrawal of Terasaki's grant, see Thomas E. Starzl, *The Puzzle People: Memoirs of a Transplant Surgeon* (Pittsburgh: University of Pittsburgh Press, 1992), 121–23.

19. Barbara Bain, Magdalene R. Vas, and Louis Lowenstein, "The Development of Large Immature Mononuclear Cells in Mixed Leukocyte Cultures," *Blood* 23 (Jan. 1964): 108–16; Fritz Bach and Kurt Hirschhorn, "Lymphocyte Interaction: A Potential Histocompatibility Test in Vitro," *Science* 143, no. 3608 (Feb. 21, 1964): 813–14. Bach used the test in the ongoing skin-graft studies in volunteers being carried out by Rapaport in the same hospital, later moved to Paris, as described earlier.

20. For an account of these immunological innovations, see Bach in *History of HLA: Ten Recollections*, ed. Paul I. Terasaki (Los Angeles: UCLA Tissue Typing Laboratory, 1990); and Terasaki, *History of Transplantation*.

21. Fritz H. Bach, R. J. Albertini, D. Bernard Amos, R. Ceppellini, P. L. Mattiuz, and V. C. Miggiano, "Mixed Leukocyte Culture Studies in Families with Known HL-A Genotypes," *Transplantation Proceedings* 1, no. 1 (Mar. 1969): 339–41; E. J. Yunis, J. M. Plate, F. E. Ward, H. F. Seigler, and D. Bernard Amos, "Anomalous MLR Responsiveness among Siblings," *Transplantation Proceedings* 3, no. 1 (Mar. 1971): 118–20; Fritz H. Bach and M. Segall, "Genetics of the Mixed Leukocyte Culture Response: A Reexamination," *Transplantation Proceedings* 4, no. 2 (June 1972): 205–8. Study of many families revealed occasional MLC stimulation by cells from siblings with identical HLA matches, pointing to a separate locus for MLC, close to HLA, with occasional crossovers possible.

22. For Jon van Rood's request to access the Catholic cousin marriage registries for such typing cells, see J. G. van den Tweel, A. B. van Oud Alblas, J. J. Keuning, E. Goulmy, A. Termijtelen, M. L. Bach, and

J. J. van Rood, "Typing for MLC (LD): I. Lymphocytes from Cousin-Marriage Offspring as Typing Cells," *Transplantation Proceedings* 5, no. 4 (Dec. 1973): 1535–38. See also J. J. van Rood, A. van Leeuwen, J. J. Keuning, and A. Blusse van Oud Alblas, "The Serological Recognition of the Human MLC Determinants Using a Modified Cytotoxicity Technique," *Tissue Antigens* 5, no. 2 (Feb. 1975): 73–79.

23. A. Ting and Peter J. Morris, "Matching for B-Cell Antigens of the HLA-DR Series in Cadaveric Renal Transplantation," *The Lancet* 311, no. 8064 (Mar. 18, 1978): 575–77. For Erik Thorsby's contributions to tissue typing at this time, see F. Vartdal, "Erik Thorsby Is 60," *Tissue Antigens* 52, no. 1 (July 1998): 96–98.

24. On the earliest detection of migration inhibition, see John R. David, S. Al-Askari, H. S. Lawrence, and L. Thomas, "Delayed Hypersensitivity in Vitro: I. The Specificity of Inhibition of Cell Migration by Antigens," *Journal of Immunology* 93, no. 2 (1964): 264–73. See also Salah Al-Askari, John R. David, H. S. Lawrence, and L. Thomas, "In Vitro Studies on Homograft Sensitivity," *Nature* 205, no. 4974 (Feb. 27, 1965): 916–17. The reaction was quantified in M. Søborg, and G. Bendixen, "Human Lymphocyte Migration as a Parameter of Hypersensitivity," *Acta Medica Scandinavica* 181, no. 2 (Feb. 1967): 247–56. The MIF story may have started earlier in the "lost era," however, and the whole story is inexplicably missing from Leslie Brent, *A History of Transplantation Immunology* (London: Academic Press, 1997). Cytokine terminology was tidied up in 1979 at the Second International Lymphokine Workshop, as reported in "Revised Nomenclature for Antigen-Nonspecific T Cell Proliferation and Helper Factors," *Journal of Immunology* 123, no. 6 (1979): 2928–29.

25. For the early promise shown by "immunological monitoring," see the complex papers given at the 1976 New York meeting of the Transplantation Society, particularly J. Miller, J. Lifton, W. C. DeWolf, B. J. Stevens, and C. Wilcox, "Efficacy of Immunologic Monitoring after Renal Transplantation," *Transplantation Proceedings* 9, no. 1 (Mar. 1977): 59–64.

26. G. Köhler and C. Milstein, "Continuous Cultures of Fused Cells Secreting Antibody of Predefined Specificity," *Nature* 256, no. 5517 (Aug. 7, 1975): 495–97.

27. The first application of monoclonal antibodies to transplantation was reported in G. Galfre, S. C. Howe, C. Milstein, et al., "Antibodies to Major Histocompatibility Antigens Produced by Hybrid Cell Lines," *Nature* 266, no. 5602 (Apr. 7, 1977): 550–52.

28. A. Benedict Cosimi, Robert B. Colvin, Robert C. Burton, Robert H. Rudin, Gideon Goldstein, Patrick C. Kung, W. Peter Hansen, Francis L. Delmonico, and Paul S. Russell, "Use of Monoclonal Antibodies to T-Cell Subsets for Immunologic Monitoring and Treatment in Recipients of Renal Allografts," *New England Journal of Medicine* 305, no. 6 (Aug. 6, 1981): 308–14.

29. Peter C. Doherty and Rolf M. Zinkernagel, "A Biological Role for the Major Histocompatibility Antigens," *The Lancet* 305, no. 7922 (June 28, 1975): 1406–9. For the historical background, see Rolf M. Zinkernagel and Peter C. Doherty, "The Discovery of MHC Restriction," *Immunology Today* 18 (1997): 14–17.

30. For a review, see Chella S. David, "The Mystery of HLA-B27 and Disease," *Immunogenetics* 46, no. 1 (1997): 73–77.

31. Thomas E. Starzl, Charles W. Putnam, Charles G. Halgrimson, Carl G. Groth, Arthur S. Booth Jr., and Israel Penn, "Renal Transplantation under Cyclophosphamide," *Transplantation Proceedings* 4, no. 4 (Dec. 1972): 461–64.

32. Joseph E. Murray, A. Birtch, and R. E. Wilson, "Thoracic Duct Drainage as an Aid for Immunosuppression," *Transplantation Proceedings* 4, no. 4 (Dec. 1972): 465–67.

33. On the use of total lymphoid irradiation (TLI), see J. Albertus Myburgh, Jacobus A. Smit, Anthony M. Meyers, J. René Botha, Selma Browde, and Peter D. Thomson, "Total Lymphoid Irradiation in Renal Transplantation," *World Journal of Surgery* 10, no. 3 (June 1986): 369–80.

34. Passenger cells were first described in David Steinmuller, "Immunization with Skin Isografts Taken from Tolerant Mice," *Science* 158, no. 3797 (Oct. 6, 1967): 127–29.

35. Mary G. McGeown, "Immunosuppression for Kidney Transplantation," *The Lancet* 302, no. 7824 (Aug. 11, 1973): 310–12. See also Peter J. Morris, "Molly McGeown and Renal Transplantation," *Nephrology Dialysis Transplantation* 13, no. 6 (1998): 1388–90.

36. An interesting account of the rise to fame of this obscure organism is found in P. D. Walzer, "*Pneumocystis carinii*: A Historical Perspective," *Seminars in Respiratory Infection* 13, no. 4 (1998): 279–82.

37. Monto Ho, Sakdidej Suwansirikul, John N. Dowling, Leona A. Youngblood, and John A. Armstrong, "The Transplanted Kidney as Source of Cytomega-

lovirus Infection," *New England Journal of Medicine*
293, no. 22 (Nov. 27, 1975): 1109–12. CMV infection
had been noticed in the early Boston cases and reported in Robert E. Kanich and John E. Craighead,
"Cytomegalovirus Infection and Cytomegalic Inclusion Disease in Renal Homotransplant Recipients,"
American Journal of Medicine 40, no. 6 (June 1966):
874–82. A single case was reported the previous year
in E. T. Hedley-Whyte and John E. Craighead, "Gener-
alized Cytomegalic Inclusion Disease after Renal Homotransplantation—Report of a Case with Isolation
of Virus," *New England Journal of Medicine* 272, no. 9
(Mar. 4, 1965): 473–75.

38. For a defense of kidney transplant biopsy at the
Second International Congress of the Transplantation
Society meeting, see Priscilla Kincaid-Smith, "Biopsy
Features of Early Acute Rejection in Cadaveric Renal Grafts," *Transplantation Proceedings* 1, no. 1 (Mar.
1969): 287–89. The work is reported in T. H. Mathew,
Priscilla Kincaid-Smith, J. Eremin, and V. C. Marshall, "Percutaneous Needle Biopsy of Renal Homografts," *Medical Journal of Australia* 1, no. 1 (Jan. 6,
1968): 6–7. For a detailed history of kidney biopsy,
see J. Stewart Cameron and Jackie Hicks, "The Introduction of Renal Biopsy into Nephrology from 1901
to 1961: A Paradigm of the Forming of Nephrology by
Technology," *American Journal of Nephrology* 17, nos.
3–4 (1997): 347–58.

39. Peter J. Morris, R. V. S. Yadav, Priscilla Kincaid-
Smith, et al., "Renal Artery Stenosis in Renal Transplantation," *Medical Journal of Australia* 1 (1971):
1255–58. On an early interventional correction, see
D. Carr, R. O. Quin, D. N. H. Hamilton, J. D. Briggs,
B. J. R. Junor, and P. F. Semple, "Transluminal Dilatation of Transplant Renal Artery Stenosis," *British
Medical Journal* 281, no. 6234 (July 19, 1980):
196–98.

40. On the use of Technetium 99mTc-DTPA, see
Donald W. Brown and Thomas E. Starzl, "Radionu-
clides in the Postoperative Management of Orthotopic Human Organ Transplantation," *Radiology* 92,
no. 2 (1969): 373–76.

41. See Patricia Morley, Ellis Barnett, P. R. F. Bell,
J. K. Briggs, K. C. Calman, D. N. Hamilton, and
A. M. Paton, "Ultrasound in the Diagnosis of Fluid
Collections Following Renal Transplantation," *Clinical Radiology* 26, no. 2 (Apr. 1975): 199–207, a paper
from Glasgow, where diagnostic ultrasound was first
introduced. For pre-ultrasound lymphocele cases,
see N. F. Inocencio, J. M. Pierce Jr., J. C. Rosenberg,
B. F. Rosenberg, P. L. Wolf, M. P. Small, and T. S. Ing,

"Renal Allograft with Massive Perirenal Accumulation of Lymph," *British Medical Journal* 3, no. 5668
(Aug. 23, 1969): 452–53.

42. For a review of the use of ultrasound at the time,
see J. Petrek, Nicholas L. Tilney, E. H. Smith, J. S. Williams, and Gordon C. Vineyard, "Ultrasound in Renal Transplantation," *Annals of Surgery* 185, no. 4
(Apr. 1977): 441–47. See also Nicholas L. Tilney, Terry
B. Strom, Gordon C. Vineyard, and John P. Merrill,
"Factors Contributing to the Declining Mortality Rate
in Renal Transplantation," *New England Journal of
Medicine* 299, no. 24 (Dec. 14, 1978): 1321–25.

43. For the interaction between the U.S. govern-
ment and early organ transplant units, see the excel-
lent review, Richard A. Rettig, "The Politics of Organ
Transplantation: A Parable of Our Time," in *Organ
Transplantation Policy: Issues and Prospects*, ed. James
F. Blumstein and Frank A. Sloan (Durham, NC: Duke
University Press, 1989), 191–227.

44. See Starzl, *Puzzle People*, 206, 257, on the two
"gold rushes"—the first when government and insurance funds started to pay for kidney replacement
costs and the second, when similar funding began for
liver transplantation. Under the U.S. fee-for-service
system, costs were uncontained. Elsewhere, surgeons
might receive a fixed salary.

45. Plans for coordinated renal replacement services
in Britain are in the *Report of the Joint Committee on
Maintenance Dialysis and Transplantation in the Treatment of Chronic Renal Failure* (London: Royal College
of Physicians, 1972).

46. The European Dialysis and Transplantation Society (EDTA) continued to accumulate reliable data on
outcomes for dialysis and transplantation. The EDTA
reports increasingly reflected the state of the art in
these services in Europe, figures that often differed
from the results reported by the pioneering units.
One of the independent reports to the British government at this time was the Office of Health Economics
pamphlet by William Laing, *Renal Failure: A Priority in Health?* (London: Office of Health Economics,
1978).

47. Thomas Starzl, John Najarian, and Sam Kountz
may have been the first to advocate the general need
for the new post of transplant coordinator.

48. Thomas E. Starzl, R. Weil, and Charles W. Putnam, "Modern Trends in Kidney Transplantation,"
Transplantation Proceedings 9, no. 1 (Mar. 1977):
1–8, 6.

49. Thomas E. Starzl, A. Francavilla, C. G. Halgrimson, F. R. Francavilla, K. A. Porter, T. H. Brown, and Charles W. Putnam, "The Origin, Hormonal Nature, and Action of Hepatotrophic Substances in Portal Venous Blood," *Surgery, Gynecology & Obstetrics* 137, no. 2 (Aug. 1973): 179–99. This study explained the necessity for liver grafts to be positioned normally (orthotopically), rather than heterotopically, as kidneys always were.

50. Frank Macfarlane Burnet, *Immunological Surveillance* (Oxford: Pergamon Press, 1970).

51. See the ferocious verdict by David Weiss on the scientific quality of these attempts at cancer immunotherapy in Andor Szentivanyi and Herman Friedman, eds., *The Immunologic Revolution: Facts and Witnesses* (Boca Raton, FL: CRC Press, 1994), 343–56.

52. For the recurring interest in Coley and his toxins, see Stephen S. Hall, *A Commotion in the Blood: Life, Death, and the Immune System* (New York: Henry Holt, 1997), esp. 65–70.

53. R. T. Prehn and J. M. Main, "Immunity to Methylcholanthrene-Induced Sarcomas," *Journal of the National Cancer Institute* 18, no. 6 (June 1957): 769–78.

54. Karl Erik Hellström and Ingegred Hellström, "Immunological Enhancement as Studied by Cell Culture Techniques," *Annual Review of Microbiology* 24 (1970): 373–98.

55. Leslie Brent, *A History of Transplantation Immunology* (London: Academic Press, 1997), 236.

56. See the excellent review in Ilana Löwy, "Experimental Systems and Clinical Practices: Tumor Immunology and Cancer Immunotherapy, 1895–1980," *Journal of the History of Biology* 27, no. 3 (1994): 403–35; and G. A. Currie, "Eighty Years of Immunotherapy: A Review of Immunological Methods Used for the Treatment of Human Cancer," *British Journal of Cancer* 26, no. 3 (June 1972): 141–53.

57. Woodruff first attempted immunotherapy of experimental tumors with allogeneic cells, and the results were encouraging enough to propose human trials of this strategy; see Michael F. A. Woodruff and M. O. Symes, "The Use of Immunologically Competent Cells in the Treatment of Cancer: Experiments with a Transplantable Mouse Tumour," *British Journal of Cancer* 16, no. 4 (Dec. 1962): 707–15.

58. J. G. Howard, "Modifications of the Graft-versus-Host Reaction by Pretreatment with *M. tuberculosis* and *C. parvum*," *Transplantation* 3, no. 2 (Mar. 1965): 170–77.

59. See June Goodfield, *The Siege of Cancer* (New York: Random House, 1975) and Hall, *Commotion in the Blood,* two of the many popular, metaphor-laden books at the time on the perennially attractive subject of stimulating the host defenses.

60. On the persistent hopes for cancer treatment via immunotherapy, see Steven A. Rosenberg and John M. Barry, *The Transformed Cell: Unlocking the Mysteries of Cancer* (New York: Putnam, 1992).

61. The first thirty of the remarkable total of two hundred patients receiving BCG immunotherapy were reported in Georges Mathé, J. L. Amiel, L. Schwartzenberg, J. Choay, P. Trolard, M. Schneider, M. Hayat, J. R. Schlumberger, and C. Jasmin, "Bone Marrow Graft in Man after Conditioning by Antilymphocytic Serum," *British Medical Journal* 2, no. 5702 (Apr. 18, 1970): 131–36. Mathé even wrote a novel on the subject: *L'Homme qui voulait être guéri* [The man who wished to be cured] (Paris: R. Laffont, 1985). Donnall Thomas also temporarily used killed leukemic cells to boost the immune response.

62. See the CIBA Foundation Symposium, *Immunopotentiation,* ed. G. E. W. Wolstenholme and Julie Knight (London: Associated Scientific Publishers, 1973).

63. See R. B. Herberman, "Counterpoint: Animal Tumor Models and Their Relevance to Human Tumor Immunology," *Journal of Biological Response Modifiers* 2, no. 1 (1983): 39–46, as well as the exchanges with Harold Hewitt in "Second Point: Animal Tumor Models and Their Relevance to Human Tumor Immunology," *Journal of Biological Response Modifiers* 2, no. 3 (1983): 210–16; and "Second Counterpoint: Animal Tumor Models and Their Relevance to Human Tumor Immunology," 217–26.

64. Weiss in Szentivanyi and Friedman, *Immunologic Revolution,* 346.

65. Rosenberg and Barry, *Transformed Cell,* 57.

66. The Issels saga is told credulously in Gordon Thomas, *Issels: The Biography of a Doctor* (London: Hodder and Stoughton, 1973).

67. Chester M. Southam and Alice E. Moore, "Individual Immunity to Cancer Cell Homografts in Man," *Annals of the New York Academy of Sciences* 73 (Oct. 1958): 635–52; E. F. Scanlon, R. A. Hawkins, W. W. Fox, and W. S. Smith, "Fatal Homotransplanted Melanoma: A Case Report," *Cancer* 18 (June 1965): 782–89. Shortly after, concerned at this and other dubious human studies, Henry K. Beecher in Boston started a debate on

the concerns surrounding human experimentation. Beecher later used his Harvard Standing Committee on Human Studies—an early ethics committee—to issue the famous brain-death report in 1968.

68. The new awareness of scientific misconduct at this time is detailed in Alexander Kohn, *False Prophets* (Oxford: Blackwell, 1989), and in William Broad and Nicholas Wade, *Betrayers of the Truth* (New York: Simon and Schuster, 1982). The Stanford case appears in Kohn, *False Prophets*, 104.

69. Full details are given in Joseph Hixson, *The Patchwork Mouse* (Garden City, NY: Anchor Press, 1976). Medawar, brought into the investigation as a Sloan-Kettering Institute trustee, gives an account in *New York Review of Books*, April 15, 1976, later reprinted in Medawar's collected essays, *The Threat and the Glory* (Oxford: Oxford University Press, 1990), 71–82, and in his *The Strange Case of the Spotted Mice: And Other Classic Essays on Science* (Oxford: Oxford University Press, 1996), 132–43.

70. The specialists involved in electroencephalography took their exclusion from the brain-death criteria badly. In Britain, Nobel Prize winner Lord Adrian and Grey Walter were pioneers of the use of the EEG technology, and these men and their "brain waves" were well known to the public; see W. Grey Walter, *The Living Brain* (London: Duckworth, 1953). When the brain-death controversy returned in 1980, the electroencephalographers had a chance to reenter the debate. The downgrading of the place of the EEG in brain-death criteria followed the study by A. Mohandas and Shelley N. Chou, "Brain Death: A Clinical and Pathological Study," *Journal of Neurosurgery* 35, no. 2 (Aug. 1971): 211–18. The large intensive care unit of the neurosurgical department at the Mayo Clinic in Minnesota refined the Harvard criteria, demoting the EEG and omitting spinal reflexes from the tests, and these became known as the Minnesota criteria. In Europe, the Institute of Neurological Sciences in Glasgow, which had done many studies in this area since 1972, also adopted the revised criteria for brain death.

71. *California Health and Safety Code*, section 7180-81 (West Supplement 1975); M. De Mere, *Report on Definition of Death from Law and Medicine Committee*, American Bar Association, adopted February 1975. The National Institutes of Health in the United States followed this lead, and, by 1981, the President's Commission for the Study of Ethical Problems had proposed the nationwide Uniform Determination of Death Act. See "Guidelines for the Determination of Death," *Journal of the American Medical Association* 246, no. 19 (Nov. 13, 1981): 2184–86. For contemporary comment, see Robert J. Joynt, "A New Look at Death," *Journal of the American Medical Association* 252, no. 5 (Aug. 3, 1984): 680–82.

72. *Commonwealth v. Golston*, 366 NE 2d 744, 1977.

73. See Russell Scott, *The Body as Property* (New York: Viking, 1981).

74. Conference of Medical Royal Colleges and Their Faculties in the United Kingdom, "Diagnosis of Brain Death," *British Medical Journal* 2, no. 6045 (Nov. 13, 1976): 1187–88, later updated as "Diagnosis of Death," *British Medical Journal* 1, no. 6159 (Feb. 3, 1979): 332.

75. See the detailed account in Christopher Pallis, "Brain Stem Death—The Evolution of a Concept," *Medico-Legal Journal* 55 (1987): 84–107.

76. See the criticisms of Paul A. Byrne, Sean O'Reilly, and Paul M. Quay, "Brain Death—An Opposing Viewpoint," *Journal of the American Medical Association* 242, no. 18 (Nov. 2, 1979): 1985–90; and D. Wainwright Evans and L. C. Lum, "Cardiac Transplantation," *The Lancet* 315, no. 8174 (Apr. 26, 1980): 933–34. David Evans continued with his criticisms and contributed to the volume *Beyond Brain Death: The Case against Brain Based Criteria for Human Death*, ed. Michael Potts, Paul Byrne, and Richard Nilges (Dordrecht, Netherlands: Kluwer Academic Publishers, 2002).

77. See *Cadaveric Organs for Transplantation: A Code of Practice Drawn up by a Working Party on Behalf of the Health Departments of Great Britain and Northern Ireland* (London 1979, revised 1983). No term other than the awkward "heart-beating cadaveric donation" had come into use, and other terminology, notably "neomort" and "biomort," was wisely dropped. "Deceased donor," a softer term, steadily replaced "cadaveric donor," but when organ donation from deceased patients without cardiac function ultimately began, the term "cardiac death" had to be revived.

78. Organ donation after diagnosis of brain death in critical care units had been common earlier, but the difference was that after ventilator switch-off, cardiac death was awaited, increasingly in the theater where organ removal took place. In this earlier phase, the time of death recorded was when the heart stopped. An intermediate phase prior to heart-beating donation was organ removal following ventilator switch-off in theater. A thorough review is found in Peter L. Abt, Carol A. Fisher, and Arun K. Singhal, "Dona-

tion after Cardiac Death in the US: History and Use," *Journal of the American College of Surgeons* 203, no. 2 (2006): 208–25.

79. Leslie Brent, "Presidential Address," *Transplantation Proceedings* 9 (1977): 1343–47, 1346.

18. The Arrival of Cyclosporine

1. Peter Morris's book *Kidney Transplantation* reached its fifth edition in 2001, signaling a certain maturity in this pioneering organ transplant service, and further editions followed. The emergence of specialist journals, notably the *Journal of Heart and Lung Transplantation* in 1981 and *Liver Transplantation* in 1998, also signaled the increasing acceptance of other procedures,

2. For the state of the art in transplantation at the turn of the twenty-first century, see Paul S. Russell's foreword to *Transplantation*, ed. Leo C. Ginns, A. Benedict Cosimi, and Peter J. Morris (Malden, MA: Blackwell, 1999), xvii–xix.

3. Jean F. Borel, in *Cyclosporin A: Proceedings of an International Conference on Cyclosporin A*, ed. D. J. G. White (Amsterdam: Elsevier, 1982), 5–18. See also Jean F. Borel, "Comparative Study of in Vitro and in Vivo Drug Effects on Cell-Mediated Cytotoxicity," *Immunology* 31, no. 4 (Oct. 1976): 631–41; and H. Stähelin, "Ciclosporin: Historical Background," *Progress in Allergy* 38 (1986): 19–27. There is now a sharp priority dispute among Sandoz company staff regarding these early events. Borel's account has been called "incomplete, misleading, and incorrect" by Stähelin in his 1996 article, "The History of Cyclosporin A (Sandimmune) Revisited: Another Point of View," *Experientia* 52, no. 1 (Jan. 16, 1996): 5–13. Borel added to his account later in "History of the Discovery of Cyclosporin and of Its Early Pharmacological Development," *Wiener Klinische Wochenschrift* 114, no. 12 (June 2002): 433–37.

4. The first relevant publications on CsA were M. Dreyfuss, E. Härri, H. Hofmann, H. Kobel, W. Pache, and H. Tscherter, "Cyclosporin A and C: New Metabolites from *Trichoderma polysporum* (Link ex Pers.) Rifai," *European Journal of Applied Microbiology* 3 (1976): 125–33; Jean F. Borel, Camille Feurer, H. U. Gubler, and H. Stähelin, "Biological Effects of Cyclosporin A: A New Antilymphocytic Agent," *Actions and Agents* 6, no. 4 (July 1976): 468–75; and A. Ruegger, M. Kuhn, H. Lichti, H. R. Loosli, R. Huguenin, C. Quiquerer, and A. von Wartburg, "Cyclosporin A, ein immunosuppressiv wirksamer: Peptidmetabolit aus *Trichoderma polysporem* Rifai," *Helvetica Chimica Acta* 59, no. 4 (1976): 1075–92. Shortly after came Jean F. Borel, Camille Feurer, C. Magnee, and

H. Stähelin, "Effects of the New Anti-Lymphocytic Peptide Cyclosporin A in Animals," *Immunology* 32, no. 6 (June 1976): 1017–25. Borel's *Agents and Actions* paper became a citation classic; see *Current Contents* 27 (1984): 16.

5. A. J. Kostakis, D. J. G. White, and Roy Yorke Calne, "Prolongation of Rat Heart Survival by Cyclosporin A," *International Research Communications System Medical Science: Cardiovascular System* 5 (1977): 243, 280; Roy Yorke Calne and D. J. G. White, "Cyclosporin A: A Powerful Immunosuppressant in Dogs with Renal Allografts," *International Research Communications System Medical Science: Cardiovascular System* 5 (1977): 595. This hard-to-find electronic journal was used for rapid publication.

6. Calne said that his unit discovered the use of oil as a solvent, but Borel (see note 3) claimed that Sandoz had already found oil to be a useful medium for administering the fungal extract.

7. Roy Yorke Calne, S. Thiru, P. McMaster, G. N. Craddock, D. J. G., White, D. B. Evans, D. C. Dunn, B. D. Pentlow, and Keith Rolles, "Cyclosporin A in Patients Receiving Renal Allografts from Cadaver Donors," *The Lancet* 312, no. 8104 (Dec. 30, 1978): 1323–27. CsA was initially used alone in a dose of 25 mg/kg extrapolated from experimental experience.

8. R. L. Powles, A. J. Barrett, H. Clink, J. Sloane, A. J. Barrett, H. E. M. Kay, and T. J. McElwain, "Cyclosporin A for the Treatment of Graft-versus-Host Disease in Man," *The Lancet* 312, no. 8104 (1978): 1327–31.

9. Roy Yorke Calne, Keith Rolles, S. Thiru, P. McMaster, G. N. Craddock, S. Aziz, D. J. G. White, D. B. Evans, D. C. Dunn, R. G. Henderson, and P. Lewis, "Cyclosporin A Initially as the Only Immunosuppressant in 34 Recipients of Cadaveric Organs," *The Lancet* 314, no. 8151 (1979): 1033–36.

10. Thomas E. Starzl, Richard Weil III, Shunzaburo Iwatsuki, Goran Klintmalm, Gerhard P. J. Schröter, Lawrence J. Koep, Yuichi Iwaki, Paul I. Terasaki, and Kendrick A. Porter, "The Use of Cyclosporin A and Prednisone in Cadaver Kidney Transplantation," *Surgery, Gynecology & Obstetrics* 151, no. 1 (July 1980): 17–26.

11. For the variable early verdicts on the drug, see J. L. Tiwari, "Cyclosporine and Kidney Graft Survival: A Review," in *Clinical Transplants*, ed. Paul I. Terasaki (Los Angeles: UCLA Tissue Typing Laboratory, 1986), 345–66.

12. The CsA complications were succinctly described as the "3 N's" (nephropathy, neurotoxicity, and neoplasia) and "8 H's" (hirsutism, hypertension, hyperplasia, hyperlipidemia, hypertrichosis, hepatotoxicity, hypersensitivity, hyperkalemia); see Ginns, Cosimi, and Morris, *Transplantation*, 1007.

13. The first report of "emotionally related" living donor transplantation is in Samuel L. Kountz, H. A. Perkins, R. Payne, et al., "Kidney Transplants Using Living Unrelated Donors," *Transplantation Proceedings* 2 (1970): 427–29. Donor-specific blood transfusion was later used in this situation; see Folkert O. Belzer, Munci Kallayoghi, and Hans Sollinger, "Donor-Specific Transfusion in Living Unrelated Donor-Recipient Combinations," *Transplantation Proceedings* 19, no. 1 (Feb. 1987): 1514–15.

14. Jerome Aroesty and Richard A. Rettig, *The Cost Effects of Improved Kidney Transplantation* (Santa Monica, CA: Rand, 1984).

15. Bartley P. Griffith, Robert L. Hardesty, G. Michael Deeb, Thomas E. Starzl, and Henry T. Bahnson, "Cardiac Transplantation with Cyclosporin A and Prednisone," *Annals of Surgery* 196, no. 3 (Sept. 1982): 324–29; Thomas E. Starzl, Göran B. G. Klintmalm, Kendrick A. Porter, Shunzaburo Iwatsuki, and Gerhard P. J. Schröter, "Liver Transplantation with Use of Cyclosporin A and Prednisone," *New England Journal of Medicine* 305, no. 5 (July 30, 1981): 266–69.

16. Kidney transplantation for cats was not accepted by Britain's Royal College of Veterinary Surgeons until 2003, and, even then, its cautious acceptance raised public concern for the rights of the donor.

17. In 2000, eight years after his heart transplant for cardiomyopathy, twenty-year-old Erik Compton, a University of Georgia student, participated in a US-PGA golf tournament. In 2001, a liver-transplanted wrestler reentered his sport, and another liver recipient won the gold medal for snowboarding in the 2002 Winter Olympics. In Scotland, two senior politicians were, respectively, long-term heart and single-lung transplant survivors. Terasaki published an interesting list of high-achieving transplanted patients; see Paul I. Terasaki and Jane Schoenberg, *Transplant Success Stories 1993* (Los Angeles: UCLA Tissue Typing Laboratory, 1993).

18. For quality of life issues, see B. J. O'Brien, N. R. Banner, S. Gibson, and M. H. Yacoub, "The Nottingham Health Profile as a Measure of Quality of Life Following Combined Heart and Lung Transplantation," *Journal of Epidemiology and Community Health* 42, no. 3 (Sept. 1988): 232–34.

19. Dale H. Cowan, *Human Organ Transplantation: Societal, Medical-Legal, Regulatory and Reimbursement Issues* (Ann Arbor: Michigan Health Administration Press, 1987). See also the preparation for establishing UNOS, in *Organ Transplantation: Issues and Recommendations; Report of the Task Force on Organ Transplantation* (Rockville, MD: U.S. Department of Health and Human Services, 1986); and Richard West, *Organ Transplantation* (London: Office of Health Economics, 1991).

20. HIV risks in transplantation are reviewed in Robert H. Rubin, Roger L. Jenkins, Byers W. Shaw Jr., David Shaffer, Richard H. Pearl, Sigfried Erb, Anthony P. Monaco, and David H. van Thiel, "The Acquired Immunodeficiency Syndrome and Transplantation," *Transplantation* 44, no. 1 (July 1987): 1–4. For an important review of other pathogens transmitted by human grafts, see T. Eastlund, "Infectious Disease Transmission through Cell, Tissue and Organ Transplantation: Reducing the Risk through Donor Selection," *Cell Transplantation* 4, no. 5 (1995): 455–77.

21. The Banff classification of the various features of rejection detected using microscopy of biopsied tissue was established in that Canadian town in 1991 at an international workshop organized by Kim Solez, an Edmonton pathologist; see Kim Solez et al., "International Standardization of Criteria for the Histologic Diagnosis of Renal Allograft Rejection: The Banff Working Classification of Kidney Transplant Pathology," *Kidney International* 44, no. 2 (Aug. 1993): 411–22.

22. Reviewed by David Hamilton in *Ultrasound of Abdominal Transplantation*, ed. Paul S. Sidhu and Grant M. Baxter (Stuttgart: Thieme, 2002), 1–12.

23. For description of the laparoscopic technique with pigs, see Inderbir S. Gill, Joseph M. Carbone, Ralph V. Clayman, Paul A. Fadden, A. Marika Stone, Bruce A. Lucas, and J. William McRoberts, "Laparoscopic Live-Donor Nephrectomy," *Journal of Endourology* 8, no. 2 (Apr. 1994): 143–48. The first human operation was reported in L. E. Ratner, L. J. Ciseck, R. G. Moore, F. G. Cigarroa, H. S. Kaufman, and L. R. Kavoussi, "Laparoscopic Live Donor Nephrectomy," *Transplantation* 60, no. 9 (Nov. 15, 1995): 1047–49.

24. See Francis D. Moore, "The History of Transplantation," in *Organ Transplantation and Replacement,* ed. G. James Cerilli (Philadelphia: Lippincott, 1988), 3–15. Moore's own early attempts at liver transplantation were unsuccessful and discouraging. A tempting comparison is from the world of music, since living composers' works are often considered unplayable but later enter the standard repertoire.

25. Roy Yorke Calne, ed., *Liver Transplantation: The Cambridge–King's College Experience* (New York: Grune & Stratton, 1983).

26. See the interesting analysis by Michael Bos, *The Diffusion of Heart and Liver Transplantation across Europe* (London: King's Fund Centre, 1991).

27. Neurosurgeon Loyal Davis, who sympathized with transplant efforts, was one of Starzl's mentors. The president got "easy ink—drama, pathos and heroism were built in; all one needed was a good face—baby, parent or politician. It didn't matter much"—the verdict of Mark Dowie in *"We Have a Donor": The Bold New World of Organ Transplanting* (New York: St. Martin's Press, 1988), 182.

28. From Clark C. Havinghurst and Nancy M. P. King, "Liver Transplantation in Massachusetts: Public Policy as Morality Play," in *Organ Transplantation Policy: Issues and Prospects,* ed. James F. Blumstein and Frank A. Sloan (Durham, NC: Duke University Press, 1989), 229–60.

29. For the advocacy at Koop's consensus development review, see Thomas E. Starzl, *The Puzzle People: Memoirs of a Transplant Surgeon* (Pittsburgh: University of Pittsburgh Press, 1992), 223.

30. Starzl, *Puzzle People,* 257.

31. Maxwell J. Mehlman, "The Oregon Medicaid Program: Is It Just?" *Health Matrix* 1, no. 2 (1991): 175–99. There was long legal debate over whether Medicaid funds could cover organ transplants at all.

32. H. Gilbert Welch and Eric B. Larson, "Dealing with Limited Resources," *New England Journal of Medicine* 319, no. 3 (July 21, 1988): 171–73.

33. The arcane, cautious funding of new developments at Boston's hospitals, remarkably similar to cautious European practice, is thoroughly dealt with in Havinghurst and King, "Liver Transplantation in Massachusetts," as it is in the Fineberg Report.

34. For the dominance of Starzl's liver unit at the University of Pittsburgh at the time, see Dowie, *"We Have a Donor."*

35. For a scholarly review of the reevaluation of the hepatic vascular supply, internal and external, and the numerous anomalies, see David A. McClusky III, Lee J. Skandalakis, Gene L. Colborn, and John E. Skandalakis, "Hepatic Surgery and Hepatic Surgical Anatomy: Historical Partners in Progress," *World Journal of Surgery* 21, no. 3 (1997): 330–42. The new views are dated to the first of three scholarly monographs by Claude Couinaud: *Le Foie: études anatomiques et chirurgicales* (Paris: Masson, 1957); none of the three volumes appeared in English.

36. The first use of a reduced cadaveric liver was reported in J. G. Fortner, D. K. Kim, M. H. Shui, S. D. Yeh, W. S. Howland, and E. J. Beattie Jr., "Heterotopic (Auxiliary) Liver Transplantation in Man," *Transplantation Proceedings* 9, no. 1 (Mar. 1977): 217–21. Later reports on split liver transplants are H. Bismuth and D. Houssin, "Reduced-Sized Orthotopic Liver Graft in Hepatic Transplantation in Children," *Surgery* 95, no. 3 (Mar. 1984): 367–72; and Cristoph E. Broelsch, P. Neuhaus, Martin Burdelski, et al., "Orthotopic Liver Transplantation," *Langenbecks Archives für Chirurgie* 369 (1984): supplement, 105–9.

37. R. Pichlmayr, B. Ringe, G. Gubernatis, J. Hauss, and H. Bunzendahl, "Transplantation einer Spenderleber auf zwei Empfänger," *Langenbecks Archiv für Chirurgie* 373, no. 2 (1988): 127–30.

38. The first reports of living-related liver donation were from Silvano Raia, José Roberto Nery, and Sergio Mies, "Liver Transplantation from Live Donors," *The Lancet* 334, no. 8661 (Aug. 26, 1989): 497; Russell W. Strong, Stephen V. Lynch, Tat Hin Ong, Hidetoshi Matsunami, Yuichi Koido, and Glenda A. Balderson, "Successful Liver Transplantation from a Living Donor to Her Son," *New England Journal of Medicine* 322, no. 21 (May 24, 1990): 1505–7. See later reviews by Christoph E. Broelsch, Peter F. Whitington, Jean C. Emond, Thomas G. Heffron, J. Richard Thistlethwaite, Larry Stevens, James Piper, Susan H. Whitington, and J. Lance Lichtor, "Liver Transplantation in Children from Living Related Donors," *Annals of Surgery* 214, no. 4 (Oct. 1991): 428–37; and Jean C. Emond, John F. Renz, Linda D. Ferrell, Philip Rosenthal, Robert C. Lim, John P. Roberts, John R. Lake, and Nancy L. Ascher, "Functional Analysis of Grafts from Living Donors: Implications for the Treatment of Older Recipients," *Annals of Surgery* 224, no. 4 (Oct. 1996): 544–54.

39. J. Wadström, X. Rogiers, M. Malago, L. Fischer, T. E. Langwieler, S. Pollock, A. Latta, Martin Burdelski, and Christoph E. Broelsch, "Experience from the

First 30 Living Related Liver Transplants in Hamburg," *Transplantation Proceedings* 27, no. 1 (Feb. 1995): 1173–74.

40. V. A. Starnes, P. E. Oyer, D. Bernstein, D. Baum, P. Gamberg, J. Miller, and Norman E. Shumway, "Heart, Heart-Lung and Lung Transplantation in the First Year of Life," *Annals of Thoracic Surgery* 53 (1992): 306–10.

41. See the excellent review by R. Margreiter, "The History of Intestinal Transplantation," *Transplantation Reviews* 11, no. 1 (1997): 9–21.

42. The Necker small bowel transplant experience is reported in Richard F. M. Wood, Paul A. Lear, Celia Ingham Clark, Otakar Stark, Vladimir Kren, Pavel Klir, and Thomas J. Gill, "First International Symposium on Small Bowel Transplantation," *Transplantation Proceedings* 22, no. 6 (1990): 2423–503.

43. D. Grant, W. Wall, R. Mimeault, R. Zhong, C. Ghent, B. Garcia, C. Stiller, and J. Duff, "Successful Small-Bowel/Liver Transplantation," *The Lancet* 335, no. 8683 (Jan. 27, 1990): 181–84. The early work is described in David White, Peter Friend, and Celia White, "Novel Approaches to Transplantation," special edition, *British Medical Bulletin* 53, no. 4 (1997).

44. Thomas E. Starzl, John Fung, Raman Venkataramanan, Satoru Todo, Anthony J. Demetris, and Ashok Jain, "FK 506 for Liver, Kidney and Pancreas Transplantation," *The Lancet* 334, no. 8670 (Oct. 28, 1989): 1000–1004; Thomas E. Starzl, Marc I. Rowe, Satoru Todo, Ronald Jaffe, Andreas Tzakis, Allen L. Hoffman, Carlos Esquivel, Kendrick A. Porter, Raman Venkataramanan, Leonard Makowka, and Rene Duquesnoy, "Transplantation of Multiple Abdominal Viscera," *Journal of the American Medical Association* 261, no. 10 (Mar. 10, 1989): 1449–57. For a patient's own account of therapy with FK 506, see Robert J. Pensack and Dwight A. Williams, *Raising Lazarus* (New York: Putnam's Sons, 1994).

45. David Grant, "Current Results of Intestinal Transplantation," *The Lancet* 347, no. 9018 (June 29, 1996): 1801–3.

46. Richard C. Lillehei, Richard L. Simmons, John S. Najarian, Richard Weil, Hisanori Uchida, Jose O. Ruiz, Carl M. Kjellstrand, and Frederick C. Goetz, "Pancreatico-Duodenal Allotransplantation: Experimental and Clinical Experience," *Annals of Surgery* 172, no. 3 (Sept. 1970): 405–36.

47. D. E. R. Sutherland, F. C. Goetz, and John S. Najarian, "Living-Related Donor Segmental Pancreatectomy for Transplantation," *Transplantation Proceedings* 12, no. 4, suppl. 2 (Dec. 1980): 19–25. For an early report on duodenocystostomy, see D. D. Nghiem and R. J. Corry, "Technique of Simultaneous Renal Pancreatoduodenal Transplantation with Urinary Drainage of Pancreatic Secretion," *American Journal of Surgery* 153, no. 4 (Apr. 1987): 405–6.

48. For a review of living-related pancreas donation, see Abhinav Humar, Rainer W. G. Gruessner, and David E. R. Sutherland, "Living Related Donor Pancreas and Pancreas-Kidney Transplantation," *British Medical Bulletin* 53, no. 4 (1997): 879–91.

49. For excellent reviews, see David E. R. Sutherland and C. G. Groth, "The History of Pancreas Transplantation," and D. W. R. Gray, "A Short History of Pancreas Transplantation," both in *History of Organ and Cell Transplantation*, ed. Nadey Hakim and Vassilios Papalois (London: Imperial College Press, 2003). An earlier review is Garth L. Warnock and Ray V. Rajotte, "Human Pancreatic Islet Transplantation," *Transplantation Reviews* 6 (1992): 195–208.

50. The pioneer paper is S. Moskalewski, "Isolation and Culture of the Islets of Langerhans of the Guinea Pig," *General and Comparative Endocrinology* 5 (June 1965): 342–53. In 2001, Ricordi won the prestigious Nessim Habif Prize for innovative surgical instruments.

51. Biohybrid devices are reviewed in Robert P. Lanza and William L. Chick, "Encapsulated Cell Transplantation," *Transplantation Reviews* 9, no. 4 (Oct. 1995): 217–30.

52. A. M. James Shapiro, Jonathan R. T. Lakey, Edmond Ryan, Gregory S. Korbutt, Ellen Toth, Garth L. Warnock, Norman M. Kneteman, and Ray V. Rajotte, "Islet Transplantation in Seven Patients with Type 1 Diabetes Mellitus Using a Glucocorticoid-Free Immunosuppressive Regimen," *New England Journal of Medicine* 343, no. 4 (July 27, 2000): 230–38.

53. John A. Hansen, Reginald A. Clift, E. Donnall Thomas, C. Dean Buckner, Rainer Storb, and Eloise R. Giblett, "Transplantation of Marrow from an Unrelated Donor to a Patient with Acute Leukemia," *New England Journal of Medicine* 303 (Sept. 4, 1980): 565–67.

54. See D. L. Confer, "Unrelated Marrow Donor Registries," *Current Opinion in Hematology* 4, no. 6 (1997): 408–12. The U.S. events are told in detail by Jeffrey McCullough, Herbert A. Perkins, and John Hansen, "The National Marrow Donor Program with Emphasis on the Early Years," *Transfusion* 46, no. 7 (2006):

1248–55. This account was added to and modified by Bart Fisher in *Transfusion* 47, no. 6 (June 2007): 1101–2.

55. Alexander Leaf, "The MGH Trustees Say No to Heart Transplants," *New England Journal of Medicine* 302, no. 19 (May 8, 1980): 1087–88.

56. Roger W. Evans, Diane L. Manninen, T. D. Overcast, et al., *The National Heart Transplantation Study: Final Report* (Seattle: Health and Population Study Center, Battelle Human Affairs Research Centers, 1984).

57. Conor M. Burke, John C. Baldwin, Adrian J. Morris, Norman E. Shumway, James Theodore, Henry D. Tazelaar, Christopher McGregor, Eugene D. Robin, and Stuart W. Jamieson, "Twenty-Eight Cases of Human Heart-Lung Transplantation," *The Lancet* 327, no. 8480 (Mar. 8, 1986): 517–19.

58. William A. Baumgartner, Thomas A. Traill, Duke E. Cameron, James D. Fonger, Irvin B. Birenbaum, and Bruce A. Reitz, "Unique Aspects of Heart and Lung Transplantation Exhibited in the 'Domino-Donor' Operation," *Journal of the American Medical Association* 261, no. 21 (Jun. 2, 1989): 3121–25. "Domino" liver grafting was used when elective liver grafting of a reasonably well patient released a liver useful to a recipient with a short life expectancy for reasons other than liver disease.

59. Leonard L. Bailey, Michael Wood, Anees Razzouk, Glen van Arsdell, and Steven Gundry, "Heart Transplantation during the First 12 Years of Life," *Archives of Surgery* 124, no. 10 (1989): 1221–25.

60. Leonard L. Bailey, Sandra Nehlsen-Canneralla, Waldo Concepcion, and Weldon B. Jolley, "Baboon-to-Human Cardiac Xenotransplantation in a Neonate," *Journal of the American Medical Association* 254, no. 23 (Dec. 20, 1985): 3321–29. Later, Loma Linda's refusal to transplant "Baby Jesse" in 1986, following a judgmental assessment of the unwed parents, refocused attention on the hospital.

61. Bailey's work and the controversies surrounding it are dealt with in the in-house brochure by Richard A. Schaefer, *Legacy—Daring to Care: The Heritage of Loma Linda* (Loma Linda, CA: Legacy Publication Association, 1990).

62. Anencephalic babies lack most of the cerebral hemisphere and, untreated, die shortly after birth. Ventilation, either as therapy or if organ donation would take place, revealed that the remaining brain stem was active, and brain stem death criteria were

thus unmet; see Medical Task Force on Anencephaly, "The Infant with Anencephaly," *New England Journal of Medicine* 322, no. 10 (Mar. 8, 1990): 669–74; and Ronald E. Cranford, "Organ Retrieval from Infants with Anencephaly," *Transplantation Proceedings* 22, no. 3 (June 1990): 1040–41.

63. This committee was but one of a remarkable array of regulatory agencies with power and oversight that arose at this time in developed nations in response to new medical and biological issues, including those arising from transplantation.

64. A letter from one government minister to another reads, "This 'mad' surgeon at Harefield is clearly trying to do transplants. How do we stop him?" Quoted in E. M. Tansey and Lois A. Reynolds, eds., *Early Heart Transplant Surgery in the UK*, vol. 3 of *Wellcome Witnesses to Twentieth Century Medicine* (London: Wellcome Trust, 1999), 53. See also Mary P. Shepherd, *Heart of Harefield: The Story of the Hospital* (London: Quiller, 1990).

65. The difficulty in Britain was that the NHS did not itemize costs and had no easy way of calculating the cost of a heart transplant in the United Kingdom. In fee-for-service health care systems, most notably that of the United States, such identification of costs was routine. The costing of pioneer heart transplants in the UK at this time marked the beginning of much wider NHS pricing.

66. Department of Health and Social Security, *Costs and Benefits of the Heart Transplant Programmes at Harefield and Papworth Hospitals* (London: Stationery Office Books, 1985).

67. Shepherd, *Heart of Harefield*.

68. See Bos, *Diffusion of Heart and Liver Transplantation across Europe*.

69. This BBC program featured poorly described cases that did not meet the usual brain-death criteria, and it favored the minority view that the EEG and cerebral angiography were necessary. The technical arguments over brain death can be followed in the letters to the *Lancet* and the *British Medical Journal* in late 1980 and early 1981, and these events are described in detail in Christopher Pallis, *An ABC of Brain Stem Death* (London: British Medical Journal, 1983). The theme of a failure of diagnosis of death in the French film *L'Amour à mort* (1984), however, failed to attract general attention.

70. The case of Ben Hardwick, featured on *That's Life*, was later described in Esther Rantzen and Shaun

Woodward, *Ben: The Story of Ben Hardwick* (London: Penguin Character, 1985). A number of supportive personal or family accounts of organ transplants appeared at this time; see the bibliographical essay for a list.

71. For the controversy in Pittsburgh, see Lee Gutkind, *Many Sleepless Nights: The World of Organ Transplantation* (Pittsburgh: University of Pittsburgh Press, 1988), 88–94; and Dowie, *"We Have a Donor,"* 35.

72. The U.S. government's support for Marcos's transplant of a kidney from one of his soldiers is detailed in Nicholas Tilney, *Transplant: From Myth to Reality* (New Haven, CT: Yale University Press, 2003), 265–66.

73. See the United Network for Organ Sharing, *Policy Proposal Statement: UNOS Policies Regarding Transplantation of Foreign Nationals and Exportation and Importation of Organs* (Richmond, 1988).

74. British Transplantation Society, "Recommendations on the Use of Living Kidney Donors in the United Kingdom," *British Medical Journal* 293, no. 6541 (July 26, 1986): 257–58.

75. Marvin Brams had a long-standing interest in organ sales; see his "Transplantable Human Organs: Should Their Sale Be Authorized by State Statutes?" *American Journal of Law and Medicine* 3, no. 2 (1977): 183–91; and "Markets for Organs to Reinforce Altruism," *Economic Affairs* 7, no. 1 (Oct. 1986): 12–14. See also H. Hansmann (1989) in Blumstein and Sloan, *Organ Transplantation Policy.*

76. Neil M. Davidson and Jean Dausset, "Markets in Kidneys," *The Lancet* 324, no. 8415 (Dec. 8, 1984): 1344.

77. See the Statement of Barry Jacobs to the Subcommittee on Health and the Environment of the Committee on Energy and Commerce, House of Representatives, 98th Cong., 1st sess., at www.organselling.com/house.htm.

78. For U.S. organ sales proposals, see Dowie, *"We Have a Donor,"* 139–43.

79. Richard A. Rettig, "The Politics of Transplantation: A Parable of Our Time," in Blumstein and Sloan, *Organ Transplantation Policy.*

80. Sales from organ banks were not affected. For the financial structure of the U.S. tissue banks, see Dowie, *"We Have a Donor,"* 121–30.

81. United Network for Organ Sharing, *Policy Proposal Statement: Policies Regarding the Listing of Patients on Multiple Transplant Waiting Lists* (Richmond, 1988). For a close analysis of prioritizing patients for liver transplantation, see Scott McCartney, *Defying the Gods: Inside the New Frontiers of Organ Transplants* (New York: Macmillan, 1994).

82. For a scholarly review, see Richard West, *Organ Transplantation* (London: Office of Health Economics, 1961).

83. For data on organ supply and demand, see the annual reports from the European Dialysis and Transplantation Association, published regularly in *Dialysis, Transplantation and Nephrology,* later renamed *Nephrology, Transplantation and Dialysis.* A decline in organ donation in Europe and the United States at this time was mirrored elsewhere, notably in Australia, where kidney donation reached a peak of fourteen donors per million in 1989 but had declined to ten per million by the mid-1990s.

84. Josep Lloveras, "Presidential Address," *Transplantation Proceedings* 29, no. 8 (1997): 3177–80, 3178.

85. In Britain, the veteran politician Tam Dalyell made many attempts to bring in "opting-out" legislation, but the failure of this approach to increase donation in Europe meant he had little support. In Britain in 2000, a series of controversies regarding the unauthorized removal and retention of human organs meant a further setback for "opting-out" schemes.

86. The legal position on donation options is reviewed in Russell Scott, *The Body as Property* (New York: Viking, 1981), 74–81.

87. For a review, see Daniel Azoulay, Guillermo Marin Hargreaves, and Henri Bismuth, "Impact of Liver Surgery on Liver Transplantation," *Current Opinion in Organ Transplantation* 5, no. 2 (2000): 57–63.

88. For what may be the first use of the term "marginal donor," see George Abouna, "Marginal Donors: A Viable Solution for Organ Shortage," *Transplantation Proceedings* 29, no. 7 (1997): 2759.

89. J. A. Van der Vliet, M. J. H. Slooff, G. Kootstra, R. A. Krom, and B. G. Rijkmans, "Non-Heartbeating Donors, Is It Worthwhile?" *Proceedings of the European Dialysis and Transplant Association* 17 (1980): 445–49. Later papers are R. M. H. Wijnen, M. H. Booster, B. M. Stubenitsy, E. Heineman, G. Kootstra, and J. de Boer, "Outcome of Transplantation of Non-Heart Beating Kidney Donors," *The Lancet* 345, no. 8957 (Apr. 29, 1995): 1067–70; and Seigo Hiraga, "An Overview of Current Non-Heart-Beating Donor Trans-

plantation," *Transplantation Proceedings* 29, no. 8 (1997): 3559–60.

90. For the return of viability tests, see the symposium in *Transplantation Proceedings* 32 (2000): 161–79.

91. Starzl remained opposed to living-related donation, citing the small but inevitable number of donor deaths; see Thomas E. Starzl, "Living Donors: Con," *Transplantation Proceedings* 19, no. 1 (Feb. 1987): 174–75.

92. For comment, see Felix T. Rapaport, "Living Donor Kidney Transplantation," *Transplantation Proceedings* 19, no. 1 (Feb. 1987): 169–73. The first report of "emotionally related" unrelated living donor transplantation was S. C. Kountz, H. A. Perkins, R. Payne, et al., "Kidney Transplants Using Living Unrelated Donors," *Transplantation Proceedings* 2 (1970): 427–29. Donor-specific blood transfusion was later used in this situation; see Folkert O. Belzer, Munci Kalayoglu, and Hans W. Sollinger, "Donor-Specific Transfusion in Living-Unrelated Renal Donor-Recipient Combinations," *Transplantation Proceedings* 19, no. 1 (Feb. 1987): 1514–15.

93. For the first such "cross-over" living-related grafting, see K. Park, "Emotionally Related Donation and Donor Swapping," *Transplantation Proceedings* 30 (1998): 3117.

94. Dowie, *"We Have a Donor,"* gives details of the early UNOS debates on sharing.

95. The debate on acceptance of alcoholics for liver transplantation is found in Alvin H. Moss and Mark Siegler, "Should Alcoholics Compete Equally for Liver Transplantation?" *Journal of the American Medical Association* 265, no. 10 (Mar. 13, 1991), 1295–98. The debate intensified in the United States when Mickey Mantle, the baseball star of the 1950s and 1960s who had battled alcoholism, was transplanted in Dallas in mid-1995 but died shortly afterward of metastatic liver cancer. The controversy also erupted in Britain when the alcoholic soccer star George Best underwent a successful liver transplant in 2002 but was publicly drinking again in 2003; the graft deteriorated and he died in 2005.

96. See the interesting review, Søren Bak-Jensen, "To Share or Not to Share? Institutional Exchange of Cadaver Kidneys in Denmark," *Medical History* 52, no. 1 (Jan. 2008): 23–46.

97. For religious attitudes and practice in Britain, see Robin Jeffrey, *Organ Donation and Transplantation:*

The Multifaith Perspective (Bradford, England: Renal Unit at the Bradford Hospitals NHS Trust, 2000). By the year 2000, nearly 40 percent of patients on dialysis in the Midlands of England had the rare blood group B. Activists successfully lobbied to divert neutral kidneys (blood group O) to this disadvantaged set of group B patients.

98. G. Randhawa, "The Impending Kidney Transplant Crisis for the Asian Population in the UK," *Public Health* 112, no. 4 (1998): 265–68. In Singapore, the stern authoritarian government barred transplantation of patients belonging to the nondonating Muslim community. The use of pig organs adapted for human transplant would also be anathema to this and other religious groups.

99. See the excellent review by Moussa, Walele, and Daar in Peter J. Morris, ed., *Kidney Transplantation: Principles and Practice,* 5th ed. (Philadelphia: Saunders, 2001), 659–92.

100. In the mid-1990s the World Bank defined less developed or "developing" nations as having a per capita income of less than $3,120. These countries are also characterized by high birth rates, high infant mortality, incomplete official health statistics, with information on medical activity often based instead on anecdotal accounts. From the growing literature on comparative ethnology, see K. S. Chugh, V. Jha, and S. Chugh, "Economics of Dialysis and Renal Transplantation in the Developing World," *Transplantation Proceedings* 31, no. 8 (Dec. 1999): 3275–77.

101. See Farhat Moazam, *Bioethics and Transplantation in a Muslim Society: A Study in Culture, Ethnography, and Religion* (Bloomington: Indiana University Press, 2006).

102. For an international perspective on organ donation and transplantation, see the Singapore Conference of the Transplantation Society in 1992, reported in *Transplantation Proceedings* 24, no. 5 (1992): 2038–85. For an international perspective on ethical problems, see *Transplantation Proceedings* 24, no. 5 (1992): 2087–129. See also the World Health Organization's *Legislative Responses to Organ Transplantation* (Dordrecht, Netherlands: Martinus Nijhoff, 1994). The kidney disease patterns were different in developing nations, and the post-transplant complications also varied. In many countries, salmonella infection and reactivation of tuberculosis and malaria were familiar post-transplant events. Even the types of post-transplant malignancies showed a curious and provocative difference, one prime example being the prevalence in Saudi Arabia of post-transplant Kaposi's sarcoma.

103. For the Middle Eastern experience, see M. S. Abomelha, ed., *Organ Transplantation: Proceedings of the Second International Middle East Symposium* (Oxford: Medical Education Services, 1986). An earlier symposium was held at Kuwait and is reported in *Current Status of Clinical Organ Transplantation*, ed. George Abouna (Boston: Martinus Nijhoff, 1984).

104. F. A. M. Shaheen, M. Z. Souqiyyeh, M. B. Attar, and A. R. al-Swailem, "The Saudi Center for Organ Transplantation: An Ideal Model for Arab Countries to Improve Treatment of End-Stage Organ Failure," *Transplantation Proceedings* 28, no. 1 (Feb. 1996): 247–49. See also Samir Johna and George M. Abouna: *The History of a Pioneer in Transplant Surgery* (Bloomington, IN: AuthorHouse, 2004).

105. In Turkey, a survey of public opinion showed that 43 percent of refusals to consider donation were on the grounds of disfigurement of the body, while only 26 percent were on religious grounds; see Halil Bilgel, Nazan Bilgel, Necla Okan, Sadik Kilicturgay, Yilmaz Ozen, and Nusret Korun, "Public Attitudes to Organ Donation: A Survey in a Turkish Community," *Transplant International* 4, no. 1 (1991): 243–45.

106. Y. I. M. El-Shahat, "Islamic Viewpoint of Organ Transplantation," *Transplantation Proceedings* 31, no. 8 (1999): 3271–74, with a list of eighteen transplant-related *fatwas* on 3272. See also Abul Fadl Mohsin Ebrahim, *Organ Transplantation: Contemporary Islamic Legal and Ethical Perspectives* (Kuala Lumpur: A. S. Noordeen, 1998).

107. Margaret Lock, "Deadly Disputes: Hybrid Selves and the Calculation of Death in Japan and North America," *Osiris* 13 (1998): 410–29.

108. See Masaya Yamauchi, "News: Transplantation in Japan," *British Medical Journal* 301, no. 6751 (Sept. 15, 1990): 507; and S. Hiraga, T. Mori, and Y. Asaura, "Current Arrangement and Activity of Organ Transplantation after New Organ Transplant Legislation in Japan," *Transplantation Proceedings* 32 (2000): 86–89. This cultural view led to an anomalous situation for American military hospitals in Japan, and they bowed to local opinion in not using brain-dead cadaveric donation on the occasions when organ donation did occur.

109. See Council of the Transplantation Society, "Commercialisation in Transplantation: The Problems and Some Guidelines for Practice," *The Lancet* 326, no. 8457 (Sept. 28, 1985): 715–16. For comments, see *Dialysis and Transplantation Today*, January 1984. See also British Transplantation Society, "Recommen-

dations on the Use of Living Donors in the United Kingdom," *British Medical Journal* 293, no. 6541 (July 26, 1986): 257–58. Sale of organs was made a crime in United States via Public Law 98-507, October 19, 1984, as it had been earlier in Ontario with its Human Tissues Gift Act in 1972, as well as by the Council of Europe in Resolution 78[29] of 1978.

110. The Islamic Council determined that sale of organs as a commodity was prohibited, and since Islam also incorporates civil law elements (the Shari'āh), penalties for such commercialism were also laid down, although small rewards for family donors were judged acceptable.

111. K. C. Kuruvila, B. N. Colabawalla, S. S. Joshi, M. H. Kamat, M. K. Mani, and F. P. Soonawalla, "Problems of Transplantation in India," *Transplantation Proceedings* 11, no. 2 (June 1979): 1296; see also M. Slapak, "Live Donors: Related and Otherwise," *Transplantation Proceedings* 17, no. 6, suppl. 4 (Dec. 1985): 13–14. In 2001, a confidential survey of 305 living kidney donors, conducted in Madras, showed an average payment of six hundred pounds had been made for the organ and that 70 percent of these operations had been arranged via a broker. Paying off debt was the motive in 96 percent of the cases, and, sadly, debt often remained or returned; see Madhav Goyal, Ravindra L. Mehta, Lawrence J. Schneiderman, and Ashwini R. Sehgal, "Economic and Health Consequences of Selling a Kidney in India," *Journal of the American Medical Association* 288, no. 13 (Oct. 2, 2002): 1589–93. For use of Indian commercial transplantation as a theme by a novelist, see Subroto Kundu, *Jehad: A Novel* (New Dehli: Lancer, 2002).

112. For the Indian defense, see A. S. Daar, "Ethical Issues—A Middle East Perspective," *Transplantation Proceedings* 21, no. 1 (Feb. 1989): 1402–3.

113. An Israeli-brokered paid kidney donor case is fully described in the *Sunday Telegraph Magazine*, June 24, 2001. See also the publications by Nancy Scheper-Hughes and Lawrence Cohen's organization, Organ Watch, set up in 1999, funded initially by the Soros Foundation's Open Society Institute. The situation in Eastern Europe was watched by the (Western) Council of Europe, which published *Trafficking in Organs in Europe*, Document 9822, June 2003.

114. See D. Reissi, A. Bardideh, B. Samadzadeh, and A. Razi, "Kidney Transplantation in Kermanshah, Iran: A 5-Year Experience," *Transplantation Proceedings* 27, no. 5 (Oct. 1995): 2765–66; and E. Ahmad, S. A. Malek Hosseini, H. Salahi, R. Javid, N. Ghahramani, and N. Nezakatgoo, "Experience with 300 Re-

nal Transplants in Shiraz, Iran," *Transplantation Proceedings* 27, no. 5 (Oct. 1995): 2767; and the fuller report in A. J. Ghods, S. Ossareh, and S. Savaj, "Results of Renal Transplantation of the Hashemi Nejad Kidney Hospital, Tehran," *Clinical Transplants* 16 (2000): 203–10; and the follow-up, A. J. Ghods, S. Ossareh, S. Abedi Azar, S. Savaj, and M. Shahroukh, "Characteristics of Patients Remaining on Chronic Dialysis after Elimination of Renal Transplant Waiting List in Iran," *Transplantation Proceedings* 34, no. 6 (2002): 2037–38. In Iran in 1999, five hundred men offered to sell one of their kidneys to raise the cash required as a bounty for the execution of Salman Rushdie, the "blasphemous" British novelist; the Iranian government discouraged this venture.

115. For doubts about the Iranian claims, see Anne Griffin, "Iranian Organ Donation: Kidneys on Demand," *British Medical Journal* 334, no. 7592 (Mar. 10, 2007): 502–7.

116. For an excellent review, see A. S. Daar and Robert A. Sells, "Living Non-Related Donor Renal Transplantation—A Reappraisal," *Transplantation Reviews* 4 (1990): 128–40.

117. J. Stewart Cameron and Raymond Hoffenberg, "The Ethics of Organ Transplantation Reconsidered: Paid Organ Donation and the Use of Executed Prisoners as Donors," *Kidney International* 55, no. 2 (1999): 724–33.

118. For changing ethical stances, see J. B. Dosseter and A. S. Daar, "Ethics in Transplantation: Allotransplantation and Xenotransplantation," in *Kidney Transplantation: Principles and Practice*, ed. Peter Morris, 5th ed. (Philadelphia: Saunders, 2001), 732–33.

119. See Ronald Guttmann, "On the Use of Organs from Executed Prisoners," *Transplantation Reviews* 6, no. 3 (1992): 189–93.

120. In the early days of transplantation, use of kidneys from executed prisoners was often suggested as a donor source. U.S. transplant units were regularly offered organs from condemned prisoners but declined them. See the interesting review by Arnold G. Diethelm, "Ethical Decisions in the History of Organ Transplantation," *Annals of Surgery* 211, no. 5 (May 1990): 505–20; and Louis J. Palmer, *Organ Transplants from Executed Prisoners: An Argument for the Creation of Death Sentence Organ Removal Statutes* (Jefferson, NC: McFarland, 1999).

121. Amnesty International began investigating China's trade in prisoners' organs in 1993, assisted by Harry Wu, a well-known dissident; see *Sunday Telegraph*, March 1, 1998. The organization estimated that 90 percent of the recent organ transplants done in China used donor organs from executed criminals. The Chinese government initially denied the accusation as an example of denigration by the West, but the arrest of two Chinese brokers offering such organs for sale in the United States confirmed the existence of such activity, which the Chinese government later admitted.

122. David J. Rothman, "The International Organ Traffic," *New York Review of Books*, March 26, 1998; and D. E. Rothman, E. Rose, T. Awaya, B. Cohen, A. Daar, S. L. Dzemeshkevich, C. J. Lee, R. Munro, H. Reyes, S. M. Rothman, K. F. Schoen, N. Scheper-Hughes, Z. Shapira, and H. Smit, "The Bellagio Task Force Report on Transplantation, Bodily Integrity and the International Traffic in Organs," *Transplantation Proceedings* 29, no. 6 (Sept. 1997): 2739–45. The gruesome dubious medical "urban myths" are found in Jan Harold Brunvand, *The Baby Train and Other Lusty Urban Legends* (New York: Norton, 1993). The Rothmans updated their studies in David J. Rothman and Sheila M. Rothman, "The Organ Market," *New York Review of Books*, October 23, 2003. See also the perceptive review by Véronique Campion-Vincent, "Organ Theft Narratives," *Western Folklore* 56, no. 1 (1997): 1–37.

123. Russell, foreword to Ginns, Cosimi, and Morris, *Transplantation*, xviii.

19. Waiting for the Xenografts

1. The upsurge in pharmaceutical company presence in clinical transplantation is dated to 1982 in Ronald Guttman, "Technology, Clinical Studies and Control in the Field of Organ Transplantation," *Journal of the History of Biology* 30, no. 3 (1997): 367–79. See also Nicholas Tilney, *Transplant: From Myth to Reality* (New Haven, CT: Yale University Press, 2003).

2. David Talbot, "The Flow Cytometric Crossmatch in Perspective," *Transplantation Immunology* 1, no. 3 (1993): 155–62.

3. Jeffrey Bidwell, "DNA-RFLP Analysis and Genotyping of HLA-DR and DQ Antigens," *Immunology Today* 9, no. 1 (1988): 18–32.

4. Thomas E. Starzl, N. Murase, S. Ildstad, C. Ricordi, A. J. Demetris, and M. Trucco, "Cell Migration, Chi-

merism and Graft Acceptance," *The Lancet* 339, no. 8809 (June 27, 1992): 1579–82; Thomas E. Starzl, Anthony J. Demetris, Noriko Murase, Massimo Trucco, Angus W. Thomson, and Abdul S. Rao, "The Lost Chord: Microchimerism and Allograft Survival," *Immunology Today* 17, no. 12 (1996): 577–84. See the following article by Kathryn Wood and David H. Sachs, "Chimerism and Transplantation Tolerance: Cause and Effect," *Immunology Today* 17, no. 12 (1996): 584–87, and the "Responses" by the authors of both articles on the following page.

5. For attempts to induce microchimerism, see K. Rolles, A. K. Burroughs, B. R. Davidson, H. G. Prentice, and M. D. Hamon, "Donor-Specific Bone Marrow Infusion after Orthotopic Liver Transplantation," *The Lancet* 343, no. 8892 (Jan. 29, 1994): 263–65.

6. The first observation of chronic kidney allograft damage is reported in Hume's pioneer 1955 paper (David M. Hume, John P. Merrill, Benjamin F. Miller, and George W. Thorn, "Experiences with Renal Homotransplantation in the Human: Report of Nine Cases," *Journal of Clinical Investigation* 34, no. 2 [Feb. 1955]: 327–82) in the study of the graft in the single patient with prolonged kidney graft function. A closer study came in 1963, again from Boston, in Joseph E. Murray, J. P. Merrill, J. Hartwell Harrison, Richard E. Wilson, and Gustave J. Dammin, "Prolonged Survival of Human-Kidney Homografts by Immunosuppressive Drug Therapy," *New England Journal of Medicine* 268, no. 24 (June 13, 1963): 1315–23.

7. Nicholas L. Tilney, "Chronic Rejection," in *Transplantation,* ed. Leo C. Ginns, A. Benedict Cosimi, and Peter J. Morris (Malden, MA: Blackwell, 1999), 43–52.

8. See David Pegg's commentary in Ginns, Cosimi, and Morris, *Transplantation,* 279–84. This focus on the condition of the kidney at the time of transplantation pleased the supporters of the perfusion machines still in use by some units, notably in the United States.

9. An alternative strategy was the simpler, cheaper, but less rigorous study of the data on outcomes of huge numbers of patients, on different therapies, held in the many national transplant registries and databases, notably the U.S. Renal Data System.

10. Elsie M. Eugui and Anthony C. Allison, "Immunosuppressive Activity of Mycophenolate Mofetil," *Annals of the New York Academy of Sciences* 685 (1993): 309–29.

11. European Mycophenolate Mofetil Cooperative Study Group, "Placebo-Controlled Study of Mycophenolate Mofetil Combined with Cyclosporin and Cor-

ticosteroids for Prevention of Acute Rejection," *The Lancet* 345, no. 8961 (May 27, 1995): 1321–25.

12. T. Ochiai, K. Nakajima, M. Nagata, T. Suzuki, T. Asano, T. Uematsu, T. Goto, S. Hori, T. Kenmochi, T. Nakagoori, et al., "Effect of a New Immunosuppressive Agent, FK 506, on Heterotopic Cardiac Allotransplantation in the Rat," *Transplantation Proceedings* 19, no. 1 (Feb. 1987): 1284–86.

13. Thomas E. Starzl, John Fung, Raman Venkataramanan, Satoru Todo, Anthony J. Demetris, and Ashok Jain, "FK506 for Human Liver, Kidney and Pancreas Transplantation," *The Lancet* 334, no. 8670 (Oct. 28, 1989): 1000–1004.

14. Thomas E. Starzl, J. J. Fung, J. P. McMichael, Satoru Todo, A. Donner, M. Eliasziw, L. Stitt, and P. Meier, "Randomised Trialomania? The Multicentre Liver Transplant Trials of Tacrolimus," *The Lancet* 346, no. 8986 (Nov. 18, 1995): 1346–50. Starzl's reanalysis supported the efficacy of the new drug and pointed out not only that a pioneer unit's increasing experience will often improve on the fixed usage and protocol necessary in any trial but also that newcomers might take time to gain experience in the art of using a new drug; see Thomas E. Starzl, *The Puzzle People: Memoirs of a Transplant Surgeon* (Pittsburgh: University of Pittsburgh Press, 1992).

15. Jun Liu, Jesse D. Farmer Jr., William S. Lane, Jeff Friedman, Irving Weissman, and Stuart L. Schreiber, "Calcineurin Is a Common Target of Cyclophilin-Cyclosporin A and FKBP-FK506 Complexes," *Cell* 66, no. 4 (1991): 807–15. The common path of cellular action in both tacrolimus and CsA proved to be calcineurin inhibition, hence their nephrotoxicity in humans.

16. Sehgal had described the antifungal properties of Rapamycin in 1975, and his group reported the immunological effects in R. R. Martel, J. Klicius, and S. Galet, "Inhibition of the Immune Response by Rapamycin, a New Antifungal Antibiotic," *Canadian Journal of Physiology and Pharmacology* 55, no. 1 (1977): 48–51. Although the drug raised lipid levels, it was not nephrotoxic like the calcineurin inhibitors, was less likely to cause insulin resistance and diabetes, and had less effect on blood pressure. Its experimental anticancer and anti-inflammatory actions were also important, raising hopes that it might lead to fewer post-transplant tumors and fibrotic lesions, thought to be part of chronic rejection.

17. A. Benedict Cosimi, Robert C. Burton, Robert B. Colvin, Gideon Goldstein, Francis L. Delmonico, Michael P. Laquaglia, Nina Tolkoff-Rubin, Robert

H. Rubin, John T. Herrin, and Paul S. Russell, "Treatment of Acute Renal Allograft Rejection with OKT3 Monclonal Antibody," *Transplantation* 32, no. 6 (Dec. 1981): 535–40.

18. These were ATGAM from Pfizer, and Lymphoglobuline and Thymoglobulin, both from Pasteur-Merieux.

19. The four-year investigation had included office raids by the Federal Bureau of Investigation and the Internal Revenue Service; see *Time* magazine, May 15, 1995. The university leadership's reputation suffered, and there was an exodus of medical faculty staff. In such cases, the FDA had powers to "grandfather," that is, approve any well-established remedies, but chose not to. In spite of the high levels of medical litigation in the United States, the pioneer transplant surgeons had remained largely free of lawsuits, in spite of their high-risk work. In Seattle in 2004, E. Donnall Thomas was cleared in a major case, one closely followed by the *Seattle Times,* alleging a lack of informed consent from some patients in his pioneering bone marrow transplant work.

20. Lloyd Ratner and Louis Kavoussi, "Laparoscopic Live Donor Nephrectomy," *Contemporary Dialysis and Nephrology* 11 (1996): 13–14.

21. Jean-Michel Dubernard, Earl Owen, Guillaume Herzberg, Marco Lanzetta, Xavier Martin, Hari Kapila, Marwan Dawahra, and Nadey S. Hakim, "Human Hand Allograft: Report on First 6 Months," *The Lancet* 353, no. 9161 (Apr. 17, 1999): 1315–20. The possibilities of hand transplants were explored in a novel by John Irving, *The Fourth Hand* (New York: Random House, 2001) and in Arthur Cheney Train's earlier *Mortmain* (New York: D. Appleton, 1907).

22. Reviewed by Johan Van den Bogaerde and David J. G. White, "Xenogeneic Transplantation," *British Medical Bulletin* 53, no. 4 (1997): 904–20; and T. Nagayasu and Jeffrey L. Platt, "Progress in Xenotransplantation," *Graft* 1 (1998): 19–24.

23. Roy Yorke Calne, "Organ Transplantation between Widely Disparate Species," *Transplantation Proceedings* 2, no. 4 (Dec. 1970): 550–56. He explained that his neologisms "concordant" and "discordant transplantation" emerged from "linguistic and taxonomic discussions" with appropriate local Cambridge University literati.

24. For the commercial lure of organ transplantation, see Thomas Okarma, "Academic-Industrial Relations in the Biopharmaceutical Sector: Complex Diplomacy in Pursuit of Value Creation," *Graft* 1 (1998): 163–64.

25. Kathryn J. Wood, "Gene Transfer," in Ginns, Cosimi and Morris, *Transplantation,* chap. 39, 814–24. The Novartis Foundation revived the earlier CIBA Foundation symposium tradition with a meeting on stem cell use, published as *Neural Transplantation in Neurodegenerative Disease: Current Status and New Directions,* ed. Derek Chadwick and Jamie Goode (Chichester, England: Wiley, 2000).

26. Rick G. Tearle, Margaret J. Tange, Zara L. Zannettino, Marina Katerelos, Trixie A. Shinkel, Bryce J. W. van Denderen, Andrew J. Lonie, Ian Lyons, Mark B. Nottle, Timothy Cox, Christiane Becker, Anita M. Peura, Peter L. Wigley, Robert J. Crawford, Allan J. Robins, Martin J. Pearse, and Anthony J. F. d'Apice, "The α-1,3-galactosyltransferase Knockout Mouse: Implications for Transplantation," *Transplantation* 61, no. 1 (1996): 13–19.

27. Clive Petience, Yasuhiro Takeuchi, and Robin A. Weiss, "Infection of Human Cells by an Endogenous Retrovirus of Pigs," *Nature Medicine* 3, no. 3 (1997): 282–86. An additional fear is that retroviruses may pass to an embryo from the mother.

28. The knocked-out gene was for alpha 1,3 galactosyltransferase.

29. D. J. G. White, G. Langford, E. E. Cozzi, and V. Young, "Production of Pigs Transgenic for Human DAF: A Strategy for Xenotransplantation," *Xenotransplantation* 2, no. 3 (1995): 213–17; David Ayares, Alan Colman, Yifan Dai, Paul Shiels, and Marilyn Moore, "Cloning Pigs Deficient in Alpha 1,3 Galactosyltransferase," *Graft* 4, no. 1 (Jan. 2001): 80–82. The double knockout later deleted alpha 1,3 galactose transferase.

30. "Guideline on Infectious Disease Issues in Xenotransplantation" (August 1996), *Federal Register,* 96-24448, September 23, 1996.

31. Great Britain Department of Health, *Animal Tissue into Humans: A Report by the Advisory Group on the Ethics of Xenotransplantation* (London: Stationery Office, 1996).

32. Walid Heneine, Annika Tibell, William M. Switzer, Paul Sandstrom, Guillermo Vazquez Rosales, Aprille Mathews, Olle Korsgren, Louisa E. Chapman, Thomas M. Folks, and Carl G. Groth, "No Evidence of Infection with Porcine Endogenous Retroviruses in Recipients of Porcine Islet–Cell Xenografts," *The Lancet* 352, no. 9129 (Aug. 29, 1998): 695–99.

33. Afzal Zaidi, Michael Schmoeckel, Farah Bhatti, Paul Waterworth, Michael Tolan, Emanuele Cozzi, Gilda Chavez, Gillian Langford, Sathia Thiru, John

Wallwork, David White, and Peter Friend, "Life Supporting Pig-to-Primate Renal Xenotransplantation Using Genetically Modified Donors," *Transplantation* 65, no. 12 (June 27, 1998): 1584–90. The control unmodified pig-to-primate organ grafts survived better than expected. Testing of altered pig organs in monkeys could be carried out only in the countries still permitting routine primate use—including the United States, Russia, Germany, and the Netherlands.

34. Karl Illmensee and Peter C. Hoppe, "Nuclear Transplantation in *Mus musculus:* Developmental Potential of Nuclei from Preimplantation Embryos," *Cell* 23, no. 1 (1981): 9–18. Investigation threw doubt on these claims, and some wondered if cloning was possible at all. The idea of human cloning had already made its way into literature; see David Rorvik, *In His Image: The Cloning of a Man* (1978), Ira Levin, *The Boys from Brazil* (1976), and Woody Allen's film *Sleeper* (1973).

35. Ian Wilmut, Keith Campbell and Colin Tudge, *The Second Creation: Dolly and the Age of Biological Control* (New York: Farrar, Straus and Giroux, 2000). Dolly was the result of creating 277 embryos, with 29 blastocysts resulting. When transferred into 13 ewes, these yielded only one pregnancy and one live birth.

36. K. McCreath, J. Howcroft, K. H. S. Campbell, Alan Colman, A. E. Schnieke, and A. J. Kind, "Production of Gene-Targeted Sheep by Nuclear Transfer from Cultured Somatic Cells," *Nature* 405, no. 6790 (June 29, 2000): 1066–69; Paul G. Shiels and Alan

G. Jardine, "Dolly, No Longer the Exception: Telomeres and Implications for Transplantation," *Cloning and Stem Cells* 5, no. 2 (2003): 157–60. Dolly was cloned from nuclei from fetal fibroblast cultures fitted with the gene for human factor X. Although nuclear transfer techniques held no immediate promise for transplantation, it was noted that telomere-shortening senescence changes persisted in the nuclei of the otherwise young Dolly. Senescence in engineered grafts would be a feature of interest to transplantation.

37. Gail R. Martin, "Isolation of a Pluripotent Cell Line from Early Mouse Embryos Cultured in Medium Conditioned by Teratocarcinoma Stem Cells," *Proceedings of the National Academy of Sciences of the United States of America* 78, no. 12 (Dec. 1981): 7634–38.

38. James A. Thomson, Joseph Itskovitz-Eldor, Sander S. Shapiro, Michelle A. Waknitz, Jennifer J. Swiergniel, Vivienne S. Marshall, and Jeffrey M. Jones, "Embryonic Stem Cell Lines Derived from Human Blastocysts," *Science* 282, no. 5391 (Nov. 6, 1998): 1145–47.

39. The U.S. Congress passed the Dickey-Wicker Amendment in 1995, preventing the use of federal funding for studies in which human embryos were destroyed. In March 2009, an executive order from President Barack Obama largely removed the restriction.

40. Kazutoshi Takahashi and Shinya Yamanaka, "Induction of Pluripotent Stem Cells from Mouse Embryonic and Adult Fibroblast Cultures," *Cell* 126, no. 4 (2006): 663–76.

Bibliographic Essay

Major Works

Substantial works on the history of transplantation include René Küss, *An Illustrated History of Organ Transplantation: The Great Adventure of the Century* (Rueil-Malmaison, France: Sandoz, 1992); Nicholas Tilney, *Transplant: From Myth to Reality* (New Haven, CT: Yale University Press, 2003); Nadey S. Hakim and Vassilios E. Papalois, eds., *History of Organ and Tissue Transplantation* (London: Imperial College Press, 2003); Leslie Brent, *A History of Transplantation Immunology* (San Diego: Academic Press, 1997); and Henk J. Klasen, *History of Free Skin Grafting: Knowledge or Empiricism?* (Berlin: Springer-Verlag, 1981). Thomas Schlich, *The Origins of Organ Transplantation* (Rochester, NY: University of Rochester Press, 2010) covers the period 1880–1930, as does Susan E. Lederer in *Flesh and Blood: Organ Transplantation and Blood Transfusion in Twentieth Century America* (Oxford: Oxford University Press, 2008). A major source on more recent times is Paul I. Terasaki, ed., *History of Transplantation: Thirty-Five Recollections* (Los Angeles: UCLA Tissue Typing Laboratory, 1991), and Paul I. Terasaki, ed., *History of HLA: Ten Recollections* (Los Angeles: UCLA Tissue Typing Laboratory, 1990). Important articles are the collected essays in *World Journal of Surgery* 24, no. 7 (2000): 755–843, which has a "Historic Landmarks" listing attached. See also Thomas E. Starzl, "Personal Reflections in Transplantation," *Surgical Clinics of North America* 58 (October 1978): 879–93. There are historical vignettes in Leslie Brent and Robert A. Sells, eds., *Organ Transplantation: Current Clinical and Immunological Concepts* (London: Baillière Tindall, 1989). The thorough text by Sir Michael Woodruff, *The Transplantation of Tissues and Organs* (Springfield, IL: Thomas, 1960), was published on the eve of rapid expansion and has a massive bibliography on the subject to that date, and a personal account of these times is found in Francis D. Moore's autobiography, *Give and Take: The Development of Tissue Transplantation* (Philadelphia: Saun-

ders, 1964), with a revised edition titled *Transplant: The Give and Take of Tissue Transplantation* (New York: Simon and Schuster, 1972). See also Rupert E. Billingham and Willys K. Silvers, eds., *Transplantation of Tissues and Cells* (Philadelphia: Wistar Institute Press, 1961), and historical accounts of tissue transplantation are found as introductions to textbooks, notably John B. de C. M. Saunders, "A Conceptual History of Transplantation," in *Transplantation,* edited by John S. Najarian and Richard L. Simmons (Philadelphia: Lea & Febiger, 1972), 3–25, and David Hamilton's introductory chapter, "Kidney Transplantation: A History," to Peter J. Morris, *Kidney Transplantation: Principles and Practice,* 6th ed., edited by Peter J. Morris and Stuart J. Knechtle (Philadelphia: Saunders, 2008), 1–8, as well as the introduction to Leo C. Ginns, A. Benedict Cosimi, and Peter J. Morris, eds., *Transplantation* (Malden, MA: Blackwell Science, 1999). Collected works of importance include the proceedings of the symposium to mark twenty-five years of transplantation at the Peter Bent Brigham Hospital, as reported in *Transplantation Proceedings* 13 (1981): supplement 1.

For individual tissue-grafting endeavors, see Benjamin W. Rycroft, *Corneal Grafts* (London: Butterworth, 1955), and, for the development of blood transfusion, see Louis K. Diamond, "A History of Blood Transfusion," in *Blood, Pure and Eloquent: A Story of Discovery, of People, and of Ideas,* edited by Maxwell M. Wintrobe (New York: McGraw-Hill, 1980), 690–717. Extensive and useful bibliographies on the history of bone grafting are found in the early volumes of *Transplantation Bulletin,* volumes 1–5, from 1954 to 1958. The development of liver transplantation is described in Thomas E. Starzl, *The Puzzle People* (Pittsburgh: University of Pittsburgh Press, 1992); in Starzl, "The Mother Lode of Liver Transplantation," *Journal of Liver Transplantation Surgery* 4, no. 1 (January 1998): 1–14; and in Thomas Starzl and John

527

J. Fung, "Themes of Liver Transplantation," *Hepatology* 51, no. 6 (June 2010): 1869–84. Bone marrow transplantation development is found in E. Donnall

Thomas, "Landmarks in the Development of Hematopoietic Cell Transplantation," *World Journal of Surgery* 24, no. 7 (July 2000): 815–18.

Immunology

Important historical texts on immunology relating to transplantation include Arthur M. Silverstein, *A History of Immunology* (San Diego: Academic Press, 1989), and Jacques F. A. P. Miller, "The Discovery of Thymus Function," in *Immunology: The Making of a Modern Science*, edited by Richard B. Gallagher, Jean Gilder, Gustav J. V. Nossal, and Gaetano Salvatore (London and San Diego: Academic Press, 1995). Debra Jan Bibel, *Milestones in Immunology: A Historical Exploration* (Madison, WI: Science Tech, 1988), has excellent reprints and comments on the classic works. See also Pauline Mazumdar, ed., *Immunology 1930–1980: Essays on the History of Immunology* (Toronto: Wall & Thompson, 1989). The rise in understanding of the lymphocyte is found in William L. Ford's careful account, "The Lymphocyte—

Its Transformation from a Frustrating Enigma to a Model of Cellular Function," in *Blood, Pure and Eloquent: A Story of Discovery, of People, and of Ideas*, edited by Maxwell M. Wintrobe (New York: McGraw-Hill, 1980), 457–508; in J. F. A. P. Miller, "Uncovering Thymus Function," *Perspectives in Biology and Medicine* 39, no. 3 (spring 1996): 338–52; and in Robert A. Good, "Runestones in Immunology: Inscriptions to Journeys of Discovery and Analysis," *Journal of Immunology* 117, no. 5 (November 1976): 1413–28. For the rapid expansion of knowledge of autoimmunity, see the important review by E. M. Tansey, S. V. Willhoft, and D. A. Christie, eds., *Self and Non-Self: A History of Autoimmunity*, volume 1, *Wellcome Witnesses to Twentieth Century Medicine* (London: Wellcome Trust, 1997).

Sources on Early Tissue Transplantation

On early "magical" tissue replacement, see Howard Clark Kee, *Medicine, Miracle and Magic in New Testament Times* (Cambridge: Cambridge University Press, 1986), and Keith Thomas, *Religion and the Decline of Magic: Studies in Popular Beliefs in Sixteenth- and Seventeenth-Century England* (London: Weidenfeld & Nicholson, 1971; repr., New York: Penguin, 1991). Medieval healing shrines are described in Ronald C. Finucane, *Miracles and Pilgrims: Popular Beliefs in Medieval England* (New York: St. Martin's, 1995). For the Cosmas and Damian iconography and other images, see B. Tosatti, "Transplantation and Reimplantation in the Arts," *Surgery* 75, no. 3 (March 1974): 389–97. A scholarly account of secular plastic surgery and of Tagliacozzi's work in particular is found in the classic work by Martha T. Gnudi and Jerome Webster, *The Life and Times of Gaspare Tagliacozzi* (Milan: Hoepli, 1939; repr., New York: Herbert Reichner, 1950). Eighteenth-century works related to transplantation are Abraham Trembley's *Mémoires pour servir* (1744), and John

Hunter's *The Natural History of Human Teeth* (1771).

For the revival of skin graft studies, see Giuseppe Baronio's thesis *Degli innesti animali* of 1804, published in English as *On Grafting in Animals*, translated by Robert M. Goldwyn and Joan Bond Sax (Boston: Boston Medical Library, 1985), and Joseph Constantine Carpue, *An Account of Two Successful Operations for Restoring a Lost Nose from the Integuments of the Forehead* (London: Longman, 1816; repr., Birmingham, AL: Classics of Medicine Library, 1991). A number of French and German texts appeared rapidly, and these and other sources on plastic surgery up to 1863 are detailed in Eduard Zeis's incomparable index: *The Zeis Index and History of Plastic Surgery 900 BC–AD 1863*, translated by Thomas J. S. Patterson (Baltimore: Williams and Wilkins, 1977). See also Charles M. Balch and Francis A. Marzoni, "Skin Transplantation during the Pre-Reverdin Era, 1804–1869," *Surgery, Gynecology & Obstetrics* 144, no. 5 (May 1977): 767–73.

Sources Covering 1860 to 1900

The French interest in transplantation in the 1860s is noted in M. J. Seghers and J. J. Longacre, "Paul Bert and His Animal Grafts," *Plastic and Reconstructive Surgery* 33 (February 1964): 178–86, and for Reverdin's role see Henri Reverdin, *Jacques-Louis Reverdin 1842–1929: Un chirurgien à l'aube d'une ère nouvelle* (Aarau, Switzerland: Sauerländer, 1971). Easily the

best early source on the "pinch" skin grafting methods is in the contemporary review John Ashhurst Jr., ed., *The International Encyclopedia of Surgery* (New York: William Wood & Co., 1881), 538–49. Thereafter, the muddled literature of skin grafting, human and experimental, is described in Henk J. Klasen, *History of Free Skin Grafting: Knowledge or Empiricism?*

(Berlin: Springer-Verlag, 1981), and the early volumes of the *Index Catalogue of the Library of the Surgeon-General's Office, United States Army* (Washington, DC, 1892) have a massive survey of the world literature on transplantation until the 1930s, now available at http://indexcat.nlm.nih.gov.

For comment on early nonskin, nonvascularized homografting, together with a list of "firsts" in each type, see Jane M. Oppenheimer, "Taking Things Apart and Putting Them Together Again," *Bulletin of the History of Medicine* 52, no. 2 (summer 1978): 149–61, and M. Borell, "Organotherapy and the Emergence of Reproductive Endocrinology," *Journal of the History of Biology* 18, no. 1 (spring 1985): 1–30. See also the important review in Chandak Sengoopta, "The Modern Ovary: Constructions, Meanings, Uses," *History of Science* 38, no. 4 (December 2000): 425–88.

Early Twentieth Century to 1920

Toni Hau, *Renal Transplantation* (Austin, TX: Silvergirl, 1987) has important translations of some of the classic papers of this time. Tissue transplantation was important at this time in Europe, and the early monographs include P. F. Marchand, *Der Process der Wundheilund mit Einschluss der Transplantation* (Stuttgart, 1901), and Georg Schöne, *Die Heteroplastiche, Homöo-* *plastische Transplantation* (Berlin, 1912). Other early works are Erich Lexer, *Die frein Transplantation* (Stuttgart, 1919); Harold Neuhof, *The Transplantation of Tissues* (New York: D. Appleton, 1923); and John S. Davis, *Plastic Surgery, Its Principles and Practice* (Philadelphia: Blakiston, 1919).

Alexis Carrel

The best notes on Alexis Carrel are John Marquis Converse, "Alexis Carrel: The Man, the Unknown," *Plastic and Reconstructive Surgery* 68, no. 4 (October 1981): 629–39, and D. Hamilton, "Alexis Carrel and the Early Days of Tissue Transplantation," *Transplantation Reviews* 2 (1987): 1–15. Carrel has attracted many admiring and uncritical biographers; see Jacques Descotes, ed., *Alexis Carrel (1873–1944), pionnier de la chirurgie vasculaire et des transplantation d'organes* (Lyon: Simep Éditions, 1966), and Robert Soupault, *Alexis Carrel 1873–1944* (Paris: Plon, 1952; repr., Paris: Les Sept Couleurs, 1972). Better accounts are Theodore I. Malinin, *Surgery and Life: The Extraordinary Career of Alexis Carrel* (New York: Harcourt Brace Jovanovich, 1969), and W. Sterling Edwards and Peter D. Edwards, *Alexis Carrel, Visionary Surgeon* (Springfield, IL: Thomas, 1974). Alexis Carrel's numerous publications are listed in Yves Christen, *Alexis Carrel: L'ouverture de l'homme* (Paris: Éditions du Félin, 1986).

The papers delivered at the symposium on the occasion of Carrel's centennial are disappointing: see Robert W. Chambers and Joseph T. Durkin, eds., *Papers of the Alexis Carrel Centennial Conference* (Washington, DC: Georgetown University Press, 1973). The recurring concerns over Carrel's scientific data are aired in Jan A. Witkowski, "Alexis Carrel and the Mysticism of Tissue Culture," *Medical History* 23, no. 3 (July 1979): 279–96. For Carrel's later work, see Alexis Carrel and Charles A. Lindbergh, *The Culture of Organs* (New York: P. B. Hoeber, 1938), and David M. Friedman, *The Immortalists: Charles Lindbergh, Dr. Alexis Carrel, and Their Daring Quest to Live Forever* (New York: Ecco, 2007).

Other Rockefeller Institute studies on transplantation immunology are examined in Ilana Löwy, "Biomedical Research and the Constraints of Medical Practice: James Bumgardner Murphy and the Early Discovery of the Role of Lymphocytes in Immune Responses," *Bulletin of the History of Medicine* 63, no. 3 (fall 1989): 356–91. The Rockefeller reductionist biology is found in Philip J. Pauly, *Controlling Life: Jacques Loeb and the Engineering Ideal in Biology* (New York: Oxford University Press, 1987). This philosophy was applauded in Sinclair Lewis's successful novel *Martin Arrowsmith* (1925), based on the Rockefeller scientists.

The Hesitant Era, 1920–1940

For the Mayo Clinic interest in transplantation in the 1920s, see S. Sterioff and N. Rucker-Johnson, "Frank C. Mann and Transplantation at the Mayo Clinic," *Mayo Clinic Proceedings* 62, no. 11 (November 1987): 1051–55, though the authors understate the Mayo Clinic's involvement. The important St. Louis interest in skin grafting is found in Eric J. Stelnicki, V. Leroy Young, Tom Francel, and Peter Randall, "Vilray P. Blair, His Surgical Descendants, and Their Roles in Plastic Surgical Departments," *Plastic and Reconstructive Surgery* 103, no. 7 (June 1999): 1990–2009, and in Bradford Cannon, Joseph E. Murray, and Elvin G. Zook, "The Influence of the St. Louis Quadrumvirate," *Plastic and Reconstructive Surgery* 95, no. 6 (May

1995): 1118–22. On Earl Padgett, see Kathryn Lyle Stephenson, "As I Remember: Earl C. Padgett," *Annals of Plastic Surgery* 6 (1981): 142–57, and Padgett's own plastic surgery text is *Skin Grafting, From a Personal and Experimental Viewpoint* (Springfield, IL: C. C. Thomas, 1942). James Barrett Brown's textbook *Skin Grafting of Burns: Primary Care, Treatment, Repair* was first published in 1943 (Philadelphia: J. B. Lippincott) and coauthored with Frank MacDowell, with a third edition in 1958.

Leo Loeb was almost alone in the 1930s in his interest in transplantation immunology, and his classic work was "Transplantation and Individuality," *Physiological Reviews* 10 (1930): 547–616, extended later in his book *The Biological Basis of Individuality* (Springfield, IL: C. C. Thomas, 1945). Loeb's own memoirs are in "Autobiographical Notes," *Perspectives in Biology and Medicine* 2, no. 1 (autumn 1958): 1–23, and for a biography see Ernest Goodpasture, "Leo Loeb, 1869–1959," *National Academy of Sciences Biographical Memoirs*, volume 35 (Washington, DC: National Academy of Sciences, 1961), 205–51, which appends Loeb's remarkable bibliography and is available online at http://www.nasonline.org/publications/biographical-memoirs/alphabetical-listing/memoirs-l.html.

Early inbred mouse development is described in Herbert C. Morse III, *Origins of Inbred Mice* (New York and London: Academic Press, 1978); Jean Holstein, *The First Fifty Years at the Jackson Laboratory* (Bar Harbor, ME: Jackson Laboratory, 1979); Clyde E. Keeler, *The Laboratory Mouse: Its Origin, Heredity and Culture* (Cambridge, MA: Harvard University Press, 1931); and Karen Rader, *Making Mice: Standardizing Animals for American Biomedical Research, 1900–1955* (Princeton, NJ: Princeton University Press,

2004). On C. C. Little, see George D. Snell, "Clarence Cook Little, 1888–1971," *National Academy of Sciences: Biographical Memoirs,* volume 46 (Washington, DC: National Academy of Sciences, 1975), 240–63, now available online at http://www.nasonline.org/publications/biographical-memoirs/alphabetical-listing/memoirs-l.html, and the excellent entry by Karen Rader in *American National Biography* (Oxford University Press, 1999), also at *American National Biography Online* (February 2000), http://www.anb.org/articles/13/13-02444.html.

The gland grafters of the 1920s are described in Gerald Carson, *The Roguish World of Doctor Brinkley* (New York: Rinehart, 1960); David Hamilton, *The Monkey Gland Affair* (London: Chatto & Windus, 1986); R. Alton Lee, *The Bizarre Careers of John R. Brinkley* (Lexington: University Press of Kentucky, 2002); and Eric S. Juhnke, *Quacks and Crusaders: The Fabulous Careers of John Brinkley, Norman Baker, and Harry Hoxsey* (Lawrence: University Press of Kansas, 2002). Satire on testis grafting is found in Bertram Gayton, *The Gland Stealers* (London: Herbert Jenkins, 1922), and Gertrude Franklin Horn Atherton, *Black Oxen* (originally published in 1923).

The first human kidney allograft, performed in the Soviet Union, is described in Yu. Yu. Voronoy, "Sobre el bloqueo del aparato reticulo-endotelial," *El Siglo Médico* 97 (1936): 296–98, and for an account of Voronoy and his work, see D. N. H. Hamilton and W. A. Reid, "Yu. Yu. Voronoy and the First Human Kidney Allograft," *Surgery, Gynecology & Obstetrics* 159, no. 3 (September 1984): 289–94. See also Tatyana I. Ulyankina, "Origin and Development of Immunology in Russia," *Cellular Immunology* 126, no. 1 (March 1990): 227–32.

Renewed Interest, 1950–1960

The mystery of the function of the lymphocyte is described in William L. Ford, "The Lymphocyte: Its Transformation from a Frustrating Enigma to a Model of Cellular Function," in *Blood, Pure and Eloquent: A Story of Discovery, of People, and of Ideas,* edited by Maxwell M. Wintrobe (New York: McGraw-Hill, 1980), 457–508. The major role of the plastic surgeons in transplantation studies in the 1950s is seen in the texts by Blair O. Rogers, "The Problem of Skin Homografts," *Plastic and Reconstructive Surgery* 5, no. 4 (April 1950): 269–82, and "Guide and Bibliography for Research into the Skin Homograft Problem," *Plastic and Reconstructive Surgery* 7, no. 3 (March 1951): 169–201. See also Bernard A. Shuster and Lloyd A. Hoffman, "An Old Friendship Revisited:

Plastic Surgery and Transplantation," *Aesthetic Plastic Surgery* 18, no. 2 (spring 1994): 135–39.

The early human kidney transplants in Paris are described in Jürgen Thorwald, *The Patients* (New York: Harcourt Brace Jovanovich, 1972), and T. E. Starzl, "France and the Early History of Organ Transplantation," *Perspectives in Biology and Medicine* 37, no. 1 (autumn 1993): 35–47. The early methods of tissue typing are found in Jean Dausset, *Immuno-hématologie biologique et clinique* (Paris: Flammarion, 1956).

The forgotten Soviet work of the time is found in N. P. Sinitsyn, *Peresadka serdtsa kak novyi metod v eksperimental'noi biologii i meditsine* [Transplantation as a new method in experimental biology and medicine] (Moscow and Leningrad, 1948), translated as Dispatch No. 763, Army Medical Library, Washington, DC. See also Vladimir Demikhov, *Peresadka zhiznenno vazhnykh organov v eksperimente* (Moscow, 1960), translated as *Experimental Transplantation of Vital Organs* (New York: Consultants Bureau, 1962).

An account of the slow genesis of heart transplantation is given in Christopher McGregor, "Evolution of Heart Transplantation," *Cardiology Clinics* 8, no. 1 (February 1990): 3–10, and in S. L. Lansman, M. A. Ergin, and R. B. Griepp, "The History of Heart and Heart-Lung Transplantation," *Cardiovascular Clinics* 20, no. 2 (1990): 3–19. An early work on cardiac replacement was Albert Brest, ed., *Heart Substitutes, Mechanical and Transplant* (Springfield, IL: Thomas, 1966), and later texts include Sara J. Shumway and Norman E. Shumway, *Thoracic Transplantation* (Cambridge, MA: Blackwell Scientific, 1995). For Christiaan Barnard's heart transplants, see Peter Hawthorne, *The Transplanted Heart: The Incredible Story of the Epic Heart Transplant Operations by Professor Christiaan Barnard and His Team* (Johannesburg: Hugh Keartland, 1968; Chicago: Rand McNally, 1968), and Marais Malan, *Heart Transplant: The Story of Barnard and the "Ultimate in Cardiac Surgery"* (Johannesburg: Voortrekkerpers, 1968). A detailed study of some events in 1968—the "Year of the Heart"—is found in E. M. Tansey and Lois A. Reynolds, eds., *Early Heart Transplant Surgery in the UK*, volume 3, *Wellcome Witnesses to Twentieth Century Medicine* (London: Wellcome Trust, 1999). Details of the Baby Fae case and the Loma Linda program are found in Richard Schaefer, *Legacy: Daring to Care; The Heritage of Loma Linda* (Loma Linda, CA: Legacy Publishing Association, 1990), reissued as *Legacy: Daring to Care; The Heritage of Loma Linda University Medical Center 1905–2005* (Loma Linda, CA: Legacy Publishing Association, 2005).

The 1960s and Beyond

Early human organ transplant experience is found in Sir Roy Yorke Calne, *Renal Transplantation* (London: Arnold, 1963); Thomas E. Starzl, *Experience in Renal Transplantation* (Philadelphia: Saunders, 1964); and Starzl's monograph (with C. W. Putnam) *Experience in Hepatic Transplantation* (Philadelphia: Saunders, 1969). Jean Hamburger, *Transplantation renales* (Paris 1971), was translated as *Renal Transplantation: Theory and Practice* (Baltimore: Williams and Wilkins, 1972; 2nd ed., 1981).

Surgical Memoirs

Francis Moore's autobiography is *A Miracle and a Privilege* (Washington, DC: Joseph Henry, 1995), and see also Roy Calne, *A Gift of Life: Observations on Organ Transplantation* (New York: Basic Books, 1970), and *The Ultimate Gift: The Story of Britain's Premier Transplant Surgeon* (London: Headline, 1998). Thomas E. Starzl, *The Puzzle People* (Pittsburgh: University of Pittsburgh Press, 1992), is of crucial importance, but Joseph Murray, *Surgery of the Soul: Reflections on a Curious Career* (Canton, MA: Science History Publications for the Boston Medical Library, 2001) is disappointing. See also John S. Najarian, *The Miracle of Transplantation: The Unique Odyssey of a Pioneer Transplant Surgeon* (Beverly Hills, CA: Medallion Publishing/Phoenix Books, 2009).

Other surgeons' recollections are Gordon Murray, *Surgery in the Making* (London: Johnson, 1964); his *Quest in Medicine* (Toronto: Ryerson, 1963); William P. Longmire Jr., *Starting from Scratch: The Early History of the UCLA Department of Surgery* (Pasadena, CA: The Castle Press, 1984); Michael Woodruff, *On Science and Surgery* (Edinburgh: Edinburgh University Press, 1977); James D. Hardy, *The World of Surgery 1945–1985: Memoirs of One Participant* (Philadelphia: University of Pennsylvania Press, 1986); and Christiaan Barnard and Curtis Bill Pepper, *One Life* (Toronto: Macmillan, 1969; New York: Bantam, 1971). Many individual reminiscences are found in *Transplantation Proceedings*, volume 6 (the David Hume Memorial Supplement, published in 1971) and in the valuable collection by Paul I. Terasaki, ed., *History of Transplantation: Thirty-Five Recollections* (Los Angeles: UCLA Tissue Typing Laboratory, 1991), which has contributions from Peter Medawar, George Snell, René Küss, Jean Hamburger, Rupert Billingham, Leslie Brent, David Hume, Joseph Murray, Thomas Starzl, Michael Woodruff, E. J. Eichwald, Willard Goodwin, Roy Calne, Willem Kolff, Sun Lee, John Dosseter, Paul Russell, Guy Alexandre, Felix Rapaport, Donnall Thomas, Dirk van Bekkum, Norman Shumway, John Najarian, Bernard Amos, Paul Terasaki, Jon van Rood, Fritz Bach, Keith Reemtsma, Christiaan Barnard, Samuel Kountz, Folkert Belzer, Anthony Monaco, Peter Morris, Rudolf Pichlmayr, and Benedict Cosimi.

Other biographical vignettes are found in Leslie Brent, "Transplantation: Some British Pioneers," *Journal of the Royal College of Physicians of London* 31, no. 4 (July–August 1997): 434–41.

Memoirs by Immunologists

For Medawar's assessment of his times, see his contribution to *The Harvey Lectures 1956–57, New York,* and his collected essays are *The Strange Case of the Spotted Mice* (Oxford: Oxford University Press, 1996). His autobiography is *Memoir of a Thinking Radish* (Oxford: Oxford University Press, 1986), added to by his wife Jean in her *A Very Decided Preference: 50 Years with Peter Medawar* (New York: W. W. Norton, 1990); see also "Advances in Immunology: A Meeting in Honor of Sir Peter Medawar," *Cellular Immunol-* ogy 62, no. 2 (August 1981): 233–310. Jacques Miller's memoirs are included in *Immunology: The Making of a Modern Science,* edited by Richard B. Gallagher et al. (London and San Diego: Academic Press, 1995), and for Sir Frank Macfarlane Burnet, see his *Changing Patterns: An Atypical Autobiography* (London: Heinemann, 1968; New York: Elsevier, 1969). Jean Dausset's memoirs are *Titres et travaux scientifiques* (Paris: Châtelaudren, 1968).

Tissue Typing

The development of the field is covered in Leslie Brent, *A History of Transplantation Immunology* (San Diego: Academic Press, 1997), and in more detail in Nancy Reinsmoen and Frances Ward, "The History of HLA and Transplantation Immunology," in *History of Organ and Cell Transplantation,* edited by Nadey Hakim and Vassilios Papalois (London: Imperial College Press, 2003), 1–54. See also Ilana Löwy, "The Impact of Medical Practice on Biomedical Research: The Case of Human Leucocyte Antigens Studies," *Minerva* 25, no. 1–2 (spring–summer 1987): 171–200. On Peter Gorer, see P. B. Medawar, *Biographical Memoirs of Fellows of the Royal Society* 7 (1961): 95–109, and D. Bernard Amos, "Recollections of Dr. Peter Gorer," *Immunogenetics* 24, no. 6 (1986): 341–44. See also P. I. Terasaki, "Longmire Lecture: My 50 Years at the University of California, Los Angeles," in "Milestones in Transplantation," *World Journal of Surgery* 24 (2000): 828–33. Paul I. Terasaki's important *History of HLA: Ten Recollections* (Los Angeles: UCLA Tissue Typing Laboratory, 1990) has memoirs by Jean Dausset, Rose Payne, Jon van Rood, Bernard Amos, Walter Bodmer, Roy Walford, Flemming Kissmeyer-Nielsen, Richard Batchelor, and Fritz Bach.

On immunosuppression, see F. O. Belzer, "Immunosuppressive Agents—A Personal Historical Perspective," *Transplantation Proceedings* 20, no. 3, suppl. 3 (June 1988): 3–7, and Robert S. Schwartz, "Immunosuppression—Back to the Future," *World Journal of Surgery* 24, no. 7 (July 2000): 783–86. Cyclosporine development is covered in H. F. Stähelin, "Ciclosporin: Historic Background," *Progress in Allergy* 38 (1986): 19–27, and in a later article, "The History of Cyclosporin A (Sandimmune) Revisited: Another Point of View," *Experientia* 52, no. 1 (January 1996): 5–13.

There is an excellent review of organ preservation in R. G. W. Johnson, "Kidney Perfusion by Continuous Perfusion," in *Organ Preservation: Basic and Applied Aspects; A Symposium of the Transplantation Society,* edited by David E. Pegg, Ib Abildgaard Jacobsen, and N. A. Halasz (Lancaster, England, 1982).

Immunotherapy for Cancer

The hopes expressed in the 1973 CIBA Symposium, *Immunopotentiation,* edited by G. E. W. Wolstenholme and J. Knight (Amsterdam: Associated Scientific Publishers, 1973) were clear, and this enthusiasm for attempted immunological control of cancer is assessed in Ilana Löwy, "Experimental Systems and Clinical Practices: Tumor Immunobiology and Cancer Immunotherapy 1895–1980," *Journal of the History of Biology* 27, no. 3 (1994): 403–35. Tumor immunotherapy attracted popular attention and was described enthusiastically in June Goodfield, *The Siege of Cancer* (New York: Random House, 1975); Stephen S. Hall, *A Commotion in the Blood: Life, Death, and the Immune System* (New York: Henry Holt, 1997); and Steven A. Rosenberg and John M. Barry, *The Transformed Cell: Unlocking the Mysteries of Cancer* (New York: Putnam, 1992). For a devastating critique, see David Weiss's chapter in *The Immunologic Revolution: Facts and Witnesses,* edited by Andor Szentivanyi and Herman Friedman (Boca Raton, FL: CRC Press, 1994), 343–56.

Experimental Transplantation

The emergence of small animal organ grafting methods is described in Sun Lee, David H. Frank, and Sang Y. Choi, "Historical Review of Small and Microvascular Surgery," *Annals of Plastic Surgery* 11, no. 1 (July 1983): 53–62, and S. Lee, "Historical Significance of Rat Organ Transplantation," *Microsurgery* 11, no. 2 (1990): 115–21.

Pathology of Organ Transplantation

General reviews are George E. Sale, ed., *The Pathology of Organ Transplantation* (Boston: Butterworths, 1990); Elizabeth H. Hammond, *Solid Organ Transplantation Pathology* (Philadelphia: Saunders, 1994); and Knut Kleesiek and Arnulf Heubner, eds., *Transplantations of Organs and Cells: Contributions of Clini-* *cal Biochemistry to Clinical Success* (Berlin: Blackwell Wissenschafts-Verlag, 1997). For historical comment on pathogens transmitted by human grafts, see T. Eastland, "Infectious Disease Transmission through Cell, Tissue and Organ Transplantation," *Cell Transplantation* 4 (1995): 455–77.

Radiology

Early x-ray studies of the human kidney are described in André Johannes Bruwer, *Classic Descriptions in Diagnostic Roentgenology* (Springfield, IL: Thomas, 1964), and the development of kidney transplant im- aging is reviewed by David Hamilton in *Ultrasound of Abdominal Transplantation*, edited by P. S. Sidhu and G. Baxter (Stuttgart: Thieme Medical Publishers, 2002).

Social and Organizational Aspects

For the first of many accounts, see Renée C. Fox and Judith P. Swazey, *The Courage to Fail: A Social View of Organ Transplants and Dialysis* (Chicago: University of Chicago Press, 1974, and the revised edition (New Brunswick, NJ: Transaction Publishers, 2002), followed by Roberta Simmons et al., *Gift of Life: The Social and Psychological Impact of Organ Transplantation* (New York: Wiley, 1977); Renée Fox and Judith P. Swazey, *Spare Parts: Organ Replacement in American Society* (New York: Oxford University Press, 1992); and Stuart J. Younger, Renée C. Fox, and Laurence J. O'Connell, eds., *Organ Transplantation: Meanings and Realities* (Madison: University of Wisconsin Press, 1996). See also Mark Dowie, *"We Have a Donor": The Bold New World of Organ Transplanting* (New York: St. Martin's, 1988); Scott McCartney, *Defying the Gods: Inside the New Frontiers of Organ Transplants* (New York: Macmillan, 1994); and Dale H. Cowan, *Human Organ Transplantation: Societal, Medical-Legal, Regulatory and Reimbursement Issues* (Ann Arbor, MI: Health Administration Press, 1987). See also an interesting analysis of the spread of new medical technology in Michael Bos, *The Diffusion of Heart and Liver Transplantation across Europe* (London: King's Fund Centre, 1991).

Governmental Issues

Historically important reviews are Richard A. Rettig, *The Federal Government and Social Planning for End-Stage Renal Disease: Past, Present, and Future* (Santa Monica, CA: Rand, 1983); Jerome Aroesty, James F. Blumstein, and Frank A. Sloan, eds., *Organ Transplantation Policy: Issues and Prospects* (Durham, NC: Duke University Press, 1989); and Richard A. Rettig, "Origins of the Medicare Entitlement," in *Biomedical Politics,* edited by Kathi Hanna (Washington, DC: National Academy Press, 1991).

Major publications from the United Network for Organ Sharing were *Policy Proposal Statement: UNOS Policies Regarding Transplantation of Foreign Nationals and Exportation and Importation of Organs* (Rich- mond, VA: UNOS, 1988); *Policy Proposal Statement: UNOS Policy Regarding the Listing of Patients on Multiple Transplant Waiting Lists* (Richmond, VA: UNOS, 1988); and Michael G. Phillips, ed., *UNOS: Organ Procurement, Preservation and Distribution in Transplantation* (Richmond, VA, 1991). In Britain, the issues appear in *Report of the Joint Committee on Maintenance Dialysis and Transplantation in the Treatment of Chronic Renal Failure* (London: Royal College of Physicians, 1972). There was later assessment by the United Kingdom Office of Health Economics in Richard West, *Organ Transplantation* (London: Office of Health Economics, 1991).

The Artificial Kidney

The best history is J. Stewart Cameron, *A History of the Treatment of Renal Failure by Dialysis* (Oxford: Oxford University Press, 2002), and important early works are W. J. Kolff, *New Ways of Treating Uraemia* (London: J. & A. Churchill, 1947), and J. P. Merrill, *The Treatment of Renal Failure: Therapeutic Principles* *in the Management of Acute and Chronic Uremia* (New York: Grune & Stratton, 1965). See also J. F. Maher, ed., *Evolution of Artificial Organs: A Festschrift to Dr. George E. Schreiner* (Cleveland: ISAO Press, 1986).

Brain Death

The Harvard Ad Hoc Committee report is "A Definition of Irreversible Coma: Report of the Ad Hoc Committee of the Harvard Medical School to Examine the Definition of Brain Death," *Journal of the American Medical Association* 205, no. 6 (August 5, 1968): 336–40. For comment, see Gary S. Belkin, "Brain Death and the Historical Understanding of Bioethics," *Journal of the History of Medicine* 58, no. 3 (July 2003): 325–61. For further discussion, see Christopher Pallis, *An ABC of Brain Stem Death* (London: British Medical Journal, 1983), and Emiko Ohnuki-Tierney, Michael V. Angrosino, Carl Becker, A. S. Daar, Takeo Funabiki, and Marc I. Lorber, "Brain Death and Organ Transplantation: The Cultural Bases of Medical Technology," *Current Anthropology* 35 (1994): 233–54.

The debate continued in Russell Scott, *The Body as Property* (New York: Viking, 1981); Margaret Lock, *Twice Dead: Transplants and the Reinvention of Death* (Berkeley: University of California Press, 2002); and Stuart J. Youngner, Robert Arnold, and Renie Schapiron, eds., *The Definition of Death: Contemporary Controversies* (Baltimore: Johns Hopkins University Press, 1999). See also Martin Pernick, "Back from the Grave: Recurring Controversies over Defining and Diagnosing Death in History," in *Death: Beyond Whole-Brain Criteria*, edited by Richard Zaner (Dordrecht, Netherlands: Kluwer Academic Publishers, 1988), 17–74, and Robert M. Arnold, Renie Schapiro, and Carol Mason Spicer, eds., *Procuring Organs for Transplant: The Debate over Non-Heart-Beating Cadaver Protocols* (Baltimore: Johns Hopkins University Press, 1995).

The Law Relevant to Transplantation

Important review articles emerged in the legal journals after the growth in use of regular dialysis and successful transplantation, notably "Patient Selection for Artificial and Transplanted Organs," *Harvard Law Review* 82, no. 6 (April 1969): 1322–42, and "Scarce Medical Resources," *Columbia Law Review* 69 (1969): 620–92. The legal position on donation is discussed in Russell Scott, *The Body as Property* (New York: Viking, 1981), 74–81, and burial practices are discussed in C. J. Polson, *The Disposal of the Dead* (London: English Universities Press, 1953; 3rd ed., 1975). For an important early discussion of brain death, see Jeffrey C. Baker, "Liability and the Heart Transplant," *Houston Law Review* 6 (1968): 85–112.

Ethical Issues

There is a good review in Arnold G. Diethelm, "Ethical Decisions in the History of Organ Transplantation," *Annals of Surgery* 211, no. 5 (May 1990): 505–20. The first in-depth airing of the wider concerns surrounding kidney transplantation and dialysis came after a critical editorial by J. Russell Elkington, "Moral Problems in the Use of Borrowed Organs, Artificial and Transplanted," *Annals of Internal Medicine* 60, no. 2 (February 1964): 309–13, and comments on his views were published shortly afterward in Irvine H. Page, "Moral Problems of Artificial and Transplanted Organs," *Annals of Internal Medicine* 61, no. 2 (August 1, 1964): 355–63.

The debate broadened at the CIBA Foundation conference, published as *Ethics in Medical Progress: With Special Reference to Transplantation*, edited by G. E. W. Wolstenholme and Maeve O'Connor (Boston: Little, Brown, 1966), later republished as *Law and Ethics of Transplantation* (London: J & A Churchill, 1968). Following the first heart transplants, a flurry of publications emerged; for an international perspective on ethical issues and organ donation, see the Singapore Conference of the Transplantation Society, as reported in *Transplantation Proceedings* 24 (1992): 2038–85, and *Transplantation Proceedings* 24, 2087–236. See also Qazi Mujahidul Islam Qasmi, *Contemporary Medical Issues in Islamic Jurisprudence* (New Delhi: Islamic Fiqh Academy, 2001), and Farhat Moazam, *Bioethics and Organ Transplantation in a Muslim Society* (Bloomington: Indiana University Press, 2006).

General concern on scientific misconduct started with a transplant scandal; see Joseph Hixson, *The Patchwork Mouse* (Garden City, NY: Anchor Press, 1976), and Medawar's insider account of the events is "The Strange Case of the Spotted Mice," review of *The Patchwork Mouse*, by Joseph Hixon, *New York Review of Books*, April 15, 1976, 6–11. Maurice Henry Pappworth's historically important *Human Guinea Pigs: Experimentation on Man* (London: Routledge & Kegan Paul, 1967; rev. ed., Harmondsworth, Middlesex: Penguin, 1969) had a brief section on transplantation.

An early investigation of organ trafficking appeared in Margaret J. Radin, *Contested Commodities: The Trouble with Trade in Sex, Children, Body Parts and Other Things* (Cambridge, MA: Harvard University Press, 1996).

Meetings and Sponsors

The International Society of Surgery meeting in 1914 had a major early symposium on transplantation, but there was nothing comparable until the 1950s, when small symposia emerged. The first of these later meetings was published as "Proceedings: Tissue Transplantation Conference New York 1952," *Journal of the National Cancer Institute* 14 (1953): 667–704, and crucially important thereafter were the New York Academy of Sciences meetings, starting in 1954, as recorded in their *Proceedings*. The CIBA Foundation, later changing its name to the Novartis Foundation, was influential in transplant and immunological matters thereafter. The first CIBA Foundation symposium, in 1953, was published as *Preservation and Transplantation of Normal Tissues*, edited by G. E. W. Wolstenholme, Margaret P. Cameron, and Joan Etherington (London: J. & A. Churchill, 1954), and many similar CIBA gatherings followed, often organized with Peter Medawar's help. Relevant symposia were *Cellular Aspects of Immunity* (1959, held in Paris); *Transplantation* (1961); *The Nature and Origin of the Immunologically Competent Cell* (1963); *The Thymus* (1965, held in Melbourne); *Ethics in Medical Prog-* *ress* (1966); *Antilymphocyte Serum* (1967); and *Immunopotentiation* (1973). There is an interesting overview in F. Peter Woodford, *The CIBA Foundation: An Analytic History 1949–1974* (Amsterdam: Associated Scientific Publishers, 1974).

The important National Academy of Sciences meeting in Washington in 1963 was convened to review the status of kidney transplantation and reported in *Transplantation*, volume 2, 147–65. The New York Academy of Sciences meetings were discontinued in 1962, giving way to the biennial meetings of the Transplantation Society from 1966 onward, with the first proceedings edited by Jean Dausset, Jean Hamburger, and Georges Mathé as *Advances in Transplantation: Proceedings of the First International Congress of the Transplantation Society, Paris, 27–30 June 1967* (Baltimore: Williams and Wilkins, 1968). Thereafter, the increasingly important meetings were reported in special issues of the journal *Transplantation Proceedings*, published from 1969. This journal also covered the many related conferences held by the growing number of societies with an interest in transplantation.

The Journals

The earliest publication dedicated to transplantation was the slim but ambitious *Transplantation Bulletin*, running from 1954 to 1958, later incorporated as a supplement within the journal *Plastic and Reconstructive Surgery* from 1958 to 1962. *Transplantation* appeared as a separate journal in 1962. Many niche journals then emerged to serve the development of various types of organ transplants. The American Society for Artificial Internal Organs was founded in 1955 and their early *Proceedings* have historic papers on the early use of the artificial kidney, as well as a valuable annual presidential address. The specialty of tissue typing was served by the annual volumes of *Histocompatibility Testing* from 1965 onward.

The European Dialysis and Transplantation Association met annually from 1964 onward and published their *Proceedings* in various forms; the *Proceedings* became *Nephrology, Dialysis and Transplantation* in 1986.

Patients' Experiences

For compilations of patient experiences, see Jürgen Thorwald's remarkable volume, *The Patients* (New York: Harcourt Brace Jovanovich, 1972), which includes recipients' accounts of the first regular dialysis and kidney transplant attempts; it is one of the earliest and best works of this type. After the San Francisco conference of the Transplantation Society, the pioneering "Symposium on the Human Aspects of Clinical Transplantation" was held, and these patients' testimonies were published in *Transplantation Proceedings*, volume 5 (1973). Paul Terasaki, with Jane Schoenberg, collected many "firsts" and uncommon cases in *Transplant Success Stories* (Los Angeles: UCLA Tissue Typing Laboratory, 1993). Lists of the longest survivors with each organ graft are in Terasaki's *Clinical Transplants*, an annual series starting in 1985.

Transplant unit life at York Columbia Presbyterian is found in Ina Yalof, *Life and Death: The Story of a Hospital* (New York: Random House, 1990), and day-to-day life in Starzl's unit at Pittsburgh is described in Lee Gutkind, *Many Sleepless Nights: The World of Organ Transplantation* (New York: Norton, 1988; repr., Pittsburgh: University of Pittsburgh Press, 1990). The numerous individual patients' narratives of kidney transplantation sold well, and typical are Kathryn Seidick, *Or You Can Let Him Go* (New York: Delacorte Press, 1984), and Elizabeth Ward,

Timbo: A Struggle for Survival (London: Sidgwick and Jackson, 1986).

A flurry of books emerged to serve the intense public interest during 1968, the "Year of the Heart," starting with the first survivor's memoirs—Philip Blaiberg, *Looking at My Heart* (New York: Stein & Day, 1968)—followed by many others, including that of Robert Casey, a governor of Pennsylvania, who wrote about his 1996 heart transplant in *Fighting for Life* (Dallas: Word Publishing, 1996). Children's heart transplantation at Loma Linda is described in Thomas Miller and Jayne Miller, *Baby James: A Legacy of Love and Family Courage* (San Francisco: Harper & Row, 1988).

Personal heart-lung recipient patients' stories include Mary Gohlke, *I'll Take Tomorrow* (New York: M. Evans, 1985). Children's transplant stories

also proved attractive to publishers, including Esther Rantzen and Shaun Woodward, *Ben: The Story of Ben Hardwick* (London: Penguin, 1985), and John B. Robbins, *Strings: The Miracle of Life* (Georgetown, MA: North Star Publications, 1998). Eric Lax's *Life and Death on 10 West* (New York: Times Books, 1984) described marrow transplants at UCLA, as did Madeline Marget, *Life's Blood* (New York: Simon and Schuster, 1992), for Boston cases. A doctor's personal account as a marrow recipient is David Biro, *One Hundred Days: My Unexpected Journey from Doctor to Patient* (New York: Pantheon, 2000).

Donation experience is described in many works, notably Leslie A. Horvitz and H. Harris Gerhard, *The Donors* (New York: New American Library, 1982), and Reg Green, *The Nicholas Effect: A Boy's Gift to the World* (London: O'Reilly, 1999).

Popular Accounts

With the early successes of kidney transplantation, the first popular texts were Francis D. Moore, *Give and Take: The Development of Tissue Transplantation* (Philadelphia: Saunders, 1964), with a revised edition titled *Transplant: The Give and Take of Tissue Transplantation* (New York: Simon and Schuster, 1972); Fred Warshofsky, *The Rebuilt Man: The Story of Spare-Parts Surgery* (New York: Crowell, 1965); Harold M. Schmeck, *The Semi-Artificial Man: A Dawning Revolution in Medicine* (London: G. G. Harrap, 1966); Donald Longmore, *Spare-Part Surgery: The Surgical Practice of the Future* (London: Aldus Books, 1968); and Albert Rosenfeld, *Second Genesis: The Coming Control of Life* (Englewood Cliffs, NJ: Prentice-Hall, 1969; rev. ed., New York: Vintage Books, 1975). See also Nikolai Mikhailovich Amosov, *The Open Heart: Heart Surgery in the Soviet Union*, translated by George St. George (New York: Simon and Schuster, 1966).

Journalists' accounts of the vivid events of early heart transplantation are found in Tony Stark, *Knife*

to the Heart: The Story of Transplant Surgery (London: Macmillan, 1996), and Thomas Thompson, *Hearts: Of Surgeons and Transplants, Miracles and Disasters along the Cardiac Frontier* (New York: McCall Publishing, 1971), reissued as *Hearts: DeBakey and Cooley, Surgeons Extraordinary* (London: Joseph, 1972). See also Harry Minetree, *Cooley: The Career of a Great Heart Surgeon* (New York: Harper's Magazine Press, 1973), and William H. Frist, *Transplant: A Heart Surgeon's Account of the Life-and-Death Dramas of the New Medicine* (New York: Atlantic Monthly Press, 1989). Other popular works include Robert Finn, *Organ Transplants: Making the Most of Your Gift of Life* (Sebastopol, CA: O'Reilly, 2000), and Calvin Stiller, with Brian C. Stiller, *Lifegifts: The Real Story of Organ Transplants* (Toronto: Stoddart, 1990).

The travails resulting from the London heart transplants in 1968 are well documented in Ayesha Nathoo, *Hearts Exposed: Transplants and the Media in 1960s Britain* (Basingstoke: Palgrave Macmillan, 2009).

Fiction

After the early twentieth-century literary interest in transplantation, there was little published with that theme until organ transplantation became a reality in the mid-1960s and each new aspect thereafter called forth its fictional shadow. Kidney transplant first merited a science-fiction role in A. E. van Vogt, *The Mind Cage* (New York: Simon and Schuster, 1957), and racketeering for organs was used in John Boyd, *The Organ Bank Farm* (New York: Weybright and Talley, 1970). Murder for the purpose of selling organs was the

theme of the best-selling *Coma*, by Robin Cook (Boston: Little, Brown, 1977), and the hepatitis epidemic of the mid-1960s features in Colin Douglas's novel *The Houseman's Tale* (Edinburgh: Canongate, 1975).

Novelists were not slow to exploit the possibility of brain transplants, the earliest offering being Leo P. Kelley, *Mindmix* (Greenwich, CT: Fawcett, 1972). The early heart transplants, starting in the late 1960s, led to a burst of related fiction, the earliest novels being Margaret Jones, *The Day They Put

Humpty Together Again (London: Collins, 1968), published in the United States as *Transplant* (New York: Stein and Day, 1968). Christiaan Barnard, with Siegfried Stander, first produced a novel titled *The Unwanted* (Cape Town: Tafelberg, 1974), and followed it up with *In the Night Season* (Cape Town: Tafelberg, 1974). Other fictional works featuring heart transplant themes include Richard Selzer, *Imagine a Woman and Other Tales* (New York: Random House, 1990), which is analyzed in Michael Potts, "Morals, Metaphysics and Heart Transplantation: Reflections on Richard Selzer's 'Whither Thou Goest,'" *Perspectives in Biology and Medicine* 41, no. 2 (winter 1998): 212–23. See also Mark Ravitch, "All Heart," *Perspectives in Biology and Medicine* 18, no. 1 (autumn 1974): 94–107. Possible transfer of personality with transplanted organs understandably attracted novelists, and this theme was used in Robert Silverberg, *To Live Again* (Garden City, NY: Doubleday, 1969); Mack Reynolds, *Looking Backward, from the Year 2000* (New York: Ace Books, 1973); and many others.

Portraits and Pictures

Many images of Cosmas and Damian and their legendary miracle are found in B. Tosatti, "Transplantation and Reimplantation in the Arts," *Surgery* 75, no. 3 (March 1974): 389–97. Portraits of those involved in early transplantation are found in René Küss, *An Illustrated History of Organ Transplantation: The Great Adventure of the Century* (Rueil-Malmaison, France: Sandoz, 1992); Terasaki's *History of Transplantation: Thirty-Five Recollections* (Los Angeles: UCLA Tissue Typing Laboratory, 1991); and also in Terasaki's *History of HLA: Ten Recollections* (Los Angeles: UCLA Tissue Typing Laboratory, 1990). See also the "Symposium on Phylogeny of Transplantation Reactions," *Transplantation Proceedings* 2 (1970): 179–341. Sir Roy Yorke Calne, tutored by a distinguished artist-patient, produced portraits of contemporaries and surgical scenes, and these are found in Anthony Monaco, *Art, Surgery and Transplantation* (London: Williams & Wilkins Europe, 1996).

For philatelic interest, see G. de Benedictis, "Transplants on Stamps," *Scalpel and Tongs* 27 (1983): 71–75. Some of the transplantation conferences stored images of their distinguished participants in their archives. The Novartis (formerly CIBA) Foundation holds valuable pictures taken at their important symposia.

Xenografts

Important reviews dealing with the use of animal organs include David K. C. Cooper and Robert P. Lanza, *Xeno: The Promise of Transplanting Animal Organs into Humans* (Oxford: Oxford University Press, 2000). For a history of the events in the rise of cellular engineering, see Ian Wilmut, Keith Campbell, and Colin Tudge, *The Second Creation: The Age of Biological Control by the Scientists Who Cloned Dolly* (London: Headline, 2000). Government reports include the Nuffield Council on Bioethics, *Animal-to-Human Transplants: the Ethics of Xenotransplantation* (London: Nuffield Council on Bioethics, 1996).

Index

Note: page numbers in italic type indicate illustrations.

A

A strain mice, 146, 157–58, 225, 240
AB blood type, 131
Abbe, Robert, 90
Abel, John, 150
About, Edmond, *Le Nez d'un notaire*, 86, 435n61, 446n75
abrin, 450n3
Abulcasis, *Chirurgia*, 13
accidents, fruitfulness of, 425–26
accommodation, of organ transplants, 284
Ackerknecht, Erwin Heinz, 433n27
Acland, Henry, 66
acquired hemolytic anemia, 485n11
acquired immunity, 186–87, 196, 198, 319, 467n37
ACTH. *See* adrenocorticotrophic hormone
actinomycin C, 277, 332, 485n8
actively acquired immunity. *See* acquired immunity
acute renal failure, 62–63
Adams, Raymond, 346
adaptation, to organ transplants, 284, 489n57
Addison, Joseph, "Noses," 30
Addison's disease, 139
adrenal gland grafting, 139
adrenal glands, 191
adrenaline, 135
adrenocorticotrophic hormone (ACTH), 192, 216, 470n10
Adrian, Lord, 513n70
adult tolerance, 253, 254, 257–58, 480n1
Advisory Group on Ethics of Xeno-transplantation (Britain), 419
Advisory Group on Transplant Problems (Britain), 354
Aesculapius, 3
afterlife, bodily integrity in, 1, 5–6, 10, 408, 433n27
Agatha, Saint, 4
age, of transplant recipients, 286, 370

Agricultural Research Institute of Animal Physiology, 329
AIDS, xvii, 489n59
air transportation, for organ collection, 326–27, 488n53, 500n37
AKA mice, 158
Albee, Fred, 131
Albert, Eduard, 88–89
Albucasis, 43
alcoholics, liver transplantation for, 520n95
Aldini, Giovanni, 56
Aldrovandi, Ulisse, 15, 435n73
alemtuzumab, 416
Alexander, Shana, 300
Alexandre, Guy, 280, 321
ALG. *See* antilymphocyte globulin
Algeria, 154–55
Algire, G. H., 229, 242, 393
Allen, Charles, 29–30, 437n27; *The Operator for the Teeth*, 43
Allen, Woody, *Sleeper*, 525n34
allografting, 18, 70, 294, 333, 492n100. *See also* homografting
alpha-1-antitrypsin, 419
alpha-1-antitrypsin deficiency, 389
ALS. *See* antilymphocyte serum
Alwall, Nils, 204, 261
American Association of Surgeons, 219
American Bar Association, 378
American Cancer Society, 241
American College of Cardiologists, 356
American College of Surgeons, 219, 282
American Legion, 248
American Medical Association, 462n5; Judicial Council, 347
American Mercury (journal), 134
American Office of Scientific Research and Development, 270
American Society for Artificial Internal Organs, 479n70
American Society of Transplant Surgeons, 397

American Surgical Association, 101, 200
American Urological Association, 210
Amnesty International, 522n121
Amos, D. Bernard, 236, 320, 323, 325, 476n20, 477n39
L'Amour à mort (film), 518n69
anatomy: contributions of transplantation history to knowledge of, xvii; Hunter and, 34–35; in India, 12
Anatomy Act (Britain, 1832), 246
Anderson, Norman F., 462n7
Androsov, P. I., 199
anencephaly, 395, 506n29, 518n62
anesthesia: duration of, 340; and skin grafting, 76; surgery without use of, 57, 60
Angell Memorial Animal Hospital, Boston, 384, 486n27
angiography, 285, 368, *368*
Anguissola of Milan, Count, 54–55
animal organ/tissue transplantation: animal-to-human, 71–72, 81, 84, 86–87, 94–96, 137, 154, 291–93, 395, 433n38, 460n79; chicken spur-to-comb experiment, 37–38, *38*, 54, 68, 435n73; controversy over, 42; early experiments in, 25–29, *26*; in eighteenth century, 55; eighteenth-century experiments in, 54; kidney transplantation, 93–95, 96; large and small animal experiments in, 329–31; limitations of, 311–12; in literature, 86–87; papal stance on, 249; pig-to-primate organ grafts, 525n33; public opinion on, 395, 417; sex glands, xix, 39; traditional belief in, 9–10, 43n9. *See also* antivivisectionism; *specific animals*
animal tumors, 106–8
Animals Act (Britain), 417
Annals of Internal Medicine (journal), 302
Anthony Nolan Registry, 393
Anthony of Padua, Saint, 6

539

Crusades, 14
crush syndrome, 204, 206, 472n31
cryopreservation, 231–32, 485n13, 488n44
CsA. *See* cyclosporine
CTAB No. 9 cream, 466n21
Curran, William, 344–45
Cushing, Harvey, 101
Cuthbertson, David, 178
cyclophosphamide, 361, 367, 485n8
cyclosporine (CsA), xx, 363, 366, 379–94, 415, 514n7, 515n12, 523n15
cyproheptadine, 367
cytomegalovirus (CMV), 367, 489n58
Czechoslovakia, 476n18

D

Da Fano, C., 111
D'Abreu, Frank, 139
daclizumab, 416
Dalyell, Tam, 519n85
Dameshek, William, 272–73, 484n1, 485n11
Damian, Saint, xiii, 5–6, *5*, *7*
Dammin, Gustave J., 217, 484n1
Danchakoff, Vera, 452n24
Dartigues, Louis, 137, *138*
Darwin, Charles, 71, 197
data charts, 280, 487n41
Dausset, Jean, 264, 316–19, *317*, 324, 398, 478n48
Davenport, Charles, 147
Davies, Lord Justice, 246, 293
Davis, Benjamin, 115
Davis, John Staige, 130–31
Davis, Loyal, 386, 465n14, 487n36, 516n27
DBA mice, 146
De Kruif, Paul, 128
dead body, ownership of, 203–4, 472n30
Dean Street Anatomy School, 56
Deanesley, Ruth, 190
death: after heart transplantation, 348, 350–51, 355, 362; after kidney transplantation, 96, 213, 215, 216, 252, 260, 262, 275, 277, 280, 282, 284, 338; after liver transplantation, 288, 387; after lung transplants, 289; cryopreservation after, 488n44; defining, 341–47, 353–55, 378–79, 406, 408, 513n70, 518n62; with dignity, 301–2, 341; legal issues concerning definition of, 341–42, 353–54, 378, 507n43; organ donation and, 343–47, 353–55, 379, 397, 505n19, 513n78; ownership of body after, 203–4, 293, 339, 371, 472n30; physical process of, 42; from renal failure, 150; tissue vitality after, 40, 42, 103. *See also* afterlife
DeBakey, Michael, 207, 351

Decastello, Alfred von, 93, 115
Deederer, Carl, 151, 461n90
Defining Death (presidential commission report), 378
Della Porta, Giovanni (Giambattista), 434n53
Demikhov, Vladimir, 199–200, 209, 289, 463n22, 471n15
Demirleau, J., 288–89
Dempster, William J. "Jim," 190, 195–98, 201, 208, 216–17, 239, 254, 274, 275, 470n9, 470n12, 485n19; *An Introduction to Experimental Surgical Studies*, 197
Denita's Bill, 401
Denmark, 397, 405
Denmark polio epidemic (1953), 340
Denver Transplant Tumor Register, 287
Denver Veterans Administration Hospital, 278–80, 285, 288
Department of Health (Britain), 379
dermatomes, 159, 462n14
Descartes, René, 33
Deterling, Ralph A., 291
developing countries, 406–11, 520n100, 520n102
devil, 8, 22
diabetes, 139, 286, 391
dialysis, 150. *See also* kidney dialysis
diathesis, 130
Dickey-Wicker Amendment (United States), 525n39
Dieffenbach, Johann, 59, 60, 61
Digby, Kenelm(e), 22–23, 25; *A Late Discourse Made in a Solemn Assembly of Nobles and Learned Men at Montpellier in France*, 22–23, *23*
DiGeorge, Angelo, 309–10, 426, 475n4
DiGeorge syndrome, 310
dignity, death with, 301–2, 341
dimethylsulfoxide (DMSO), 232
dinitrochlorobenzene, 116
Dionysus, 2
diphtheria, 105
discovery, 426
disease: bodily manifestations of, 62; chemical/quantitative approach to, 150–51
disease transmission: kidney transplantation as source of, xvii; skin grafts as source of, xvii, 86; tooth transplantation as source of, xvii, 46–47
disintegration, of skin grafts, 187
dissection: animal, 36
DNA transfers, 418–19
dogs: experiments using, 25–29; heart transplantation for, 199–201; kidney transplantation for, 93, 195, 198, 266, 274–76, *276*, 486n27,

487n34; liver transplantation for, 278, 288; radiation response of, 198; skin grafts using, 81, 433n38; two-headed dog experiments, 243, 479n69
Doherty, Peter, 366, 497n7
Dolly (cloned sheep), 421, *421*, 525n35, 525n36
domino liver grafting, 395, 518n58
Donald, Hugh P., 221–22
Donath, J., 118, 453n47
donations. *See* organ donation; tissue donation
donor cards, 370–71, 401–2
donors: black, 5, 75, 79; in Britain, 370–71; for corneal grafting, 244–46; demographic characteristics of, 405; emotionally-related, 383, 398, 404, 520n92; hypothermic treatment of, 483n31; intrafamilial, 143–44, 212–13, 277–78, 314, 466n32, 483n33, 520n91; multiple, for single patient, 132, 134; of ovaries, 85; payment of, 44–45, 80, 134, 383, 398, 409–11, 521n111; programs for, 370–71, 386, 401–3; related (*see* intrafamilial); servants as, 19, 21, 43–44, 75; shortage of, 400–405, 412, 519n83; in Soviet Union, 161, 244–45; in Spain, 401; sympathetic between recipient and, 21–24, 75; tissue typing and, 365; in United States, 370; unrelated, 75, 259–60, 264, 321, 361, 364–65, 383, 393, 398, 404, 409–10. *See also* organ donation; tissue donation
Doran, George H., *The Talkers*, 141
Dossetor, John B., 286, 410
Dougherty, Thomas, 270
Douglas, Colin, *The Houseman's Tale*, 495n27
Downstate Medical Center, Brooklyn, 306
Drinker, Cecil, 169
dropsy, 62
drug combinations, 469n77
Dubernard, Jean-Michel, 336
Dubost, Charles, 211, 470n1
Duhamel de Monceau, Henri-Louis, 37, *38*
Dunphy, J. Engelbert, 500n41
duodenum, 391
Dutrochet, Henri, 61, 441n37

E

Eady, Robin, 298, 493n6
ears, 10–11, *133*, 134
Eason, John, 118, 453n47
East Grinstead hospital, England, 176, 465n11
East India Company, 49

Easter Island, 415
Eastlick, Herbert, 224
Ebeling, Albert, 116
Ebert, James, 452n24
Ebert, Robert H., 344–46
Eck, Nikolai, 90
Ecuador, 43
Edgewood Arsenal research, 270, 271
Edinburgh, Scotland, 51–53, *266*
EDTA. *See* European Dialysis and
    Transplant Association
education: plastic surgery and, 51–53;
    in Renaissance period, 14, 16
Egorov, Igor, 476n20
Egyptian medicine, skin grafts in,
    433n34
Ehrlich, Paul, 106, 108, 110, 115, 152,
    450n3, 451n12
Eichwald, E. J., 241, 244, 267, 295,
    323, 479n60, 479n61
eighteenth century, 31–48; bone graft-
    ing in, 38–39; gland grafting in, 39;
    horticultural model in, 40; Hunt-
    er's work in, 34–48; nature of life
    and the soul in, 40–42; regenera-
    tion experiments in, 31–34; tissue
    adhesion in, 36, 39–40; Trembley's
    work in, 31–33
Elanskii (Soviet scientist), 161
electrocardiogram, 357
electroencephalography, 513n70
electrolytes, 328–29, 442n16
Elion, Gertrude "Trudy," 276, *276*,
    486n24
Elkinton, J. R., 302, 494n21
Emanuel, Victor R., *The Messiah of the
    Cylinder*, 141
emotionally-related donors, 383, 398,
    404, 520n92
empiricism. *See* theory and laboratory
    research vs. empiricism and clini-
    cal practice
empirics, 433n40. *See also* artisans,
    surgery practiced by
en bloc technique, *96, 292*
Enderlen, Eugen, 97–98, *97, 98*
Enders, John, 474n63
endocrinology, xix
Endocrinology (journal), 137, 139,
    457n36
end-stage renal failure, 294, 295, 297,
    300, 301, 304, 406
engineered organs, 418–20
England: eighteenth-century ex-
    perimentation in, 31–48; plastic
    surgery in, 56–58; tooth transplan-
    tation in, 43–48. *See also* Britain;
    Royal Society of London; United
    Kingdom
English, Terence, 396–97
enhancement, 234–35, 331, 373

epsilon aminocaproic acid (EACA),
    491n79
errors, fruitfulness of, 425
ethics: "bioethics" coined, 494n13;
    of blood transfusions, 29–30, 47;
    criminal organ removal, 411; and
    defining death, 343–47; in devel-
    oping countries, 407–11; folklore
    dilemmas concerning, 2; growing
    significance of, xviii, 300; of hu-
    man experimentation, 377, 503n2,
    512n67; of kidney treatments,
    xviii, 298–303, 503n2; and life-
    support treatment, 341, 343–47;
    of liver transplantation, 520n95;
    in miraculous replacements, 6; of
    organ distribution, 404–6; origins
    of medical, 85; of ovarian trans-
    plantation, 85; of patient eligibility/
    selection, 299–301, 306, 404–6,
    520n95; and quality of life/death,
    301–2, 341; of resuscitation, 302–3;
    scarce resource issues for, 300–
    301, 404, 503n2; of tooth trans-
    plantation, 47–48; of vaccinations,
    306; and volunteers, 498n18; of
    xenografting, 419
ethics committees, 344
Ethics in Medical Progress (Wolsten-
    holme and O'Connor, eds.), 504n8
Ethics Law (France), 403
ethylene oxide, 202
Eugenic Records Office, 147
eugenics, 141, 147, 148, 168–69
"Eureka" moments, 309–10, 426
Euro-Collins solution, 329
European Dialysis and Transplant
    Association (EDTA), 282, 488n50,
    511n46
Eurotransplant, 326, 336
Evans, Herbert, 135
experimental organ transplantation,
    195–220; artificial kidney ma-
    chines, 204–5; heart transplanta-
    tion, 199–200; kidney transplanta-
    tion, 195–98, 207–20; Korean War
    and, 206–7; temperature as factor
    in, 199–202; tissue banks, 202–4
experimentation: in eighteenth cen-
    tury, 31–48; in nineteenth-century
    Paris, 65–76; replicability and, 66;
    rise of, 20–21; Royal Society and,
    25–30; in surgical field, 34–36; in
    transplantation, 37–38. *See also*
    human experimentation
experiments of nature, 223, 309, 373,
    426, 475n4, 496n38
Eye Bank Association of America, 248
Eye-Bank for Sight Restoration, Inc.,
    247–48
eyeless needles, xx

France-Soir (newspaper), 210
Franchescetti, Albert, 246
Franco-Prussian War, 76
Frankenstein, xiv, 58–59, 432n22, 440n25, 494n18
fraud, 126, 424
free market theory of organ donation, 398
freemartin female cattle, 36, 221, 222, 223
Fresenius, 335
Friedman, Eli, 306
Friedman, Milton, 398
frog larvae, 34
frog skin, grafts using, 81
Fujisawa Pharmaceutical Company, 415
funding. See costs and funding
fungal infections, 367
fungal products, for immunosuppression, 380–81, 415

G

Gaillard, Pieter, 241–42
Galen, 13, 22
Galton, Francis, 470n6
Galvani, Luigi, 56
Ganesha, 2–3
Gassendus, Petrus, 435n73
Gayton, Bertram, The Gland Stealers, 141
Gelin, Lars-Erik, 329
Gell, Philip, 228
General Medical Council (Britain), 398
genetic engineering, 418–20
genetics: and antigens, 322; and cancer, 147; as factor in transplantation, 111; graft success affected by, 143–44, 232–34; and inbreeding, 148–49, 157–58, 224, 235, 462n6, 462n7; mice breeding and, 145–46; transmission of acquired traits as theory in, 154–55, 227. See also eugenics
Gentleman's Magazine, 49–50, 52
Gerdy, Pierre Nicolas, 65–66
Germany: plastic surgery in, 59–60, 443n34; postwar medical and scientific decline in, 126–27; tooth transplantation in, 438n50; transplantation in, 88–89
Gey, George, 241
Gibson, Thomas "Tom," 173, 178–84, 181, 185, 466n19, 466n22, 467n37, 467n39
Gillies, Harold, 176–77, 179, 246, 465n9; Plastic Surgery of the Face, 176
Gilman, Alfred, 270, 271, 484n6, 484n7

gland grafting: assessment of, 83–84, 445n61; literary treatments of, 141; in 1920s, 135, 139; in nineteenth century, 83–86; placement concerns, 83. See also sex gland grafting
Glasgow Medical Journal, 79
Glasser, Herbert, 170
Glazer, Shep, 304
Glick, Bruce, 309, 425
Gliedman, Marvin, 391
glycerol, 232
glycogen storage disease, 389
goats, 94–95, 139–40, 271
Godber, George, 356
Golanitzky, J., 122
golden era in medicine, 452n27
Golden Legend, The, 6
Golgi, Camillo, 115
Golston case, 378
Good, Robert, 219, 309, 361, 377–78, 462n6, 475n4, 484n1, 485n12
Goodman, Louis S., 270, 484n7
Goodwin, William, 278, 279, 280, 487n33, 487n39, 499n30
Gordon, Yaakov, 85
Gore, Al, 386–87, 394, 398, 399
Gorer, Peter, 154, 225, 232–37, 233, 294, 315, 318, 320, 467n47, 470n4, 475n8, 477n39, 481n9, 498n13
Gosselin, Leon, 71, 72, 73
Gottschalk, Carl W., 494n23
Gottschalk Report, 303–4, 494n23
Gowans, James, 174, 238, 239, 256, 465n2, 473n44, 478n53
Grabar, Pierre, 259
graft loss. See tissue rejection
graft tolerance, Hunter's cattle dissections and, 36
grafting: intrafamilial, 143–44; routine, 244–46. See also autografting; bone grafts; corneal grafting; gland grafting; homografting; skin grafts; tissue grafts
graft-versus-host (GvH) reaction, 112–13, 118, 196, 238–40, 258, 360–61, 427, 452n23, 452n24, 470n5, 478n56, 508n6
Graham, Evarts, 158
Graham, Thomas, 63, 63, 150, 441n43
Graiai, 2
Grant, David, 390
grants, for transplantation research, 95
grave robbers, 44, 56, 246
grave signs, of death, 342, 344
Graves, Robert, 393–94
Greek medicine, plastic surgery in, 12–13
Greenwood, John, 46
Gregory, James, 52–53, 55

Grey, Zachary, 435n64
Grimm brothers, 2, 86
Grondin, Pierre, 351
Groote Schuur Hospital, 347, 505n27
Groth, Carl-Gustav, 336
Gudov, V. F., 199
Guilmet, Daniel, 362
Guthrie, Charles C., 100–103, 100, 158, 170, 199, 202, 289, 449n41, 462n10
Guttmann, E., 467n40
Guttmann, Ludwig, 467n40
GvH reaction. See graft-versus-host (GvH) reaction

H

Haas, Georg, 150
Al-Hakam II, 13
Haldane, J.B.S., 225, 232, 460n74, 468n56
Halloran Hospital, Staten Island, New York, 188
Hallowell (Yorkshire surgeon), 89–90
Halpern, B. N., 374
Halsted, William S., 99, 127, 129, 130, 134–35
Halsted's Law, 99
Hamburg International Living Donor Liver Transplant Registry, 389
Hamburger, Jean, 195, 201, 211, 212, 213, 262, 279, 318, 483n33, 484n35, 492n101
Hamel, Henri-Louis du, 37, 38
Hamilton, Frank, 76–77
Hammersmith Hospital, London, 196–99, 204
Hammond, Levi J., 98, 136, 449n30
Hanau, Arthur N., 107
hand transplantation, 141, 291
haplotypes, 322
Harbison, S. P., 129
Hardwick, Ben, 518n70
Hardy, James D., 289, 292–93, 342, 347–48
harpies, 3
Harris, H. A., 206
Harrison, Hartwell, 250, 484n1
Harvard criteria for brain death, 345–47, 378, 513n70
Harvard Law Review, 300
Harvard Medical School, 101; Ad Hoc Committee on Brain Death, 342, 345–47; Research Laboratories, 249; Standing Committee on Human Studies, 344–45, 512n67
Harwell, Britain. See Radiobiology Research Unit, Harwell, Britain
Hašek, Milan, 226–27, 226, 267, 294
Hastings Institute, 401
Hauschka, Theodore, 241
headhunters of Borneo, 365

heart transplantation: in Britain, 356, 395–97; complications of, 506n37; costs and funding of, 396, 518n65; criticisms of, 351–52, 352; death of patient and, 343–44; experimental, 199–200; in folklore, 2; funding of, 355–56, 362; mortality after, 348, 350–51, 355, 362; pediatric, 395, 396; public opinion on, 351–52, 355; resumptions of, 362, 394–95; rise of, 347–48, 350–51; routinization of, 383; temperature in, 200–201; "Year of the Heart," 340–58

heart-beating donation, 343–44, 346, 353, 355, 379, 504n7, 505n16, 506n29, 507n41, 508n52, 513n77

heart-lung bypass pump, 199, 201

heart-lung machines, 327, 500n43

Heinlein, Robert, *I Will Fear No Evil*, 508n54

Heister, Lorenz, *Chirurgie*, 30

Hejinian, John, *Extreme Remedies*, 508n54

Hektoen, Ludvig, 119, 120, 120, 121, 454n52

hemodialysis. *See* kidney dialysis

hemolysin, 67, 442n10

Hench, Philip S., 191

Henry VIII, king of England, 43

heparin, 218

hepatitis, 305–6, 418, 495n27

Herbert, Johnston, 80

Heredity (journal), 223

heterografting, 69–70, 78–79, 81, 84, 294, 333, 492n89, 492n100. *See also* xenografting

Heyde, M., 118

Hildemann, Bill, 231

Hill, Rolla B., 285; "Transplantation Pneumonia," 489n59

Hinduism, 405, 408

Hingston, W. H., 77

Hippocrates, 13

Hippocratic Oath, xviii

hirudin, 150

histocompatibility, 234, 316, 325, 366, 498n13

Histocompatibility Testing, 498n10

historical change and progress, xv, 424–30

historiography, xv, 423–30

Hitchcock, C. R., 291–92

Hitchings, George, 276, 276, 293, 486n24

Hitler, Adolf, 176

HIV. *See* human immunodeficiency virus

HLA tissue typing system, 325, 363–66, 509n21

HLA-D, 364–65, 508n10

HMS Furious, 174

Hoare, James, 28

holism, xviii, 65, 128–30, 151, 193, 205, 271

Holman, Emile, 134–35

Holmes, Joseph, 337

Homan, Emile, 468n49

homografting: abandonment of term, 294; auto- vs., 18–19; defined, 18, 69–70; evidence against, 75, 88, 110–11, 152, 156, 159, 171, 173, 177, 183, 189–91, 468n54; in gland grafting, 97–98; supporters of, 19, 21–23, 78–81, 130–31, 172, 176–78, 182, 190–91, 229, 468n59, 468n60

homosexuality, 136

Hooke, Robert, 28–29

Hopewell, John, 274–75, 486n22

Hôpital Necker, Paris, 211

Horder, Lord, 151

Horsley, Victor, 84

horticulture, as model for skin grafts, 17–18, 40, 434n49

Hoskins, R. G., 139

hospitals, cooperation between, 489n54

Howard, Hector, 201

Howard, J. G., 374

Hua T'o, 2

Huette, Charles, 67; *Précis iconographique de médecine opératoire et d'anatomie chirurgicale* (with Bernard), 442n8

Hufnagel, Charles, 214–15

human experimentation, 377, 503n2, 512n67

human immunodeficiency virus (HIV), 385

Human Organ Transplant Act (Britain), 398

Human Tissue Act (Britain), 339, 354

humanism, 14

Hume, David, 162, 214–17, 214, 242, 258, 275, 277, 279, 285, 286, 321, 325, 336, 347, 463n29, 468n49, 474n59, 483n34, 509n15

humoral theory of immunity, 88, 105–6, 236–37, 256, 257, 406, 426–27

Hunt, H. L., 137, 156, 457n36

Hunter, John, xiv, xvii, 27, 30, 34–48, 35, 53, 54, 58, 67, 69, 82, 83, 84, 136, 142, 160, 426, 427, 437n23, 437n27; *Natural History of the Human Teeth*, 46

Hunter, William, 34, 36, 53, 90

Huxley, Aldous, *Brave New World*, 300

Hyatt, George W., 202

hydra, 31, 231

hyperbaric oxygen tanks, 500n43

hyperparathyroidism, 285

hypothermia: donor, 483n31; in surgery, 200–201, 471n18

I

Iambulus, 2

Iamia, 3

Ibuka, Kenji, 151

identical twins: bone marrow transplantation between, 267; kidney transplantation between, 249–52; lessons learned from, 426; skin grafts between, 171–72, 172, 189, 221–22, 222

Illingworth, Charles, 178, 466n19

imaging, 285, 368, 385

Immune Tolerance Network, 414

immunity: ancient awareness of, 105; athrepsia (exhaustion) theory of, 105, 108, 110; auto-, 118; cell-mediated, xv–xvi, 106, 116, 227–31, 236–37, 257, 287, 296, 308–9, 426–27; contributions of transplantation history to knowledge of, xvi–xvii; humoral theory of, 88, 105–6, 236–37, 256, 257, 426–27; proteins and, 450n13. *See also* acquired immunity

immunological tolerance. *See* tolerance

immunologically competent cells, 238, 240

immunology, 88, 185, 306–7, 365–66. *See also* transplantation immunology

immunosuppression: combined regimen for, 278–80, 284, 288, 312–13, 382; early work on, 118–19, 198; emergence of, 269; for growth of exotic organisms, 452n26; kidney transplantation and, 260; new agents of, 414–16; pregnancy after, 286; radiation for, 254–68; use of term, 294, 484n1. *See also* chemical immunosuppression

immunosuppression therapy, xvi

immunotherapy, 117–18, 371–76, 416, 512n57

Imperial Cancer Research Fund, 451n17

Imuran. *See* azathioprine

in vitro tests, 365–66

inbred animals, 143–49, 157–58, 224, 228, 235, 462n6, 462n7

Index-Catalogue of the Library of the Surgeon-General's Office, 443n34

India, kidney donation and transplantation in, 407, 409–11, 521n111

Indian medicine, plastic surgery and skin grafting in, xv, 10–12, 14, 23, 49–50, 52, 55

individuality: biological, 71; fingerprints as manifestation of, 87; graft success and, 18; matching and, 122–23; skin grafts and, 189; super-, 157; supergenetic, 149; tissue, 314–15

orchometer, 139, *139*
Oregon: liver transplantation debate in, 387–88; organ donation in, 401
organ distribution, ethics of, 404–6
organ donation: in Australia, 519n83; in Britain, 401–2, 519n85; crossover, 404; death criteria and, 343–47, 353–55, 379, 397, 505n19, 513n78; demographic factors in, 405; in developing countries, 406–9; legal issues concerning, 293, 338–39, 353–54, 371, 401; promotion of, 386, 401–3, *402*; public opinion and, xiii, 245–49, 353, 400–401, 472n28, 521n105; termination of life support and, 343; in United States, 401. *See also* donors; heart-beating donation; tissue donation
organ perfusion, 169–71, *170, 171*
organ preservation: criteria for, 170; duration of, 103; intracellular fluid flush for, 328–29; perfusion and, 170–71, 327, 403–4; temperature and, 199–202; tests for, 328
organ sharing agencies, 370, 400–401
organ supply and demand, 282–83, 403–4
organ trafficking, 411
organ transplantation: assessments of, 87; attitudes toward, 265–66; Carrel's vision for, 124; challenges in using, 488n53; conferences on, 241–44, 479n63, 479n70; contributions of, to other fields, xvi–xx; costs of, 384; criticisms of, 357; custom-built units for, *266*; early history of, 8–30; experimental, 195–220, 287–91; global reception of, xviii; high achievers after, 515n17; matching and, 318–19; in 1970s, 359; 1960s pioneers of, 357; nomenclature of, 242; papal stance on, 249; patient eligibility/ selection for, 400; regression in mid–twentieth century in, 125–53, 456n1; in seventeenth century, 20–30; sites where performed, 384; twentieth-century origins of, 88–104. *See also specific organs*
organ viability. *See* organ preservation
Organ Watch, 521n113
organs, engineered, 418–20
Oribasius, 13
Orr, Thomas, 156
Orthodox Jews, 405–6
O'Shaughnessy, William, 63
Osler, William, 128
Ottesen, J., 238
Oudot, J., 195, 470n2
Ovalicin, 380
ovarian transplantation, 85, 139

Owen, Ray D., 222–23, 226, 476n17, 481n12
oxalosis, 286
Oxford University, 174, 176

P
Padgett, Earl, 142, 159, 172
Page, Irvine, 301
Pain, Barry, *The Octave of Claudius*, 141
painted mice case, 377–78
Pakistan, 411
Palenzke v. Bruning, 203
Palmer, James F., 48
pancreas grafting, 139
pancreas transplantation, 290, 383, 391–93
pancreatic islet grafting, 290, 392–93, *392*
Panorama (television program), 397, 518n69
Pappenheimer, Alwin M., Jr., 116, 117, 332
parabiosis, 118
paradigm shifts, 426–27
Paré, Ambroise, 20, 43
parenteral nutrition, 390
Paris, France, 65–76, 211–13, 262–64, 265, 483n33, 484n35
Paris Transplant, 326
Parke Davis & Company, 279
Parkes, A. S., 190, 232, 468n58
partial-thickness skin grafts, 12
Pasteur, Louis, 105
Pasteur Institute, 66
patient eligibility/selection: criteria for, 286, 299–301, 400; fairness and equity in, 404–6; health behaviors as factor in, 520n95; for hepatitis vaccine, 306; for kidney treatments, 299–301, 337, 370; lay input on, 299; for liver transplantation, 520n95; sharing schemes and, 325
Paton, Townley, 245–48
Paufique, Louis, 246
Pauling, Linus, 484n5
Paulus Aegineta, 13
Pavlov, Ivan, 209
Payne, Rose, 317, 500n41
Payr, Erwin, 91, *91*, 93, 127
Pearson, Karl, 460n76
pediatrics: heart transplants, 395, *396*; intestinal transplants, 291; kidney transplants, 286; liver transplants, 388
Peer, Lyndon, 242
Pegasus, 2
Pélikan (French physician), 71
penicillin, 16, 174, 178, 465n3, 467n43
Penn, Israel "Sol," 287
perfusion: heart transplantation and,

201; machines for, 327–29; organ viability and, 169–71, 327, 403–4; Soviet surgeons and, 500n39; tissue viability and, 67–68
Perrin (Lyon surgeon), 97
Persian medicine, 433n38
Perthes, Georg, 111
Peru, 410
Peter, Saint, 4
Peter Bent Brigham Hospital, Boston, 188–89, 213–17, 261, 279, 306, 488n51, 489n54
Pettigrew, Gavin, 38
phagocytes, 106
phantom limb sensation, 432n20
pharmaceutical industry: costs in, xx, 382; involvement of, xx, 312, 335, 380, 414–15
Philippines, 410, 411
physiology, origins of, 35
Pichlmayr, Rudolf, 387, 389
Pien Ch'iao, 2
pigs: genetic engineering of, 419–20; as kidney donors, 94–95; pig-to-primate organ grafts, 525n33; religious scruples concerning, 520n98; skin grafts using, 81; transplantation experiments on, 329
pinch grafts, 73–75, 77
Pirogov, Nikolay, 73
Pittsburgh Liver Transplant Registry, 399
Pius XII, Pope, 249, 341
Plant, O. H., 327
plasma cells, 196
plastic, first use of term, 59
Plastic and Reconstructive Surgery (journal), 188, 191, 244, 295
plastic surgery: in ancient history, xiii; Indian practice of, 10–12, *11*, 49–50, 52, 55, 434n47; in medieval period, 13; in nineteenth century, xiv, 56–61; Renaissance revival of, 13–20; Tagliacozzi and, 15–19, *17*; in United States, 60–61, 187–88. *See also* skin grafts; tissue transplantation
plastics, xix–xx
Pliny the Elder, 4
poison gases, 484n3. *See also* mustard gas
Poisson, Jacques, 326
Polidori, John, 58–59; *The Vampyre*, 59
Polley, Howard, 191
Pollock, George, 75
polyps (coelenterate hydra), 31–33, *32*
Poncet, Antonin, 81
Porter, Kendrick "Ken," 273–74, 321, 470n5, 485n13
positive cross-matches, 323

potassium, 328–29, 442n16
Poultry Science (journal), 309
prednisolone, 382
prednisone, 382
pregnancy: after kidney transplantation, 252, 286, 490n70; antibodies resulting from, 317; technology to support, 494n19
Prehn, Richmond, 242, 256, 373, 481n10, 481n11
preservation: after-death cryopreservation, 488n44; of cells, 231–32; of kidneys, 325; of organs, 103, 170–71, 199–202, 327–29, 403–4
Prévot, A. R., 374
Primate Center, Rijswijk Radiobiological Institute, Netherlands, 335, 503n73
prisoners, organ removal from, 411, 522n120, 522n121
privileged sites, for grafts, 112, 185, 229, 452n22, 477n25, 477n28
progress. *See* historical change and progress
prosthetic devices, noses as, 20
proteins, and immunity, 450n3
Prynne, William, 20
psychoneuroimmunology, 209
Public Law No. 92-603, 304
public opinion: on animal-to-human transplantation, 395, 417; on heart transplantation, 351–52, 355; importance of, xiii; on military experiments, 497n6; on organ donation, xiii, 245–49, 353, 400–401, 521n105; on surgical profession, 357–58; on tissue donation, 472n28; on xenografting, 420
purgative phenolsulfthalein (PSP), 150
Pusey, Nathan, 346
Pybus, F. C., 139, 457n40

Q
quackery, 135, 139–40, 156
quality of life, 301–2

R
Rabbinical Council of America, 406
rabbit bone graft story, 26, 27
Rabelais, François, 8, 9, 62
race and racism: black donors and white recipients, 5, 75, 79, 141; races as species, 72
radiation: controlled release of, 454n53; experiments with, 119, 198; protection against, 255–57; and skin grafts, 470n9; sterilization using, 202
radiation therapy, xix; low-dose, 262, 264–65, 483n33; and marrow replacement, 253, 256–62, 484n37; selective, 332, 367

radiation tolerance, 253–68
radiation-chimera, 257
radioactive isotopes, xix, 255
Radiobiology Research Unit, Harwell, Britain, 240, 255, 256, 259
radiology, 285, 368, 385
radiotherapy, 118
Rae, John, 45
Rae, William, 47
Raff, Martin, 309
rainwater worms, 34
Ramón y Cajal, Santiago, 115
Rapa Nui (Easter Island), 415
Rapamycin (Rapamune), 392, 415, 523n16
Rapaport, Felix, 243, 316, 319, 466n32, 509n19
RASt. *See* renal artery stenosis
rats: eye transplantation claims for, 126; lymphocyte studies on, 174; organ transplantation in, 330–31, 331; research uses of, 144–46; skin grafts using, 78; tissue grafts using, 70–71, 124, 142–44, 157
Read, Alexander, 24, 435n66, 439n7
Reader's Digest (magazine), 169, 248
Reagan, Nancy, 465n14
Reagan, Ronald, 386, 394, 398, 399
Réaumur, René Antoine Ferchault de, 32
Reconstruction Hospitals, 131
red blood cells, transplantation of, 67
Redi, Francesco, 24–25
reduced grafts, 389
reductionism, 65, 127, 168–69, 231, 307
Reemtsma, Keith, 280, 292, 311, 492n90
reflexes, 209
regeneration, 33–34, 54
regulations, 416, 419–20
Reid, Stephen E., 468n59
Reinherz, E. L., 366
rejection crisis, 262, 278, 294, 492n101
rejection of foreign tissue. *See* tissue rejection
religion: attitudes influenced by, xviii, 433n27; and organ donation, 405–8; and restoration of body parts, 1, 405–6. *See also* Christianity
renal artery stenosis (RASt), 285, 489n60
renal failure: acute, 62–63; chemical/quantitative approach to, 151; dietary and fluid regimen for, 204–5; ethical issues concerning, xviii; and hepatitis, 305–6; Korean War and, 206–7; nineteenth-century study of, 62–63; novel instances of, 204; peak of, in 1920s, 150. *See also* artificial kidney machines

renal function tests, 150–51
Renard, Marius, *213*
replacement of body parts, attitudes toward; attitudes toward, 1, 431n2; fingertips, 441n35; in folklore, 1–2; misconceptions concerning, 61
resistance to novelty, 429
respiration, assisted, 303, 340–44
restoration of body parts. *See* replacement of body parts
restriction, 366
resurrection. *See* afterlife, bodily integrity in
resuscitation, 42, 302–3, 340–41
reticuloendothelial system, 106, 122
retroviruses, 419, 524n27
Reverdin, Jacques-Louis, 72–75, *73*, 77, 79, 84
reverse incompatibility, 167, 464n30, 474n64
Reynolds, Joshua, 35, 38
Rhazes, 13
rheumatoid arthritis, 191
rhinoplasty. *See* noses
Rhoads, Cornelius P. "Dusty," 270, 451n12
Rich, Arnold, 238
Richards, Alfred Newton, 169, 327
Richards, Victor, 484n1
ricin, 450n3
Ricordi, Camillo, 392, 517n50
Rifkind, David, "Transplantation Pneumonia," 489n59
Ripley, Sherman, 475n5
Riteris, J. M., 262
rituximab, 416
Robbins, Frederick, 474n63
Rockefeller Institute, 101, 102, 112, 127–28, 169, 188
Roger, Noëlle, *Le Nouvel Adam*, 141
Roger II, 14
Rogers, Blair, 188, 219, 225, 227, 242, 243, 319, 468n50
Roitt, Ivan, 309
Roman medicine, plastic surgery in, 13
Romantic movement, 59
Röntgen, Wilhelm, 119
Roosevelt, Eleanor, 188
Rosenberg, Steven, 376
rotation flaps, 10–12
Rous, Peyton, 112
Rowlands, David T., "Transplantation Pneumonia," 489n59
Rowlandson, Thomas, 44, *45*
Rowntree, Leonard, 150, 152
Royal College of Surgeons of England, 219
Royal College of Veterinary Surgeons (Britain), 515n16
Royal Infirmary, Glasgow, 173, 178–80
Royal National Institute for the Blind, 248

Tilney, Nicholas, 332
Time (magazine), 170
Times (London) [newspaper], 150, 352
Ting, Alan, 321, 365, 509n15
tissue: individuality of, 314–15; properties of, 66
tissue adhesion, 36, 39–40, 69
tissue banks, 104, 202–4
tissue donation: legal issues concerning, 203–4, 246, 353–54, 472n28; public campaigns for, 247–49, 402. *See also* donors; organ donation
tissue grafts, xvi. *See also* skin grafts
tissue recognition, 142
tissue rejection: adumbrations of, in Renaissance period, 18–19; biologists' work on, xv–xvi; challenge presented by, xiv; early awareness of, 110–11; enhancement and, 234–35; features of, 414; genetics of, 232–34; homografting and, 82; immunological causes of, 111, 173, 183; as modern notion, 9–10; use of term, 187, 217, 294, 468n49
tissue transplantation: earliest photograph of, 79; in nineteenth-century Paris, 67–76; terminology of, 48n9. *See also* plastic surgery; skin grafts
Tissue Transplantation Conference (New York, 1952), 241–42
tissue typing: adumbrations of, 122–23; and antibodies, 323; benefits and shortcomings of, 363–64, 366; bone marrow transplantation and, 360–61; early work on, 104, 154; graft success affected by, 144, 237; kidney transplantation and, 318–23; methods of, 318, 364; significance of, xvi; Terasaki and, 189, 363, 509n17; terminology of, 497n7, 498n10, 498n13; workshops for, 323–24. *See also* matching
tissue viability/vitality: blood perfusion and, 67–68; early experiments on, 36, 40–41, 41, 69; living graft required for, 144; organ perfusion and, 170; temperature and, 103, 133–34, 450n44, 450n45
Tit-Bits (magazine), 142
Todd, Charles, 122–23
tolerance: in absence of medication, 284, 489n57; adult, 253, 254, 257–58, 480n1; of grafts, 36; GvH reaction and, 240; in kidney transplantation, 284; Medawarian, 253, 257, 480n1, 485n15; Medawar's discovery of, 194, 220, 225–26, 296, 467n44; neonatal, in mice, 225–26; in outbred animals, 475n10; radiation, 253–68; use of term, 223, 475n8

tolerance induction, xvi, 105, 220, 226, 240–41, 253, 254, 258, 260, 264, 267, 269, 272, 328, 333, 379, 414
toluene, 120
tooth transplantation, 43–48; to cock's comb, 44, 48, 438n35; disease transmission through, xvii, 46–47; donors for, 43–45, 45, 438n50, 439n52; ethical issues concerning, 47–48; history of, 43; Hunter's work in, xvii, 36, 43–45; later attitudes toward, 48; outside of England, 45–46
Topsell, Edward, *Historie of Fourefooted Beastes*, 3
total lymphoid irradiation (TLI), 367
tourism, transplant, 410–11
Toussait, Charles, 321
trafficking, organ, 411
Train, Arthur, *Mortmain*, 141, 524n21
training. *See* education
transnational issues, 388, 397–98
transplant coordinators, 370, 511n47
Transplant Games, 384
transplant management. *See* clinical management; surgical management
Transplant Regulatory Authority (Britain), 396
transplant tourism, 410–11
transplantation: criticisms of, 357; in nineteenth-century Paris, 65–76; in twentieth century, 88–104; use of term, 27, 437n27, 438n32. *See also* specific types
Transplantation (journal), 295, 375, 479n61
Transplantation Bulletin (journal), 479n61
transplantation immunology: animal studies, 106–8; autoimmunity, 118; bursa of Fabricius role, 309–10; cellular mechanisms, 106; chemical immunosuppression, 120–21; in early 1960s, 306–10; fundamental advances in, 307–10; Gibson-Medawar Report on, 181–84; graft loss, 110–11; humoral theory, 105–6; immunosuppression, 118–21; immunotherapy, 117–18; lost era of, 105–25, 452n27; lymphocyte role, 112–16, 143, 151–52, 182–83, 307; midcentury advances in, 173–94; origins of, 88, 110; radiation, 119; Rockefeller Institute and, 112; terminology of, 186–87, 293–95, 492n89, 492n97, 492n99, 492n100; thymus gland role, 308–10
Transplantation Journal, 244
Transplantation of Normal Tissues conference (London, 1954), 242

Transplantation Proceedings (journal), 295, 378, 479n70
Transplantation Society, 295, 354, 358, 360, 363, 372, 377, 378, 409
Trapeznikov (Russian scientist), 116, 229
Traub, E., 223
Trembley, Abraham, 30–33, 40, 231; *Mémoires*, 32
Trentin, John J., 257, 481n11
trinitrobenzene, 228
tris-nitrogen mustard, 270
trypsin, 465n13
tuberculosis, 86
Tuffier, Théodore, 94
tumor enhancement, 118
tumors, transplant-related, 286–87
Turkey, 105, 410, 521n105
twins. *See* identical twins
twisted-neck myth, 1, 6, 432n18, 432n22
tyrosinemia, 389
Tyzzer, Ernest, 147

U

UK Code, 379
Ukrainian Experimental Institute for Eye Diseases, 244–45
ulcers, skin grafts for, 73–76
Ullmann, Emerich, 91, 93, 123
ultrasound, xix, 368, 369, 385
umbilical cord, 41, 41
uncertainty principle, 65
Underwood, H. L., 111, 451n16
Unger, Ernst, 95–96, 96, 160, 448n21
Uniform Anatomical Gift Act (United States), 338–39, 353–54, 370, 401
Uniform Determination of Death Act (United States), 354, 378
United Kingdom, medical costs in, 495n25
United Kingdom Transplant Service (UKTS), 326
United Network for Organ Sharing (UNOS), 325–26, 399–400, 509n17
United States: border-crossing issues in, 397; donation campaigns in, 247–48; donors in, 370; kidney dialysis funding in, 303–5; kidney transplantation in, 213–18, 368–69; literature featuring transplantation in, 141; organ donation in, 401; plastic surgery in, 60–61, 187–88; postwar medicine and science in, 128, 130–31; skin grafting in, 76–77; tooth transplantation in, 45–46
University College, London, 224, 225
University of Birmingham, 186
University of California at Los Angeles School of Medicine, 189